Part 1 MRCOG Revision Notes and Sample SBAs

This concise yet comprehensive guide is focused on the curriculum and current exam style of the MRCOG Part 1 examination. It integrates clinical knowledge with basic science, providing readers with a deeper understanding of pathophysiology of medical disorders in obstetrics and gynaecology. The lead editor is a member of the Part 1 Examination Committee and her insights are skilfully woven into the book's revision notes, sample Single Best Answer (SBA) question and answer explanations, and tips on exam technique. The book encourages a structured thought process to develop, making it easier for clinicians to make differential diagnoses and conduct relevant investigations and treatment plans. The focus on basic sciences also endows readers with the ability to develop research ideas and evaluate findings. Featuring easy-to-read text, highlighted key points, colour illustrations, and plenty of practice papers, this succinct guide is essential preparation reading for trainee obstetricians and gynaecologists taking the challenging Part 1 MRCOG exam.

Dr Neelanjana Mukhopadhaya, DGO, DCRM, PGcert (Med Education), FICOG, FRCOG is Consultant Obstetrician and Gynaecologist, Luton and Dunstable University Hospital; Honorary Senior Lecturer, University College London; and Chair of the Part 1 MRCOG subcommittee, Royal College of Obstetricians and Gynaecologists, London, UK.

Dr Jyotsna Pundir is Consultant Gynaecologist and Sub-Specialist in Reproductive Medicine and Surgery, St Bartholomew's Hospital, Barts Health NHS Trust, London, and Honorary Senior Lecturer, Queen Mary University, London, UK.

Dr Mala Arora FRCOG (UK), FICOG (India) FICMCH, DA (UK) D Obst (Ire) is Director of Noble Health Care Services Private Limited, Faribadad, Haryana, India. She became Chairperson of the Indian College of Obstetrics and Gynecology in 2017 and Vice President of FOGSI in 2011.

Part 1 MRCOG Revision Notes and Sample SBAs

Edited by

Neelanjana Mukhopadhaya
Bedfordshire Hospitals NHS Foundation Trust

Jyotsna Pundir
St Bartholomew's Hospital

Mala Arora
Noble IVF Centre, Faridabad

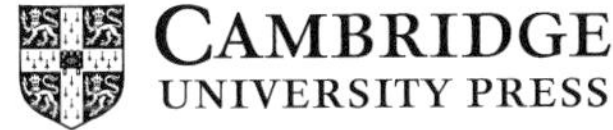

CAMBRIDGE
UNIVERSITY PRESS

University Printing House, Cambridge CB2 8BS, United Kingdom

One Liberty Plaza, 20th Floor, New York, NY 10006, USA

477 Williamstown Road, Port Melbourne, VIC 3207, Australia

314–321, 3rd Floor, Plot 3, Splendor Forum, Jasola District Centre, New Delhi – 110025, India

79 Anson Road, #06–04/06, Singapore 079906

Cambridge University Press is part of the University of Cambridge.

It furthers the University's mission by disseminating knowledge in the pursuit of education, learning, and research at the highest international levels of excellence.

www.cambridge.org
Information on this title: www.cambridge.org/9781108714082
DOI: 10.1017/9781108644396

First published 2020

Printed in the United Kingdom by TJ Books Limited, Padstow Cornwall

A catalogue record for this publication is available from the British Library.

ISBN 978-1-108-71408-2 Paperback

Firstly, to my parents who inculcated the values of perseverance, commitment and the assiduity for doing my best at all times.

Secondly, to my husband and children for the credence that they had in me and for motivating me during the many hours of preparation and writing.

Finally, to my juniors and students who are the future, and a source of inspiration to me.

Neelanjana Mukhopadhaya

This book is dedicated to budding obstetricians and gynaecologists attempting MRCOG part 1 examination. This will certainly help to build a solid foundation of basic sciences to support their practical skills and clinical management in the future.

Mala Arora

To my mother for everything I am today, to my husband and two lovely boys for their patience and endless support, to my brothers and in-laws for their faith and encouragement, and finally to my father for his wisdom.

Jyotsna Pundir

Contents

Contributors

Mala Arora
FRCOG, FICOG, FICMCH, DA, D Obst
Director of Noble Health Care Services Private Limited
Faribadad, Haryana, India

Sheetal Barhate
MBBS, MS, MRCOG
Clinical Fellow
Centre for Reproductive Medicine
St Bartholomew's Hospital, London

Jane Ding
BSc, MPhil, PhD, BMBCh, MRCOG, DFSRH
ST7 Trainee
Obstetrics and Gynaecology
Royal London Hospital

Siddharth Dutta
MBBS, MD (Pharmacology)
Senior Resident
Department of Pharmacology
All India Institute of Medical Sciences, Jodhpur

Kahkashan Jeelani
Senior Resident
Department of Anatomy
Maulana Azad Medical College, New Delhi, India

Bhupinder Kalra
MBBS, MD (Pharmacology)
Associate Professor Department of Pharmacology
Maulana Azad Medical College, New Delhi, India

Kamalpreet Kaur
Senior Resident
Department of Anatomy
Maulana Azad Medical College, New Delhi, India

Smita Kaushik
MBBS, MD (Medical Biochemistry)
Director Professor
Department of Biochemistry
Maulana Azad Medical College and Lok Nayak Hospital, New Delhi, India

Nita Khurana
MBBS, MD (Pathology)
Director Professor and Head Department of Pathology
Maulana Azad Medical College, New Delhi, India

Sahil Kumar
MBBS, MD
Senior Resident
Department of Pharmacology
Maulana Azad Medical College, New Delhi, India

Jodie Lam
MRCOG
Consultant in Obstetrics and Gynaecology
Bedfordshire Hospitals NHS Trust

Varuna Mallya
MBBS, MD (Pathology)
Associate Professor Department of Pathology
Maulana Azad Medical College, New Delhi, India

Tanuja Mokashi
MRCOG
Specialty Doctor
Department of Obstetrics and Gynaecology
Bedfordshire Hospitals NHS Trust

Neelanjana Mukhopadhaya
MBBS, DGO, FRCOG
Consultant Obstetrician and Gynaecologist
Bedfordshire NHS Hospitals Foundation Trust
Honorary Senior Lecturer, University College, London

Anita Pawar
MBBS, MD, PhD
Professor Physiology

Lady Hardinge Medical College, New Delhi, India

Deepika Poonia
Senior Resident
Department of Anatomy
Maulana Azad Medical College, New Delhi, India

Jyotsna Pundir
MBBS, MD, DNB, MRCOG, DFSRH
Consultant Reproductive Medicine and Surgery
Centre for Reproductive Medicine, St Bartholomew's Hospital, London
Honorary Senior Lecturer, Queen Mary University, London

Renuka Sharma
MBBS, MD
Director Professor Physiology
VMMC and Safdarjung Hospital, New Delhi, India

Rachana Shukla
Consultant Radiologist
Department of Radiology
Bedfordshire Hospitals NHS Trust

Vandana Tayal
MBBS, MD (Pharmacology)
Associate Professor
Department of Pharmacology
Maulana Azad Medical College, New Delhi, India

Swati Tiwari
Assistant Professor
Department of Anatomy
Maulana Azad Medical College, New Delhi, India

Vandana Tiwari
Senior Resident
Department of Anatomy
Maulana Azad Medical College, New Delhi, India

Neelam Vasudeva
Director Professor
Department of Anatomy
Maulana Azad Medical College, New Delhi, India

Sabah Yaseen
Senior Resident
Department of Anatomy
Maulana Azad Medical College, New Delhi, India

Introduction

Part 1 MRCOG is a UK-based examination for postgraduate trainees in obstetrics and gynaecology. It is the first step in a series of three examinations, which leads to the award of membership of the Royal College of Obstetricians and Gynaecologists (RCOG) in the UK. This examination is based on basic sciences related to obstetrics and gynaecology. Historically, the examination paper was focused on molecular biology, cellular mechanisms and other aspects of basic sciences, which did not quite have relevance in current clinical practice. Over the years, the examination has transitioned into a new style with questions that are relevant to clinical practice. The questions are currently SBAs and there are two papers, which aim to assess knowledge in all areas of obstetrics and gynaecology, consisting of 100 questions each, over two-and-a-half hours. The examination in future will be conducted electronically. Each question has five options and one of the options is the best answer for that question. The questions will be based on the new syllabus that RCOG has introduced recently and will be linked to the Capabilities in Practice (CiPs) in 15 core knowledge areas. Many of the questions will have images, tables, blood results, ultrasound findings, and so on, and the candidate will need to recognise or make a diagnosis. All questions are aimed at assessing knowledge at ST1/ST2 level of training in the UK.

This book will help doctors make a clear correlation between the basic sciences and clinical application of the knowledge in routine obstetrics and gynaecology practice. Hence, I would recommend this book to all obstetricians and gynaecologists who would like to refresh their basic science knowledge and not just those who are aiming to sit the Part 1 MRCOG exam. The papers are differentiated into various topics.

Paper 1 will cover the following topics:

- Anatomy
- Embryology
- Physiology
- Biochemistry
- Genetics
- Statistics/epidemiology
- Endocrinology

Paper 2 will cover the following topics:

- Biophysics
- Clinical Management
- Data interpretation
- Immunology
- Microbiology
- Pathology
- Pharmacology

Finally, I hope this book has covered all areas that are relevant to this examination in a succinct and concise manner, which will be easy to remember and retain. There are three practice papers at the end of this book, which will help the candidate practise examination-style questions.

I wish all my readers aiming to sit the part 1 MRCOG examination success, and to all others who are reading for knowledge acquisition, that you will rediscover basic understanding of clinical conditions, which will start to make more sense. I hope that this will enable you to become a better clinician.

Part 1 Syllabus (RCOG)

Part 1 MRCOG, which covers the basic and applied sciences relevant to the clinical practice of obstetrics and gynaecology, is focused on the summative assessment of CiP 6. This is because, by achieving Part 1 MRCOG, the candidate/trainee will have demonstrated an active participation in acquiring the fundamental scientific knowledge that underpins the development of clinical expertise. They will have demonstrated an early indication of self-development beyond the experiential learning within the clinical environment.

CiP 6: the doctor takes an active role in helping himself or herself and others to develop.

Part 1 MRCOG assesses the Scientific Platform for Clinical Practice. It examines the 15 core knowledge areas in four domains of understanding. There is inevitably overlap between knowledge areas and requirements, and not all domains are relevant to a particular knowledge requirement. This is assessed using SBA questions.

1. Understanding cell function: this incorporates physiology, endocrinology and biochemistry
2. Understanding human structure: this incorporates anatomy, embryology and genetics
3. Understanding measurement and manipulation: this incorporates biophysics, epidemiology and statistics, data interpretation and pharmacology
4. Understanding illness: this incorporates immunology, microbiology, pathology and clinical management

Knowledge Area 1: Clinical Skills

Summary Knowledge Requirements: Part 1 MRCOG

- Patterns of symptoms and the importance of risk factors
- Pathological basis for physical signs and clinical investigation
- How to interpret results of clinical investigations

Knowledge Area 2: Teaching and Research

Summary Knowledge Requirements: Part 1 MRCOG

- Principles of screening, clinical trial design (multicentre, randomised controlled trials, and so on) and the statistical methods used in clinical research
- Levels of evidence, quantification of risk, power of study, level of significance, informed consent and ethical and regulatory approvals in research
- Principles of safe prescribing, quality control in medicine and the accuracy of tests

Knowledge Area 3: Core Surgical skills

Summary Knowledge Requirements: Part 1 MRCOG

- Demonstrate an understanding of the issues surrounding informed consent, including knowledge of complication rates, risks and likely success rates of different gynaecological operations, together with an understanding of diagnostic methods and treatment of complications
- Demonstrate familiarity with surgery by discussing common operations, together with common surgical instruments and sutures
- Demonstrate detailed knowledge of the basic surgical procedures in obstetrics and gynaecology, including diagnostic laparoscopy, hysteroscopy, gynaecological laparotomy for ovarian cysts, ectopic pregnancy, hysterectomy and vaginal surgery for prolapse, incontinence and vaginal hysterectomy
- Know the principles and procedures involved in more complex gynaecological surgery for cancer and endometriosis
- Have good knowledge of the principles of safe surgery, surgical instruments and sutures, and the management of the common complications of surgery
- Be aware of the principles of surgical teamworking, risk management and risk reduction

Knowledge Area 4: Postoperative Care

Summary Knowledge Requirements: Part 1 MRCOG

- Applied clinical science related to the postoperative period, including physiological and biochemical aspects of fluid balance, the metabolism of nutrients after surgery and the biochemistry of enzymes, vitamins and minerals
- Organisms implicated in postoperative infections and the therapies used to treat them
- Therapeutic drugs used perioperatively, including analgesics and thromboprophylactic agents

- Histopathology of the pelvic organs, the breast and the endocrine organs, including the pituitary and the hypothalamus
- Classification systems of gynaecological and obstetric conditions

Knowledge Area 5: Antenatal Care

Summary Knowledge Requirements: Part 1 MRCOG

- Maternal anatomical, endocrine and physiological adaptations occurring in pregnancy
- Pathology of major organ systems, including the common haemoglobinopathies and connective tissue disorders as applied to pregnancy
- Screening tests commonly performed in pregnancy
- Fetal anatomy, including abnormalities, embryology, endocrine function and physiology
- Normal fetal physiology and development, together with the aetiology of fetal malformations and acquired problems, including abnormalities of growth; this will include regulation of amniotic fluid volume and fetal interaction with the amniotic fluid
- Development and function of the placenta in pregnancy, with specific knowledge of how the placenta handles drugs
- Principles of inheritance and features and effects of common inherited disorders
- Basic ultrasound findings in pregnancy
- How to define and interpret data on maternal, neonatal and perinatal mortality
- Impact of maternal health and other variables (e.g. social deprivation) on pregnancy outcome

Knowledge Area 6: Maternal Medicine

Summary Knowledge Requirements: Part 1 MRCOG

- Epidemiology and pathological processes that underlie common maternal diseases in pregnancy, including diabetes and endocrine, respiratory, cardiac and haematological disease
- Pathophysiology and presentation of common infections that affect pregnant women and the treatments and interventions used for these infections
- Drugs used to treat maternal disease, and the potential maternal and fetal complications associated with their use
- Imaging methods used to screen for maternal and fetal complications of maternal disease (e.g. ultrasound, X-ray and magnetic resonance imaging) and how to interpret their results

Knowledge Area 7: Management of Labour

Summary Knowledge Requirements: Part 1 MRCOG

- Physiology, biochemistry and endocrinology of parturition, including maturation of the fetal endocrine system, the influence of hormones on signalling pathways in the myometrium and the biochemistry of myometrial contractility
- Principles of tocolysis and stimulation of uterine contraction
- Fetal physiology in late pregnancy
- Fetal assessment in late pregnancy and labour, and how to interpret the results
- Placentation and the implications of infection on labour, and the optical therapeutic options

Knowledge Area 8: Management of Delivery

Summary Knowledge Requirements: Part 1 MRCOG

- Labour and the mechanism and physiology of childbirth and the third stage of labour
- Aetiology and pathology of congenital and bone malformations of the genital tract
- Mode of action of drugs used in labour, at delivery and in the third stage of labour
- Indications for, and risks of, operative delivery
- Biochemical basis of acid–base balance, normal fetal physiological changes in labour and how to interpret fetal and cord blood analysis
- Female perineum and principles underlying the management of perineal repair

Knowledge Area 9: Postpartum Problems

Summary Knowledge Requirements: Part 1 MRCOG

- Physiology and structural changes in the neonate
- Physiology of lactation, uterine involution and the pathology and management of puerperal sepsis and infection
- Common puerperal complications, including mental health issues
- Postpartum contraception and other drugs used postpartum and during lactation

Knowledge Area 10: Gynaecological Problems

Summary Knowledge Requirements: Part 1 MRCOG

- Anatomy, physiology and histopathology of the pituitary gland and female reproductive tract, including an understanding of changes at puberty, at menopause and during the menstrual cycle, including ovulation
- Epidemiology, microbiology and therapeutics of benign gynaecological conditions, including infection
- How to interpret results of commonly performed investigations for benign gynaecological conditions
- Principles of medical and surgical management of gynaecological problems

Knowledge Area 11: Subfertility

Summary Knowledge Requirements: Part 1 MRCOG

- Epidemiology of subfertility and treatment
- Anatomy, development, function and cell biology of the organs of the male and female reproductive tracts in the context of their relevance to fertility and its disorders
- How to interpret results of investigations commonly performed as part of the investigation of subfertility

Knowledge Area 12: Sexual and Reproductive Health

Summary Knowledge Requirements: Part 1 MRCOG

- Physiology, endocrinology, epidemiology and pharmacology of contraception
- Epidemiology and serology of sexually transmitted infections (STIs), the microorganisms involved, the drugs used in their treatment and the pathological features of STIs
- Termination of pregnancy, including assessment, Fraser competency, surgical management and the drugs used in medical termination of pregnancy

Knowledge Area 13: Early Pregnancy Care

Summary Knowledge Requirements: Part 1 MRCOG

- Basic sciences pertaining to early pregnancy and its loss, including the endocrine aspects of the maternal recognition of pregnancy, the luteal maintenance of early pregnancy and the physiology of fetomaternal communication
- Aetiology and histopathology of miscarriage, ectopic pregnancy and trophoblastic disease
- Diagnostic features of ultrasound used in early pregnancy, the epidemiology of pregnancy loss and the medical agents used to manage pregnancy loss (miscarriage, ectopic pregnancy and trophoblastic disease)
- How to interpret the results of investigations used in early pregnancy problems

Knowledge Area 14: Gynaecological Oncology

Summary Knowledge Requirements: Part 1 MRCOG

- Surgical anatomy of the abdomen and pelvis
- Cellular biology of cancer, genetic origins of cancer and principles of diagnosis and screening for gynaecological cancer

- Pain pathways, transmission of pain centrally and pathology of pain in gynaecological malignancy
- Epidemiology and aetiology of cancers affecting women
- Pathology of and classification systems for gynaecological cancer and premalignant gynaecological conditions
- Principles of radiotherapy and chemotherapy in the management of gynaecological cancer and their effects on gonadal function

Knowledge Area 15: Urogynaecology and Pelvic Floor Problems

Summary Knowledge Requirements: Part 1 MRCOG

- Structure of the bladder and pelvic floor, and their innervation
- Mechanisms of continence and micturition, and principles of pelvic floor support
- How congenital anomalies, pregnancy and childbirth, disease, infection and estrogen deficiency affect these mechanisms
- Principles underlying the treatment of bladder and pelvic floor problems and the impact of other drugs on bladder function

Section 1

Anatomy

Neelam Vasudeva and Mala Arora

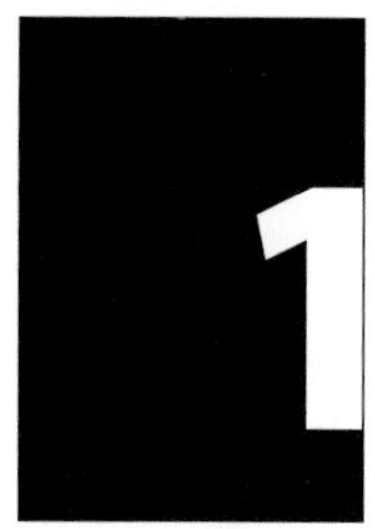

Surgical Anatomy of the Female Pelvis and Abdominal Wall

Kahkashan Jeelani

1 Anterior Abdominal Wall

The anterior abdominal wall is a multilayered structure. The layers are:

- skin
- subcutaneous layer (superficial fatty or Camper's fascia and deep membranous or Scarpa's fascia)
- musculoaponeurotic layer (rectus abdominis with rectus sheath)
- muscle layer
- fascia transversalis
- extraperitoneal fat and parietal peritoneum

Function:

- helps increase intra-abdominal pressure
- accommodates abdominal expansion caused by ingestion, pregnancy, fat deposition or pathology

1.1 Skin and Subcutaneous Tissue

- The direction of fibres is predominantly transverse with curving concave upwards in the dermal layer of skin, so vertical incision on skin generates more tension and a wider scar.
- The subcutaneous tissue above the umbilicus is a single layer, but below the umbilicus, the deepest part of subcutaneous tissue is reinforced by elastic and collagen fibres, so there are two layers: superficial fatty layer and deep membranous layer.
- The membranous layer is continuous inferiorly into the perineal region as superficial perineal fascia or Colles' fascia.
- The Camper's fascia and Scarpa's fascia are not well-defined layers. Scarpa's fascia is best developed laterally, but not seen as a well-defined layer during vertical incision.

1.2 Musculoaponeurotic Layer

The musculoaponeurotic layer is a layer of muscle and fibrous tissue, and consists of two groups of muscles:

- vertical: rectus abdominis and pyramidalis
- oblique flank muscles: external oblique, internal oblique and transverse abdominis
  - Each rectus abdominis has three or more tendinous intersections. These intersections are above the umbilicus, but when found below it, then rectus sheath is attached to rectus muscle and the two structures become difficult to separate during a Pfannenstiel incision.
  - The direction of internal oblique is perpendicular to the direction of fibres of external oblique muscle, but in the lower abdomen, fibres of internal oblique arch more caudally and run in a direction similar to external oblique muscle.
  - The lower portion of transverse abdominis muscle is fused with the internal oblique, and during transverse incision of the lower abdomen, only two layers are discernible at the lateral margin of incision.
  - The direction of fibres of the flank muscles are transversely oriented. This is the reason that a vertical incision is more prone to tension and subsequently dehiscence compared to a transverse incision.

1.3 Rectus Sheath

- The rectus sheath is a strong, incomplete fibrous compartment of rectus abdominis and pyramidalis muscles formed by the conjoined aponeurosis of the flat muscles of the abdomen.

- For surgeons, the lower quarter of the rectus sheath is entirely anterior to the rectus muscles. Above this, it splits and encloses both ventral and dorsal aspect of the rectus sheath. This transition point is called the arcuate line (one-half of the distance between the umbilicus and pubic symphysis).
- At the arcuate line, the midline ridge of the rectus sheath towards the umbilicus needs sharp dissection during a Pfannenstiel incision.
- The linea alba transmits only small vessels and nerves to the skin, so a midline incision is relatively bloodless and avoids nerves.

2 Abdominal Incisions

Principles governing abdominal incision:

- The incision must give ready access to the area of investigation and must allow extension if required.
- The muscles must split in the direction of their fibres.
- The incision must not divide nerves.
- The rectus muscles may be cut transversely without weakening of the abdominal wall.
- Drainage tubes should be inserted through separate, small incisions as their presence in a main wound hampers the strength of the ultimate scar.

2.1 General Laparotomy Incisions

- incision on the anterior abdominal wall follows cleavage line/Langer's line in skin
- type of incision (see Figure 1.1):
  - longitudinal: median/midline
    - paramedian
  - oblique and transverse
  - high-risk incision
  - minimally invasive/endoscopic surgery

2.1.1 Midline Incision

- The incision runs along any length of linea alba from xiphoid to pubic symphysis, either above and below the umbilicus or both skirting the umbilicus.
- This incision divides skin, linea alba, fascia transversalis, extraperitoneal fat and peritoneum.
- The linea alba above the umbilicus is dense, strong, and 1 cm wide, so holds sutures well, but in the lower abdomen, the linea alba is very narrow, so poor suture technique predisposes to incisional hernia.
- For laparoscopic surgery, insertion of the Veress needle is through the umbilicus followed by midline intra- or subumbilical port. Lateral laparoscopic ports (lateral to rectus sheath) should be made under transillumination and placed low to avoid damage of inferior epigastric vessels.

2.1.2 Paramedian Incision

- Paramedian incision may extend from the costal margin to the pubic hairline.
- It is a vertical incision; 2–2.5 cm away from, and parallel to, the midline.
- The structures cut by a paramedian incision are the skin, anterior rectus sheath, rectus abdominis, posterior rectus sheath (above arcuate line), fascia transversalis, extraperitoneal fat and peritoneum.

2.1.3 The Lower Abdominal Transverse Incision

2.1.3.1 Pfannenstiel Incision/Suprapubic Incision

- This incision is commonly used in most gynaecological laparotomies and obstetric surgery such as caesarean section for approaching pelvic organs.
- Incision is horizontal, approximately 10–15 cm long, with slight convexity and made above the pubic symphysis, but just below the hairline (2 cm above the pubic symphysis).
- The linea alba and anterior layer of rectus sheath are divided in the line of skin incision.
- During this incision, injury to bladder, ilioinguinal and iliohypogastric nerves must be avoided.

2.1.3.2 Kustner Incision

- The Kustner incision is also known as a modified Pfannenstiel incision.
- Incision line is slightly curved, beginning below the level of the anterior superior iliac spine and extending just below the pubic hairline.
- The incision is more time consuming and extensibility is limited, and there may be

a chance of damage to inferior epigastric vessels.

2.1.3.3 Joel-Cohen Incision

- A Joel-Cohen incision is sometimes used to perform caesarean sections.
- It is a straight transverse incision through skin, 3 cm below the level of the anterior superior iliac spine, but higher than the Pfannenstiel incision.

2.1.3.4 Cherney Incision

- A Cherney incision involves transection of the rectus muscles at their insertion with upwards retraction.
- It can be used for urinary incontinence procedures like Burch colposuspension to access the space of Retzius.

2.1.3.5 Maylard Incision

- A Maylard incision is a transverse incision in which a cut is made through the rectus muscle transversely for wider access to pelvic organs; for example, gynecological malignancies.

2.1.3.6 Rutherford Morison

- A Rutherford Morison is an oblique incision in the lower abdomen along the inguinal ligament.

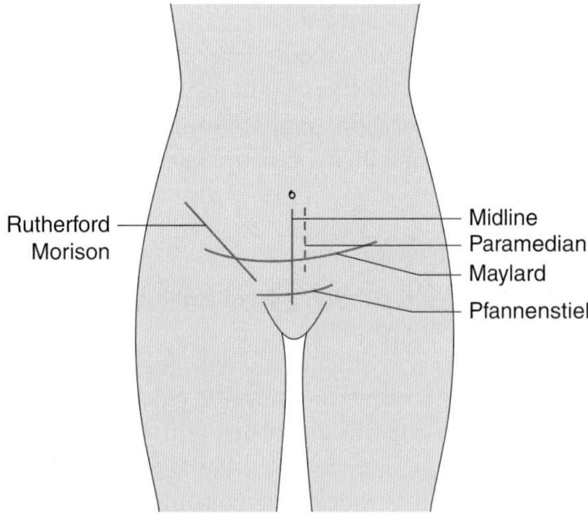

Figure 1.1 Incisions of the anterior abdominal wall.

3 Types of Caesarean Section

3.1 Lower Segment Caesarean Section (LSCS)

- The incision on skin may be vertical or transverse. The vertical incision is rarely used. The commonest incision is the transverse incision, i.e. Pfannenstiel or Joel-Cohen incision.
- Incision on uterus: the peritoneum of the utero-vesical pouch is cut transversely about 1.25 cm below its attachment to the uterus. The uterine incision is a transverse incision on the muscles of the uterus starting at the midline.

3.2 Classical Caesarean Section

- The incision on the abdomen is usually transverse and rarely longitudinal.
- The incision on the uterus is about 12.5 cm long and is longitudinally placed in the midline of the anterior uterine wall.
- Indications for a classical caesarean section are previous myomectomies, lower segment fibroids, placenta praevia anterior and extreme preterm delivery.

4 Female Pelvis

- The pelvic cavity is funnel shaped with posterior angulation, and is continuous with the abdominal cavity at the pelvic inlet.
- The pelvic cavity has an antero-inferior wall, two lateral walls, a posterior wall and a floor. The antero-inferior wall is formed by the body and rami of pubis, and the two lateral walls include the right and left hip bone, along with obturator foramen closed by obturator membrane and obturator internus muscles. The posterior wall consists of a bony wall (sacrum and coccyx) and musculoligamentous part (ligaments of sacroiliac joints and piriformis).
- The pelvic floor consists of levator ani muscles and their fascia, along with perineal membrane (urogenital diaphragm). See Figure 1.2.
- The pelvis is divided into the anterior and posterior triangle by an imaginary line two between ischial tuberosities. The anterior triangle is a layered structure. From superficial to deep is skin, subcutaneous tissue, perineal membrane,

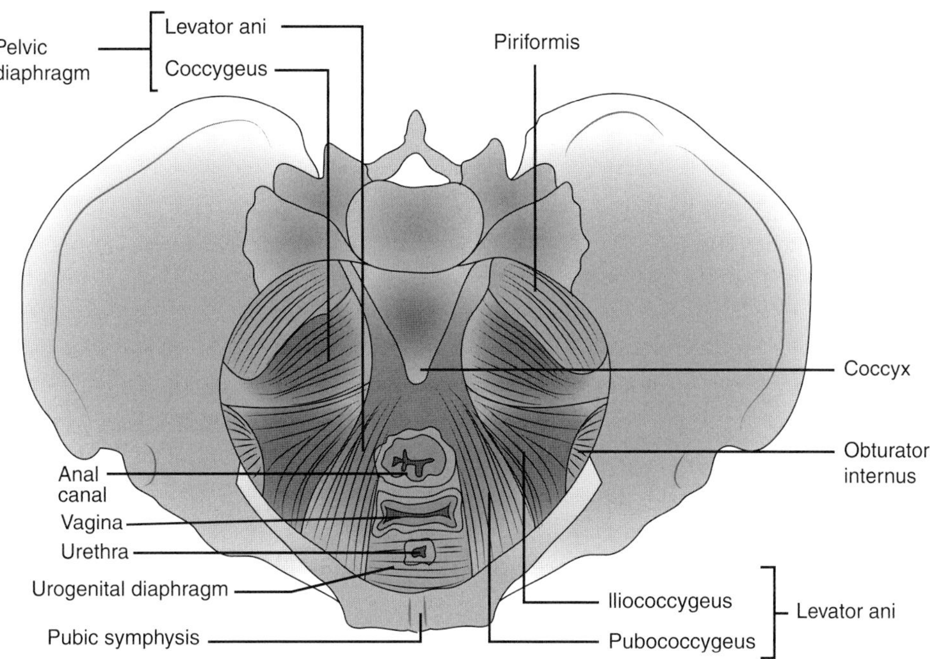

Figure 1.2 The pelvic cavity. Used with permission from Benjamin-Cummings, an imprint of Addison Wesley Longman, Inc.

muscle layer (i.e. levator ani) and, in the posterior triangle, the ischiorectal fossa lies between the pelvic wall and levator ani.

- The perineal membrane is a triangular sheet of dense fibromuscular tissue, which spans in the anterior half of the pelvic outlet and forms the anterior portion of the pelvic floor.
- The perineal body is also called the central tendon of perineum. It is a mass of connective tissue bounded by the lower vagina and anus.
- It is 1.25 cm in front of the anal margin in the median plane.
- The ten muscles of the perineum converge and interlace in the perineal body. The muscles are as follows:
  - bulbospongiosus (two)
  - superficial transverse perinei (two)
  - deep transverse perinei (two)
  - levator ani (two)
  - external anal sphincter
  - longitudinal muscle coat of rectum
- The perineal body indirectly supports pelvic organs and, when damaged during parturition, leads to prolapse of the bladder, uterus and rectum.

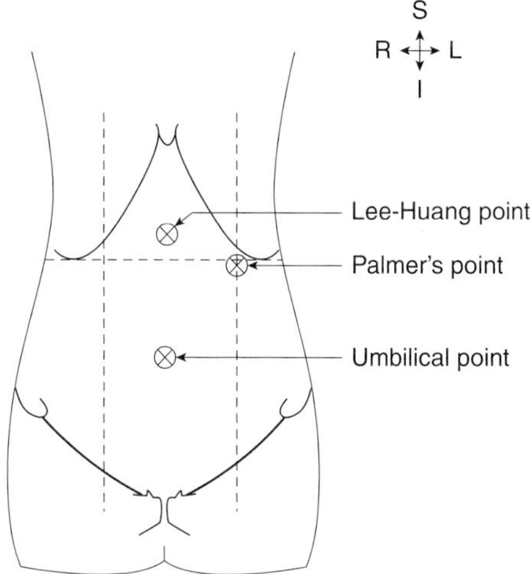

Figure 1.3 Laparoscopic entry points. S: superior; L: left; I: inferior; R: right

5 Clinical Procedures on Pelvis

5.1 Episiotomy

- Episiotomy is the surgically planned incision on the perineum and posterior vaginal wall during the second stage of labour.
- Types: mediolateral, median, lateral and J-shaped.

- Right mediolateral incision is the commonly performed procedure. The incision is diagonally outwards and downwards from the midpoint of the fourchette, about 2.5 cm away from the anus (midpoint between the anus and ischial tuberosity).
- Median or left lateral incision can cause higher risk of damage to the anal sphincter and the rectum; hence this is not done.

The incised structures are:

- posterior vaginal wall
- superficial and deep transverse perinei msucles
- bulbospongiosus and part of levator ani
- fascia covering over muscle
- transverse perineal branch of pudendal nerve and vessels
- subcutaneous tissue and skin

5.2 Culdocentesis and Culdoscopy

Culdocentesis is a procedure to drain a pelvic abscess in the recto-uterine pouch through the posterior fornix of vagina. It is possible due to the proximity of the peritoneal cavity to posterior fornix.

The needle should pass through:

- mucous membrane of vagina
- muscular coat of vagina
- connective tissue wall of vagina
- visceral layer of pelvic fascia
- visceral layer of peritoneum

5.3 Injury to the Pelvic Floor

- During childbirth, usually the pelvic floor supports the descending fetal head.
- During this process, the muscles of the pelvic floor (mainly the pubococcygeus, puborectalis and medial part of levator ani) are damaged along with injury to the ligaments. This weakens the support of pelvic organs, leads to their prolapse and alters the position of the bladder neck and urethra.

Blood Supply and Lymphatic Drainage of the Anterior Abdominal Wall –– Knowledge of the blood supply of the anterior abdominal wall is important in planning any operative procedure of the anterior abdominal wall (e.g. abdominal incisions, mucocutaneous flap formation, reconstruction of the abdominal wall during ventral hernia repair, and laparoscopic procedures).

Vascular Supply of the Anterior Abdominal Wall ––

- superior epigastric artery and vein
- inferior epigastric artery and vein
- posterior intercostal, subcostal and lumbar arteries
- femoral artery branches:
  - superficial epigastric artery
  - superficial circumflex iliac artery
  - superficial external pudendal artery
  - deep circumflex iliac artery

Superior epigastric artery and vein:

- arises at the level of sixth costal cartilage as one of the terminal branches of internal thoracic artery
- course: after its origin, descends between the costal and xiphoid slips of diaphragm accompanied with two veins; it passes anterior to transversus thoracis and upper fibres of transversus abdominis muscle and enters the rectus sheath; in the rectus sheath, superior epigastric artery anastomoses with the inferior epigastric artery, usually above the level of umbilicus
- branches of superior epigastric artery supply rectus abdominis and perforate the anterior lamina of the rectus sheath to supply the abdominal wall skin

Inferior epigastric artery/deep inferior epigastric artery and vein:

- originates from external iliac artery, accompanied by two veins, which join to form a single vein and drains into the external iliac vein
- course: it ascends along the medial margin of deep inguinal ring; pierces the fascia transversalis and enters the rectus sheath anterior to arcuate line and finally anastomoses with superior epigastric artery; insertion of laparoscopic ports or abdominal drains at this site leads to disruptions of the artery and haematoma formation
- the branches of the inferior epigastric artery are the cremasteric artery, pubic branch, muscular branch and cutaneous branch

Posterior intercostal, subcostal and lumbar arteries:

- the tenth and eleventh posterior intercostal arteries (branches of thoracic aorta), the subcostal artery, and the lumbar arteries pierce the aponeurosis of transversus abdominis to enter the neurovascular plane; knowledge of these arteries and accompanied segmental nerve is important for making myofascial flaps in abdominal wall reconstruction

Lymphatic Drainage of Anterior Abdominal Wall -- The lymphatic vessels of the anterior abdominal wall are arranged in two sets: superficial and deep. Superficial lymphatics of the anterior abdominal wall follow its subcutaneous blood vessels. Lymphatics from the lumbar and gluteal regions run with circumflex iliac vessels, and those from the infra-umbilical skin run along superficial epigastric vessels. Finally, lymphatics running along the circumflex iliac vessels and superficial epigastric vessels drain into the superficial inguinal lymph node. The supraumbilical region is drained by axillary and parasternal lymph nodes.

The deep lymphatics accompany the deeper arteries. Laterally, these lymphatics run along with intercostal and subcostal arteries or may follow lumbar arteries and drain into the posterior mediastinal or lateral aortic lymph node. From the upper anterior abdominal wall, lymphatics drain into parasternal nodes along with the superior epigastric artery, while from the lower abdominal wall they drain into external iliac nodes via the inferior epigastric artery and deep circumflex artery.

Nerve Supply of the Anterior Abdominal Wall -- The skin and muscles of the anterior abdominal wall are supplied by the ventral rami of the sixth to eleventh intercostal nerves, the subcostal nerve, and the first lumbar nerve (iliohypogastric and ilioinguinal nerve). These nerves run anteriorly within the neurovascular plane formed between the transversus abdominis and internal oblique muscle. The transversus abdominis plane (TAP) block is a regional anaesthetic technique for abdominal surgery, in which local anaesthetic agent is injected into the neurovascular plane (between the internal oblique and transversus abdominis muscles) under ultrasound guidance.

6 Laparoscopic Port Entry Techniques and Potential Injuries

Today, laparoscopic procedures are more popular and are more commonly practised.

Access and port placement: to create working space in the abdomen, the peritoneal cavity of the patient must be distended by insufflation of CO_2, which is called pneumoperitoneum. This is created through an open or closed technique.

6.1 Entry Techniques

- The open (Hasson) technique: in this method, an incision is made in the anterior abdominal wall under direct vision. Injuries related to the blind insertion of the Veress needle and the primary trocar can be avoided by this technique.
- The closed (Veress) technique: in this method, the Veress needle punctures the layer of anterior abdominal wall at the umbilicus because there is little or no fat or muscle between the skin and peritoneum.
- Direct trocar entry technique: through this technique, laparoscopic entry is initiated by only one blind step instead of two steps (i.e. Veress needle, insufflation and then trocar). In this method, the anterior abdominal wall is sufficiently elevated by hand or by towel clip and then the trocar is directly inserted into the peritoneal cavity. The most common site of primary entry is through an infraumbilical or subumbilical skin incision.
- Optical (direct vision) access technique: in this method, the peritoneal cavity is accessed by specialised trocar, which allows each layer of the abdominal wall to be visualised.
- Radially expanding access technique: in this method, the abdomen is first insufflated by Veress needle, the needle is removed and the sleeve acts as a tract through the abdominal wall.

6.2 Access Locations

- Umbilical point: this is the most common site for Veress needle insertion.
- Left upper quadrant (Palmer's) point: the needle is inserted 3 cm below the left subcostal margin in the midclavicular line. This point is mainly used in obese patients and patients with previous laparotomy scars.
- Middle upper abdomen (Lee-Huang) point: the site for Veress needle and primary port insertion is midway between xiphoid process and umbilicus.
- Jain point: paraumbilical left lateral to the umbilicus on a line drawn 2.5 cm medial to anterior superior iliac spine.

6.3 Complications of Laparoscopic Surgery

No surgical procedure is without risks and, despite the minimal invasive nature of laparoscopic surgery, it can lead to some complications. Complications during laparoscopic surgery include the following (see Chapter 50 for further reading):

- Vascular injury: this type of injury mainly occurs in the closed insertion technique. The needle and the first trocar are inserted blindly.
- Bowel injury: incidence of bowel injury is rare (0.06–0.14%).
- Solid organ injury: this is very rare.
- Abdominal wall bleeding: this generally occurs when there is injury of the abdominal wall vessels during trocar insertion. Bleeding is noticed either by blood dribbling from the trocar into the abdomen or bleeding around the trocar site during a procedure or after trocar removal. This complication can be prevented by identifying the epigastric vessels through transillumination of the abdominal wall with a laparoscope.
- Nerve damage: abnormal stretching and compression of a nerve may cause peripheral damage during laparoscopic procedure.
- Thermal injury: thermal damage by electrocautery and lasers may cause thermal injury to viscera and abdominal vessels.

2 The Breast

Kamalpreet Kaur

1 Anatomy of the Breast

- The mammary gland rests on a bed that extends from the lateral border of the sternum to the midaxillary line, and vertically from the second to sixth ribs. Two-thirds of the breast rests on a bed formed by pectoral fascia overlying the pectoralis major; the other third over the fascia covering the serratus anterior muscle.
- The retromammary space is a potential space between the breast and the pectoral fascia, and contains loose connective tissue. This allows some degree of movement of the breast on the pectoral fascia.
- A small part of mammary gland may extend along the inferolateral edge of the pectoralis major towards the axillary fossa (armpit), forming an axillary process or tail (of Spence).
- The mammary gland is firmly attached to the dermis of overlying skin by suspensory ligaments (of Cooper), which are fibrous condensations of connective tissue that help support the lobes and lobules of the mammary gland.
- The mammary gland consists of glandular and supporting fibrous tissue embedded within a fatty matrix, together with blood vessels, lymphatics and nerves.
- The amount of fat surrounding the glandular tissue determines the size of nonlactating breasts. During pregnancy, breast size increases because of the formation of new glandular tissue.
- Each breast consists of 15–20 lobules, which radiate out from the nipple.
- The lactiferous duct from each lobule opens separately on the summit of the nipple and possesses a dilated lactiferous sinus just before its termination.
- The base of the nipple is surrounded by a circular pigmented area of skin, the areola. The areola contains numerous sebaceous glands, which enlarge during pregnancy and secrete an oily substance, which acts as a protective lubricant for the areola and nipple, and protects them from chafing and irritation as mother and baby begin the nursing experience.
- The nipples are conical or cylindrical prominences in the centre of the areola. They have no fat, hair or sweat glands. The tips of the nipples are fissured with the lactiferous ducts opening into them. The nipples are composed mostly of circularly arranged smooth muscle fibres, which compress the lactiferous ducts during lactation and erect the nipples in response to stimulation, as when a baby begins to suckle. See Figure 2.1.

1.1 Age Changes in Mammary Glands

- Before puberty, the breast tissue consists of a system of ducts embedded in connective tissue, which does not extend beyond the margin of the areola.
- At puberty, breasts gradually enlarge under the influence of ovarian hormones. The duct system elongates and undergoes branching. Peripheral branches form solid, spheroidal masses of cells, which are precursors of alveoli.

1.2 Changes During Pregnancy

- In early months, there is rapid increase in the length and branching of the duct system.
- The connective tissue becomes filled with budding and expanding secretory alveoli (which develop at the end of smaller ducts).
- Vascularity of connective tissue increases to provide adequate nourishment for the developing gland.
- The nipple enlarges and the areola becomes darker.

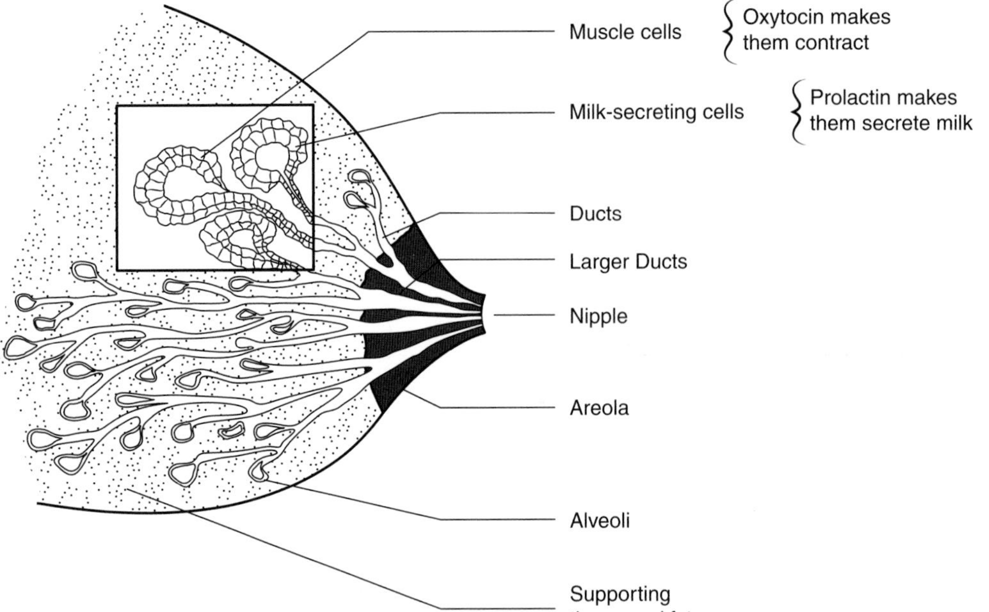

Figure 2.1 Anatomy of the mammary gland.

- During the second half of pregnancy, the breasts continue to enlarge because of distension of secretory alveoli with fluid secretion called colostrum.
- Postweaning, the breasts return to an inactive state (almost to the original size). Any remaining milk is absorbed, and secretory alveoli shrink and disappear.

1.3 Changes During Menopause

- Following menopause, the breast atrophies. Most of the secretory alveoli disappear, leaving behind the ducts and fibrofatty tissue. The atrophy is caused by the absence of ovarian Estrogens and progesterone. See Figure 2.2.

1.4 Development of the Mammary Gland

- In the young embryo, a linear thickening of ectoderm appears, known as the milk ridge, which extends from the axilla obliquely to the inguinal region.
- Later, this ridge disappears except for a small part in the pectoral region.
- The localised area thickens and sends off 15–20 solid cords, which grow into the underlying mesenchyme.
- Depressed ectodermal thickening becomes raised to form the nipple.
- At the fifth month, the areola is recognised as a circular pigmented area of skin around the nipple.
- Polythelia (supernumerary nipples) occur along a line corresponding to the position of the milk ridge. They are liable to be mistaken for moles. See Figure 2.3.

2 Blood Supply

- arteries:
  - perforating branches of the internal thoracic artery
  - intercostal arteries
  - lateral thoracic and thoracoacromial branches of the axillary artery
- veins: correspond to the arteries

3 Lymphatic Drainage

The lymph drainage is important because of the risk of development of cancer in the gland and subsequent dissemination of malignant cells along the lymph vessels to lymphatic nodes.

- Approximately 60% of carcinomas of breast occur in the upper lateral quadrant.

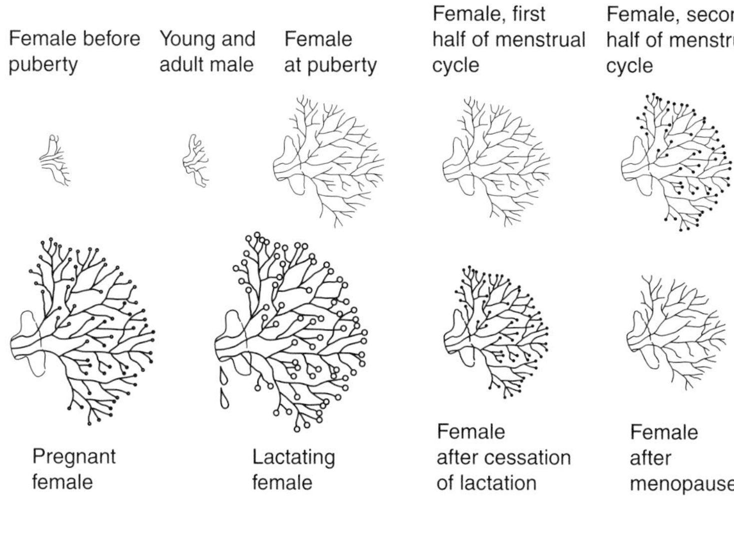

Figure 2.2 Extent of development of the ducts and secretory alveoli in the breasts in both sexes at different stages of activity.

Figure 2.3 The milk lines of the developing breast.

- In patients with localised cancer of the breast, simple mastectomy or lumpectomy is most commonly undertaken, followed by radiotherapy to the axillary lymph nodes and/or hormone therapy.
- In patients with localised breast cancer with early metastasis in the axillary lymph nodes, radical mastectomy offers the best chances of cure.
- Radical mastectomy removes the primary tumour, along with the associated lymph vessels and lymph nodes en-bloc. The axillary blood vessels, the brachial plexus and the nerves to the serratus anterior and latissimus dorsi are preserved.

4 Breast Examination

- With the patient undressed to the waist and sitting upright, the breasts are inspected for symmetry and any localised swelling.
- The nipples should be carefully examined for evidence of retraction.
- The patient is asked to lie down so that the breasts can be palpated against the underlying thoracic wall in a clockwise manner.
- Finally, the patient is asked to sit up and raise both arms above her head to check for dimpling of the skin or retraction of nipple.

5 Mammography

- Mammography is the radiographic examination of the breast using extremely low doses of X-rays.
- It is used for the screening of benign and malignant tumours and cysts.

5.1 Sonomammography

- Sonomammography is performed as an adjunct to mammography.
- It can differentiate solid masses from cystic masses, as well as their vascularity.
- It can be helpful in guiding fine needle aspiration procedures for cytology.
- Complete breast imaging should utilise both mammography and sonomammography.

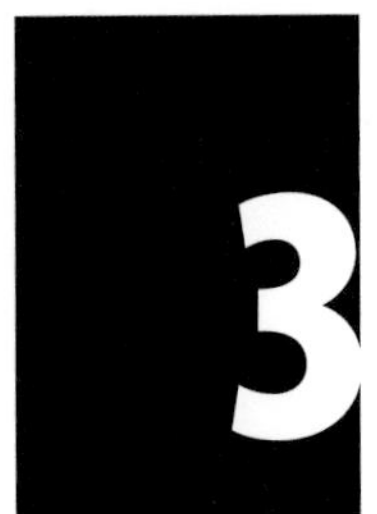

Anatomy of the Pelvis in Obstetrics

Kahkashan Jeelani

1 Bony Pelvis

The bony pelvis consists of four bones (two iliac (innominate) hip bones, sacrum and coccyx), and four joints in the articulated pelvis (i.e., two sacroiliac joints, pubic symphysis and sacrococcygeal joint). Both the anterior superior iliac spines and the upper end of the pubic symphysis lie in the same coronal plane, and the tip of the coccyx corresponds with the upper margin of the pubic symphysis. The pelvic surface of the body of pubis is directed more upwards than backwards, and the pelvic surface of the sacrococcygeal curve faces more downwards than forwards.

The female pelvis has been classified into four types according to its shape by Caldwell and Moloy. See Figure 3.1 and Table 3.1.

1.1 Effects of Hormones on Pelvic Joints in Pregnancy

- Increased levels of estrogen, progesterone and relaxin in the latter half of pregnancy leads to increased movement of pelvic joints (due to the softening of the ligaments of the sacroiliac and sacrococcygeal joints and increase in size of the interpubic disc).
- Relaxation of the sacroiliac joints and pubic symphysis permits 10–15% increase in transverse diameter).
- Relaxation of ligaments leads to less effective interlocking mechanism of sacroiliac joints. This causes greater rotation of the pelvis and the lordotic posture during pregnancy.

1.2 Effect of Age

- Obliteration of the cavity in the sacroiliac joint occurs in both sexes after middle age.

2 Function

The primary function of the pelvis is to transfer the body weight from the axial skeleton to the appendicular skeleton for standing and walking. In the female, it is also adapted for childbearing.

Anatomically, the pelvis is divided into greater or false pelvis and lesser or true pelvis. The entrance to the lesser pelvis or the pelvic brim is bounded by the upper part of the pubic symphysis, pubic crest, pubic tubercle, pectineal line, iliopubic eminence, arcuate line of ilium, anterior margin of ala of sacrum, sacral promontory. See Figure 3.2 and Figure 3.3.

Android Gynaecoid Platypelloid Anthropoid

A

B

C

Figure 3.1 Classification of pelvic shape. (Caldwell and Moloy)
A Pelvic inlet
B Mid pelvis
C Pelvic outlet

Table 3.1 Classification of the pelvis (Caldwell and Moloy classification) based on shape of inlet

	Gynaecoid	Anthropoid	Android	Platypelloid
Occurrence	50%	25%	20%	Approx. 5%
Shape of inlet	Round	Oval anteroposterior	Triangular	Transversely oval
Sacrum	Well curved from above, downwards and side to side	Long and narrow	Straight and inclined forwards	Short, straight and inclined posteriorly
Sacrosciatic notch	Wide and shallow	More wide and shallow	Shallow	Small and narrow
Cavity	Wide and shallow	Wider	-	-
Pelvic side wall	Straight or slightly curved	Straight	Convergent	Divergent
Ischial spine	Not prominent	Prominent	Prominent	Not prominent
Subpubic angle	Wide (85 degrees)	Short and narrow	Narrow	Wide with short pubic arch
Bituberous diameter	Normal	Short and narrow	Short	Spacious
Outcome	Good for obstetric outcome	High incidence of face to pubis delivery	Pelvic delivery is difficult with higher incidence of perineal tear	Outcome is generally good

Android is most common in males
Anthropoid and android are more common in white Women
Anthropoid and gynaecoid are common in black Women
Platypelloid is observed in osteomalacia or rickets

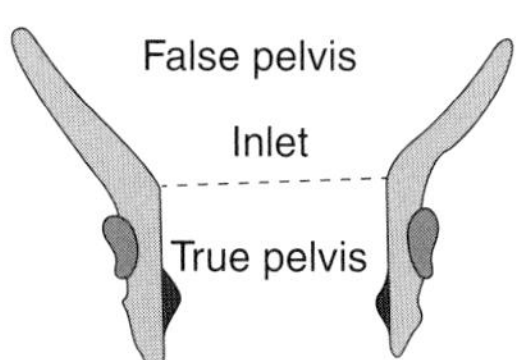

Figure 3.2 The pelvis: greater or false pelvis; lesser or true pelvis.

- An inlet/pelvic brim
- Pelvic cavity
- An outlet

3 The Pelvic Inlet/Pelvic Brim

- The shape of the pelvic inlet/pelvic brim in adult Women is almost round (the anteroposterior diameter being the shortest).
- The plane of inlet slopes downwards and forwards. The angle of inclination between the plane of inlet and the horizontal plane is approximately 50 to 60 degrees.
- High inclination is caused by sacralisation of the fifth lumbar vertebra and leads to a delay in engagement of the fetal head, while low inclination is seen in lumbarisation of the first sacral vertebra and favours early engagement.
- The axis is a line drawn perpendicular through the plane of inlet. This coincides with the axis of the uterus, so that the force of uterine contractions will propel the fetal head to pass through the pelvic brim. See Figures 3.3 and 3.4.

3.1 The Pelvic Cavity

The pelvic cavity lies between the pelvic inlet and outlet, and the wall of the cavity is formed by the pubic symphysis, the body of pubis with two rami, the pelvic surface of ilium and ischium, as well as the pelvic surface of the sacrum and coccyx.

The axis of the cavity points downwards. The baby's head's travel trajectory, through the axis of cavity, is from the axis of inlet to the axis of outlet.

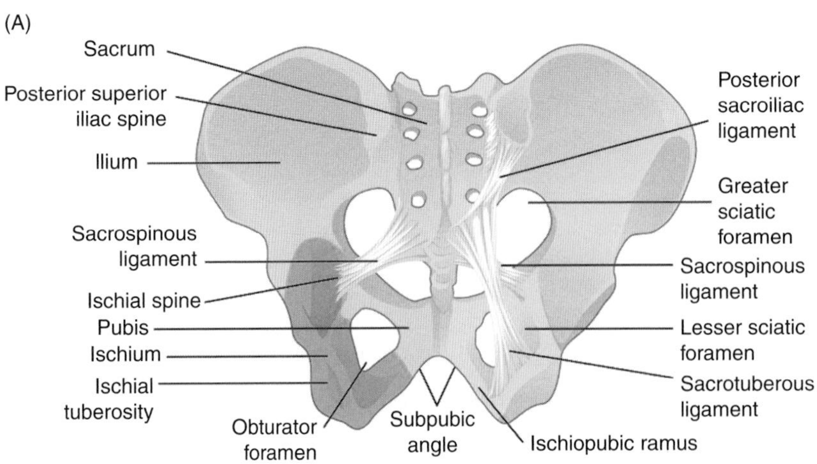

Figure 3.3 The greater pelvis only supports the gravid enlarged uterus. The lesser pelvis is adapted for parturition by forming birth canal. Used with permission from Lumen.

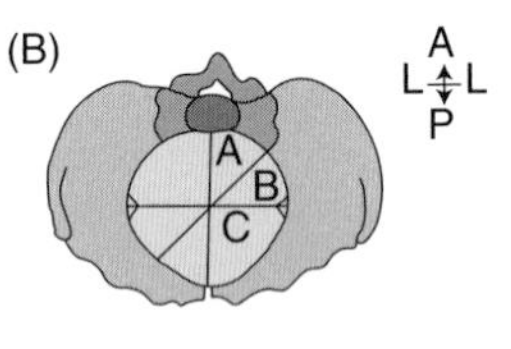

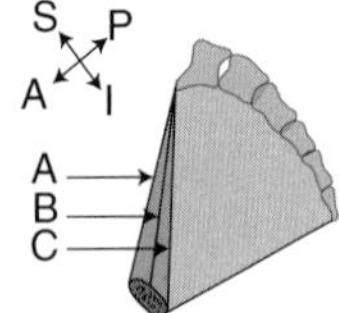

Figure 3.4 The axis of inlet corresponds to A and the axis of outlet coincides with B.

A Uterine axis
B Vaginal axis

A anterior; P posterior; L lateral; S superior; I inferior

The diameters and boundaries of the pelvic inlet and the pelvic cavity are elaborated on in Tables 3.2 and 3.3.

3.2 The Pelvic Outlet

- The pelvic outlet is roughly diamond shaped.
- The plane of the pelvic outlet extends from the tip of the coccyx to the lower border of the pubic symphysis. It does not lie in one plane as the tip of the coccyx is at a lower plane than the pubic symphysis.
  - When extended forwards, it makes an angle of about 10–15 degrees with horizontal.
  - The axis of the pelvic outlet is directed downwards and forwards, and coincides with the axis of the vaginal canal.

The pelvic outlet diameters are elaborated on in Table 3.4.

4 The Fetal Skull

The fetal skull is the largest part of the fetal body to negotiate the maternal pelvis. The skull is made up of:

- frontal bones that make the forehead
- two parietal bones, on either side of skull
- two temporal bones above the ears on either side
- one occipital bone that forms the back and base of skull

The *sutures* between these bones can allow the bones to overlap during the passage of the head through the maternal pelvis. The sutures are:

- sagittal suture – joins the two parietal bones in the midline
- coronal suture – joins the frontal bone with the parietal bones
- lambdoid suture – joins the occipital and parietal bones
- frontal suture – lies in between the two frontal bones

These sutures enclose two membranous areas called *fontanelles*:

- Anterior fontanelle, also called *bregma*, is larger and shaped like a diamond. It lies at the junction of frontal, coronal and sagittal sutures.
- Posterior fontanelle, also called *lambda*, is smaller and triangular in shape. It lies at the junction of lambdoid and sagittal sutures. See Figure 3.5.

The diameters of the fetal skull are depicted in Table 3.5.

The presenting part of the fetal skull during vaginal delivery may be:

Table 3.2 Diameters of the pelvic inlet

Diameter	Extent	Value (female)
Anteroposterior diameter/anatomical conjugate/true conjugate	Middle of sacral promontory to upper margin of pubic symphysis	11 cm
Oblique diameter	Sacroiliac joint of one side to the iliopubic eminence	12–12.5 cm
Transverse diameter	• Widest measurement across inlet • The line crosses the true conjugate in its middle third, usually posterior to centre	13 cm
Obstetric conjugate	Middle of sacral promontory to middle of the posterior surface of pubic symphysis	10 cm
Diagonal conjugate	• Middle of sacral promontory to the lower margin of pubic symphysis • Measured clinically during pelvic examination	12 cm

Table 3.3 Diameters of the pelvic cavity

Diameter	Extent	Value (female)
Anteroposterior diameter	• From the centre of the posterior surface of the pubic symphysis to the junction of the second and third sacral vertebrae • It is the plane of the greatest pelvic dimension	13 cm
Oblique diameter	• Lower end of sacroiliac joint to the centre of opposite obturator membrane • It is the longest diameter	13.1 cm
Transverse diameter	Widest transverse distance across the lateral bony walls of the pelvic cavity	12.5 cm

Table 3.4 Diameters of the pelvic outlet

Diameter	Extent	Value (female)
Anteroposterior diameter	Lower border of pubic symphysis to the tip of coccyx (or* the sacrococcygeal joint)	12.5–13 cm
Oblique diameter	Between the ischiopubic rami of one side to the middle of the opposite sacrotuberous ligament	11 cm
Transverse diameter	Between the inner borders of the ischial tuberosities	11 cm

* The coccyx is normally mobile, so is not considered in obstetric measurements.

- *Vertex:* the area between the anterior and posterior fontanelle and the two parietal bones. This is the presenting part when the head is fully flexed in a normal delivery. The presenting diameter is suboccipitobregmatic, which is the smallest diameter.
- *Brow*: the area between the anterior fontanelle and the upper margin of the eyes. This is the presenting part when the head is partially extended, and the presenting diameter is suboccipto frontal, which is a larger diameter of the fetal skull.
- *Face*: the area between the eyebrow and the fetal chin. This is the presenting part when the head is fully extended and the presenting diameter is submento bregmatic. This presentation is risky for both mother and baby.

To allow the passage of the fetal skull through the bony pelvis, the following mechanisms come into play:

- Alignment of the smallest diameter of the fetal skull to the largest diameter of the maternal pelvis at the inlet and outlet.
- Presence of anterior and posterior fontanelle, which allow some degree of skull compression.

Table 3.5 Diameters of the fetal skull

Biparietal diameter	9.5 cm largest	One parietal boss to the other	
Suboccipitobregmatic	9.5 cm	Occiput to anterior fontanelle	Engages in vertex presentation
Occipitofrontal	11.5 cm	Occiput to eyebrows	
Submentobregmatic	10.5 cm	Chin to anterior fontanelle	Engages in face presentation
Occipitomental	13.5 cm largest	Occiput to chin	Engages in brow presentation

- Moulding of the fetal skull; that is, overriding of the skull bones at suture lines will reduce the fetal skull diameter if required.

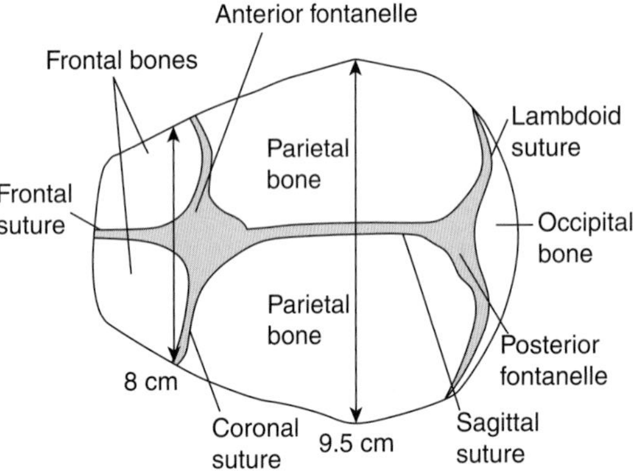

Figure 3.5 Fetal skull bones, sutures and fontanelles. Source: www.open.edu/openlearncreate/mod/oucontent/view.php?id=36§ion=6.5.2

5 Clinical Anatomy

- Spondylolisthesis:
  - Spondylolisthesis is the bilateral separation of the vertebral body from its vertebral arch, and leads to the anterior sliding of the vertebral body on the sacrum.
  - It reduces the diameter of pelvic inlet and interferes with the engagement of the fetal head.
- Osteomalacia:
  - Osteomalacia is when the pelvis becomes platypelloid in type.
  - There is difficulty in engagement of the fetal head at the inlet of the pelvis, but the outlet is roomy, so further descent of the head takes place normally.

It is important to be familiar with the anatomy of the pelvic inlet, cavity and outlet to understand the reasons for arrest in the descent of the fetal head through the birth canal.

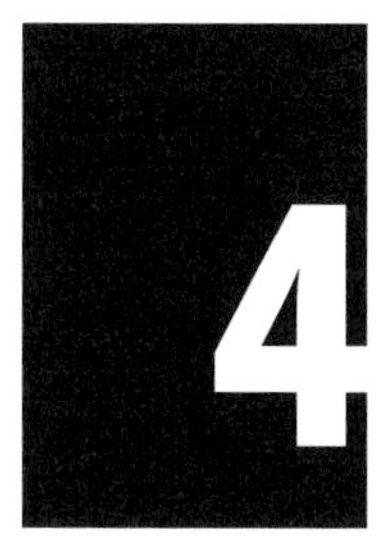

Anatomical Adaptation to Puberty, Pregnancy and Menopause

Swati Tiwari

1 Puberty

- Puberty refers to the transition period from childhood to adulthood.
- It begins at around 10–11 years of age in girls. It is completed by 15–17 years when Women attain sexual maturity.
- It begins under the influence of hormonal signalling to the ovaries in Women (gonads in males).
- This stimulates libido and the growth, function and transformation of the brain, bones, muscle, blood, skin, hair, breasts and sexual organs.

2 Menopause

- Menopause refers to the permanent cessation of menstruation as a result of loss of ovarian follicular activity.
- Climacteric refers to the period of time on either side of menopause, during which the female passes from the reproductive to non-reproductive stage (about 5–10 years).
- Age of menopause:
  - Genetically predetermined.
  - Occurs around 45–55 years of age; the average being 50 years
  - Cigarette smoking, severe malnutrition and thin body habitus predispose to early menopause.
  - Clinical relevance: due to today's longer lifespan, Women spend considerable time in estrogen deprivation, causing long-term symptomatic and metabolic complications.
- Important symptoms of menopause:
  - Cessation of menstruation.
  - Urogenital atrophy.
  - Osteoporosis and fracture.
  - Cardiovascular disease.
  - Psychological changes.
  - Vasomotor symptoms: hot flushes (cutaneous vasodilation and perspiration).
  - Sexual dysfunction.
  - Skin and hair: loss of collagen, thinner skin.
  - Dementia and cognitive decline.

3 Mammary Glands

3.1 Newborn

- Newborn breasts contain lactiferous ducts, but no alveoli.
- Witch's milk: some secretions may occur from newborn breasts under the influence of maternal hormones that cross the placenta and enter the fetal circulation.

3.2 Puberty

1. Thelarche is defined as development of breast. It is characterised by the following:
   - First noticeable sign of puberty, and occurs anywhere between 10 and 16 years of age (peak time: 13 years of age).
   - Occurs under the influence of increase in sex steroids.
   - Increase in adipose tissue content.
   - Inactive gland with sparse glandular component.
   - Proliferation of duct system.
   - Terminal part of ducts has polyhedral cells but very few alveoli are seen at this stage.

Table 4.1 describes the Tanner stages of development.

Table 4.1 The Tanner stages of breast development in girls

Stage I	Elevation of papilla
Stage II	Breast bud and papilla elevated, enlargement of sides of areola (around 9.8 years)
Stage III	Enlargement of entire breast tissue
Stage IV	Secondary mound of areola and papilla projecting above breast (12.1 years)
Stage V	Areola recessed to general contour of breast

2. Pubarche:
   - Pubarche is the growth of pubic and underarm hair, oil and sweat glands, especially in the axilla).
3. Menarche:
   - Menarche is the onset of first menstrual period.
   - Blind girls have late menarche.
   - Cyclic changes begin in the mammary gland.
   - In the follicular phase (estrogen influence): intralobular stroma is less dense. Terminal ductules appear as cords lined by cuboidal cells. There is little or no lumen.
   - In the luteal phase (progesterone influence): lining epithelial cells are taller. Small amounts of secretions appear in the lumen. Oedematous intralobular stroma. Women perceive tenderness and increase in breast tissue mass.
   - Last few days of menstrual cycle: there is involution and apoptosis.

3.3 Pregnancy

Serial changes in the breast during pregnancy are described in Table 4.2.

3.3.1 Lactation

- During lactation, milk is produced by the epithelial cells of the alveoli and accumulates in their lumens and inside the lactiferous ducts.
- Colostrum: in the first two or three days after birth, a protein-rich thick fluid called colostrum is secreted. This high-protein secretion, rich in vitamin A, sodium and chloride also contains lymphocytes and monocytes, minerals and lactalbumin. It contains less fat and more protein than regular milk and is rich in antibodies (predominantly secretory immunoglobulin A (IgA)), which provide some degree of passive immunity to the newborn, especially within the gut lumen.
- Milk: usually produced by the fourth day after parturition, this is a fluid that contains minerals, electrolytes, carbohydrates (including lactose), immunoglobulins (mostly IgA), proteins (including caseins) and lipids.

Table 4.2 Breast changes during pregnancy

First trimester	• Elongation and branching of terminal ductules • Proliferation and differentiation of lining epithelial cells • Hyperpigmented areola, appearance of Montgomery tubercles and secondary areola
Second trimester	Differentiation of alveoli lined by flat to low columnar cells
Third trimester	• Maturation of alveoli: lining epithelium becomes cuboidal • Cells develop extensive rough endoplasmic reticulum (rER) with lipid droplets • Hypertrophy of secretory cells • Accumulation of secretions in alveoli

3.4 Menopause

- Reabsorption of fat.
- Atrophy of glandular component.
- Nipples decrease in size.
- Breasts become flat and pendulous.

4 Vagina and Labia

4.1 Newborn

- Vagina is 2.5–3.5 cm long and 1.5 cm wide at fornices.
- Cervix extends into vagina for about 1 cm.
- It is lined by thin, stratified epithelium.
- Labia are thin.

4.2 Puberty

- Vagina is lined by stratified epithelium, comprising many layers compared to that in childhood.
- Cells are rich in glycogen.

- Döderlein's bacilli appear: convert glycogen into lactic acid; hence, vaginal pH becomes acidic (pH 4–5).

4.3 Pregnancy

- Chadwick's sign is violet discoloration of the vagina due to increased vascularity and hyperaemia.
- Varicose veins may develop due to pressure from enlarged uterus.
- Labia become thicker.

4.4 Menopause

- Vaginal dryness and loss of elasticity causes narrowing.
- Epithelium becomes thinner.
- Maturation index (parabasal, intermediate and superficial cells) is 10/85/5.
- Lack of estrogen causes changes in local pH, thereby affecting normal flora. This predisposes to urinary tract infections and dyspareunia.
- Labia and skin become thinner and prone to tears with mild friction.
- Scantier pubic hair.
- Increased risk of uterovaginal prolapse.

5 Uterus, Cervix and Fallopian Tubes

5.1 Newborn

- Uterine body:cervix ratio = 1:2.

5.2 Puberty

- Uterine body:cervix ratio = 1:1.
- Uterus weight: average 70 gm; cavity: about 10 ml.
- Uterus is pear shaped.
- Cyclic changes in the endometrium with each menstrual cycle. See Figure 4.1.
- Increased vascularity and hyperplasia of muscles.
- Hypertrophy of cervix and increased secretions.
- Watery secretions with less protein and more electrolytes to favour penetration of sperm during midcycle.

5.3 Pregnancy

5.3.1 Uterus

- Increase in size and weight of the uterus. It weighs 1100 g at term.
- Uterus is globular in shape. By 12 weeks, the uterus enters the abdominal cavity and pushes intestines laterally and upwards. Undergoes dextrorotation.
- Enlargement is more marked at the fundus: fundus becomes dome shaped. Thus, fallopian tubes, round ligament and ligament of ovary appear to attach in the middle of the uterus.
- Uterine enlargement is attributed more to stretching and marked hypertrophy of muscle cells rather than formation of new myocytes. Increase in supporting fibrous and elastic tissue.
- Three muscle layers become distinct. Prominent intermediate layer with criss-cross pattern arranged like a figure of '8': forming a living ligature for arrest of haemorrhage from the placental bed after delivery.
- Uterine walls become thicker early in pregnancy, but thin out as pregnancy advances. Walls are thin and soft such that palpation of fetus is possible through the walls.
- The uterus undergoes infrequent Braxton-Hicks contractions.
- Remodelling of uterine vessels, especially the veins, show increased calibre and distensibility to accommodate increased uteroplacental blood flow.
- Decidual reaction: active cell proliferation in endometrium, increased secretory activity. Three layers: superficial compact layer (decidual cells, gland ducts and capillaries), intermediate spongy layer (dilated uterine glands, blood vessels and decidual cells) and thin basal layer (basal part of uterine glands, regenerative layer).

5.3.2 Cervix

- Goodell's sign: softening of cervix and cyanosis due to increased vascularity and oedema.
- Rearrangement of collagen tissue to aid dilation during delivery and subsequent repair.
- Significant proliferation of cervical glands: they form almost half of cervical mass.

- Large amount of tenacious mucous plug closes the entry of cervical canal after conception. It gets expelled during delivery.
- Basal cells near squamocolumnar junction become prominent in size, shape and staining. Endocervical mucosa extends beyond squamocolumnar junction.

5.3.3 Fallopian Tubes

- Slight hypertrophy of fallopian tube musculature and flattening of lining epithelium.

5.4 Menopause

- Uterus becomes smaller due to muscle atrophy.
- Ratio of uterine body:cervix reverts to 1:1.
- Endometrium is thinner.
- Cervical secretions are scanty.
- Fallopian tubes show signs of atrophy: thinner muscle coat, lack of cilia, less prominent plicae.

6 Ovaries

6.1 Newborn

- Primordial follicles.
- Most of them undergo atresia.

6.2 Puberty

- Ovaries enlarge in size.
- Follicular phase: luteinising hormone induces ovaries to produce androgens (androstenedione and testosterone).
- Androgens are aromatised in granulosa cells to Estradiol and Estrone.
- Around 400 000 primordial follicles are present at puberty.
- Cyclic changes:
  - Proliferative phase: 15–20 follicles mature each month: from primary to secondary to tertiary stage, but only one attains full maturation (25 mm diameter) in each cycle. Surface of the ovary bulges and a stigma appears (avascular spot) from where ovum is extruded.
  - Secretory phase: formation of corpus luteum.
  - Menstrual phase: degeneration of corpus luteum.

6.3 Pregnancy

- Cessation of ovulation and further maturation of follicles.
- Enlargement of corpus luteum in early pregnancy (6–7 weeks of gestation) to secrete progesterone to support the pregnancy.
- Increased calibre of ovarian vascular pedicle.

6.4 Menopause

- Ovaries shrink and appear white.
- Thinner cortex and prominent medulla.
- Abundant stromal cells.
- Most follicles have undergone atresia, and a scar with hyaline streaks develops.

7 Pelvis

7.1 Newborn

- Until puberty, the female pelvis resembles a male pelvis.

7.2 Puberty

- After puberty, the female pelvis starts to become wider to allow for childbirth. Thus, it attains an evolutionary compromise between childbirth and bipedal locomotion.

7.3 Pregnancy

- Relaxation of pubic symphysis begins in early pregnancy and increases during the last three months.
- This process reverses soon after delivery and regression is completed in 3–5 months.
- Width of the pubic symphysis increases, particularly in multiparous Women and regresses to normal soon after delivery.
- Increased mobility of sacroiliac joint, especially in the dorsal lithotomy position. Hence, this position is preferred during vaginal delivery.

7.4 Menopause

- Loss of muscle tone, with pelvic relaxation.

- Pelvic cellular tissue becomes scant.
- Ligaments supporting the uterus and vagina lose their tone.

8 Bones

8.1 Puberty

- Estrogen and insulin-like growth factor 1 lead to the growth of bones and gain in height.
- Adult stature is achieved by the end of puberty.

8.2 Pregnancy and Lactation

- Increased demand for calcium in the fetus leads to transfer of calcium from the maternal to the fetal body. This predisposes to maternal bone loss, despite increased calcium absorption in the female during pregnancy.
- Women tend to lose 3–7% of bone density during lactation, which is regained after weaning.

8.3 Menopause

- Deficiency of estrogen causes a loss in bone mass by 3–5% per year.
- Osteoporosis sets in with reduction in bone mass, but mineral:matrix ratio is normal.
- High risk of bone fractures.

Bibliography

Carpenter, S. E. K., Rock, J. A. (2000). *Pediatric and Adolescent Gynecology*, 2nd ed., Lippincott Williams & Wilkins Publishers.

Hoffman, B. L., Schorge, J. O., Bradshaw, K. D., et al. (2014). *Williams Gynecology*, 3rd ed., McGraw-Hill Education.

Howkins and Bourne. (2014). *Shaw's Textbook of Gynaecology*, 16th ed., Elsevier.

Huseynov, A., Zollikofer C. P. E., Coudyzer, W., et al. (2016). Developmental evidence for obstetric adaptation of the human female pelvis. *PNAS*, **113**(19), 5227–32.

Kalkwarf H. J., Specker B. L. (2002). Bone mineral changes during pregnancy and lactation. *Endocrine*, **17**(1), 49–53.

Konar, H. *DC Dutta's Textbook of Obstetrics*, 9th ed., Jaypee.

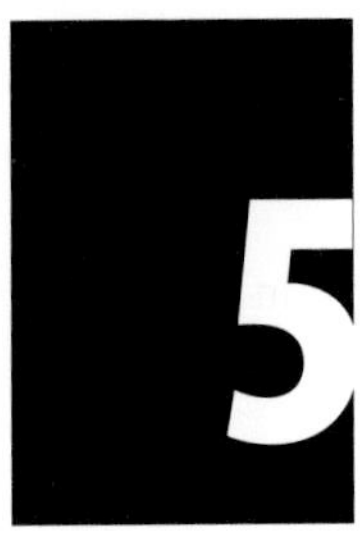

Anatomy of the Endocrine Glands: Thyroid and Pituitary

Sabah Yaseen

1 Thyroid Gland

- Highly vascular endocrine gland, situated at the level of fifth cervical to first thoracic vertebrae. It usually weighs 25 g, but is slightly heavier in Women and enlarges during menstruation and pregnancy.
- The thyroid gland consists of two lobes and interconnecting isthmus.
- Blood supply: superior thyroid and inferior thyroid artery. In 10% of the population there is a thyroid ima artery, which has a variable origin. Superior, inferior and middle thyroid veins form a thyroid plexus of veins on the anterior surface of the gland. Fourth thyroid vein of Kocher may be present sometimes. See Figure 5.1.
- Microstructure:
    - The thyroid gland consists of a number of follicles, which are the functional units of thyroid.
    - The follicles consist of a central colloid core surrounded by epithelium, which varies from squamous to cuboidal to columnar, depending on their level of activity.
    - Follicular cells secrete thyroid hormones triiodothyronine (T3) and tetraiodothyronine (T4) . These hormones regulate tissue basal metabolism and heat production, and also regulate the development of the nervous system in the fetus.
    - C cells in the thymus secrete calcitonin, which helps to lower the blood calcium.
- Applied:
    - Goitre is enlargement of the thyroid gland, caused either due to hypothyroidism or hyperthyroidism.
    - Hypothyroidism can be due to insufficient dietary iodine causing iodine deficiency/ endemic goitre, or it can be an autoimmune disease such as Hashimoto's thyroiditis.
    - Adolescent goitre/puberty goitre: enlargement of thyroid gland during puberty induced by increase in hormone requirement. It often resolves spontaneously as the period of maximal hormonal activity passes.
    - Hyperplasia of the thyroid gland occurs during pregnancy, due to which there may be slight enlargement of the gland but the hormone secretion is normal.
    - Hypothyroidism leads to menorrhagia and polymenorrhoea. However, in some cases, irregular periods or even amenorrhoea can occur. This occurs because low T3 and T4 stimulates the hypothalamus to produce thyrotropin-releasing hormone, which in turn stimulates thyroid stimulating hormone (TSH) and prolactin production in the pituitary. Hence, increased prolactin inhibits gonadotropin-releasing hormone release needed for luteinising hormone (LH) and follicle stimulating hormone (FSH) production, causing abnormal ovarian function.
    - Congenital hypothyroidism (also referred to as cretinism): caused by extreme hypothyroidism during childhood. In normal pregnancy, thyroid hormones cross the placental barrier and are critical in the early stages of fetal brain development. The fetal thyroid starts functioning at 14 weeks of gestation. If maternal hypothyroidism is present before the development of the fetal thyroid gland, the intellectual disability is severe. Thyroid hormones also stimulate gene expression of growth hormone in somatotrophs. Therefore, generalised stunted body growth is seen in hypothyroidism.

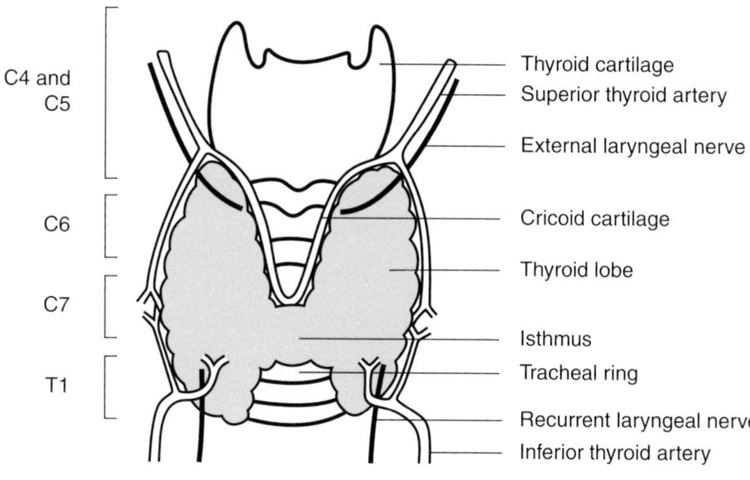

Figure 5.1 The thyroid gland and its relations.

2 Pituitary Gland

- The pituitary gland is a pea-sized endocrine gland located centrally at the base of the brain and lies in a depression called the pituitary fossa in the sphenoid bone, also known as sella turcica.
- The pituitary gland is a short stalk, and the infundibulum and vascular network connects the gland to the hypothalamus. The pituitary gland has two functional components:
  - Anterior lobe (adenohypophysis): the glandular tissue.
  - Posterior lobe (neurohypophysis): neurosecretory tissue.
    - The anterior lobe consists of:
      - the pars distalis, which makes up the bulk of this lobe
      - pars intermedia: located behind the pars distalis
      - pars tuberalis, which forms a sheath around the infundibulum
    - The posterior lobe consists of:
      - the pars nervosa, which contains neurosecretory axons and their ending
      - the infundibulum, which connects the gland to the hypothalamus
- Arterial supply: superior hypophyseal and inferior hypophyseal arteries.
- The primary capillary plexus is formed by arteries around the infundibulum, from where the hypophyseal portal vessels arise. These run along the pars tuberalis and form the secondary capillary plexus. This system of vessels carries the neuroendocrine secretions of hypothalamic neurons to release this in the pars distalis. See Figure 5.2.
- Microstructure:
  - Adenohypophysis: consists of epithelial cells of varying size and shape arranged in cords or irregular follicles, between which lies sinusoids. Five functional cell types are identified in the pars distalis based on immunocytochemical reaction.
  - Somatotrophs: secrete growth hormones.
  - Lactotrophs: secrete prolactin.
  - Corticotrophs: secrete adrenocorticotropic hormone.
  - Gonadotrophs: secrete FSH and LH.
  - Thyrotrophs: secrete TSH.
  - Neurohypophysis: stores and releases secretory products from the hypothalamus. These neurohormones are vasopressin or antidiuretic hormone and oxytocin from the supraoptic and paraventricular nuclei of the hypothalamus.
- Applied:
  - Panhypopituitarism: decreased secretions of all anterior pituitary hormones. It may be seen in Sheehan's syndrome associated with postpartum haemorrhage. It may also be congenital or acquired due to craniopharyngiomas, chromophobe tumours or thrombosis of pituitary blood vessels. The

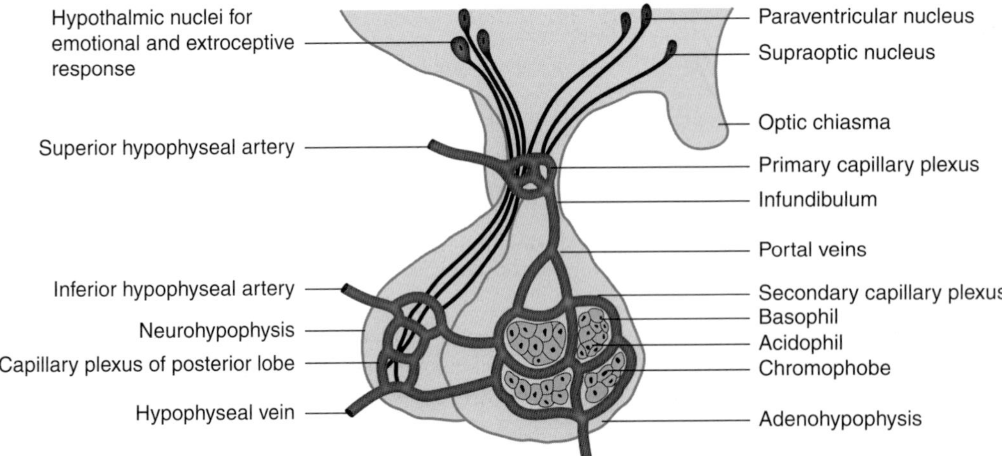

Figure 5.2 The pituitary gland showing hypophyseal portal system.

general effects are hypothyroidism and decreased production of glucocorticoids and gonadotropic hormones.

- During normal pregnancy, the pituitary gland enlarges by 30–50% in weight due to hyperplasia of lactotrophs. Sometimes the enlarged gland may press on the optic chiasma, causing bitemporal hemianopia.
- Hormonally active tumours originating from somatotrophs are associated with hypersecretions of growth hormones and cause gigantism in children and acromegaly in adults.
- Lactotroph adenomas (prolactinomas) are common types of secretory pituitary adenomas. They cause infertility because of the inhibitory effect of elevated prolactin on gonadotropin secretion, resulting in anovulation.
- Gonadotroph adenomas cause menstrual irregularities, ovarian hyperstimulation syndrome and precocious puberty.
- The pituitary gland may become infarcted after shock due to postpartum haemorrhage. This leads to development of postpartum necrosis of the pituitary known as Sheehan's syndrome.

6 Structural Changes in the Newborn

Kamalpreet Kaur

The first four-week period after birth is referred to as the neonatal period. At the moment of birth, the baby suddenly has to make drastic physiological adjustments for changes from intrauterine to extra-uterine life. The care of the child during this critical period and the understanding of the fundamental changes that are taking place within its body are essential.

1 Changes that Take Place at Birth

1.1 Respiratory System

- During labour, as soon as the placental circulation ceases, the respiratory system must function to take over the activity of gaseous exchange from the placenta.
- During labour, the oxygen tension of the fetal blood is lowered, carbon dioxide tension rises and the blood becomes acidotic.
- There appear to be two phases in the respiratory efforts. The first phase requires considerable exertion to achieve expansion of the lungs with air. During this phase, the baby exhibits strong gasping movements.
- The second phase is the establishment of rhythmic breathing movements. This is usually followed quickly by a lusty cry. A normal baby establishes rhythmic breathing movements within one minute after delivery.
- The respiratory centre in the medulla oblongata responds to a number of subliminal stimuli, such as:
    - stimulation through chemoreceptor reflexes from the aortic and carotid bodies due to acidosis after tying of umbilical cord
    - cutaneous stimulation and exposure to cold
- The amniotic fluid present within the respiratory tree before birth is expelled through the mouth in vertex deliveries by compression of the thorax by the birth canal. Any residual fluid is expelled through the pulmonary lymphatics.

1.2 Circulatory System

- The interruption of umbilical flow when the cord is tied results in immediate fall in blood pressure in the inferior vena cava.
- The closure of the ductus arteriosus by muscular contraction of its wall increases the blood flow through the lung vessels, with subsequent increase in pressure in the left atrium.
- Due to the above changes, the foramen ovale is functionally closed by apposition of the septum primum with the septum secundum as the neonate takes its first breath. Permanent closure occurs in about one year.
- The diminished pulmonary vascular resistance associated with inflation of the lungs causes the direction of blood flow from left to right. Later, the ductus becomes fibrosed to form the ligamentum arteriosum.
- Closure of the umbilical arteries is caused by thermal and mechanical stimuli, and change in oxygen tension. The distal part of the umbilical arteries form median umbilical ligaments and proximal portions remain open as superior vesical arteries.
- Closure of the umbilical vein and ductus venosus occurs shortly after that of the umbilical arteries. After obliteration, they form ligamentum teres hepatis and ligamentum venosum respectively. See Figure 6.1.

1.3 Blood Changes

- At birth, the infant has a large number of erythrocytes – 5–6 million mm^3 – and a high haemoglobin level, 15–20 g/100 ml of blood. The

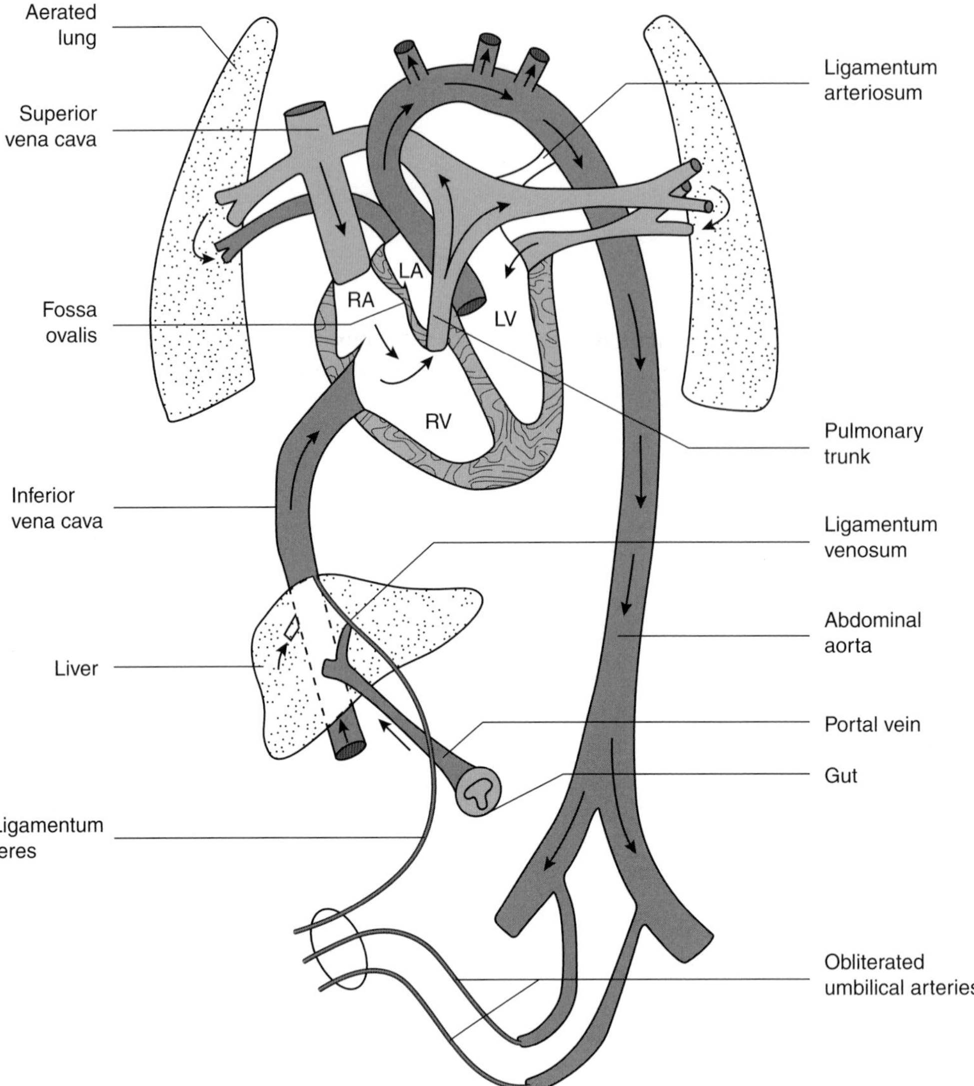

Figure 6.1 Changes taking place at birth.
RA: right atrium; LA: left atrium; LV: left ventricle: RV: right ventricle

high values are as a result of the need to provide adequate amounts of oxygen in the fetus in utero.

- At the end of the first week, the high values begin to fall until, by the end of the first month, all infants develop physiological anaemia. This is asymptomatic and recovery is spontaneous.
- The normal leucocyte count in a newborn is 10 000 to 35 000 mm^3. Most of the cells are polymorphonuclear neutrophils. After the third week, there is a predominance of lymphocytes, which persists until the fourth year.

1.4 Body Temperature

- In a newborn, the heat regulating mechanism is in an immature state.
- Immediately after birth, temperature falls by 3° Fahrenheit, but increased muscular activity, increased metabolic activity and improved vasomotor control results in a rise in temperature, which stabilises within eight hours.
- Brown adipose tissue plays an important role in heat regulation and is found in the root of the

neck, axilla, between the scapulae, around vessels and the organs in the thorax and posterior abdominal wall.

1.5 Skin

- At birth, the newborn's skin is slightly cyanotic, but within a few minutes becomes pink.
- Slight circumoral cyanosis and cyanosis of hands and feet may persist for a few hours until peripheral circulation opens up.
- Newborn skin will vary depending on the length of the pregnancy. Premature infants have thin, transparent skin. The skin of a full-term infant is thicker.

1.6 Icterus Neonatorum (Physiological Jaundice)

- In nearly half of all healthy babies, the bilirubin content of blood is raised to cause a slight degree of jaundice as a result of temporary impairment of excretion of bilirubin by the liver and increased destruction of erythrocytes.
- It is asymptomatic and usually occurs during the second or third day, and disappears after two weeks.

1.7 The Gastrointestinal System

- By the fourth month of intrauterine life, the fetus begins to swallow large quantities of amniotic fluid, and faecal material known as meconium begins to form.
- After birth, the baby shows signs of hunger by becoming restless, crying fretfully and sucking on its fingers.
- Sense of smell is acute, and the mouth is turned towards the source of milk.
- Sucking is assisted by the presence of transverse corrugations of mucous membrane of the palate, and the buccal pad of fat that prevents indrawing of the cheeks.
- Sucking is accomplished by the combined action of the tongue, cheeks and palate. Lips play a small part. Therefore, babies with a cleft palate find it impossible to suck, whereas babies with a cleft lip suck quite well.
- Digestion of proteins and carbohydrates takes place at birth, but starch is poorly tolerated.
- Meconium is sticky, dark green, odourless material consisting of a mixture of digestive secretions, bile pigments, desquamated cells and lanugo and vernix caseosa swallowed with amniotic fluid. These are the first stools passed by infant.
- After 3–4 days, meconium ceases and greenish-yellow stools are passed. After the fifth day, yellow milk stools appear.

1.8 The Renal System

- At birth, the biochemical characteristics of the urine are the same as in utero; that is, urine is acidic, hypotonic to plasma and contains very little sodium or chloride, and no phosphate.
- Large amounts of uric acid are excreted by the newborn.
- Infant kidneys may have difficulty in excreting excessive amounts of water and electrolytes (this fact should be remembered when instituting intravenous therapy).
- The total amount of urine passed per day varies from 30 ml to 60 ml, and at the end of the first week, this rises to about 200 ml per day.

1.9 The Umbilical Cord

- The cord stump shrivels, dries and sloughs off by the sixth to tenth day.
- At the site of separation, a small granulating surface persists for several days.
- Later, fibrosis of thrombosed umbilical vessels occurs, and they contract and invaginate the skin at the root of the cord, producing the typical umbilicus.

1.10 Weight Loss

- The average weight of a normal, full-term baby is about 3500 g.
- During the first 3–5 days, up to 10% of birthweight is lost due to loss of fluid from the body and relatively low fluid intake.
- By the eighth to the fourteenth day, this weight is regained and, during the next three months, the baby gains approximately 30 g per day.

1.11 Posture

- The baby who has had a normal cephalic presentation, when placed on its back, turns its head to one or the other side, and the arms and legs are semiflexed.

- The infant is unable to raise its head.
- Hip joints are partially abducted, externally rotated and semiflexed.
- At the end of the first month, the position of flexion decreases.

1.12 Behaviour

- The infant often yawns and stretches, may sneeze and often has hiccups after feeding.
- A newborn cries vigorously without tears; the first cry is heard immediately following delivery.
- A newborn usually sleeps most of the time.

1.13 Reflex Movements

- Certain reflexes are well developed at birth:
    - sucking reflex
    - rooting reflex
    - grasp reflex
    - plantar reflex (Babinski's reflex)
    - knee jerk
    - superficial abdominal reflexes
    - tonic neck reflex
    - startle reflex

1.14 Eyes and Ears

- A newborn perceives light and closes its eyes whenever there is bright light. Eye movements are uncoordinated at first and the eyes may squint.
- The iris is light in colour and the permanent darker colour does not appear until between three months and one year of age.
- The lacrimal glands do not function at birth and tears do not appear with crying until the end of the third or fourth week.
- A newborn can hear at birth and responds to loud noises.

1.15 The Skeleton

- The head of a newborn is large and accounts for one-fourth of the body length.
- The vault of the skull has areas of residual membranes called fontanelles.
- The face may be asymmetrical at birth, caused by fetal posture and pressure in utero, and this usually disappears within a few days after birth.

1.16 Changes After Withdrawal of Maternal Hormones

- The mammary glands of infants of both sexes may become enlarged and tense during the first week of life, and a milky fluid called witch's milk may be expressed from the nipples.
- The female external genitalia show congestion and moisture. As the hormonal levels in the blood become reduced, there may be uterine bleeding, vaginal desquamation and a mucoid vaginal discharge.

1.17 Defence Against Infection

- The newborn lacks specific antibodies, and the ability to form new antibodies is slow during the first few months of life.
- The newborn is also susceptible to certain organisms that are nonpathogenic to adults; for example, skin commensals.

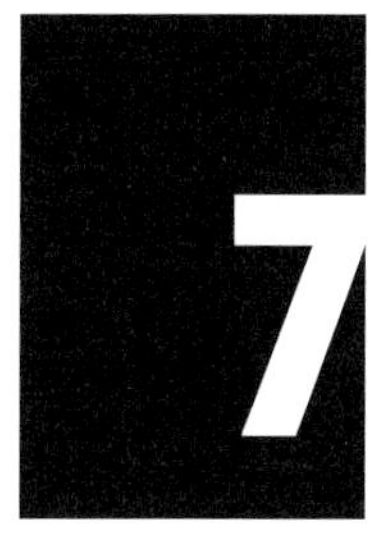

The Male and Female Reproductive Tracts and the Müllerian Anomalies

Vandana Tiwari

1 The Male Reproductive Tract

1.1 Development

- The male reproductive tract is developed from the intermediate mesoderm, which forms a urogenital ridge that gives rise to testicular stroma and the mesonephric (Wolffian) duct.
- Mesodermal (coelomic) epithelium gives rise to Sertoli cells and the paramesonephric duct.
- Primordial germ cells migrate from the yolk sac and give rise to the spermatogonia.

The anatomy of the male reproductive tract is shown in Figure 7.1.

1.2 Scrotum

- The scrotum is located outside of the abdominal cavity.
- It comprises a thin layer of smooth and skeletal muscle and skin.

1.3 Testis

- The testis contains 200 to 300 lobules, and each lobule contains two to three highly coiled seminiferous tubules.
- At puberty, the seminiferous tubules begin to produce about 400 million sperm.
- The spermatogenic cells are protected by a blood–testis barrier, which keeps the cells protected from activating the immune system.

1.4 Epididymis

- Sperm completes maturation and gains the ability to swim and fertilise.

1.5 Ductus Deferens

- The ductus deferens runs superior to the testicles and enters the abdominopelvic cavity, runs posterior to the bladder, passes by the seminal vesicle, forms the ampulla and ejaculatory duct, and finally leads into the prostatic urethra.

1.6 Clinical Implications

- In vasectomy, part of the ductus deferens is ligated and excised through an incision in the superior part of the scrotum. Hence, the subsequent ejaculated fluid from the seminal glands, prostate and bulbourethral glands contain no sperm. Any sperm not expelled degenerates in the epididymis and proximal part of the ductus deferens.
- Abscesses of the seminal glands may rupture, and pus can enter the peritoneal cavity.
- Benign hypertrophy of the prostate is a common cause of urethral obstruction, cystitis and kidney damage.

2 The Female Reproductive Tract

The anatomy of the female reproductive tract is shown in Figure 7.2.

2.1 Ovaries

- The ovaries are supported along the lateral pelvic sidewalls by the ovarian ligaments (attaching to the posterolateral aspect of the uterus), the mesovarium (the anastomotic region of the uterine and ovarian vessels), and the infundibulopelvic ligament, which are reflections of the broad ligament attaching the ovaries to the lateral pelvis.

- The ovaries rest in the ovarian fossa, immediately adjacent to the iliac vessels and the ureters.
- They contain three distinct cell populations:
  - germ cells
  - stromal cells, which are tightly packed around developing follicles and which secrete hormones
  - epithelium

2.2 Fallopian Tubes

- Each fallopian tube is 7–12 cm in length and <1 cm in diameter.
- Parts of fallopian tubes (medial to lateral) include:
  - interstitial (narrowest)
  - isthmus: 1 mm in diameter; the perfect spot for tubal ligation
  - ampulla: 6 mm in diameter; fertilisation of the ovum occurs here, and most ectopic pregnancies occur in the ampulla
  - fimbria (infundibulum)
- The fallopian tubes are covered by peritoneum and connected to the upper margin of broad ligament through the mesosalpinx.
- Blood supply is by the uterine and ovarian arteries.
- They are innervated by the uterovaginal and ovarian plexus.

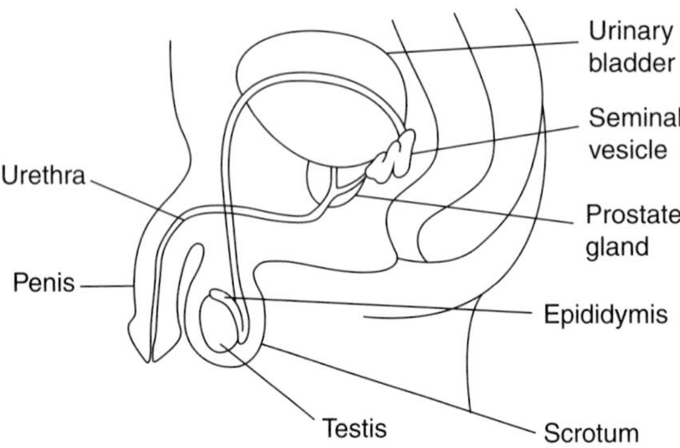

Figure 7.1 Anatomy of the male reproductive tract.

2.3 Uterus

- The uterus is a thick, muscular organ. It is derived from the fusion of two paramesonephric (müllerian) ducts.
- These ducts also form the upper two-thirds of the vagina and the fallopian tubes.
- It is divided into three segments: fundus, lower segment and cervix. At birth, the cervix and corpus are equal in size. In adult women, the corpus grows to two to three times the size of the cervix.
- Flexion is the angle between the long axis of the uterine corpus and cervix.
- Version is the angle of the junction of the uterus with the upper vagina.

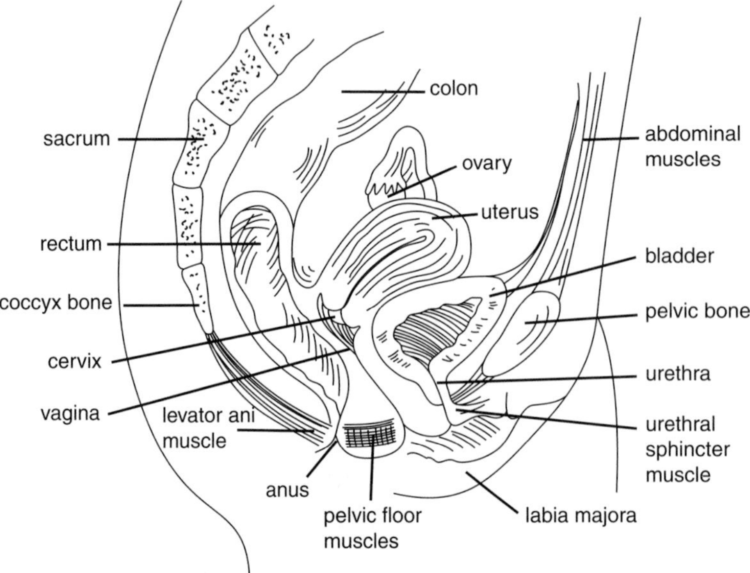

Figure 7.2 Female reproductive tract.

- The three layers of the uterus are the serosa, myometrium (smooth muscle), and endometrium.
  - The muscular layer of the uterus is the myometrium, which consists of interlacing smooth muscle fibres and connective tissue.
  - Interlacing myometrial fibres which surround the myometrial vessels control the bleeding from the placental site during the third stage of labour.
  - The uterine junctional zone is a region representing the inner myometrium and is a very important imaging feature in pelvic magnetic resonance imaging for interpretation of various pathologies. It is usually visualised as a low T2 signal layer beneath the endometrium. This low signal intensity is thought to be from closely packed compact smooth muscle cells with little extracellular matrix and water content. Disruption or alteration of the junctional zone can be caused by various pathological conditions:
    - uterine adenomyosis: makes the junctional zone thicker and hazy
      - a junctional zone of <8 mm is considered unlikely to represent adenomyosis
      - a junctional zone of >12 mm very likely represents adenomyosis
    - a feature of myometrial invasion with endometrial carcinoma
    - a feature of myometrial invasion by an invasive mole in the spectrum of gestational trophoblastic disease
    - uterine lymphoma, which is not thought to disrupt the junctional zone
- Blood supply: uterine artery anastomoses with the ovarian and vaginal artery (for this reason, during myomectomy surgeons place tourniquets at both the infundibulopelvic ligament and uterine isthmus to decrease blood flow from the ovarian and uterine arteries respectively).
- Innervations: uterovaginal plexus comprises sympathetic and parasympathetic fibres. Sympathetic fibres come from T10 to L1, while the parasympathetic fibres come from sacral 2, 3 and 4.

2.3.1 Uterine Supports

- The levator ani forms the pelvic floor, which supports the weight of the uterus.

2.3.1.1 Cardinal Ligament

- The cardinal ligament is found at the base of the broad ligament.
- It provides the main support for the uterus and cervix.
- It attaches to the cervix and extends laterally, connecting to the endopelvic fascia.

2.3.1.2 Uterosacral Ligaments

- The uterosacral ligaments provide minor cervical support.
- They originate from the upper posterior cervix, travel around the rectum bilaterally, and fan out to attach to the first to fifth sacral vertebrae.
- The rectum lies medial to the uterosacral ligament and ureter along with sidewall vessels in close proximity to this ligament. During pelvic reconstruction, surgeons use the uterosacral ligament as attachment sites for the vaginal apex as the above-mentioned structures are vulnerable to injury.

2.3.1.3 Round Ligament

- The round ligament is made of fibrous and musclar tissue.
- It is anterior to the fallopian tubes. (It assists the surgeon during tubal sterilisation in minilaparotomy incision. Division of the round ligament is an initial step in abdominal and laparoscopic hysterectomy. This opens the broad ligament and allows direct visualisation of the ureter and safe ligation and division of the uterine artery.)
- It correlates with the male gubernaculum.
- The round ligament extends laterally, crosses the external iliac vessels, enters the internal inguinal ring, and is inserted into the labia majora.
- The Sampson's artery is a branch of the uterine artery that runs along the length of the round ligament.

2.3.1.4 Broad Ligament

- Double reflection of the peritoneum is draped over the round ligaments.

2.3.2 Pregnancy-induced Uterine Changes

- During pregnancy, there is remarkable uterine growth due to hypertrophy of the muscle fibres.
- Weight changes from 70 g to approximately 1100 g at term.
- Its total volume increases to 5 L.
- Flattening of the fundal convexity between the tubal insertions occurs to become dome-shaped.
- The round ligament attaches to the junction of the middle and upper third of the uterus.
- The fallopian tubes elongate.
- The ovaries appear grossly unchanged.

2.3.3 Lymphatic Drainage

- Cervical cancer: drains first to the parametrial nodes, which drain to the obturator nodes, then to the pelvic nodes and finally to the paraaortic nodes.
- Uterine cancer: drains first to the pelvic nodes or paraaortic nodes.
- Ovarian cancer: can metastasise to either the pelvic or paraaortic nodes, but shows peritoneal spread at an early stage.

2.3.4 Key Points of Ureteric Relation in the Pelvis

- In the pelvis, the ureter runs medial to and parallel with the internal iliac artery.
- The uterine artery crosses over the ureter (water under the bridge).
- The remaining 2–3 cm of the ureter passes through the cardinal ligament into the bladder.

2.4 Vagina

- The vagina is a hollow fibromuscular tube.
- It extends from the vulvar vestibule to the uterus.
- It is attached at a higher point posteriorly than anteriorly, so the posterior vaginal wall is 3 cm longer than the anterior wall.
- Recesses within the vaginal lumen in front of, behind and at the sides of the cervix are known as anterior, posterior and lateral fornices respectively.
- Blood supply: the vaginal artery branches from the uterine, middle rectal and internal pudendal arteries.
- Innervations: upper vagina: uterovaginal plexus, which is mainly sympathetic, and lower vagina and labia by the pudendal nerve, which is somatic.

Anomalous development of the müllerian ducts is elaborated on in Table 7.1.

Table 7.1 Müllerian duct anomalies in males and Women

Müllerian duct anomalies		
Source	**Male**	**Female**
Paramesonephric ducts (müllerian ducts) • Unfused part • Uterovaginal primordium	• Most of the ducts disappear; the remaining form the appendix of testis • Prostatic utricle	• Fallopian tubes • Uterus • Cranial part of vagina
Anomalies • Müllerian agenesis • True duplication of the müllerian ducts • Incomplete müllerian fusion • Vascular accident or torsion after completion of gonadal and ductal differentiation • Persistence of müllerian derivatives	• Uterus and fallopian tubes may persist • Normal male external genitalia, Wolffian (mesonephric) derivatives, and testes • Pubertal virilisation occurs	• Absence of the uterine corpus, the uterine cervix and the upper portion of the vagina • Primary amenorrhea • Secondary sexual development is normal • Uterine remnants may exist in the form of bilateral cords • Associated renal anomalies may be pelvic kidney, renal ectopia and unilateral aplasia • Skeletal anomalies, especially vertebral anomalies • Two separate uteri; each of which may have two fallopian tubes

Table 7.1 (cont.)

Müllerian duct anomalies		
Source	**Male**	**Female**
		• Unicornuate uterus • Arcuate uterus • Septate uterus • Bicornuate uterus • Didelphic uterus with a septate vagina • Isolated absence of fallopian tubes
Paraovarian cysts (POCs) Origin: • Mesothelium covering the peritoneum (mesothelial cysts) 68% • Paramesonephric (paramesonephric cysts or müllerian cysts) 30% • Mesonephric remnants (mesonephric cysts or Wolffian cysts) 2%		• In women aged 20–40 years old • Accounts for ~10–20% of adnexal masses • Single cysts can be bilateral • Vary greatly in size • Small lesions: asymptomatic • Large lesions: present with pelvic pain, dysmenorrhoeal infections, vaginal discharge and urinary incontinence Examples: • Gartner's duct cyst (benign vaginal cyst) • Paratubal cysts or hydatid cysts of Morgagni • Paramesonephric cyst

8 Functional Anatomy of the Urinary Tract

Deepika Poonia

1 The Pelvic Floor

The pelvic floor (Figure 8.1) plays an important role in providing bladder and bowel control, and assists in parturition by promoting the rotation of the fetal head. It also supports the pelvic viscera including the enlarged gravid uterus. It is weakened during pregnancy, childbirth and menopause. This can lead to:

- anterior vaginal wall prolapse: cystocele and urethrocele
- central prolapse: uterine prolapse and vaginal vault prolapse
- posterior vaginal wall prolapse: rectocele and enterocele

The pelvic floor is formed by two important muscles:

- levator ani
- coccygeus/ischiococcygeus

1.1 Clinical Significance

- Levator ani contracts to occlude levator hiatus or urogenital hiatus. This action occludes the vaginal canal and prevents the prolapse of pelvic organs.
- Constant baseline contraction of the levator ani holds the load of pelvic viscera.
- The puborectalis creates the anorectal angle; thus maintaining anal continence and reinforcing the external anal sphincter.

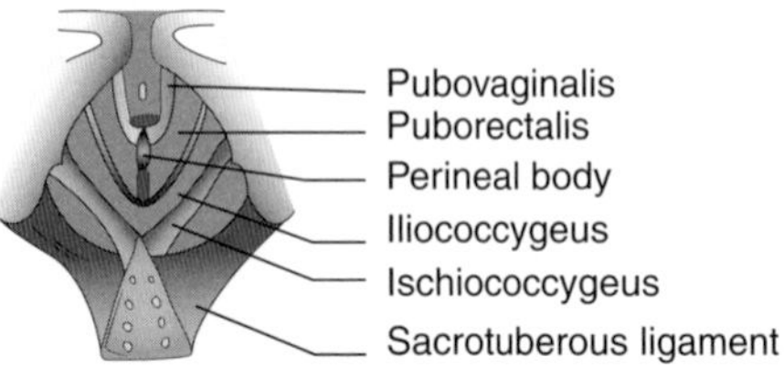

Figure 8.1 The pelvic floor.

- Relaxation of the levator ani permits micturition and defecation.
- During parturition, when the head reaches the pelvic floor, the levator ani contracts to rotate the fetal head. As a result, the fetal head entering the pelvic brim in the transverse axis rotates to the anteroposterior axis of the pelvic cavity. Next, the anterior fibres of the levator ani relax to enlarge the size of the urogenital hiatus and birth canal. After parturition, the levator ani recoils to acquire normal position.
- Laceration of the perineal body results in pelvic floor weakness.
- Kegel's exercises should be advocated postpregnancy and postmenopause to strengthen the levator ani muscles.

2 Ureter

The ureter is 25–30 cm long and 3 mm in diameter, and runs through the retroperitoneal space. It shows three sites of constriction where a calculous may obstruct the lumen:

- pelviureteric junction
- brim of lesser pelvis
- ureterovesical junction

2.1 Course of the Pelvic Ureter

Initially, the direction is posterolateral along the anterior border of the greater sciatic notch. At the level of the ischial spine, it turns anteromedially to reach the base of the urinary bladder. At this point, it lies in proximity to the uterine artery and passes under the cervical (Mackenrodt) ligament. This is where it is most vulnerable to injury. See Figure 8.2.

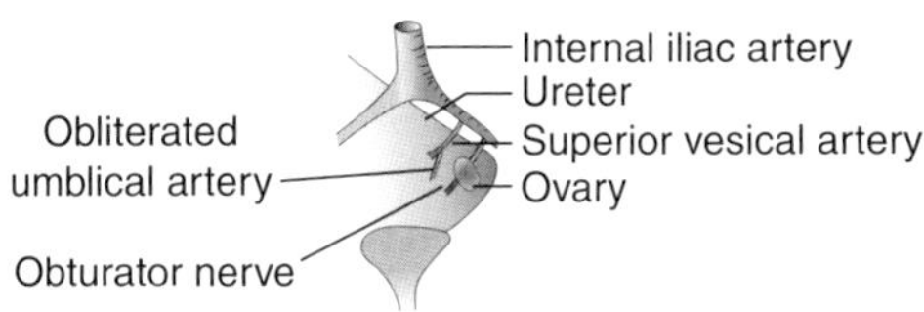

Figure 8.2 Ovarian fossa.

2.2 Common Sites of Ureteric Injury

- The ureter lies retroperitoneally and crosses the bifurcation of the internal iliac artery. It may be stripped off with the peritoneum during abdominal hysterectomy. It is very likely to be injured during internal iliac artery ligation for postpartum haemorrhage.
- At the level of the ischial spine, the ureter lies deep to the uterine artery, 2 cm lateral to the supravaginal part of the cervix. It can be injured while ligating the uterine arteries. The ureter takes a turn anteriorly lateral to the lateral vaginal fornix. It can be ligated while closing the vaginal vault or it may be damaged by electrocautery while controlling haemorrhage from the descending vaginal branch of the uterine artery. This is the most common site of injury. The proximity of the ureter to the uterine artery and vaginal vault warrants caution during vaginal vault interventions.
- At the base of the infundibulopelvic ligament as the ureters cross the pelvic brim at the ovarian fossa.
- At the level of uterosacral ligaments.

2.2.1 Steps to Prevent Ureteric Injury

During surgery, the ureter is seen as a whitish cord, which is nonpulsatile and shows peristaltic activity when gently pinched with forceps.

- Visualisation of peristaltic activity is the best method of identifying the ureter.
- Placement of ureteric catheters via cystoscopy helps to identify the ureters in cases of dense pelvic adhesions and distorted pelvic anatomy.
- Placement of infrared ureteric catheters illuminates the ureters, thus safeguarding accidental injury.
- In cases of ureteric injury during surgery, immediate reimplantation of the ureter into the bladder and placement of a ureteric stent will ensure complete recovery.

2.2.2 Further Points of Clinical Interest

- As the uterus is deviated to one side, commonly left, the left ureter is closer to the vagina compared to the right ureter.
- During surgery on the left-hand side, the apex of the sigmoid mesocolon is the guide to the ureter as it enters the pelvis.
- The ureter may get compressed by large myomas, ovarian cysts, aortic aneurysm and retroperitoneal masses.
- On radiograph, the ureter lies medial to the tip of the transverse processes of lumbar vertebrae, and crosses the pelvic brim at the sacroiliac joint.
- Congenitally anomalous ureter may present as double ureter or ectopic ureteric insertion. See Table 8.2.

3 Kidney

- Location: the right kidney is slightly lower than the left kidney (due to the right lobe of liver).
- Both kidneys move in a vertical direction of about 1 inch with respiration.
- Structures present in the hilum: from front to back, the renal vein, renal artery and ureter.
- Coverings of the kidney: fibrous capsule, perirenal fat, renal fascia and pararenal fat.
- Nerve supply: renal sympathetic plexus (afferents from T10, 11 and 12 spinal nerves).
- Important relations of the kidney are shown in Table 8.1.

4 Urinary Bladder

The urinary bladder is located in the pelvis, immediately behind the pubic bone. It is a pelvic organ but, when distended, it may become an abdominal organ and may also push the uterus and cervix out of the pelvis. The empty bladder is pyramidal in shape, but when distended it is ovoid, and its superior surface bulges upwards into the abdominal cavity. The peritoneum gets reflected to the anterior abdominal wall such that the bladder comes in direct contact with the anterior abdominal wall. Acute

Table 8.1 Relations of the kidney

	Anterior	Posterior
Right kidney	• Suprarenal gland • Liver • Second part of duodenum • Right colic flexure	• Diaphragm • Costodiaphragmatic recess • Twelfth rib • Psoas major, quadratus lumborum, transversus abdominalis
Left kidney	• Suprarenal gland • Spleen • Stomach • Pancreas • Left colic flexure • Coils of jejunum	• Diaphragm • Costodiaphragmatic recess • Eleventh and twelfth ribs • Psoas major, quadratus lumborum, transversus abdominalis • Subcostal, iliohypogastric, ilioinguinal nerves

anteversion of the uterus may be corrected by simply allowing the bladder to distend.

Table 8.2 Renal anomalies

Renal anomalies	Ureteric anomalies
Unilateral renal agenesis	Partial duplication of ureter
Unilateral renal hypoplasia	Complete duplication of ureter
Pelvic kidney	
Supernumary kidney	

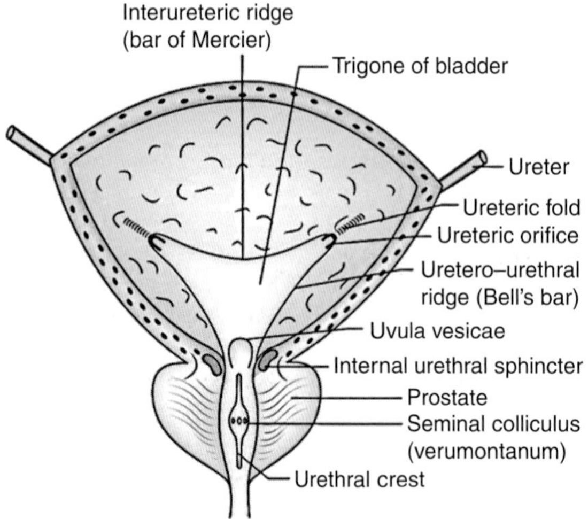

Figure 8.3 Anatomical structures in the bladder.

Anatomically it consists of the following parts: (see Figure 8.3)

- The apex is directed anteriorly, and lies at the level of the upper margin of the pubic symphysis.
- The base is directed posteriorly. The upper part is covered with peritoneum (vesicouterine pouch).
- The superior surface is covered with peritoneum, and is related to coils of ileum and the sigmoid colon.
- Nerve supply: supplied by the autonomic nervous system:
  - Inferior hypogastric plexus: L1, L2 (sympathetic fibres) promote bladder relaxation.
  - Pelvic splanchnic nerves S2, S3, S4 (parasympathetic fibres) promote bladder contraction and micturition.

- Overactive bladder is an entity that results in urge incontinence. It affects older Women. It occurs due to overactive parasympathetic nerves and is treated with anticholinergic drugs.

Bibliography

Copel, J. A., D'Alton, M. E. (2018). *Obstetric Imaging: Fetal Diagnosis and Care*, 2nd ed., Elsevier.

9 Fetal and Maternal Imaging

Deepika Poonia

1 X-Rays

Exposure of the abdomen and pelvis to ionising radiation should be minimised in women of childbearing age due to its effect on the reproductive organs such as the ovary. The fetus is particularly susceptible to inadvertent exposure to X-rays. Hence, if the last menstrual period is not definitely known, the abdomen should be shielded with a lead apron when performing X-rays of the head and neck, chest and limbs. If imaging of the abdomen and pelvis is mandatory, an ultrasound scan (USS) or a magnetic resonance imaging (MRI) scan is far safer than a computed tomography (CT) scan in reproductive-age women where a pregnancy history is not available.

1.1 Prerequisites for X-Rays

- Minimum X-ray dose (<5 rad; i.e., 0.05 Gy) to be used.
- Fetal shielding is required.
- First trimester X-rays must be avoided. Hence, every woman should provide the date of her last menstrual period to avoid inadvertent X-rays in early pregnancy.
- USS/MRI scan must be considered as an alternative investigation in comorbid conditions.

1.2 Indications

With the advent of high-resolution USS and MRI, there is almost no role of an X-ray in fetal and maternal imaging.

- Intrauterine fetal death (IUFD): is easily diagnosed by the absence of cardiac activity by USS. However, certain bony signs are suggestive of IUFD and would be visualised on an X-ray.
    - Spalding sign: irregular overlapping of the cranial bones due to liquefaction of brain matter and softening of ligaments. Appears seven days after death.
    - Hyperflexion of the spine.
    - Crowding of ribs.
    - Roberts sign: appearance of gas shadow in the heart chambers and great vessels. Appears within 12 hours of intrauterine fetal death.
- Ossification centres of lower end of the femur appears at 32 weeks and that of the upper end of the tibia appears at 36 weeks and this may give an indication of fetal maturity.
- Secondary abdominal pregnancy: presence of an empty endometrial cavity and the presence of a fetus in the abdomen confirms an abdominal pregnancy. Again, with USS being widely available, even in developing countries, an abdominal radiograph would rarely be used. Where further imaging is indicated, an MRI scan is more useful as it can also delineate the placental position and attachments.

1.3 Maternal Indications

- X-Ray pelvimetry is occasionally performed in cases of pelvic deformity or pelvic fractures.

2 Ultrasound Scans

For further information on this subject, see Section 12, Chapter 71.

The clinical application of USS in pregnancy was introduced by Ian Donald in Glasgow, UK, in 1958. Ultrasound waves are generated by an alternating current, which passes through piezoelectric crystals in a transducer to generate high-frequency sound waves. These sound waves reflect from the tissue back to the transducer, which converts them back to an alternating current and generates an image on the screen. The principles of ultrasound imaging are as follows:

- The degree of reflection of sound is directly proportional to the difference between acoustic impedance of the two structures.
- Water-soluble gel between the transducer and the skin acts as a coupling agent.
- Solid viscera appear echogenic.
- Acoustic enhancement or dark colour is shown by hollow viscera and cysts.
- Acoustic shadowing is produced by bones and calcified structures like stones.

2.1 Modes of Ultrasound Imaging in Obstetrics and Gynaecology

- Transabdominal sonography.
- Transvaginal sonography.
- Transrectal and transperineal sonography.
- Doppler interrogation of arteries and veins to ascertain blood flow.
- Saline infusion sonography to visualise the endometrial cavity.
- Endoscopic ultrasound probes are being developed to ascertain the degree of tissue invasion and vascularity of dense adhesions.

2.2 Standard Ultrasound Images

- B-mode: a two-dimensional ultrasound image display composed of bright dots representing the ultrasound echoes. Using brightness mode display, two-dimensional images are obtained, in greyscale.
- M-mode: to study moving organs; for example, fetal heart rate.
- 3D imaging refers to reconstruction of a three-dimensional picture after capturing an ultrasound image.
- 4D is the viewing of three-dimensional images in motion.
- Colour Doppler is used to map and study blood flow in arteries and veins. If the blood is flowing towards the transducer, the vessels will appear red (artery) and if the blood is flowing away from the transducer, the vessels will appear blue (vein).
- Pulse wave Doppler study reveals that systolic and diastolic blood flow patterns in arteries are consistent and can be studied to calculate the systolic:diastolic ratio, pulsatility index and resistance index of a vessel.
- Pulse Doppler index shows the capillary perfusion in a structure.

2.3 Transabdominal Sonography

Transabdominal sonography is the preferred mode of imaging in the second and third trimesters of pregnancy. It utilises a 3–5 MHz curvilinear transducer. A distended urinary bladder provides a good reference point for pelvic structures and acts as an acoustic window to improve transmission of ultrasound waves. It also pushes the uterus upwards for clear imaging and displaces the small intestine from the field of view. However, it does not allow accurate assessment of cervical length.

Fetal anomaly scans, growth scans, echocardiography, placental localisation and Doppler assessments are performed transabdominally. All invasive procedures during pregnancy (such as fetal reduction, amniocentesis, cordocentesis and drainage of obstructive lesions like hydronephrosis and ventriculomegaly) are performed under abdominal ultrasound guidance.

2.4 Transvaginal Sonography

Transvaginal sonography employs a multifrequency 5–10 MHz transducer. It provides clear images of the pelvic organs such as the uterus and ovaries when the urinary bladder is empty. The probe is positioned in each fornix for visualisation of the ovary.

- Undertaken in the first trimester. Early anomaly scan between 10 and 14 weeks, followed by a detailed anomaly scan between 18 and 20 weeks.

2.5 Transperineal Scan

Transperineal scan is used to image pelvic organs in preadolescent girls. The abdominal probe is covered and placed on the perineal region. It is also used in adults for real-time imaging of the pubic symphysis, urethra and bladder neck.

2.6 Transrectal Ultrasound

This can be a useful modality to:

- assess anal sphincter morphology after childbirth
- view lesions in the rectovaginal septum
- view vesicovaginal fistulous tracts

- assess the integrity of repair of fourth-degree perineal tears

2.7 Indications for Ultrasound in Pregnancy

- diagnosis of pregnancy
- confirm viability of pregnancy
- assessment of gestational age
- localisation of placenta
- assessment of liquor volume
- diagnosis of cervical incompetence
- diagnosis of uterine malformations
- diagnosis of multiple pregnancy, IUFD, ectopic pregnancy, placental abruption, molar pregnancy
- anomaly scan
- assessment of intrauterine growth restriction (IUGR)
- diagnosis of presentation

2.8 First Trimester Scan

This is preferably done by transvaginal scanning. The gestation sac appears at 4–5 weeks as a hypoechoic structure with an echogenic rim. It is placed eccentrically in the uterine cavity. Its rate of growth in the first trimester is 1.1 mm in diameter per day until it attains a diameter of 20–25 mm. If it is <0.6 mm per day, this indicates abnormal fetal development.

A healthy gestational sac is characterised by:

- eccentric location
- regular outline
- double decidual sign
- at five weeks it contains a yolk sac and by six weeks a fetal pole with cardiac activity
- echogenic rim of choriodecidual reaction

The first ultrasound scan is performed between five and eight weeks of gestation. It is useful for the following:

- Confirming an intrauterine pregnancy and diagnosing an ectopic pregnancy, if no gestational sac is visible on transvaginal scan with a serum beta hCG level of 1500 IU/L.
- Number of sacs/fetuses and their chorionicity and amnionicity in cases of multifetal pregnancy.
- Presence of cardiac activity. This appears between six and seven weeks and confirms viability.
- Period of gestation or dating is most accurate when performed in the first trimester by measuring the crown–rump length.
- Early pregnancy complications like anembryonic sac or threatened, missed or incomplete miscarriage.
- Nuchal translucency is assessed between 11 and 13 weeks of gestation. If greater than 3 mm, chances of congenital anomalies are higher.
- Diagnosis of hydatidiform mole.
- Diagnosis of adnexal masses like ovarian cysts and ovarian torsion.
- Diagnosis of uterine anomalies like myomas and bicornuate uterus.

2.9 Early Anomaly Scan

Also called the nuchal scan, an early anomaly scan is performed between 10 and 14 weeks of gestation by the transvaginal route. It is the earliest assessment of fetal anatomy. This should include the study of the following structures:

- Fetal head: this is well formed and allows the visualisation of midline structures like the falx cerebri and the posterior fossa. Anencephaly can be diagnosed. Intracranial translucency is increased in trisomy 21.
- Fetal face and the appearance of the nasal bone is an important sign to rule out trisomy 21.
- Fetal spine is visualised in its entire length to rule out spina bifida.
- Nuchal translucency is measured at the region of the neck. If increased to greater than 3 mm it is associated with congenital anomalies.
- Fetal thorax appears symmetric and diaphragm completely separates it from the abdominal structures. The fetal heart shows formation of four chambers.
- Fetal abdomen may show deficient development in gastroschisis and omphalocele.
- The stomach bubble appears at this time and the urinary bladder and kidneys are visible.
- Fetal limbs can be studied including visualisation of the foot and digits of the hand.

Besides the anatomical study, this scan should also assess the following:

- The cervical canal. The normal length should be 3–5 cm. If shorter than 2.5 cm, it signifies cervical incompetence, for which remedial measures can be taken at this stage.
- Placental location. This is mandatory in patients with previous uterine scars like caesarean section/

myomectomy to rule out a morbidly adherent placenta. It is also helpful in patients who may require invasive diagnostic procedures later.
- Adnexal masses like ovarian cysts, particularly theca lutein cysts, which may be associated with hydatidiform mole.
- Uterine artery Doppler indices. This is the time that the uterine artery blood flow starts to increase during the diastole; thereby reducing the pulsatility index and resistive index values. If the diastolic flow does not increase, it may be a heralding sign for pregnancy complications like preeclampsia, and fetal growth restriction.

2.10 Second Trimester Anomaly Scan

This is performed transabdominally between 20 and 24 weeks. It is to rule out most structural fetal anomalies:

- Anomalies of the head and spine like hydrocephalus, ventriculomegaly, spina bifida and other neural tube defects. A fetus with spina bifida has cranial signs like small biparietal diameter, frontal bone scalloping (lemon sign), and elongation and downwards displacement of cerebellum (banana sign).
- Face anomalies like cleft lip and cleft palate.
- Fetal neck anomalies like goitre.
- Abdominal defects like congenital diaphragmatic hernia and abdominal wall defects.
- Fetal renal anomalies like polycystic kidney disease and hypoplastic kidneys, which are usually accompanied by oligohydramnios.
- Cardiac defects are better visualised at this scan and fetal echocardiographic assessment is possible.
- Limb defects like talipes equinovarus and anomalies of the digits can be identified.

This opportunity should also be used to assess the amniotic fluid volume, placental location and grading, uterine artery Doppler indices and cervical length. The latter is preferably done by a transvaginal scan with an empty bladder.

2.11 Indications for Second and Third Trimester Scan

Transabdominal scans are performed at monthly intervals in multifetal pregnancy to assess fetal growth. In a singleton pregnancy, if the abdomen appears smaller or larger than the gestational age, ultrasound scan is needed to assess fetal growth.

- gestational age and fetal growth
- fetal presentation
- discrepancy in gestational age and uterine height, for fetal growth restriction and IUFD
- cervical incompetence
- multiple gestation
- suspected pelvic mass
- biophysical profile
- volume of liquor
- placental location, abruption of placenta, placenta praevia
- congenital anomalies that appear late; for example, polycystic kidneys, posterior urethral valves:
  - fetal weight estimation
  - to assist invasive procedures like amniocentesis and fetal therapy
  - in Rh-isoimmunisation cases, assessment of middle cerebral artery Doppler to assess fetal hypoxia

2.12 Doppler Ultrasound in Obstetrics

- Pulsed wave Doppler is used in obstetrics.
- Indices measured are:
  - systolic:diastolic ratio
  - resistance index (RI) = (systole–diastole)/ systolic peak velocity
  - pulsatility index (PI) = (systole–diastole)/ mean
- Commonly examined vessels are:
  - maternal uterine arteries
  - fetal umbilical artery and vein, middle cerebral artery, ductus venosus, inferior vena cava and superior vena cava
- Indications are shown in Table 9.1.
- Uterine artery: if PI >1.45 at 18–22 weeks with diastolic notching, this implies preeclampsia and IUGR.
- Umbilical artery: normally, umbilical artery resistance decreases with gestational age.
  - If flow decreases and end diastolic velocity decreases, this implies IUGR.

Table 9.1 Indications for Doppler assessment

Indication	Vessel studied	Observation
IUGR (most important indication)	• Umbilical artery • Ductus venosus • Middle cerebral artery	Absent or reversal of flow
Rh-isoimmunised pregnancy	Middle cerebral artery	Initially flow increases; later reduces
Multiple pregnancy	Umbilical artery	Twin-to-twin transfusion can be detected
Ectopic pregnancy	• Uterine artery • Ovarian artery	Decreased flow to endometrium and increased flow to adnexa
Gestational trophoblastic disease	Uterine artery	Increased flow to endometrium
Secondary postpartum haemorrhage	Uterine artery	Abnormal arteriovenous malformation

  - If absent end diastolic velocity (AEDV) is zero, this implies reduced fetal blood flow, which could lead to fetal distress.
  - Reversal of diastolic flow (REDF) implies severe reduction in fetal blood flow, which could be a terminal event.
- Middle cerebral artery: this is indicated in Rh-isoimmunisation during pregnancy that leads to fetal anaemia and hypoxia.
  - Fetal hypoxia: increased flow due to decreased resistance in the middle cerebral artery (brain-sparing effect).
  - Continued hypoxia leads to decrease in flow.
  - Severe fetal distress shows reversal of brain-sparing effect and decreased flow in diastole.

3 MRI scans in Obstetrics

This is a safe modality in pregnancy and is occasionally indicated.

- MRI scans distinguish between placenta accreta, increta and percreta
- detects any viable fetal pole in gestational trophoblastic disease.
- detects pelvic masses in pregnancy and red degeneration of uterine leiomyoma in pregnancy
- diagnoses ectopic pregnancy in the ovary and other rare locations
- detects fetal location, presentation and anatomy in secondary abdominal pregnancy
- diagnoses postpartum complications like abscess, haematoma and pelvic vein thrombosis, as well as other comorbid conditions
- detects uterine arteriovenous malformation postsurgery

USS is indicated in every pregnancy for the detection of congenital anomalies and to detect pregnancy complications. In some cases, MRI scan may be indicated. However, X-rays and CT scans should be avoided during pregnancy, particularly of the abdomen and pelvis.

Section 2

Embryology

Sheetal Barhate

10 Gametes and Fertilisation

Sheetal Barhate

1 Oogenesis

- Oogenesis begins in the ovary during the embryonic period at around six to eight weeks. Gametes are derived from primordial germ cells.
- After rapid mitotic division of the primordial germ cells, the number of oocytes reach up to 6–7 million by 16–20 weeks. This number falls to 1–2 million by birth. The process of atresia continues and, until the onset of puberty, this number reduces to 300 000 to 500 000.
- In the next 35–40 years, 400 to 500 will be selected to ovulate and only a few hundred will remain until menopause.
- This process is called apoptosis (programmed cell death).
- At birth, all the primary oocytes enter the prophase of first meiotic division and remain suspended.
- At puberty around 15 to 20 follicles are recruited each month.
- The flat cells surrounding the oocyte proliferate, forming stratified epithelium called granulosa cells.
- Granulosa cells are surrounded by a basement membrane separating them from the surrounding the ovarian tissue called theca folliculi.
- As the follicle continues to grow, these theca folliculi differentiate into theca interna cells and an outer fibrous capsule called theca externa.
- Oocyte and granulosa tissues also secrete a layer of glycoprotein on the surface of the oocyte called the zona pellucida.
- Under the influence of hormones, the follicle continues to grow, leading to ovulation.
- meiosis I is completed just before ovulation, forming a secondary oocyte and polar body.
- The cell then enters into meiosis II and arrests in the metaphase.
- meiosis II is completed only after fertilisation, giving rise to a fertilised ovum and a second polar body. See Figure 10.1.

2 Spermatogenesis

- The germ cells in a male infant are situated in the sex cord of the testis.
- At puberty, primordial germ cells give rise to spermatogonial stem cells.
- At regular intervals, type A spermatogonia are developed from these stem cells. These further undergo several mitotic divisions, giving rise to type B spermatogonia, which in turn divide and give rise to primary spermatocyte.
- Primary spermatocyte undergoes meiosis I to form secondary spermatocyte, which further undergoes second meiotic division, forming haploid spermatids.
- This spermatid undergoes several changes to form mature spermatozoa.
- The approximate time taken for development of spermatozoa from spermatogonia is 74 days. An additional 12–20 days are spent in travelling through the epididymis. See Figure 10.2.

2.1 Semen Analysis

Table 10.1 shows the World Health Organization reference values for semen analysis.

2.2 Structure of Human Sperm

A mature human sperm consists of four parts:

1. Head:
   a. The head of the sperm consists of an acrosome, which is a cap-like structure just in front of the nucleus proper.
   b. The acrosomal cap is formed from the Golgi complex of spermatid.

c. The main function of the acrosome is secretion of a lytic enzyme called hyaluronidase, which helps in the penetration of the ovum.

Table 10.1 World Health Organization reference values for semen analysis

Semen volume	1.5 ml or more
pH	7.2 or more
Sperm concentration	15 million per ml or more
Total sperm number	39 million per ejaculate or more
Total progressive motility	32% or more
Total non-progressive motility	40% or more
Vitality	58% or more live
Sperm morphology (percentage of normal forms)	4% normal or more

d. The nucleus consists of condensed chromatin and is the source for genetic information.

2. Neck:
   a. The neck consists of two centrioles: the proximal and distal centrioles
   b. The proximal centriole helps the zygotic division by forming the first meiotic spindle.
   c. The distal centriole is responsible for the formation of the axial filament of the tail
3. Middle piece:
   a. The middle piece consists of mitochondria and is known as the powerhouse of the sperm.
   b. This provides the energy for the sperm to travel through the female genital tract.
4. Tail:
   a. This is the terminal part of the sperm and consists of axial filaments.

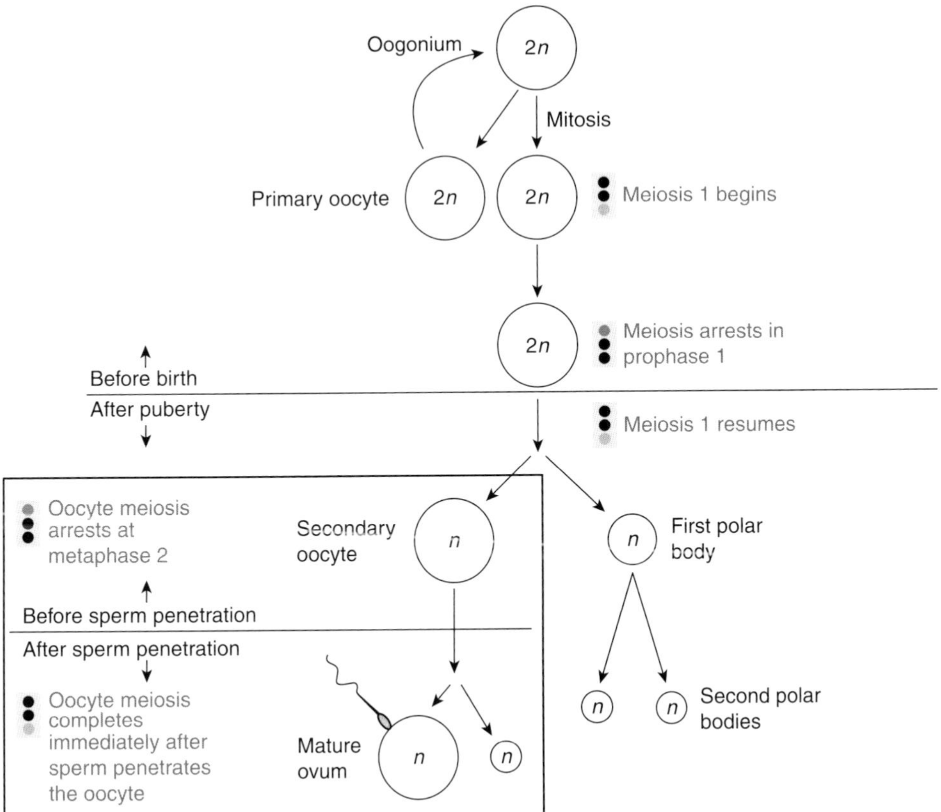

Figure 10.1 Oogenesis. Used with permission from Lumen.

b. This is responsible for the movement of the sperm in the genital tract. See Figure 10.3.

3 Fertilisation

- Fertilisation takes place in the ampullary portion of the fallopian tube.
- Capacitation: the process that occurs during the sperm's journey through the cervix, leading to acquisition of ability of sperm to undergo acrosome reaction. This in turn helps to increase its motility and aids its ability to bind to the zona pellucida.
- Egg transport: after ovulation, the oocyte and its cumulus are transported to the ampullary portion of the fallopian tube with the help of smooth muscle contractions and ciliary-induced flow of secretory fluid.
- Around 200 to 300 million sperm are deposited in the vagina, but only a few hundred reach the egg, and only one fertilises the egg. However, other sperm aid in the fertilisation process.
- The life of a fertilisable egg is approximately 12 to 24 hours; whereas the lifespan of a fertilisable sperm is approximately 48 to 72 hours. However, sperm can live in the female genital tract for seven days.
- Key steps in fertilisation:
  1. Receptors on the sperm head bind to ligands on the zona pellucida, inducing the acrosome reaction, which in turn releases enzymes essential for fusion of the sperm and oocyte membranes.
  2. Fertilisation immediately leads to the release of a substance from the cortical granules (cortical reaction), leading to the hardening of the zona and inactivation of ligands of sperm receptors avoiding polyspermy.
  3. Immediately after entry of spermatozoa, the oocyte finishes the second meiotic division and releases the second polar body, leading to the formation of the female pronucleus.
  4. The sperm loses its tail and swells, forming the male pronucleus.
  5. Both maternal and paternal chromosomes intermingle, leading to the formation of the zygote, which further undergoes mitotic division, leading to the two-cell stage.

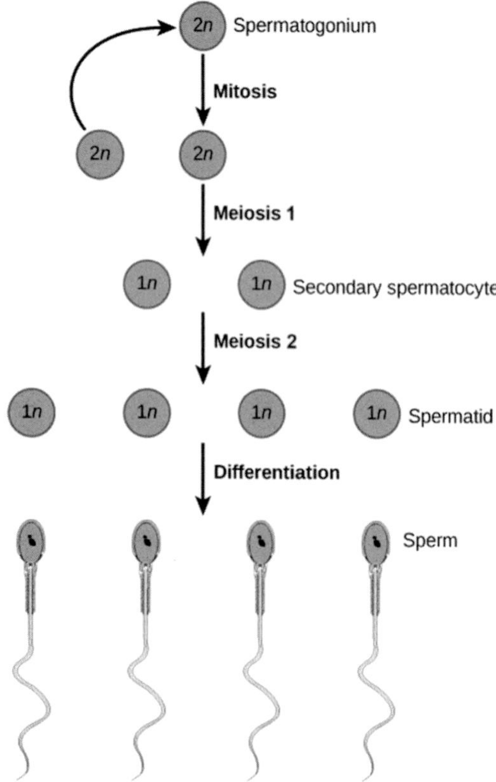

Figure 10.2 Spermatogenesis.

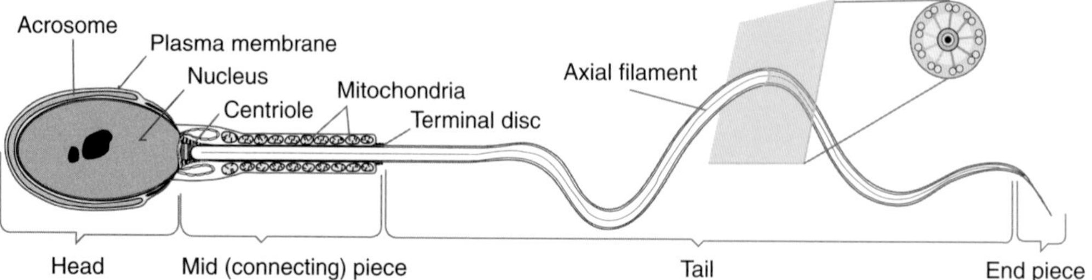

Figure 10.3 Structure of human sperm.

3.1 First week

- The zygote undergoes a series of mitotic divisions, resulting in the formation of the morula (16-cell embryo) in three days.
- Each cell is called a blastomere, which is smaller and pluripotent.
- The inner cells of the morula are called the inner cell mass and this gives rise to the embryo proper. Outer cells are called the outer cell mass, which contributes to the formation of the placenta.
- At this stage, the morula reaches the uterine cavity.
- A fluid-filled cavity appears in the morula forming a blastocyst.
- Cells of the inner cell mass move to one pole and are now called embryoblasts. The outer cell mass flattens and forms the epithelial wall of the blastocyst.
- The zona pellucida disappears at this stage.
- Implantation occurs in secretory phase of the menstrual cycle at around the sixth day of fertilisation in the endometrium along the anterior or posterior wall.

Early Fetal Embryology and Placental Development

Sheetal Barhate

1 Formation of the Uteroplacental Circulation and Bilaminar Embryonic Disc

- Day 8:
  1. Blastocyst is partially embedded in the endometrial stroma.
  2. Trophoblast has differentiated into the inner cytotrophoblast and outer syncytiotrophoblast.
  3. Formation of the bilaminar embryonic disc: differentiation of the inner cell mass into the hypoblast layer adjacent to the blastocyst cavity and epiblast layers adjacent to the amniotic cavity.
- Day 9:
  1. Blastocyst is completely embedded in the endometrium and the surface defect is closed by fibrin coagulum.
  2. Exuberant growth of trophoblast occurs at the embryonic pole.
  3. Large lacunae form in the syncytiotrophoblast (lacunar stage).
  4. Primitive yolk sac is formed.
- Days 11 and 12
  1. Blastocyst is completely embedded in the endometrium and the defect is closed by surface epithelium.
  2. At the embryonic pole, the syncytiotrophoblast erodes the epithelial lining of the maternal capillaries (sinusoids).
  3. Maternal blood enters the lacunar system, leading to formation of the uteroplacental circulation.
  4. There is formation of extraembryonic somatic mesoderm in between the cytotrophoblast and the amnion.
  5. There is formation of extraembryonic splanchnic mesoderm in between the cytotrophoblast and the yolk sac.
  6. The extraembryonic mesoderm develops from yolk sac cells.
- Day 13:
  1. Primary villi are formed (cellular columns of cytotrophoblast surrounded by syncytiotrophoblast).
  2. Secondary or definitive yolk sac develops.
  3. There is formation of the chorionic plate from the extraembryonic mesoderm, which lines the inner aspect of the trophoblast.
  4. The connecting stalk develops, which is the future umbilical cord.

2 Formation of the Trilaminar Embryonic Disc and Mesoderm

- Gastrulation is the process of formation of the trilaminar germ disc, giving rise to three layered embryonic discs (ectoderm, mesoderm and endoderm).
- Gastrulation begins with the formation of the primitive streak, which occurs at around the fifteenth to sixteenth day.
- The cephalic end of the primitive streak is known as the primitive node, which is a slightly elevated area surrounding the small primitive pit.
- Cells of epiblast (ectoderm) migrate towards the primitive streak and invaginate between the bilaminar embryonic disc (between the epiblast and hypoblast), giving rise to mesoderm.
- The epiblast develops into the ectoderm and the hypoblast develops into the endoderm.

- The mesoderm is absent in two locations where the original two germ layers stay together, which are as follows:
  1. Prechordal plate at the cephalad end on the disc, which is soon replaced by buccopharyngeal membrane.
  2. Cloacal plate at the caudal end, which is replaced by cloacal membrane in future.

Box 11.1 Germ layer derivatives

Endoderm

- epithelium of the gastrointestinal tract
- liver
- pancreas
- urachus
- urinary bladder

Epithelial portions of

- pharynx
- thyroid
- trachea, bronchi, lungs
- tympanic cavity
- pharyngotympanic tube
- tonsils
- parathyroids

Mesoderm

- skeleton (head and body)
- muscle
- connective tissue
- circulatory system
- cardiovascular system
- lymphatic system
- urinary system
- spleen
- adrenal cortex
- genital system
- dermis
- dentine of teeth

Ectoderm

Nervous Tissue

- central nervous system
- retina
- posterior pituitary
- pineal gland

Neural crest:

- pineal gland
- adrenal medulla
- cranial and sensory ganglia and nerve

Box 11.1 (cont.)

Epidermis

- hair
- nails
- mammary glands
- cutaneous glands
- anterior pituitary
- teeth enamel
- inner ear
- eye lens

3 Notochord Formation

- Cells from the primitive node migrate towards the buccopharyngeal membrane, forming the notochordal plate.
- This plate further folds, forming the notochord.
- It forms a longitudinal axis for the embryo and nuclei pulposi of the intervertebral disc.

4 Neurulation

- On the nineteenth day, the cranial end of the ectoderm forms the neural plate, which in turn folds to form the neural tube. This process is known as neurulation.
- Neural crest cells are formed at the edges of the neural tube.
- The neural crest cells give rise to the structures shown in Table 11.1.

Table 11.1 Structures arising from neural crest cells

Connective tissue and bones of the face and skull
Cranial nerve ganglia
C cells of the thyroid gland
Conotruncal septum in the heart
Odontoblasts
Dermis in the face and neck
Spinal (dorsal root) ganglia
Sympathetic chain and preaortic ganglia
Parasympathetic ganglia of the gastrointestinal tract
Adrenal ganglia
Schwann cells
Glial cells
Meninges (forebrain)
Melanocyte
Smooth muscle cells to blood vessels of the face and forebrain

Table 11.2 Development of pharyngeal arches

Pharyngeal arch	Muscle	Skeletal	Nerve	Artery	Ligaments
First	• Muscles of mastication • Mylohyoid • Tensor tympani • Anterior belly of digastric	• Maxilla • Mandible • Malleus • Incus	Trigeminal nerve	Maxillary artery (terminal branches)	• Anterior ligament of malleus • Sphenomandibular ligament
Second	• Muscles of facial expression • Stapedius • Stylohyoid • Posterior belly of digastric	• Stapes • Styloid process • Lesser cornu of hyoid • Upper part of body of hyoid	Facial nerve	• Stapedial (embryonic) • Caroticotympanic (adult)	Stylohyoid ligament
Third	Stylopharyngeus	• Greater cornu of hyoid • Lower part of body of hyoid bone	Glossopharyngeal nerve	• Common carotid artery • Internal carotid artery	
Fourth	• Cricothyroid • Soft palate muscles	• Thyroid • Cricoid • Arytenoid • Corniculate and cuneiform cartilages	• Vagus • Laryngeal branch of vagus	• Superior part of aortic arch (left) • Subclavian artery (right)	
Sixth	Laryngeal intrinsic muscles (not cricothyroid)	• Thyroid • Cricoid • Arytenoid • Corniculate and cuneiform cartilages	Recurrent laryngeal nerve	Part of right pulmonary artery	

Table 11.3 Derivatives of the pharyngeal pouches

Pharyngeal pouch	Derivatives
First	• Tympanic cavity • Eustachian tube
Second	• Palatine tonsils • Tonsillar fossa
Third	• Inferior parathyroid gland • Thymus
Fourth	• Superior parathyroid gland • Ultimobranchial body • Parafollicular cells of thyroid gland

5 Development of the Pharyngeal Arches and Pharyngeal Pouches

Development of the pharyngeal arches is shown in Table 11.2.

The derivatives of the pharyngeal pouches are shown in Table 11.3.

6 Development of the Trophoblast and Placenta

- The trophoblast continues to develop from the third week.
- After formation of the mesodermal layer, the mesoderm penetrates the primary villi, giving rise to secondary villi.
- By the end of the third week, the mesodermal cells in the secondary villi give rise to blood vessels, forming the villus capillary system and leading to the formation of tertiary or definitive placental villi.
- This capillary system connects the capillaries in the chorionic plate and the connecting stalk; thus establishing contact with the embryonic circulatory system.
- With further proliferation of cytotrophoblasts through syncytiotrophoblasts, there is formation of the stem or anchoring villi.
- These villi extend from the chorionic plate to the decidua basalis (the part of the endometrium that forms placenta).
- Until the beginning of the eighth week, the entire chorionic sac is covered with villi.
- As the gestational sac grows, the only part that is associated with the decidua basalis retains its villi, forming the chorion frondosum.
- The villi on the abembryonic side degenerate, giving rise to smooth chorion laeve.
- By the beginning of the second month, these villi undergo extensive branching.
- Endovascular invasion occurs: the process by which cytotrophoblasts invade the terminal ends of spiral arteries.
- These cells replace maternal endothelial cells in the spiral arteries, creating hybrid vessels containing both fetal and maternal cells.
- The small-diameter, high-resistance, spiral vessels are converted into large-diameter, low-resistance vessels, resulting in increased quantities of maternal blood into the intervillous space.
- By the beginning of the fourth month, the cytotrophoblastic cells and some connective tissue disappear. This leaves behind only a thin membrane of syncytium and endothelial walls of the vessels, facilitating the exchange of oxygen and nutrients between fetus and mother.
- Subsequently, chorion laeve fuses with the opposite uterine wall, obliterating the uterine cavity.

12 Fetal Development

Sheetal Barhate

1 The Gastrointestinal System

- The primitive gut is formed by incorporation of the portion of the endoderm lining the yolk sac during cephalocaudal and lateral folding of the embryo around the fourth week of the embryonic period.
- As the gut tube develops, the endoderm proliferates rapidly and temporarily occludes the lumen of the tube around the fifth week. At around the seventh week, recanalisation of the tube starts due to apoptosis of the endoderm, such that by the ninth week, the lumen is open again.

The primitive gut is divided into three main parts:

1. Foregut:
   - The foregut extends from the caudal end of the pharyngeal tube to the liver outgrowth.
   - Derivatives of the foregut:
     - oesophagus
     - trachea and lung bud
     - stomach
     - duodenum proximal to the entrance of the common bile duct
     - liver, biliary apparatus and pancreas
   - Blood supply of the foregut:
     - branches of coeliac trunk
2. Midgut:
   - The midgut develops from the part of the primitive duct from the liver bud to the junction of the right two-thirds of the transverse colon to the left one-third of the transverse colon in adults.
   - Derivatives of the midgut:
     - duodenum distal to the opening of the common bile duct
     - small intestine
     - caecum and appendix
     - ascending colon and two-thirds of transverse colon
   - Blood supply:
     - branches of superior mesenteric artery
3. Hindgut:
   - The hindgut develops from the part of the primitive duct from the left third of the transverse colon to the cloacal membrane.
   - Derivatives of the hindgut:
     - distal third of the transverse colon
     - descending colon
     - sigmoid colon
     - rectum
     - upper anal canal
   - Blood supply:
     - branches of the inferior mesenteric artery

1.1 Physiological Herniation of the Gut

- Due to the differential growth of the cranial part of the midgut as compared to the caudal part, and development of various other organs in the abdominal cavity, the midgut herniates through the umbilical opening into the umbilical cord at around the sixth week of gestation.
- At around the tenth week, when the abdominal cavity has sufficiently enlarged, organs begin to return in a specific manner.
- During this process, the midgut rotates a total of 270 degrees counterclockwise (90 degrees during herniation and 180 degrees during return).
- The plane of rotation is through the superior mesenteric artery.

1.2 Clinical Embryology

- Meckel's diverticulum:
  - A Meckel's diverticulum occurs due to the persistence of a small portion of the vitelline duct.
  - It occurs in 2–4% of the population.
  - The vitelline duct sometimes communicates with the anterior abdominal wall, giving rise to a vitelline duct fistula. This can lead to faecal discharge through the umbilicus.
- Omphalocele:
  - An omphalocele is a condition that occurs due to the failure of a reduction of physiological herniation during the embryonic period.
  - The herniated gut is covered by a translucent membrane comprising of peritoneum and amniotic membrane.
  - The umbilical cord is attached to the top of the omphalocele.
  - The content of the sac is bowel. There is no evidence of other organs in the hernia sac.
  - It is associated with chromosomal abnormalities 50% of the time.
  - Cardiac abnormalities are associated in 50% of cases, and 40% have associated neural tube defects.
  - Prognosis depends on associated abnormalities.
- Gastroschisis:
  - Gastroschisis occurs due to a developmental defect in the anterior abdominal wall.
  - The umbilical cord is attached to one side of the defect, usually on the right side.
  - The herniated sac may contain other abdominal organs like the liver and gall bladder.
  - It is rarely associated with chromosomal abnormalities or any other abnormality.
  - Gastroschisis usually has a good prognosis.

2 The Cardiovascular System

2.1 Formation of the Heart Tube

- This process begins by the sixteenth day of embryonic life.
- The heart progenitor cells, which originate from epiblasts, migrate through the primitive streak, forming the primary heart field (which gives rise to part of the atria, left ventricle and part of the right ventricle) and secondary heart field (which gives rise to part of the right ventricle, part of the atria, conus cordis and truncus arteriosus).
- Some of the heart progenitor cells develop into endothelial cells, forming an endothelial tube and others form myoblasts, which surround the tube.
- With the folding of the body walls, two loops of the tube fuse, forming a single heart tube.
- During the fourth week, this heart tube folds on itself (cardiac looping) and the heart achieves its normal position with the atria posterior and ventricles in a more anterior position.
- The smooth wall portion of the right atrium is formed by incorporation of the sinus venosus, whereas the smooth wall of the left atrium is formed by the incorporation of the root of the pulmonary vein.
- The ventricles of the heart are formed by the bulbus cordis and the primitive ventricles.
- The ascending aorta and pulmonary trunk are developed from the truncus arteriosus, whereas venous drainage of the heart arises from the sinus venosum and sinus venarum. See Figure 12.1.

2.2 Formation of the Atrial Septum

- The atrial septum formation occurs between the fourth and sixth week.
- This starts with formation of the septum primum, which is a thick crescent-shaped membranous structure. It grows from the roof of the atrium towards the endocardial cushion, leaving a gap called the ostium primum.
- With further development of the septum primum, the ostium primum closes, but at the same time cells in the ostium primum undergo programmed cell death, forming the ostium secundum.
- A thick septum develops to the right side of the septum primum, which acts like a flap narrowing the septum, leaving only a small gap known as the foramen ovale, which remains patent until birth.

2.3 Formation of the Ventricular Septum

- The ventricular septum consists of a muscular part, which develops from the floor of the ventricle

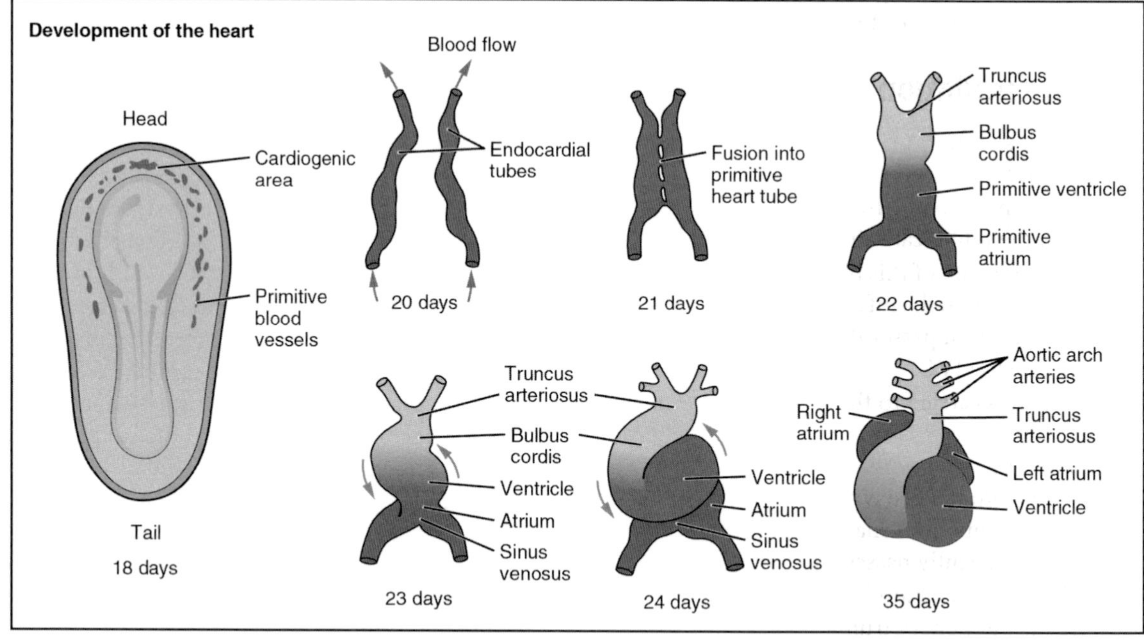

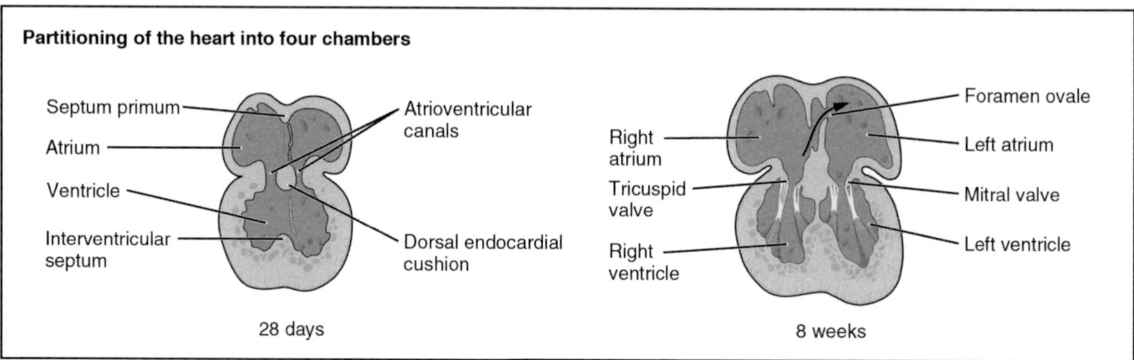

Figure 12.1 Development of the heart. Used with permission from https://commons.wikimedia.org/wiki/File:2037_Embryonic_Development_of_Heart.jpg

and grows towards the endocardial cushions and membranous part, which arises from the endocardial cushions and the aortopulmonary septum.

- The ventricular septum contains the atrioventricular conducting bundle.

2.4 Development of the Aortic Arches

- The first arch disappears (leaving the maxillary artery).
- The second arch disappears (leaving the stapedial artery).
- The third arch gives rise to the common carotid artery and the first part of the internal carotid artery. The external carotid artery arises as a direct branch from the third arch.
- The fourth arch on the left side gives rise to the portion of the aortic arch from the left common carotid to the left subclavian arteries, and on the right side it gives rise to the right subclavian artery (the proximal portion).
- The fifth arch disappears.
- The sixth arch on the left side gives rise to the left pulmonary artery and ductus arteriosus, and on the right side gives rise to the right pulmonary artery.

The distal part of the right side disappears, and the distal part of the left side forms the ductus arteriosus.

3 Fetal Circulation

- The main source of oxygenated blood to the fetus is the placenta.
- This oxygenated blood from the placenta is carried through the umbilical vein to the fetus.
- A greater portion of this blood passes through the ductus venosus to the inferior vena cava (IVC) and a smaller portion passes through the substance of the liver to the IVC.
- This blood is carried to the right atrium by the IVC. Most of this passes through the foramen ovale into the left atrium and the rest of it gets mixed up with the deoxygenated blood returning through the superior vena cava to the right atrium, which subsequently passes to the right ventricle.
- The deoxygenated blood from the right ventricle enters the pulmonary trunk, the greater part of which is shunted by the ductus arteriosus into the aorta. Only a small portion of blood that reaches the lungs passes to the left atrium.
- The left atrium receives oxygenated blood from the right atrium via the foramen ovale and a small amount of deoxygenated blood from the lung.
- This oxygenated blood passes into the left ventricle and then into the aorta. Some of this passes into the carotid and subclavian arteries. The rest of the blood mixes with the deoxygenated blood from the ductus arteriosus.
- The deoxygenated blood is then carried by the aorta to the placenta via the umbilical arteries.

3.1 Changes in Circulation at Birth

- The umbilical arteries contract immediately after birth, which prevents loss of fetal blood into the placenta.
- When the infant breathes for the first time, resistance of the pulmonary vasculature drops, leading to an increase in the pressure in the left atrium as compared to the right atrium, which leads to closure of the foramen ovale. Additionally, increase in oxygen concentration in the blood leads to a decrease in prostaglandin, causing closure of the ductus arteriosus.
- Due to these closures, blood is prevented from bypassing the pulmonary circulation and the newborn's blood is oxygenated in the newly operational lung.

Table 12.1 Vessel remnants after birth

Umbilical artery	Medial umbilical ligament
Left umbilical vein	Ligamentum teres of the liver
Ductus venosus	Ligamentum venosum
Ductus arteriosus	Ligamentum arteriosum

3.2 Remnants After Birth

The vessel remnants after birth are shown in Table 12.1.

4 The Respiratory System

- At around the fourth week, the respiratory diverticulum appears (lung bud), which develops as an outgrowth of the ventral wall of the foregut.
- With the formation of the tracheoesophageal septum, the foregut is divided into the oesophagus dorsally and the trachea and lung bud ventrally.
- Development of the larynx:
  - Laryngeal epithelium is developed from endoderm.
  - Laryngeal muscles and cartilages are developed from the fourth and sixth pharyngeal arches.
- Development of the trachea and bronchial tree:
  - The lung bud gives rise to the trachea and the two main bronchi. The right main bronchus further develops into three secondary bronchi and three lobes, and the left main bronchus develops into two secondary bronchi and two lobes.
  - By the seventh week, 10 tertiary bronchi are formed on the right side and eight on the left side.
  - The tracheal epithelium and glands develop from the endoderm and tracheal connective tissue. Smooth muscles and cartilages are developed from the splanchnic mesoderm.
- Development of the lungs:
  - The terminal bronchioles further divide into respiratory bronchioles and primitive alveolar sacs. This process starts at the fifth week.
  - The development of lung tissue is divided into the following four stages:
    1. Pseudoglandular stage. This stage lasts from the fifth to the sixteenth week. During

this stage, the tertiary bronchi continue branching and form terminal bronchioles. No respiratory bronchioles or alveoli are present.

2. Canalicular period stage. This stage lasts from the sixteenth to the twenty-sixth week. During this stage, each terminal bronchiole divides into two or more respiratory bronchioles, which further divide into three to six alveolar ducts.
3. Terminal sac period. This stage lasts from the twenty-sixth week to birth. During this stage, primitive alveoli and capillaries establish close contact.
4. Alveolar period. This stage lasts from the eighth month to childhood. During this stage, mature alveoli develop and they have well established epithelial and endothelial contacts.
    - Type 1 alveolar cells lining the alveolar cavity are responsible for gas exchange. Type 2 alveolar cells are responsible for the secretion of surfactant.

4.1 Clinical Embryology

Tracheoesophageal fistula (TEF):

- This abnormality develops due to a defect in the formation of the tracheoesophageal septum.
- TEF occurs in around 1 in 3000 births.
- Ninety percent of the time, there is formation of a blind oesophageal pouch from the upper portion of the oesophagus, and the lower portion forms a fistula with the trachea.
- Isolated oesophageal atresia and H type of tracheoesophageal fistula is present in 4% of cases, whereas other variations form 1% each.
- Associated cardiac anomalies occur in 33% of cases.
- Sometimes TEF occurs as a component of VACTERL association (vertebral anomalies, anal atresia, cardiac defects, TEF, oesophageal atresia, renal anomalies and limb defects).

5 The Genitourinary System

5.1 Development of the Urogenital System

The urogenital system arises from the intermediate mesoderm, which forms a urogenital ridge on either side of the aorta and the primitive urogenital sinus, which is part of the cloaca.

5.2 Intermediate Mesoderm

The intermediate mesoderm forms a bulge on the posterior abdominal wall lateral to the attachment of the dorsal mesentery of the gut. This bulge is known as the urogenital ridge or nephrogenic cord. Its surface is covered by the coelomic epithelium lining the peritoneal cavity. The urogenital ridge forms:

- excretory tubules: development of the kidneys
- nephric duct: later becomes the mesonephric duct
- paramesonephric duct is formed lateral to the nephric duct
- gonads (testis/ovary): develop from the coelomic epithelium lining the medial side of the nephrogenic cord

5.2.1 Cloaca

The terminal part of the hindgut ends in the cloaca, which is an endoderm-lined chamber that contacts the surface ectoderm at the cloacal membrane and communicates with the allantois. The allantois is a membranous sac, which extends into the umbilicus alongside the vitelline duct.

The cloaca is then divided by the urorectal septum:

- The dorsal (inferior) portion develops into the rectum and anal canal.
- The ventral (superior) portion develops into the bladder and urogenital sinus.
- The urogenital sinus gives rise to the bladder and lower urogenital tracts (prostatic and penile urethrae in males; urethra and lower vagina in women). See Figure 12.2.

6 Development of the Kidneys

The urogenital ridge develops into three sets of tubular nephric structures:

1. Pronephros, which mostly regress
2. Mesonephros:
    - mesonephric tubules: these tubules carry out some kidney function at first, but many of the tubules then regress
    - mesonephric duct (Wolffian duct): persists and opens to the cloaca at the tail of the embryo
3. Metanephros: gives rise to adult kidneys.

The adult kidneys arise from two sources:

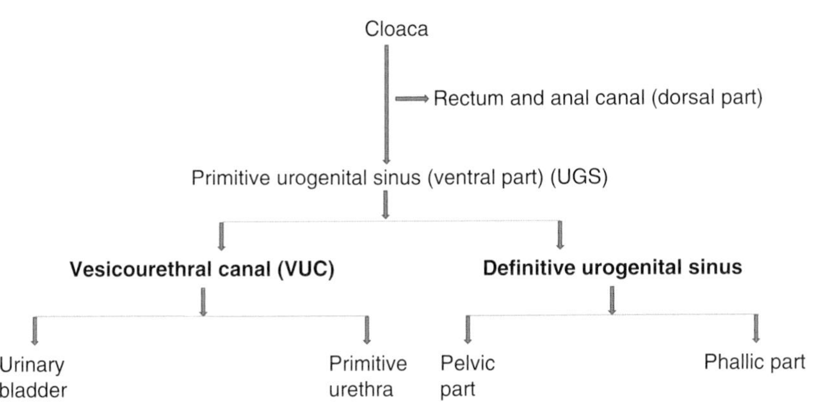

Figure 12.2 Primitive urogenital sinus.

- The metanephric blastema: a condensation of nearby renogenic intermediate mesoderm from the lowest part of the nephrogenic cord. It forms glomerular capillaries, proximal convoluted tubules, the loops of Henle and distal convoluted tubules.
- The ureteric bud develops from an outgrowth of the caudal mesonephric duct, and forms the collecting tubules and ducts, minor and major calyces and the ureters.

6.1 Ascent of the Kidneys

The kidneys initially form near the tail of the embryo. Growth of the embryo in length causes the kidneys to 'ascend' to their final position in the lumbar region. Malformations related to the ascent of the kidneys include:

- pelvic kidney: one or both kidneys stay in the pelvis
- horseshoe kidney: two developing kidneys fuse ventrally into a single, horseshoe shape, which gets trapped in the abdomen by the inferior mesenteric artery
- supernumerary arteries: there can often be more than one renal artery per kidney, which is often asymptomatic but can sometimes cause hydronephrosis

6.2 Rotation of the Kidneys

The hilum of the kidney at first faces anteriorly, which gradually rotates to face medially.

7 Development of the Ureters

The ureters are derived from the part of the ureteric bud that lies between the pelvis of the kidney and vesicourethral canal.

8 Development of the Bladder

The lower end of the mesonephric ducts open into primitive urogenital sinus (UGS; part of the cloaca). The ureteric buds arise from the mesonephric ducts a little cranial to their opening in the UGS. The parts of the mesonephric ducts caudal to the origin of the ureteric buds are absorbed into the vesicourethral canal, resulting in separate openings for mesonephric ducts and the ureteric buds. The openings of the ureteric buds move cranially and laterally. The triangular area between their openings is derived from the absorbed ducts and is therefore mesodermal in origin and forms the trigone of bladder and the posterior wall of part of the urethra.

The developing bladder is continuous cranially with the allantois. The allantois atrophies and is seen as the urachus (a fibrous band), extending from the apex of the bladder to the umbilicus.

9 Development of the Female Urethra

The female urethra develops from the caudal part of the vesicourethral canal (VUC) (endodermal, but the posterior wall of it is derived from absorbed mesonephric ducts; hence, it is mesodermal in origin) and may receive slight contribution from the pelvic part of the urogenital sinus.

10 Development of the Male Urethra

- The part extending from the bladder to the openings of the ejaculatory ducts (original openings of the mesonephric ducts) is derived from the caudal part of the VUC (endodermal, but the posterior wall of it is derived from absorbed mesonephric ducts; hence, it is mesodermal in origin).
- The rest of the prostatic urethra and the membranous urethra develop from the pelvic part of the definitive UGS.
- Except for the terminal part, the penile urethra develops from the phallic part of the definitive UGS.
- The terminal part of the urethra that lies in the glans is derived from ectoderm.

11 Development of Gonads

- The indifferent stage: at the initial stages of gonadal development, it is not possible to distinguish between the male and female gonad. The gonads begin as genital ridges: a pair of longitudinal ridges derived from the intermediate mesoderm and overlying epithelium.
- Fourth week: germ cells begin to migrate from the endoderm lining of the yolk sac to the genital ridges, via the dorsal mesentery of the hindgut, and reach the genital ridges in the sixth week.
- Simultaneously, the epithelium of the genital ridges proliferates and penetrates the intermediate mesoderm to form the primitive sex cords. The combination of germ cells and primitive sex cords forms the indifferent gonad.
- Male: the SRY gene on the Y chromosome stimulates the development of the primitive sex cords to form testis (medullary) cords. The tunica albuginea, a fibrous connective tissue layer, forms around the cords. A portion of the testis cords breaks off to form the future rete testis. The remaining cords contain two types of cells: germ cells and Sertoli cells (derived from the surface epithelium of the gland). At puberty, these cords acquire a lumen and become the seminiferous tubules, where sperm is produced. Located between the testis cords are the Leydig cells (derived from the intermediate mesoderm), which begin production of testosterone by the eighth week; this drives differentiation of the internal and external genitalia.
- Female: in the absence of the SRY gene, the primitive sex cords degenerate and do not form the testis cords. Instead, the epithelium of the gonad continues to proliferate, producing cortical cords. In the third month, these cords break up into clusters, surrounding each oogonium (germ cell) with a layer of epithelial follicular cells, forming a primordial follicle.

11.1 Development of the Internal Genitalia

- Indifferent stage: in the first weeks of urogenital development, all embryos have two pairs of ducts, both ending at the cloaca. These are the mesonephric (Wolffian) ducts and paramesonephric (müllerian) ducts.
- Male: in the presence of testosterone produced by the Leydig cells, the mesonephric ducts develop to form the primary male genital ducts and give rise to the efferent ductules, epididymis, vas deferens and seminal vesicles. Meanwhile, paramesonephric ducts degenerate in the presence of anti-müllerian hormone produced by Sertoli cells. Its developmental remnant is the appendix testis; a small portion of tissue located on the upper pole of each testicle, which has no physiological function. Some testosterone is converted into dihydrotestosterone (DHT), which supports the development of the prostate gland, penis and scrotum.
- Female: in the female, in the absence of testosterone, the mesonephric ducts degenerate, leaving behind only a vestigial remnant, Gartner's duct. The absence of anti-müllerian hormone allows for development of the paramesonephric ducts. These ducts can be described as having three parts:
  - cranial: becomes the fallopian tubes
  - horizontal: becomes the fallopian tubes
  - caudal: fuses to form the uterus, cervix and upper one-third of the vagina
- The lower two-thirds of the vagina is formed by sinovaginal bulbs derived from the pelvic part of the urogenital sinus.

11.2 Development of the External Genitalia

- Indifferent stage: development of the external genitalia begins in the third week. Mesenchymal cells from the primitive streak migrate to the cloacal membrane to form a pair of cloacal folds. Cranially, these folds fuse to form the genital tubercle. Caudally, they divide into the urethral folds (anterior) and anal folds (posterior). Genital swellings develop on either side of the urethral folds.

- Male: development of male external genitalia is under the influence of androgens from the testes, DHT. There is rapid elongation of the genital tubercle, which becomes the phallus. The urethral folds are pulled to form the urethral groove, which extends along the caudal aspect of the phallus. The folds close over by the fourth month, forming the penile urethra. The genital swellings become the scrotal swellings, moving caudally to eventually form the scrotum.
- Female: estrogens in the female embryo are responsible for external genital development. The genital tubercle only elongates slightly to form the clitoris. The urethral folds and genital swellings do not fuse, but instead form the labia minora and labia majora, respectively. The urogenital groove remains open, forming the vestibule into which the urethra and vagina open.
- The urogenital sinus contributes to the formation of the bulbourethral glands and the lower two-thirds of the vagina.
- The uterovaginal canal and the UGS are soon separated from each other by the formation of a solid plate of cells called the vaginal plate. The vagina is formed by the development of a lumen within the vaginal plate.
- The hymen is situated at the junction of the lower end of the vaginal plate with the UGS.

11.3 Descent of the Gonads

- While the gonads arise in the upper lumbar region, they are each tethered to the scrotum or labia by the gubernaculum: a ligamentous structure formed from mesenchyme.
- Testes: as the body of the fetus grows, the testes become more caudal. They pass through the inguinal canal around the twenty-eighth week, and reach the scrotum by the thirty-third week. During their descent, the testes retain their original blood supply, with the testicular arteries branching from the lumbar aorta. The scrotal ligament is the adult remnant of the gubernaculum.
- Ovaries: the ovaries initially migrate caudally in a similar fashion to the testes from their origin on the posterior abdominal wall. However, they do not travel as far, reaching their final position just within the true pelvis. The gubernaculum becomes the ovarian ligament and round ligament of the uterus. See Figure 12.3 and Table 12.2.

12 Disorders of Sex Development

Disorders of sex development (DSD) are congenital conditions with atypical development of chromosomal, gonadal or anatomic sex.

12.1 Background and Prevalence

- DSD is defined as genital ambiguity at birth or late onset.
- The incidence is 1 per 4500, although some degree of male undervirilisation or female virilisation may be present in as many as 2% of live births.
- Psychosexual development is influenced by multiple factors such as exposure to androgens and sex chromosome genes, as well as social circumstance and family dynamics. See Table 12.3.

12.2 History

- Obstetric history: any evidence of endocrine disturbance during pregnancy: a history of maternal virilisation may suggest a maternal androgen-secreting tumour or aromatase deficiency; use of any drugs in pregnancy that may cause virilisation of a female fetus.
- Any previous neonatal deaths (which might suggest an undiagnosed adrenal crisis).
- Family history:
  - consanguineous parents mean an increased risk of autosomal recessive condition
  - a history of genital ambiguity, abnormal pubertal development or infertility (X-linked recessive condition such as androgen insensitivity)
- Gestation of the baby: in preterm girls, the clitoris and labia minora are relatively prominent, and in boys, the testes are usually undescended until about 34 weeks of gestation.

12.3 Features That Suggest DSD

Most causes of DSD are recognised in the neonatal period:

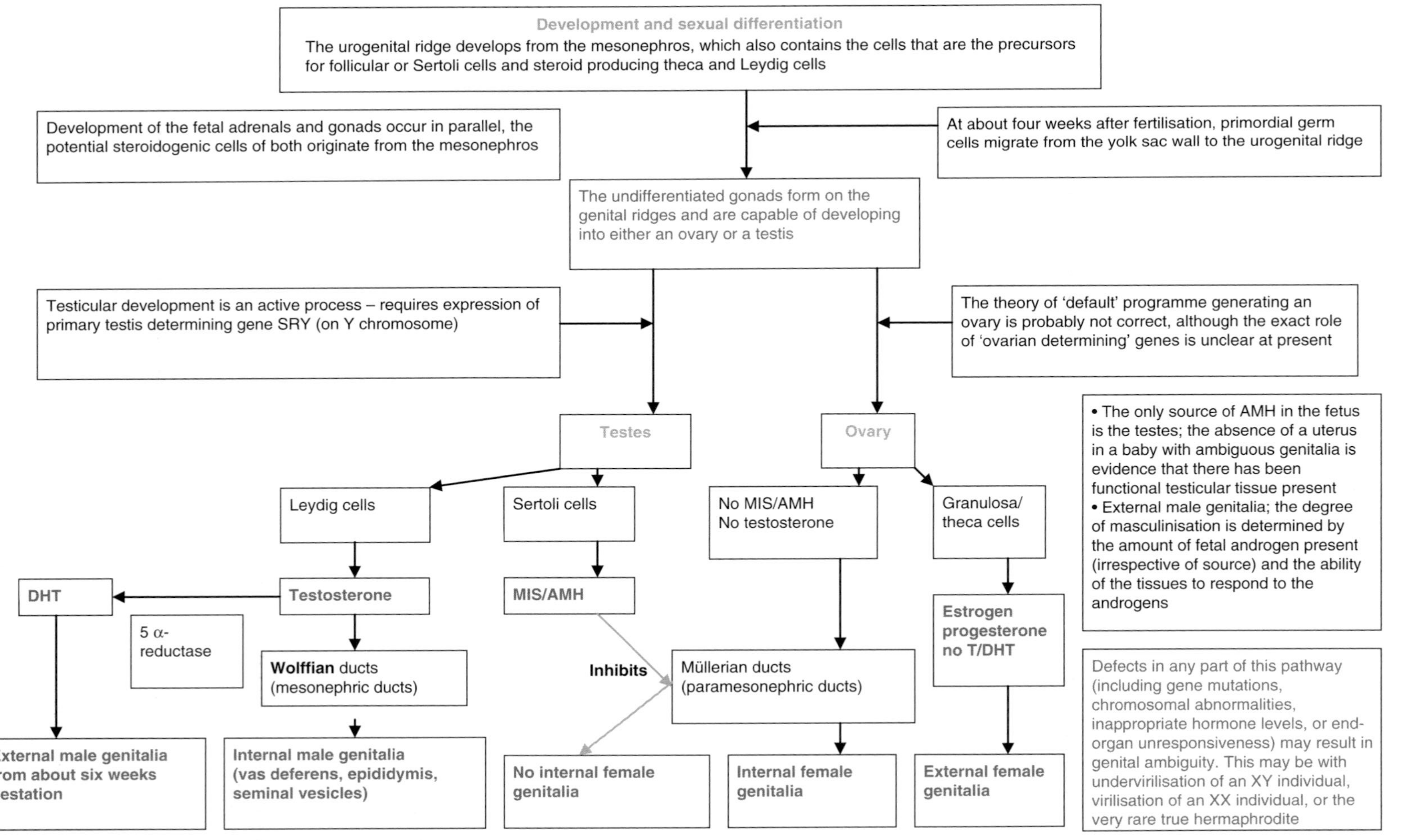

Figure 12.3 Development and sexual differentiation.
T: testosterone
DHT: dihydrotestosterone
MIS: müllerian inhibitory substance
AMH: antimüllerian hormone

Table 12.2 Development of male and female genitalia

	Female	Male
Ureteric bud	Ureter	Ureter
Mesonephric ducts	Trigone of bladder Gartner's duct	Rete testis, efferent ducts, epididymis, vas deferens, seminal vesicle, trigone of bladder
Paramesonephric ducts	Oviduct, uterus, upper one-third of vagina	Appendix testis
Urogenital sinus	Bladder (except trigone), bulbourethral gland, urethra, lower two-thirds of vagina	Bladder (except trigone), prostate gland, bulbourethral gland, urethra
Genital tubercle	Body and glans of clitoris	Body and glans of penis Corpora cavernosum and spongiosum
Genital folds	Labia minora	Ventral aspect of penis Penile raphe
Genital swellings	Labia majora Mons pubis	Scrotum Scrotal raphe
Gubernaculum	Ovarian ligament and round ligament of the uterus	Scrotal ligament

Table 12.3 Nomenclature

• Male pseudohermaphrodite, undervirilisation/undermasculinisation of XY male	• 46,XY DSD
• Female pseudohermaphrodite, overvirilisation/masculinisation of XX female	• 46,XX DSD
• True hermaphrodite	• Ovotesticular DSD
• XX male or XX sex reversal	• 46,XX testicular DSD
• XY sex reversal	• 46,XY complete gonadal dysgenesis

International consensus conference, 2006, Nomenclature

- overt genital ambiguity
- apparent female genitalia with an enlarged clitoris, posterior labial fusion or an inguinal/labial mass
- apparent male genitalia with bilateral undescended testes in a full-term infant, micropenis, isolated perineal hypospadias or mild hypospadias with undescended testis, hypospadias associated with separation of the scrotal sacs
- discordance between genital appearance and a prenatal karyotype

12.4 Later Presentations in Older Children and Young Adults

- previously unrecognised genital ambiguity
- inguinal hernia in a female
- virilisation in a female
- delayed or incomplete puberty
- primary amenorrhea (see Figure 12.6)
- breast development in a male
- gross and occasionally cyclic haematuria in a male

12.5 General Physical Examination

- Any dysmorphic features (syndromes associated with ambiguous genitalia).
- Hypoglycaemia: cortisol deficiency secondary to hypothalamic-pituitary or adrenocortical insufficiency.
- State of hydration and blood pressure: various forms of congenital adrenal hyperplasia (CAH) can be associated with differing degrees of salt loss or hypertension. Although the cardiovascular collapse with salt loss and hyperkalaemia in CAH does not usually occur until between the fourth to fifteenth day of life, it should be anticipated until CAH has been excluded.
- Jaundice (both conjugated and unconjugated) may be caused by concomitant thyroid hormone or cortisol deficiency.
- Urine for protein as a screen for any associated renal anomaly.
- Hyperpigmentation, especially of the genital skin and nipples, occurs in the presence of excessive

adrenocorticotropic hormone (ACTH) and proopiomelanocortin, and may be apparent in CAH.

12.6 Examination of External Genitalia

- The palpability of the gonads and the degree of virilisation should be determined.
- Gonads: if both gonads are palpable, they are likely to be testes (or ovotestes), which may be normal or dysgenetic. They may be situated high in the inguinal canal, so careful examination is required.
- Penis: the length of the phallus should be determined. A well-developed phallus indicates that significant levels of circulating testosterone were present in utero.
- Chordee should be noted as this may decrease the apparent length of the phallus and the penis may be 'buried' in some cases.
- Urethral meatus: the presence of hypospadias and the position of the urethral meatus should be determined.
- The degree of fusion and rugosity of the labioscrotal folds should be noted and the presence or absence of a separate vaginal opening determined.

12.7 Investigations

Investigations to ascertain whether the child is an undervirilised male or a virilised female include the following:

- Karyotype with SRY detection: full karyotype for confirmation and exclusion of mosaicism. The latter may be tissue specific and may not be apparent from blood, but only from skin or gonadal biopsies.
- Human chorionic gonadotropin (hCG) stimulation test: this is undertaken to determine whether functioning Leydig cells are present, to delineate a block in testosterone biosynthesis from androstenedione (17b-hydroxysteroid dehydrogenase deficiency) or conversion of testosterone to DHT (5 α-reductase deficiency).
- Anti-müllerian hormone (AMH) and inhibin B levels: AMH and inhibin B are secreted by the Sertoli cells. AMH is undetectable in female serum until the onset of puberty. AMH may be a more sensitive marker for the presence of testicular tissue than serum testosterone levels. Basal inhibin B gives reliable information about both the presence and function of the testes.
- Determination of internal anatomy of uterus, ovaries:
    - ultrasound scan: also helps to exclude renal anomalies, to visualise the adrenal glands and locate inguinal gonads, although it is not sensitive for intra-abdominal gonads
    - examination under anaesthetic/cystoscopy or urogenital sonogram/MRI scan
    - laparoscopy: to confirm the anatomy of the internal genitalia and to take gonadal biopsies
- 17-hydroxyprogesterone and testosterone.
- Serum and urine electrolytes.
- gonadotropin: raised basal gonadotropin are consistent with primary gonadal failure.
- Adrenal steroid biosynthesis: ACTH stimulation tests.
- Urinary steroid analysis: output of adrenal steroids will be low in adrenal insufficiency. In CAH, specific ratios of metabolites will be altered, depending on the level of the enzyme block.
- Skin and gonadal biopsies:
    - genital skin biopsies to establish cell lines for androgen receptor binding assays and analysis of 5 α-reductase activity
- Gonadal biopsies are essential for dysgenesis and true hermaphroditism. See Figures 12.4 and 12.5.

12.8 Management

General concepts of care:

- Multidisciplinary team: paediatric subspecialists in endocrinology, surgery, urology, genetics, neonatology, psychology/psychiatry, gynaecology, nursing and medical ethics.
- Psychosocial management to promote positive adaptation.
- Gender assignment in newborns:
    - Gender assignment should be avoided before expert evaluation of the newborn. However, it should be made as quickly as thorough diagnostic evaluation permits.
    - Factors that influence gender assignment: diagnosis, genital appearance, therapeutic options, need for lifelong replacement therapy, potential for fertility, views of the family and, sometimes, circumstances relating to cultural practices.

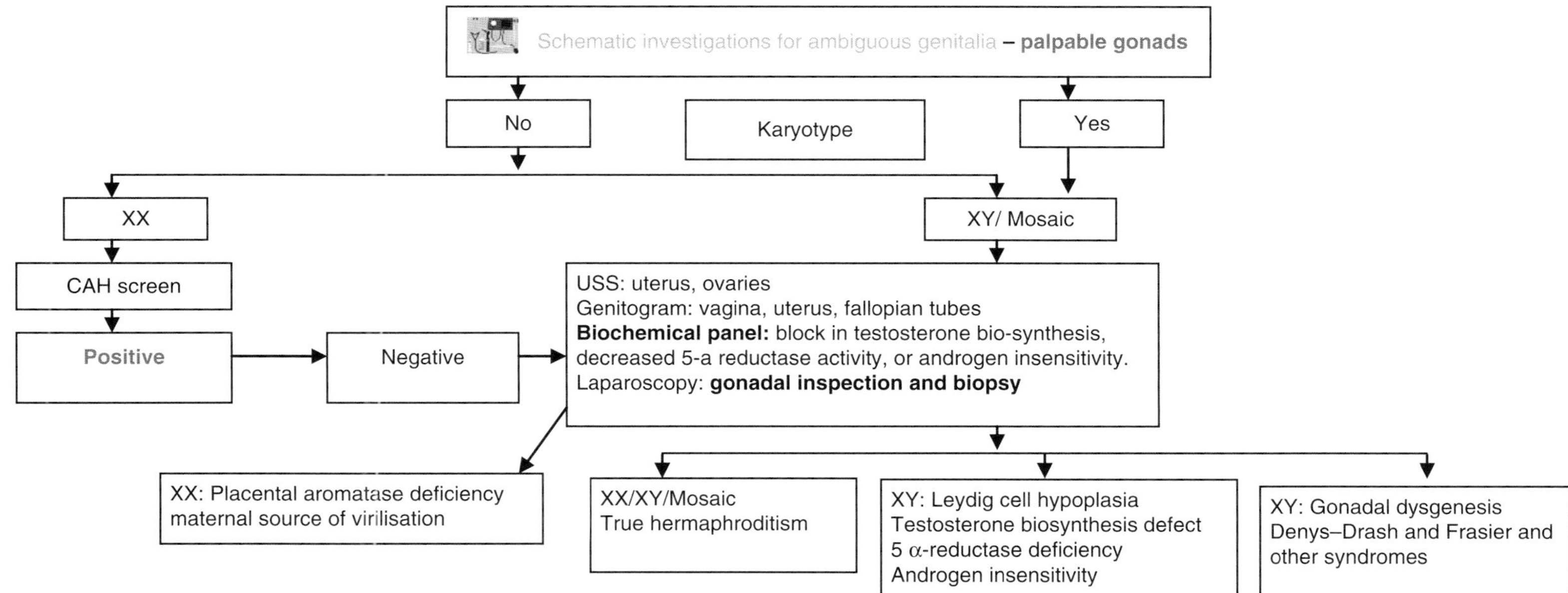

Figure 12.4 Schematic investigations for ambiguous genitalia.

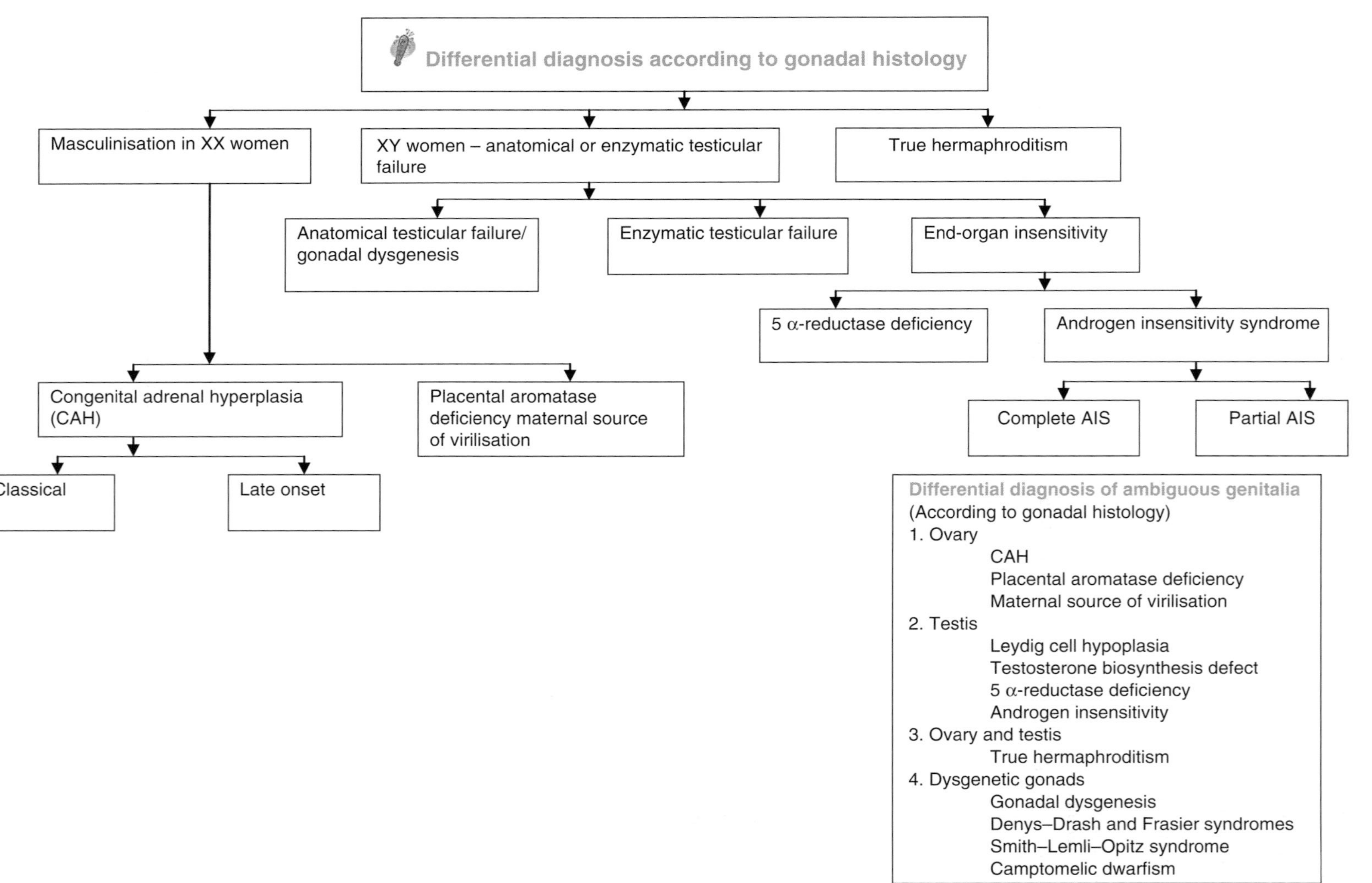

Figure 12.5 Differential diagnosis according to gonadal histology.
AIS - Androgen insensitvity syndrome

- The recommendations are to raise infants as follows:
  - 46,XY complete androgen insensitivity (CAIS) and 46,XX CAH: raise as women
  - 5 α-reductase or 17β-hydroxysteroid dehydrogenase-3 deficiency: raise as males.
- Surgical management:
  - The emphasis is on functional outcome rather than a cosmetic appearance. The rationale for early reconstruction includes the beneficial effects of estrogen on infant tissues, avoiding complications from anatomic anomalies, minimising family concern and distress, and mitigating the risks of stigmatisation and gender-identity confusion of atypical genital appearance.
  - However, surgical reconstruction in infancy may need to be refined at the time of puberty.
- Masculinising genital surgery: involves more surgical procedures and difficulties than feminising genitoplasty:
  - Repair involving hypospadias includes chordee correction, urethral reconstruction and judicious testosterone supplementation.
  - If needed, adult-sized testicular prostheses may be inserted after sufficient pubertal scrotal development.
- Feminising genital surgery:
  - External genitalia reconstruction and vaginal exteriorisation, with early separation of the vagina and urethra.
  - Clitoral reduction may be considered in severe virilisation and performed in conjunction with common urogenital sinus repair.
  - Vaginal dilatation should not be advised during childhood. Vaginoplasty should be performed in the teenage years: it has potential for scarring, which would require modification before sexual function.
- Risk of gonadal tumour: germ-cell malignancy only occurs in patients who have Y-chromosomal material. The highest risk (up to 60%) is in patients with gonadal dysgenesis and partial androgen insensitivity syndrome (AIS) with intra-abdominal gonads. Intra-abdominal gonads of high-risk patients should be removed at diagnosis. The lowest risk (<5%) is found in ovotestis and genetically confirmed CAIS. Gonadal biopsy should be performed at puberty in patients with DSD, raised as males with scrotal gonads.
- Sex steroid replacement: hypogonadism is common in patients with dysgenetic gonads, defects in sex steroid biosynthesis and resistance to androgens:
  - hormonal induction of puberty to induce secondary sexual characteristics, a pubertal growth spurt and optimal bone mineral accumulation
  - route: intramuscular depot injections, oral and transdermal
  - partial androgen insensitivity (PAIS) may need supraphysiologic doses of testosterone for optimal effect
  - women with hypogonadism: estrogen should be supplemented to induce pubertal changes and menses; a progestin should be added after breakthrough bleeding develops or within one to two years of continuous estrogen.
- Fertility: women with an adequately formed uterus and males with evidence of functional seminiferous tubules may have fertility potential with assisted-reproduction techniques. Fertility-potential considerations include:
  - expected fertility in virilised women with a well-developed uterus and ovaries
  - unlikely fertility in undermasculinised males without assisted-reproduction techniques
  - fertility in some patients with ovotesticular DSD

12.9 True Hermaphrodite

- Varying degrees of sexual ambiguity: maleness predominates in some; femaleness in others.
- In the majority, a uterus and a vagina are present.
- Karyotypes: 46,XX (60%), 46,XX/XY (13%), 46,XY (11%), 46,XY/47,XXY (6%) and other mosaics (10%).
- Distribution of the gonads: combination of an ovotestis on one side and an ovary on the other; a testis on one side and an ovary on the other. Ovotestis may be bilateral or combined with a testis.
- Diagnosis: gonadal biopsy showing both ovarian and testicular tissue.
- Sex of rearing should be determined based on the functional capability of the external genitalia, after which inappropriate organs should be removed. In some cases, it may be possible to identify the ovarian and testicular portions of an ovotestis for certain and

to remove only the part that is unwanted. If this is not possible, both must be removed.

- Replacement hormone therapy at puberty.

12.10 Gonadal Dysgenesis/Anatomical Testicular Failure

- Failure of normal testicular differentiation and development may be the result of a chromosome mosaicism affecting the sex chromosomes or possibly associated with an abnormal isochromosome, but usually the sex chromosomes appear to be normal and the condition is referred to as pure gonadal dysgenesis.
- It has variable features depending on how much testicular differentiation is present. Since differentiation is often poor, most patients have mild masculinisation or none at all, and the uterus, fallopian tubes and vagina are generally present.
- Management: reconstruction of the external genitalia and removal of the streak or rudimentary gonad. The degree of masculinisation is often minimal and, if it is limited to a minor degree of clitoral enlargement with little or no fusion of the genital folds, surgery need not be undertaken.
- The risk of malignancy in the rudimentary testes is about 30%. Therefore, the gonads should be removed during childhood. Around the age of puberty, start estrogen–progestogen replacement therapy to produce secondary sexual development and menstruation.

12.11 Enzymatic Testicular Failure

- A number of biosynthetic defects can occur at each stage of testosterone biosynthesis process.
- Clinical features are varied, but, since such enzyme defects are generally incomplete, there is external genital ambiguity of varying degrees.
- The uterus, fallopian tubes and upper vagina are absent as the production of Müllerian inhibitory substance (MIS) is normal.
- Decision on the sex of rearing depends on the degree of masculinisation of the external genitalia, but the female role is often chosen.
- hCG stimulation with measurement of various androgens helps to determine the site of the enzyme block.

12.12 5 α-reductase Deficiency

- Autosomal recessive; history of other affected family members.
- Normal masculinisation of the external genitalia requires the conversion of testosterone to dihydrotestosterone by 5 α-reductase. The Wolffian structures respond directly to testosterone. Therefore, the internal organs will be male. The uterus, fallopian tubes and upper vagina will always be absent since MIS production is normal. There is deficient or absent breast development, yet normal or increased pubic and axillary hair.
- Male infants will have poor masculinisation of external genitalia.
- As a rule, the degree of genital masculinisation is small or, at worst, moderate, and most children are initially placed in the female role. At puberty, however, the testes produce increased amounts of testosterone and there is greater virilisation.
- Penis size: barely adequate and the female gender role is often preferred.
- Test: hCG stimulation of the gonad: elevated testosterone to DHT ratio.

12.13 Androgen Insensitivity

- Incidence: 1:60 000 male births.
- X-linked recessive.
- Karyotype: 46, XY.
- Testosterone levels are normal, but there is insensitivity to secreted androgens due to complete absence of the gene for the androgen receptor or due to mutations in the gene. The condition may be complete in patients who have an absent androgen receptor or, in some cases, where the androgen receptor mutation is not complete, some receptivity may persist and partial androgenisation may occur.
- Patients present at or after puberty, but may be sometimes seen earlier in childhood if the defect is incomplete or when a testis is found to occupy a hernial sac.

Complete androgen insensitivity

- Present at or after puberty, with primary amenorrhoea despite normal breast development. Absent or scanty pubic and axillary hair; normal vulva, but a short blind vagina with no cervix. Anti-müllerian factor prevents the development of müllerian structures: therefore, there is no uterus or fallopian tubes. External genitalia appear female.

- The Wolffian structures also fail to develop because of the insensitivity to testosterone.

Partial androgen insensitivity

- In about 10% of patients, the defect is incomplete. The external genitalia may be ambiguous at birth, and virilisation may occur before puberty.
- Management: depends on the age at which the patient is seen.
- If seen after puberty when breast development is complete, gonadectomy should be undertaken due to the increased risk of cancer (5%). Hormone replacement therapy (HRT) should be provided with estrogen; this does not need to be cyclical since the uterus is absent.
- If the patient is seen for the first time in childhood, feminisation will occur at puberty and nothing needs to be done until that time. If, however, there are heterosexual features, it is very likely that masculinisation will occur to some extent at puberty. This will have a profound psychological effect on the patient when she has been brought up in the female role. In these circumstances, gonadectomy should be advised in childhood and induction of puberty with HRT at the appropriate time.
- Surgery is seldom necessary to elongate the vagina as it is usually functional, but, if required, graduated dilatation using Frank's procedure is the treatment of choice.
- Phenotypic males with 46,XX karyotype are rarely found. Those who have been appropriately examined have been shown to be H-Y antigen-positive and there is little clinical ambiguity in this group, the external genitalia being generally normal, although underdeveloped. Hypospadias may be present.
- Isolated deficiency of müllerian inhibition has also been reported, but such cases do not present clinically as examples of doubtful sex unless some unrelated surgical procedure reveals the surprising presence of müllerian structures in an otherwise normal or near normal male.

13 Cholesterol Synthesis Pathway

13.1 Congenital Adrenal Hyperplasia

- The most common cause of female intersex.
- Autosomal recessive.
- Congenital adrenal hyperplasia (CAH) is an enzyme deficiency related to the biosynthesis of cortisol and aldosterone.
- Severe enzyme deficiency: ambiguous genitalia in the newborn due to virilisation.
- Partial enzyme deficiency: presents in adolescence with virilisation in the female and (precocious puberty in the male).
- Newborn with ambiguous genitalia: enlarged clitoris and excessive fusion of the labioscrotal folds, which obscure the vagina and urethra, with a single opening at some point on the perineum, usually near the base of the clitoris, although sometimes along its ventral surface and rarely at the tip. Thickening and rugosity of the labia majora with some resemblance to a scrotum. The uterus, fallopian tubes and vagina are always present, and the vagina opens at some point in the urogenital sinus.
- Late onset: accounts for up to 2–20% of women presenting with hirsutism and oligomenorrhoea. May mimic polycystic ovarian syndrome (PCOS). 17-OH progesterone levels are less elevated. Test for confirmation: adrenocorticotropic hormone (ACTH) stimulation test with measurement of 17-OH progesterone.

Treatment

- Glucocorticoids: replace glucocorticoids deficit and decreases ACTH secretion. Overtreatment should be avoided as it may cause linear growth restriction, delayed puberty and Cushingoid signs. Infants: hydrocortisone twice daily. Adults: prednisolone.
- Mineralocorticoid replacement with fludrocortisone.
- Clitoral reduction and vaginoplasty with correction of labial fusion and anomalous urethral position. It is advised that timing of surgery is delayed until adolescence.
- Women are fertile with adequate replacement therapy. There is a risk of autosomal recessive condition being passed on to the next generation.

13.2 Congenital Adrenal Hyperplasia: Enzyme Defects

21-hydroxylase deficiency (90% of cases)

- Incidence: 1 in 5000 to 1 in 15 000.

- Gene: on the short arm of chromosome 6.
- Results in a failure of conversion of 17α-hydroxyprogesterone to desoxycortisol and progesterone to deoxycorticosterone, leading to increased progesterone and 17α-hydroxyprogesterone (raised 50–400 times), which is therefore converted to androstenedione and subsequently to testosterone.
- Also results in insufficient cortisol production, stimulating increased production of corticotropin-releasing hormone and ACTH. High ACTH levels lead to adrenal hyperplasia and production of excess androgens.
- Symptoms of excessive androgens are found in varying degrees as a result of the severity of the enzyme defect.
- Severe deficiency: adrenal aldosterone secretion is insufficient to stimulate sodium reabsorption by the distal renal tubules, resulting in salt wasting (seen in one-third cases), as well as cortisol deficiency in addition to androgen excess. The child may die of wasting and vomiting within a few weeks of life due to this salt-losing syndrome.
- Prenatal treatment with daily dexamethasone has been shown to reduce the virilisation process.

11β-hydroxylase deficiency

- Second commonest.
- Gene on chromosome 8.
- May present with virilisation, hypertension and hypokalaemia. Hypertension (HT) is secondary to an increase in 11-deoxycortisol and deoxycorticosterone (mineralocorticoid).
- High levels of 17-OH progesterone, 11-deoxycortisol and deoxycorticosterone.

3β-hydroxysteroid dehydrogenase deficiency

- Decreased synthesis of glucocorticoids, mineralocorticoids, androgens and estrogen.
- Newborns are unwell at birth, and frequently fail to survive.
- May be a mild genital ambiguity due to very high levels of dehydroepiandrosterone (androgenic at extremely high levels).

17 α-hydroxylase deficiency

- Failure of production cortisol, androgens and estradiol.
- Gene is located on chromosome 10.
- Presents with HT, hypokalaemia.
- Female: infantile female external genitalia and absent secondary sexual characteristics at puberty with primary amenorrhoea and raised gonadotropin.
- Male: genital ambiguity at birth.
- Increased levels of 11-deoxycorticosterone.

Desmolase deficiency

- Prevents production of any active steroid, with inevitable death.
- The internal and external genitalia are female.

Section 3

Physiology

Neelanjana Mukhopadhaya

13 Female Physiology

Renuka Sharma

1 The Ovaries

- The ovaries are located within the broad ligament, close to the lateral wall of the pelvic cavity, and extend onto the peritoneal cavity.
- Each ovary is divided into an outer cortex and inner medulla.
- The dense cellular stroma of the cortex houses the ovarian follicles, which are the functional units, performing both gametogenic and endocrine function.
- The stages in the development of the follicle are shown in Figure 13.1.
- During fetal development, the ovaries contain over 7 million primordial follicles, which reduces to a million at birth and around 300 000–400 000 at puberty.
- They undergo part of the first meiotic division at birth and survive in prophase arrest until adulthood. Just before ovulation, the first meiotic division is completed. One of the daughter cells, the secondary oocyte, receives most of the cytoplasm, and immediately begins the second meiotic division, but this division stops at metaphase and is completed only when a sperm penetrates the oocyte and forms a haploid ovum.

2 The Menstrual Cycle

- The reproductive system of women shows regular cyclic changes, which teleologically may be regarded as periodic preparations for fertilisation and pregnancy. See Figure 13.2.
- In humans and other primates, the cycle is a menstrual cycle, and its most conspicuous feature is the periodic vaginal bleeding that occurs with the shedding of the uterine mucosa (menstruation).
- The length of the cycle is roughly 28 days, divided into the following phases:
  - days 1–5 (menstrual phase)
  - days 6–14 (follicular/preovulatory phase)
  - days 14–28 day (luteal/postovulatory phase)

3 Ovarian Cycle

3.1 Follicular Phase

- At the start of each cycle, several follicles enlarge, and a cavity forms around the ovum (antrum formation), filled with follicular fluid.
- Usually one of the follicles (dominant follicle) grows rapidly from day six, which is related to the ability of the follicle to secrete the estrogen needed for maturation, while the others regress, forming atretic follicles.
- When women are injected with highly purified human pituitary gonadotropin preparations, many follicles develop simultaneously.
- Ovarian (graafian) follicle: is lined by theca interna cells, which produce estrogen as they secrete androgens that are aromatised to estrogen by the granulosa cells.

Resting primordial follicle (0.03–0.04 mm)
Primary follicle (0.04–0.06 mm)
Secondary preantral follicle (0.06–2 mm)
Large antral follicle (2–5 mm)
Dominant follicle (15–20 mm)
Corpus luteum (20–30 mm)
Atretic follicles (0.01–2 mm)

Figure 13.1 Stages in the development of a follicle.

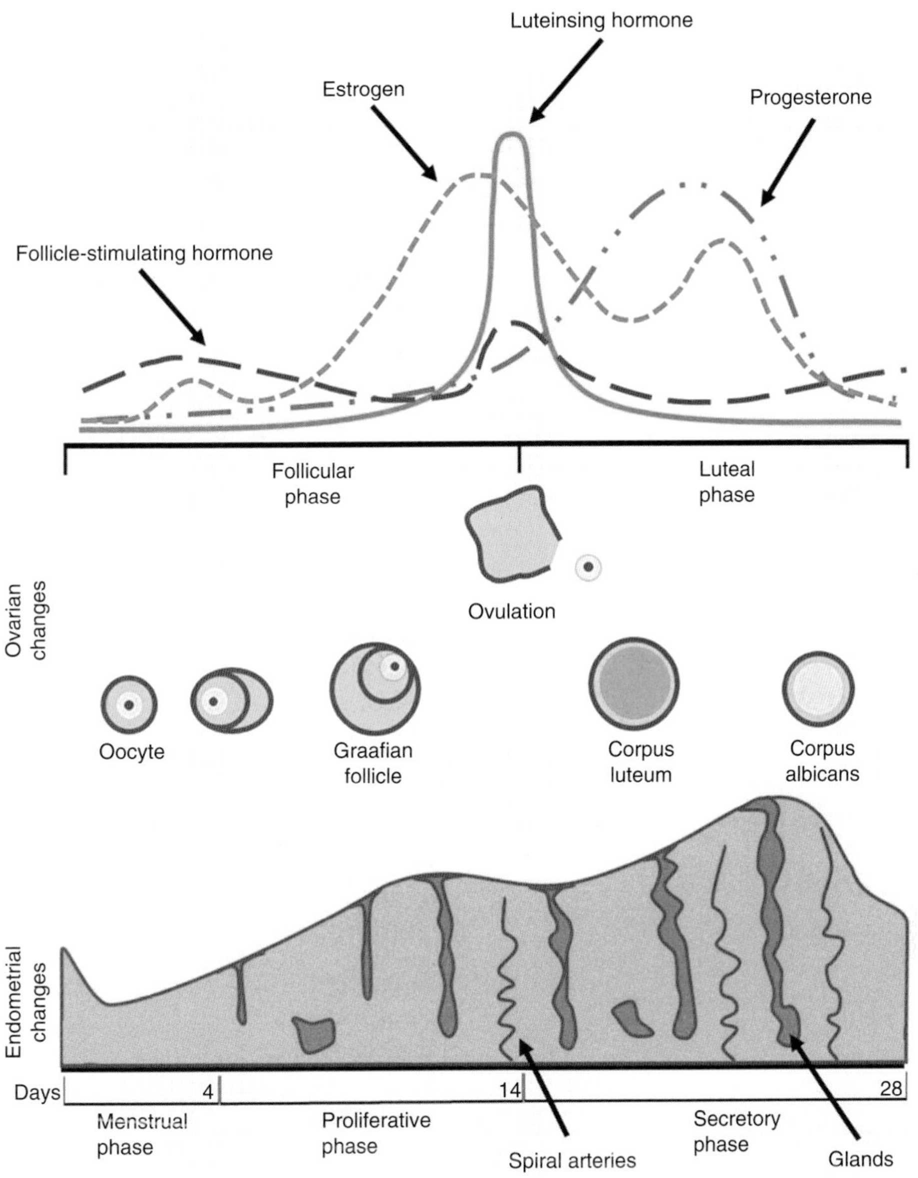

Figure 13.2 The menstrual cycle. Copyright © 2019 Lineage Medical, Inc. All rights reserved.

3.2 Ovulation

- On the fourteenth day of the cycle, the distended follicle ruptures and the ovum is extruded into the abdominal cavity, picked up by the fimbriated ends of the uterine tubes, and transported to the uterus.
- The follicle that ruptures at the time of ovulation promptly fills with blood, forming a corpus haemorrhagicum. Minor bleeding from the follicle into the abdominal cavity may cause peritoneal irritation and transient lower abdominal pain (mittelschmerz).

3.3 Luteal Phase

- The granulosa and theca cells of the follicle lining rapidly proliferate, and the clotted blood is replaced with yellowish, lipid-rich luteal cells, forming the corpus luteum, which secretes estrogen and progesterone.
- An adequate blood supply is crucial for the growth of the corpus luteum, in which the vascular endothelial growth factor plays an important role.
- If pregnancy occurs, the corpus luteum persists; whereas if it does not, the corpus luteum begins to degenerate around the twenty-fourth day of the cycle) and is eventually replaced by scar tissue, forming a corpus albicans.

4 Uterine Cycle

- The uterine cycle is divided into the menstrual phase followed by the proliferative phase (fifth to fourteenth day) when a new endometrium regrows under the influence of estrogens from the developing follicle.
- The endometrium increases rapidly in thickness and simultaneously the uterine glands are drawn out so that they lengthen.
- Also called the preovulatory or follicular phase of the cycle.

Secretory or luteal phase: represents preparation of the uterus for implantation of the fertilised ovum.

- The length of this phase is remarkably constant at about 14 days.
- After ovulation, the endometrium becomes very highly vascularised and slightly oedematous, and the glands become coiled and tortuous, and begin secreting a clear fluid.
- The endometrium is supplied by two types of arteries. The superficial two-thirds of the endometrium that is shed during menstruation (the stratum functionale) is supplied by long, coiled spiral arteries, whereas the deep layer that is not shed (the stratum basale) is supplied by short, straight basilar arteries.
- When fertilisation fails to occur during the secretory phase, the endometrium is shed and a new cycle starts.
- Regression of the corpus luteum leads to withdrawal of hormonal support for the endometrium, which reduces in thickness, causing the coiling of the spiral arteries, leading to spasm and degeneration of walls. The vasospasm is produced by prostaglandin F2 (PGF2) released by the secretory endometrium.

5 Normal Menstruation

- Seventy-five percent of menstrual blood is arterial in origin.
- It contains tissue debris, prostaglandins and relatively large amounts of fibrinolysin from endometrial tissue.
- The usual duration is three to five days.
- The average amount of blood lost is 30 ml, which can be affected by various factors, including the endometrial thickness, medication and clotting disorders.

6 Anovulatory Cycles

- In such cycles, ovulation fails to occur during the menstrual cycle.
- It is common for the first 12 to 18 months after menarche and again before the onset of the menopause.

7 Cyclical Changes in the Uterine Cervix

- The cervical mucosa does not undergo cyclical desquamation, but there are regular changes in the cervical mucus.
- estrogen makes the mucus thinner and more alkaline. These changes promote the survival and transport of sperms.
- The mucus is thinnest at the time of ovulation, and its elasticity, or spinnbarkeit, increases so that, by

midcycle, a drop can be stretched into a long, thin thread, which may be 8 to 12 cm or more in length. In addition, it dries in an arborising, fern-like pattern when a thin layer is spread on a slide.

- Progesterone makes it thick, tenacious and cellular; hence, after ovulation and during pregnancy, it becomes thick and fails to form the fern pattern.

8 Cyclical Changes in the Breasts

- Cyclical changes also take place in the breasts during the menstrual cycle.
- estrogens cause proliferation of mammary ducts, whereas progesterone causes growth of lobules and alveoli.
- The breast swelling, tenderness, and pain experienced by many women during the 10 days preceding menstruation are probably due to distention of the ducts, hyperaemia and interstitial oedema, which regress during menstruation.

9 Indicators of Ovulation

It is important to know when ovulation occurs to plan management for fertility or contraception.

- A convenient indicator of the time of ovulation is the rise in the basal body temperature, which starts one to two days after ovulation and can be recorded using a digital thermometer in the morning before getting out of bed. The cause of the temperature change is probably the increase in progesterone secretion, since progesterone is thermogenic.
- A surge in luteinising hormone (LH) secretion triggers ovulation, and ovulation normally occurs about nine hours after the peak of the LH surge at midcycle.
- Ultrasound examination is an accurate, noninvasive method.

10 Ovarian Hormones

10.1 Biosynthesis

- The naturally occurring estrogens are 17-estradiol, (E2) (most potent), estrone (E_1) (less potent and predominant in menopause), and Estriol (E_3) (least potent and predominant in pregnancy), which are C18 steroids and secreted primarily by the granulosa cells of the ovarian follicles, corpus luteum and placenta.
- Their biosynthesis depends on the enzyme aromatase (CYP19), which converts testosterone to estradiol and androstenedione to estrone.
- Theca interna and mature granulosa cells have many LH receptors, and LH acts via cAMP to increase conversion of cholesterol to androstenedione.
- The theca interna cells supply androstenedione to the granulosa cells, which make estradiol when provided with androgens, which is secreted into the follicular fluid.
- Granulosa cells have many follicle stimulating hormone (FSH) receptors, and FSH facilitates their secretion of estradiol by acting via cAMP to increase their aromatase activity.

10.2 Metabolism

- Of the circulating estradiol, 98% is bound to protein, 60% to albumin, and 38% to gonadal steroid-binding globulin, or sex-hormone-binding globulin which also binds testosterone.
- In the liver, estradiol, estrone and Estriol are converted to glucuronide and sulphate conjugates, and excreted in the urine with some amount also entering the enterohepatic circulation.

10.3 Secretion

- Almost all plasma estrogen comes from the ovary, and two peaks of secretion occur: one just before ovulation and one during the midluteal phase.
- The estradiol secretion rate is 36 g/d in the early follicular phase, 380 g/d just before ovulation, and 250 g/d during the midluteal phase, which declines to very low levels after menopause.

10.4 Effects on the Female Genitalia

- estrogens facilitate the growth of the ovarian follicles and increase the motility of the uterine tubes.
- They increase uterine blood flow and develop uterine smooth muscle and their contractile proteins, making the muscle more active, excitable and sensitive to the action of oxytocin.

- Chronic treatment with estrogens causes the endometrium to hypertrophy and discontinuation causes sloughing withdrawal bleeding.

10.5 Effects on Endocrine Organs

- estrogens decrease FSH secretion, but have a variable effect on LH. They can inhibit LH secretion (negative feedback) and, in other circumstances, they increase LH secretion (positive feedback).
- estrogens also cause increased secretion of angiotensinogen and thyroid-binding globulin.
- estrogens cause epiphysial closure in humans

10.6 Effects on the Central Nervous System

estrogens are responsible for oestrous behaviour in animals, and they increase libido in humans via a direct action on hypothalamic neurons.

10.7 Effects on the Breasts

- estrogens produce duct growth in the breasts and are largely responsible for breast enlargement at puberty.
- estrogens cause pigmentation of the areola.

10.8 Female Secondary Sex Characteristics

estrogens are responsible for the body changes in girls at puberty, in addition to enlargement of the breasts, uterus, and vagina:

- Narrow shoulders and broad hips, thighs that converge, and arms that diverge (wide carrying angle).
- The larynx retains its prepubertal proportions and the voice stays high-pitched.
- Less body hair and more scalp hair, and the pubic hair generally has a characteristic flat-topped pattern (female escutcheon).

10.9 Other Actions

- Along with aldosterone, estrogen leads to salt and water retention and weight gain, just before menstruation.
- estrogens have a significant plasma cholesterol lowering action, and they rapidly produce vasodilation by increasing the local production of nitric oxide.
- Sebaceous gland secretions become more fluid and inhibit information of comedones and acne.

10.10 Mechanism of Action

- There are two principal types of nuclear estrogen receptors: estrogen receptor ER-alpha, (chromosome 6) and ER-beta (chromosome 14).
- ER-alpha is found mainly in uterus, kidneys, liver and heart, whereas ER-beta is found in the ovaries, prostate, lungs, gastrointestinal tract, haemopoietic system and central nervous system (CNS).
- After binding estrogen, they form homodimers, which cause DNA transcription as well as heterodimers with ER-alpha binding to ER-beta.
- Most of the effects of estrogens are genomic, which are mediated by transcriptional processes by its action on nuclear receptors. However, some rapid actions like feedback effects on gonadotropin secretion are mediated via production of mRNAs and this is called the non-genomic action.

10.11 Synthetic and Environmental estrogens

Natural estrogens have both undesirable and desirable effects (e.g., they preserve bone in osteoporosis, but can cause uterine and breast cancer). They have poor oral efficacy due to hepatic metabolism.

10.11.1 Synthetic estrogens

Synthetic estrogens include:

- ethinyl derivative of estradiol, which is a potent estrogen
- tamoxifen and raloxifene, which are selective estrogen receptor modulators, and which have the bone-preserving effects of estradiol without stimulation of breast or uterus.

10.11.2 Environmental estrogens

Environmental estrogens include some nonsteroidal substances, plant estrogens and dioxins, which are produced by a variety of industrial processes, and can activate estrogen response elements on genes.

11 Progesterone

Biosynthesis: progesterone is a C21 steroid, secreted by the corpus luteum, the placenta, and (in small amounts) the follicle.

11.1 Metabolism

- Of the circulating progesterone, 98% is bound: 80% to albumin and 18% to corticosteroid-binding globulin.
- Progesterone has a short half-life and is converted in the liver to pregnanediol, which is conjugated to glucuronic acid and excreted in the urine.

11.2 Secretion

In women, the level of progesterone is approximately 0.9 ng/mL during the follicular phase of the menstrual cycle, secreted by the ovarian follicles, and 18 ng/mL in the luteal phase as the corpus luteum produces large quantities of progesterone via activation of the adenylyl cyclase mechanism.

11.3 Actions

The principal target organs of progesterone are the uterus, the breasts and the brain.

- Progesterone is responsible for the progestational changes in the endometrium and the cyclic changes in the cervix and vagina described above.
- It has an antiestrogenic effect on the myometrial cells, decreasing their excitability, their sensitivity to oxytocin and their spontaneous electrical activity, while increasing their membrane potential.
- It also decreases the number of estrogen receptors in the endometrium and increases the rate of conversion of 17-estradiol to less active estrogens.
- In the breast, progesterone stimulates the development of lobules and alveoli. It induces differentiation of estrogen-prepared ductal tissue and supports the secretory function of the breast during lactation.

11.4 Other Actions

- The feedback effects of progesterone are complex and are exerted at both the hypothalamic and pituitary levels.
- Large doses of progesterone inhibit LH secretion and potentiate the inhibitory effect of estrogens, preventing ovulation.
- Progesterone is thermogenic and is probably responsible for the rise in basal body temperature at the time of ovulation.
- It stimulates respiration, and the alveolar partial pressure of carbon dioxide in women during the luteal phase of the menstrual cycle is lower than that in men.
- Large doses of progesterone produce natriuresis, probably by blocking the action of aldosterone on the kidney.

11.5 Mechanism of Action

- The effects of progesterone, like those of other steroids, are brought about by an action on DNA to initiate synthesis of new mRNA.
- The progesterone receptor is bound to a heat shock protein in the absence of the steroid, and progesterone binding releases the heat shock protein, exposing the DNA-binding domain of the receptor.
- The synthetic steroid mifepristone (RU486) binds to the receptor, but does not release the heat shock protein, and it blocks the binding of progesterone.
- As the maintenance of early pregnancy depends on the stimulatory effect of progesterone on endometrial growth and its inhibition of uterine contractility, mifepristone combined with a prostaglandin can be used in the medical termination of pregnancy.
- There are two isoforms of the progesterone receptor (PRA and PRB), which are produced by differential processing from a single gene.
- Substances that mimic the action of progesterone are sometimes called progestational agents, gestagens or progestins. They are used along with synthetic estrogens as oral contraceptive agents.

12 Relaxin

- Relaxin is a polypeptide hormone, which is produced in the corpus luteum, uterus, placenta and mammary glands in women.
- During pregnancy, it relaxes the pubic symphysis and other pelvic joints, and softens and dilates the uterine cervix, hence facilitating delivery.

- It also inhibits uterine contractions and may play a role in the development of the mammary glands.
- In men, it is found in semen, where it may help maintain sperm motility and aid in sperm penetration of the ovum.

13 Control of Ovarian Function

- Follicle-stimulating hormone (FSH) from the pituitary is responsible for the early maturation of the ovarian follicles, and FSH and LH together are responsible for their final maturation.
- A burst of LH secretion is responsible for ovulation and the initial formation of the corpus luteum.
- LH stimulates the secretion of estrogen and progesterone from the corpus luteum.

13.1 Hypothalamic Components

The hypothalamus occupies a key position in the control of gonadotropin secretion.

- Hypothalamic control is exerted by gonadotropin-releasing hormone (GnRH) secreted into the portal hypophyseal vessels, which stimulates the secretion of FSH as well as LH.
- GnRH is normally secreted in episodic bursts, which produce the peaks of LH secretion that are essential for normal secretion of gonadotropins.
- In addition, fluctuations in the frequency and amplitude of the GnRH bursts are also important in generating the other hormonal changes responsible for the menstrual cycle.
- GnRH frequency is increased (1 pulse/60–90 min) by estrogens and also in the late follicular phase of the cycle, culminating in the LH surge decreased by progesterone and testosterone. The sensitivity of the gonadotropes to GnRH is greatly increased because of their exposure to GnRH pulses of the frequency that exist at this time (self-priming effect)
- Decreased GnRH frequency (1 pulse/120 min) leads to promotion of FSH production.
- The downregulation of pituitary receptors and the consequent decrease in LH secretion produced by constantly elevated levels of GnRH has led to the use of long-acting GnRH analogues to inhibit LH secretion in precocious puberty and in prostate cancer.

14 Feedback Effects

14.1 Follicular Phase

- Initially, inhibin B is low and FSH is modestly elevated, fostering follicular growth.
- LH secretion is low due to the negative feedback effect of the rising plasma estrogen level.
- In the 36 to 48 hours before ovulation, the estrogen feedback effect becomes positive, and this initiates the burst of LH secretion (LH surge) that produces ovulation after about nine hours.
- FSH secretion also peaks, despite a small rise in inhibin, probably because of the strong stimulation of gonadotropes by GnRH.

14.2 Luteal Phase

- LH and FSH levels are low because of the elevated levels of estrogen, progesterone and inhibin.
- It has been demonstrated that, when circulating levels of progesterone are high, the positive feedback effect of estrogen is inhibited.
- Similarly, both the negative and the positive feedback effects of estrogen are exerted in the mediobasal hypothalamus, but exactly how negative feedback is switched to positive and back to negative feedback in the luteal phase remains unknown.

14.3 Control of the Cycle

- Regression of the corpus luteum (luteolysis), possibly due to the combined action of PGF2 (prostaglandin) and ET-1 (endothelin), which are both vasoconstrictors, is the key to the start of the menstrual cycle.
- Once luteolysis begins, the estrogen and progesterone levels fall and the secretion of FSH and LH increases.
- A new crop of follicles develops, and then a single dominant follicle matures as a result of the action of FSH and LH.
- Near midcycle, estrogen secretion from the follicle rises, which augments the responsiveness of the pituitary to GnRH and triggers a burst of LH secretion.
- The resulting ovulation is followed by formation of a corpus luteum. Although estrogen secretion drops, progesterone and estrogen levels rise together, along with inhibin B.

- The elevated levels inhibit FSH and LH secretion for a while, but luteolysis again occurs and a new cycle starts.

15 Abnormalities of Ovarian Function

15.1 Menstrual Abnormalities

Some women who are infertile have anovulatory cycles; that is, they fail to ovulate but have menstrual periods at fairly regular intervals.

- Amenorrhoea is the absence of menstrual periods and, if menstrual bleeding has never occurred, the condition is called primary amenorrhoea.
- Cessation of cycles in a woman with previously normal periods is called secondary amenorrhoea. The most common cause of secondary amenorrhoea is pregnancy. Some other causes include emotional stimuli, environmental changes, hypothalamic diseases, pituitary disorders and primary ovarian disorders.
- Hypomenorrhoea and menorrhagia refers to scanty and abnormally profuse flow, respectively, during regular periods.
- Metrorrhagia is bleeding from the uterus between periods.
- Oligomenorrhoea is reduced frequency of periods.
- Dysmenorrhoea is painful menstruation, commonly seen in young women due to the accumulation of prostaglandins in the uterus, and treated with inhibitors of prostaglandin synthesis.
- Premenstrual syndrome: some women develop irritability, bloating, oedema, decreased ability to concentrate, depression, headache, and constipation during the last 7 to 10 days of their menstrual cycles due to salt and water retention. The antidepressant, fluoxetine and the benzodiazepine, alprazolam, produce symptomatic relief, as do GnRH-releasing agonists in doses that suppress the pituitary–ovarian axis.

15.2 Polycystic Ovarian Syndrome

- Overall, polycystic ovarian syndrome accounts for 75% of anovulatory infertility.
- Key features are chronic anovulation with high circulating levels of androgen, estrogen and LH, obesity and insulin resistance.
- Diagnostic criteria include amenorrhea, hyperandrogenism (evidenced by acne, hirsutism and raised androgens) and polycystic ovaries detected by ultrasonography.
- Lifestyle measures like weight loss, exercise and metformin therapy are the mainstays of treatment.

16 Genetic Defects Causing Reproductive Abnormalities

A number of single-gene mutations cause reproductive abnormalities when they occur in women:

1. Kallmann syndrome, which causes hypogonadotropic hypogonadism.
2. GnRH resistance, FSH resistance and LH resistance, which are due to defects in the GnRH, FSH and LH receptors, respectively.
3. Aromatase deficiency, which prevents the formation of estrogens.

An interesting gain-of-function mutation causes McCune–Albright syndrome, in which genes become constitutively active in certain cells, but not others (mosaicism) because a somatic mutation after initial cell division has occurred in the embryo. It is associated with multiple endocrine abnormalities, including precocious puberty and amenorrhoea with galactorrhoea.

17 Fertilisation

Fertilisation involves the following:

- Substances produced by the ovum chemoattract approximately 50–100 sperm.
- Sperm adhere to the zona pellucida (the membranous structure surrounding the ovum).
- Sperm bind to a sperm receptor in the zona and initiate the acrosomal reaction, releasing enzymes like acrosin.
- Only one sperm fuses with the membrane of the ovum mediated by fertilin and releases its nucleus into the cytoplasm of the ovum.
- Fusion sets off a reduction in the membrane potential of the ovum, which prevents polyspermy (the fertilisation of the ovum by more than one sperm).
- It takes three days for a blastocyst (the developing embryo) to move down the fallopian tube into the uterus reaching an 8- or 16-cell stage.

- Once in contact with the endometrium of the uterus, the blastocyst becomes surrounded by an outer layer of syncytiotrophoblast (a multinucleate mass with no discernible cell boundaries) and an inner layer of cytotrophoblast made up of individual cells.
- The syncytiotrophoblast erodes the endometrium, and the blastocyst burrows into it (implantation), usually at the dorsal wall of the uterus.
- It is followed by the development of the placenta, and the trophoblast remains associated with it.

18 Early Nutrition of the Embryo

- Uterine changes occurring under the effect of progesterone secreted by the ovarian corpus luteum are responsible for supplying nutrition to the conceptus (the embryo and its adjacent parts or associated membranes).
- When the conceptus implants in the endometrium, endometrial cells swell further and store even more nutrients. These cells are now called decidual cells, and the total mass of cells is called the decidua.
- During the first week after implantation, decidua is the only means by which the embryo can obtain nutrients. Thereafter, it contributes a part of nutrition to the embryo up to eight weeks.
- In addition, the placenta also begins to provide nutrition after about the sixteenth day beyond fertilisation (a little more than one week after implantation).

14 Male Physiology

Renuka Sharma

1 The Male Reproductive System

- The male reproductive system consists of a pair of testes, accessory sex glands and a system of tubules, which collect their secretions and pour them into the prostatic part of the urethra, beyond which the passage is common for urine and seminal fluid.
- The testis has two major functions: spermatogenesis and endocrine secretions.
- Gonadal hormones are responsible for maintenance of the male reproductive tract, semen production, maintenance of secondary sex characteristics and libido.

1.1 Scrotum

- The scrotum is a muscular sac that lies behind the penis.
- It is the location for sperm production.
- The temperature in the scrotum is about 2–4 degrees less than the body core temperature.
- The dartos muscle forms from the subcutaneous layer of the scrotum.
- The dartos muscle divides the scrotum into two compartments in the middle, each housing one testis.
- The cremaster muscle is the continuation of the internal oblique muscle and forms a muscular net around the entire scrotum.

1.2 Structure of the Testes

See Figure 14.1.

- Each testis is 4–5 cm in length.
- They are located in the scrotum.
- The scrotum is lined with connective tissue:
    - the outer lining is the tunica vaginalis, and has a parietal and visceral layer
    - the tunica albuginea is a dense, tough, white, connective tissue
    - the tunica albuginea invaginates into the testes to form septa, which divide the testes into 300–400 lobules
    - within the lobules are the seminiferous tubules
    - tightly coiled seminiferous tubules form the bulk of the testes
- Spermatozoa develop from the primitive germ cells (spermatogenesis) in the walls of the seminiferous tubules.
- From the lumen of the seminiferous tubules, the sperm moves into the meshwork of tubules called the rete testis in the head of the epididymis.
- From there, spermatozoa pass through the tail of the epididymis into the vas deferens.
- Fifteen to twenty efferent ductules cross the tunica albuginea and leave the testes.
- The ductules enter through the ejaculatory ducts into the urethra in the body of the prostate at the time of ejaculation.
- Between the tubules in the testes are nests of cells containing lipid granules, the interstitial cells of Leydig, which secrete testosterone into the bloodstream.
- The spermatic arteries that drain into the testes are tortuous, and blood in them runs parallel, but in the opposite direction to blood in the pampiniform plexus of spermatic veins. This anatomic arrangement may permit countercurrent exchange of heat and testosterone.
- The testes move down the abdominal cavity and into the scrotal cavity through the inguinal canal.
- Cryptorchidism is a failure of the testes to descend into the scrotal cavity.

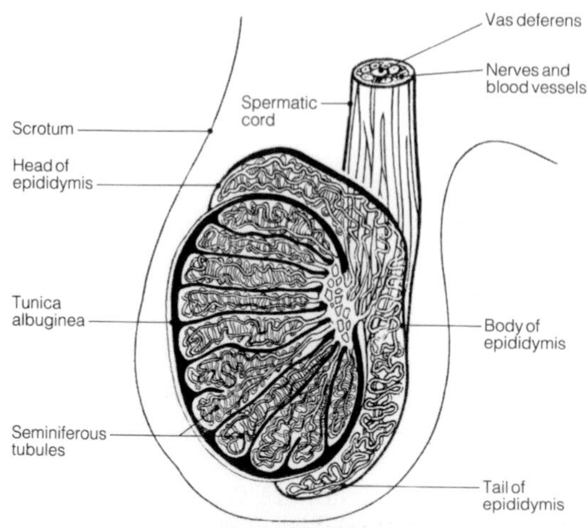

Figure 14.1 Cross section of the testis. Used with permission from https://visualsonline.cancer.gov/details.cfm?imageid=1769

1.3 Embryological Origin of the Male Reproductive Tract

The embryological origin of the male reproductive tract is covered in detail in Section 2, Embryology.

- Paramesonephric ducts give rise to the:
  - testes
  - epididymis
  - vas deferens
- Mesonephric ducts give rise to the accessory glands:
  - prostate
  - bulbourethral or Cowper's gland
  - seminal vesicle
- Developing tubules within the testes secrete a polypeptide müllerian inhibitory factor, which causes the regression of the paramesonephric ducts 60 days after fertilisation.

1.4 Sertoli Cells

- Elongated branching cells are supporting cells called sustentacular cells (typically found in the epithelium).
- The walls of the seminiferous tubules are lined by primitive germ cells and Sertoli cells: large, complex glycogen-containing cells, which stretch from the basal lamina of the tubule to the lumen.
- Tight junctions between adjacent Sertoli cells near the basal lamina form a blood–testis barrier, which prevents passage of molecules from interstitial tissue and the basal compartment to the lumen.
- The barrier is penetrated by the maturing germ cells by progressive breakdown of the tight junctions above the germ cells, with concomitant formation of new tight junctions below them.
- Sertoli cells secrete the following
  - androgen binding protein (testosterone binding protein)
  - Anti-müllerian hormone (AMH): secreted in early stages of fetal life
  - inhibin and activin: generally produced after puberty; this regulates follicle stimulating hormone (FSH) by positive and negative feedback
  - estradiol: aromatase from the Sertoli cell converts testosterone to 17β estradiol
  - transferrin: blood plasma protein helps to transport iron
- FSH stimulates the androgen binding protein produced by Sertoli cells and formation of blood–testes barrier.
- FSH also increases spermatozoa by preventing the apoptosis of type A spermatozoa and helps with maturation.
- Inhibin acts as a negative feedback to reduce the release of FSH and GnRH.
- Testosterone levels in the testes is 20–50 times higher than in the blood.

1.5 Functions of the Blood–Testis Barrier

- The blood–testis barrier maintains the composition of the fluid in the lumen of the seminiferous tubules, which contains very little protein and glucose, but is rich in androgens, estrogens, K^+, inositol, glutamic and aspartic acid.
- Protects the germ cells from blood-borne noxious agents.
- Prevents antigenic products of germ-cell division from entering the circulation and generating an autoimmune response.
- Helps establish an osmotic gradient, which facilitates the movement of fluid into the tubular lumen.

1.6 Leydig Cells

- Also called interstitial cells of Leydig, which lie adjacent to the seminiferous tubules.
- Leydig cells have an eosinophilic cytoplasm.
- Leydig cells produce testosterone in the presence of luteinising hormone (LH): LH binds to the Leydig cells to stimulate testosterone secretion and androgen production.
- Contain lipofuscin pigment and inclusions called Reinke crystals (rod-like structures measuring 3–20 μm). These are seen in <50% of Leydig cells and have no function. Typically used to diagnose Leydig cell tumours histologically.
- Leydig cell tumours are usually benign, but can be hormonally active and produce testosterone.

1.7 Germ Cells

- Spermatogonia (least mature) line the basement membrane.
- Spermatogonia are stem cells and can differentiate into different cell types (2 n).
- Primary spermatogonia (2 n=46 chromosomes).
- Secondary spermatogonia (n=23 chromosomes): first meiosis.
- Spermatids (n=23 chromosomes): second meiosis.
- Sperm.

1.8 Epididymis

- The epididymis is nearly 6 m long, but lies in a tightly coiled state.
- It takes roughly 12 days for the immotile sperm to traverse through the epididymis into the head, predominantly moved by the contraction of the smooth muscles lining the epidydimal tubules.
- It consists of three parts: caput, corpus and cauda and is the main site of storage.
- Mature sperm are stored in the tail (cauda) of the epididymis.
- Individual ducts join to make the vas deferens.

1.9 Vas Deferens

- The vas deferens is a thick muscular tube bundled together with connective tissue, blood vessels and nerves in the spermatid cord
- It is easily accessible and hence vasectomy is performed by cutting and sealing a small portion of it.

1.10 Seminal Vesicle

- The seminal vesicle is a tubular gland that lies behind the urinary bladder.
- The secretions from this gland comprise nearly 60% of the fluid in the semen.

1.11 Structure of a Sperm

- Each sperm contains a head, midpiece and a tail.
- This distinctive head contains a compact haploid nucleus with very little cytoplasm, hence the head measures only 5 μm long.
- The acrosome covers most of the head of the sperm and is filled with lysosomal enzymes.
- The midpiece contains tightly packed mitochondria. The adenosine triphosphate (ATP) produced by mitochondria helps the flagellum to enable the sperm to move. See Figure 14.2.

1.12 Effect of Temperature

- As spermatogenesis requires a temperature considerably lower than that of the body interior,

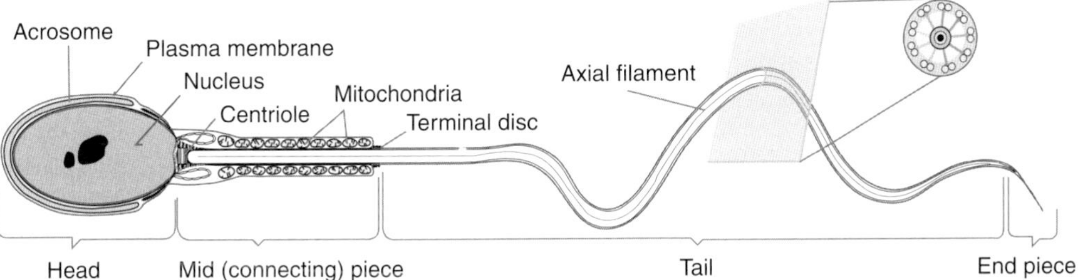

Figure 14.2 Structure of the sperm.

the testes are normally maintained at a temperature of about 32 °C.

- They are kept cool by air circulating around the scrotum and by heat exchange in a countercurrent fashion between the spermatic arteries and veins.
- When the testes are retained in the abdomen, it results in degeneration of the tubular walls and sterility.
- Similarly, hot baths (43–45 °C for 30 min per day) and insulated athletic supporters reduce the sperm count in humans; in some cases by 90%.

1.13 Capacitation

- Once ejaculated into the female, the spermatozoa move up the uterus to the isthmus of the uterine tubes, where they slow down and undergo capacitation.
- This further maturation process involves two components: increasing the motility of the spermatozoa and facilitating their preparation for the acrosome reaction.
- However, the role of capacitation appears to be facilitatory, rather than obligatory, because fertilisation is readily produced in vitro.
- This is the penultimate step in the maturation of the sperm that occurs in the female reproductive tract and prepares the sperm for fertilising the oocyte.
- There is destablisation of the acrosomal membrane in the sperm head. Chemical changes in the tail allows greater mobility of sperm.
- More fluid in the membrane leads to increased permeability to calcium.
- The uterus aids by secreting albumin, lipoproteins, proteolytic and glycosidic enzymes in the process of capacitation.
- From the isthmus, the capacitated spermatozoa move rapidly to the tubal ampulla, where fertilisation takes place.

2 Testosterone Synthesis and Function

- Testosterone is the main androgen and is a 19-carbon compound with a hydroxyl (-OH) group in the 17 position.
- Other androgens are androstenedione and dehydroepiandrosterone.
- LH increases cholesterol desmolase activity (converts cholesterol to pregnenolone) and then to testosterone.
- Testosterone is synthesised mainly in the testes (95%) and the remaining in the adrenals (5%).
- It is synthesised from cholesterol in the Leydig cells and is also formed from androstenedione secreted by the adrenal cortex.
- Free cholesterol is generated by a cholesterol hormone sensitive lipase and transferred to mitochondrial membrane in a steroidogenic acute regulatory protein (StAR) dependent manner.
- Cholesterol is converted to pregnenolone, which is hydroxylated in the 17 position by 17-hydroxylase and then subjected to side-chain cleavage to form dehydroepiandrosterone.
- Dehydroepiandrosterone and androstenedione are then converted to testosterone.
- Testosterone is converted in the liver to inactive metabolites. Immediate metabolites are 5α dihydrotestosterone (DHT) and estradiol.
- Of the testosterone, 98% is bound to plasma-binding globulin (65% bound to sex hormone-binding globulin and 33% bound weakly to albumin) and 2% is free.

2.1 Secretion

- Small amounts of testosterone are also secreted in women, from the ovary (major source) and adrenal gland.
- The plasma testosterone level (free and bound) is 8.7–29 nmol/L in adult males and 0.2–1.7 nmol/L in adult women.
- Testosterone and its metabolites are excreted primarily in the urine as urinary 17-ketosteroids, conjugated androgens and diol or triol derivatives.

2.2 Function of Testosterone

- In addition to their actions during development, testosterone and other androgens exert an inhibitory feedback effect on pituitary LH secretion.
- Testosterone develops and maintains the male secondary sex characteristics.
- It exerts an important protein-anabolic, growth-promoting effect
- Along with FSH, it maintains spermatogenesis.

2.3 Androgenic Effects of Testosterone

- Development of male reproductive organs.
- Promotes secondary sexual characteristics.
- Maturation of sex organs.
- Deepening of voice.
- Growth of body hair: facial, axillary and pubic hair.

2.4 Anabolic Effects of Testosterone

- Promotes protein synthesis and muscle mass: increases the synthesis and decreases the breakdown of protein, leading to an increase in the rate of growth.
- Promotes bone density and bone maturation.
- Regulates thromboxane A_2 receptors on megakaryocytes and platelets.
- Moderate sodium (Na^+), potassium (K^+), water (H_2O), calcium ($Ca2^+$), sulphate ($SO4^-$) and phosphate (PO4) retention; they also increase the size of the kidneys.

3 Anabolic Steroids and Their Effects

3.1 Negative Effects on Men

- reduced sperm count
- enlarged prostate
- shrinkage of testes
- baldness
- headaches
- breast enlargement
- liver damage
- acne
- high blood pressure and heart disease
- impotence
- joint pain
- aggressive behaviour

3.2 Negative Effects in Women

- reduced breast size
- enlarged clitoris
- increase in facial and body hair
- deepened voice
- menstrual disorders

3.3 Mechanism of Action

- Like other steroids, testosterone binds to an intracellular receptor, and the receptor–steroid complex then binds to DNA in the nucleus, facilitating transcription of various genes.
- In addition, testosterone is converted to DHT by 5 α-reductase in some target cells, and DHT binds to the same intracellular receptor as testosterone.
- Testosterone–receptor complexes are less stable than DHT–receptor complexes in target cells. DHT formation is a way of amplifying the action of testosterone in target tissues.
- Humans have two 5 α-reductase: type 1 is present in the skin and scalp, whereas type 2 is present in genital skin, the prostate and other genital tissues.
- Testosterone–receptor complexes are responsible for the maturation of Wolffian duct structures and for the formation of male internal genitalia, but DHT–receptor complexes are needed to form male external genitalia.
- DHT–receptor complexes are also primarily responsible for enlargement of the prostate and penis at the time of puberty, as well as for the facial hair, acne and the temporal recession of the hairline.
- Conversely, the increase in muscle mass and the development of male sex drive and libido depend primarily on testosterone rather than DHT.

4 Testicular Production of estrogens

- In men, the plasma estradiol level is 17 and 70 ng/dL.
- Over 80% of estradiol and 95% of the estrone in the plasma of adult men is formed by extragonadal and extra-adrenal tissues.

5 Control of Testicular Function

- The testes are regulated by an endocrine axis involving hypothalamic gonadotropin-releasing hormone (GnRH) secreting neurons and pituitary gonadotropes, which produce both LH and FSH.

6 Regulation of Leydig Cell Function

- Leydig cells express the LH receptor, which is coupled to a cAMP-dependent protein kinase A signalling pathway. Effects include hydrolysis of cholesterol esters and new expression of StAR protein.

- LH is a tropic hormone and acts on Leydig cells and stimulates the secretion of testosterone, which in turn feeds back to inhibit LH secretion by acting directly on the anterior pituitary and by inhibiting the secretion of GnRH from the hypothalamus.

7 Regulation of Sertoli Cell Function

- FSH is a tropic hormone and stimulates Sertoli cells and FSH and androgens maintain the gametogenic function of the testes.
- FSH also stimulates the secretion of androgen binding protein (ABP) and inhibin.
- Inhibin is a factor of testicular origin, which inhibits FSH secretion by a direct action on the pituitary.
- Inhibin is produced by Sertoli cells (males) and granulosa cells (women).

8 Semen

- The seminal fluid mixes with the fluids from the prostate, and the bulbourethral glands provide nutrition and protection to sperm during its journey in the female reproductive tract.
- The seminal fluid coagulates in the vagina due to the acidity.
- After 15–30 minutes, the prostate-specific antigen causes the de-coagulation of the seminal coagulate to allow the sperm to move.
- Seminal fluids contain proteolytic enzymes, fructose and amino acids.
- The bulbourethral glands secrete a clear fluid to lubricate the lumen of the urethra.
- The seminal fluid is alkaline.

Normal WHO criteria for normal seminal parameters are shown in Table 14.1.

Other components are shown in Table 14.2.

Table 14.1 WHO criteria for normal seminal parameters

Volume	2 ml or more
pH	7.2–8.0
Sperm concentration	20 x 10^6 spermatozoa/ml
Sperm count	40 x 10^6 spermatozoa/ ejaculation
Motility	50% or more within 60 minutes of ejaculation

Table 14.2 Components of seminal fluid

Fructose (1.5–6.5 mg/mL)	Phosphorylcholine
Ergothioneine	Ascorbic acid
Flavins	Prostaglandins
Spermine	Citric acid
Cholesterol, phospholipids	Fibrinolysin, fibrinogenase
Acid phosphatase	Phosphate buffers
Bicarbonate	Hyaluronidase

9 Erection

- An erection is caused by the stimulation of the parasympathetic division of the autonomic nervous system.
- An increase in nitric oxide takes place, which causes vasodilatation mainly in the corpus cavernosa and less in the corpus spongiosa. Nitric oxide synthase, which catalyses the formation of nitric oxide, which activates guanylyl cyclase, results in increased production of cyclic guanosine 5' monophosphate (cGMP), a potent vasodilator.
- The efferent parasympathetic fibres are in the pelvic splanchnic nerves (nervi erigentes). The fibres presumably release acetylcholine and the vasodilator vasoactive intestinal polypeptide as co-transmitters.
- The drugs sildenafil, tadalafil and vardenafil all inhibit the breakdown of cGMP by phosphodiesterases (PDEs) and have gained worldwide fame for the treatment of impotence.
- The multiple PDEs are divided into seven isoenzyme families, and these drugs are all most active against PDE V, found in the corpora cavernosa.
- PDE VI is found in the retina, and one of the side effects of these drugs is a transient loss of the ability to discriminate between blue and green.
- Normally, erection is terminated by sympathetic vasoconstrictor impulses to the penile arterioles.

10 Ejaculation

- Ejaculation is a two-part spinal reflex that involves emission, the movement of the semen into the urethra and ejaculation proper: the propulsion of the semen out of the urethra at the time of orgasm.

- The afferent pathways are mostly fibres from touch receptors in the glans penis, which reach the spinal cord through the internal pudendal nerves.
- Emission is a sympathetic response, integrated in the upper lumbar segments of the spinal cord and effected by contraction of the smooth muscle of the vasa deferentia and seminal vesicles in response to stimuli in the hypogastric nerves.
- Sympathetic stimulation of the spinal nerves S2–4 via the pudendal nerve leads to rhythmic contraction of the bulbospongiosus and ischiocavernosus muscle. The pubococcygeus muscle also helps with this. This leads to movement of sperm into the vas deferens and urethra, and then ejaculation.

11 Prostate Specific Antigen

- The prostate produces and secretes into the semen and the bloodstream a 30 kDa serine protease generally called prostate specific antigen (PSA).
- PSA hydrolyses the sperm motility inhibitor semenogelin in semen, and it has several substrates in plasma, but its precise function in the circulation is unknown.
- An elevated plasma PSA occurs in prostate cancer and is widely used as a screening test for this disease, although PSA is also elevated in benign prostatic hyperplasia and prostatitis.

12 Vasectomy

- Bilateral ligation of the vas deferens (vasectomy) has proven to be a relatively safe and convenient contraceptive procedure.
- However, it has proven difficult to restore the patency of the vas deferens in those wishing to restore fertility, and the current success rate for such operations, as measured by the subsequent production of pregnancy, is about 50%.

13 Associated Disorders

13.1 Cryptorchidism

- Testicular descent from the abdomen to the inguinal region during fetal development depends on müllerian inhibitory substance.
- Out of newborn males, 10% are reported to have incomplete descent, with the testes remaining in the abdominal cavity or inguinal canal.
- Cryptorchidism may lead to development of malignant tumours or irreversible damage to the spermatogenic epithelium.
- Treatment: gonadotropic hormone and/or surgery.

13.2 Klinefelter Syndrome

- Presence of an extra X chromosome, with the commonest phenotype being 47, XXY.
- At puberty, low androgen production results in fibrotic testes and the destruction of seminiferous tubules, leading to infertility.
- Associated features include gynaecomastia, behavioural problems and decreased bone growth and density.

13.3 Male Hypogonadism

- Hypergonadotropic hypogonadism is due to testicular disease in adults. Circulating gonadotropin levels are elevated.
- Hypogonadotropic hypogonadism is secondary to disorders of pituitary or hypothalamus (e.g., Kallmann syndrome) and circulating gonadotropin levels are depressed
- Eunuchoidism is seen in cases of early Leydig cell deficiency. These individuals are characteristically tall, have narrow shoulders, small genitalia and a high-pitched voice.

13.4 Androgen-Secreting Tumours

- Androgen-secreting Leydig cell tumours are rare and cause detectable endocrine symptoms only in prepubertal boys, who develop precocious pseudopuberty.

13.5 Congenital 5 α-reductase Deficiency

For further information on this subject, see Section 5, Endocrinology.

- Individuals with this syndrome are born with male internal genitalia including testes, but they have female external genitalia and are usually raised as girls.
- At puberty, LH secretion and circulating testosterone levels are increased. Consequently, they develop male body contours and male libido. At this point, they usually change their gender identities and 'become boys'.

15 Fetal Physiology

Anita Pawar

1 Introduction

Initial development of the placenta and fetal membranes precedes the development of the fetus. During the first two to three weeks after implantation of the blastocyst, the fetus remains almost microscopic, but thereafter, the length of the fetus increases almost in proportion to the gestational age.

2 Development of the Organ Systems

2.1 Circulatory System

- After fertilisation, the human heart starts to beat at a rate of about 65 beats per minute (BPM) during the fourth week of pregnancy. The rate rapidly increases to about 140–170 BPM at 6–7 weeks, and drops to 120–160 BPM in the second and third trimesters.
- The placenta acts as the point of gas exchange. The umbilical vein transports oxygenated blood from the placenta away from the high-resistance pulmonary circuit to the low-resistance systemic circuit via the foramen ovale and ductus arteriosus.
- The fetal blood is relatively hypoxaemic with a partial pressure of oxygen (pO_2) of 20–30 mmHg and oxyhaemoglobin concentration saturation of 75–85%.
- The fetal circulation is a parallel system, while after birth the circulatory system is a series system.

2.2 Formation of Blood Cells

- Formation of blood cells starts in the yolk sac and mesothelial layers of the placenta at about the third week of fetal development. Thereafter, the fetal mesenchyme and the endothelium of the fetal blood vessels take over, followed by the liver (by six weeks) and then the spleen and other lymphoid tissues (by the third month). Finally, from the third month onward, the bone marrow gradually becomes the principal source of the red blood cells, as well as most of the white blood cells, except for lymphocyte and plasma cell production, which occurs mainly in the lymphoid tissue.
- The blood of the human fetus normally contains fetal haemoglobin (haemoglobin F). Its structure is similar to that of haemoglobin A except that the β chains are replaced by γ chains; that is, haemoglobin F is $\alpha_2\ \gamma_2$.
- fetal haemoglobin is normally replaced by adult haemoglobin soon after birth.
- The fetal haemoglobin has a higher affinity for oxygen. The oxygen content at a given pO_2 is greater than that of adult haemoglobin because it binds to 2,3-diphosphoglyceric acid (2,3 DPG) less avidly. Haemoglobin F is critical to facilitate movement of oxygen from the maternal to the fetal circulation, particularly at later stages of gestation where fetal oxygen demand increases.
- Respiratory system: respiration does not occur during fetal life and the lungs remain almost completely deflated. This prevents the filling of the lungs with fluid and debris from the meconium excreted by the fetus's gastrointestinal tract into the amniotic fluid.
- Nervous system: the reflexes of the fetus involving the spinal cord and even the brain stem are present by the third to fourth months of pregnancy. However, those nervous system functions that involve the cerebral cortex are still only in the early stages of development, even at birth. Indeed, myelinisation of some major tracts of the brain is complete only after about one year of postnatal life.

2.3 The Gastrointestinal Tract

- By midpregnancy, the fetus begins to ingest and absorb large quantities of amniotic fluid, and during the last two to three months, gastrointestinal function approaches that of the normal neonate. In addition, meconium starts to form from the thirteenth week onwards and is excreted into the amniotic fluid from around 16 weeks.

- Meconium is composed of 98% water and 2% residues (mucus, epithelial cells, and other residues of excretory products from the gastrointestinal mucosa and glands) from the fetus. In addition, there are proteins, carbohydrates, lipids, phospholipids and urea; all of which aid in the growth of the fetus.

2.4 Amniotic Fluid

- Normal pH is 7.0–7.5.
- Amniotic fluid index (AFI) is the sum of the deepest vertical pools of amniotic fluid in four quadrants of the abdomen during scanning. The normal value is 5–25 and a median AFI is 14.
- Oligohydramnios is when the AFI is <5. This can cause fetal abnormalities such as limb contractures, hypoplastic lungs and other deformities.
- Severe oligohydramnios can cause Potter sequence characterised by clubbed feet, low-set ears, parrot-beak nose, cranial abnormalities, pulmonary hypoplasia and adrenal and genital hypoplasia.

2.5 The Renal System

- fetal kidneys begin to function at about 16 weeks and the fetal urine contributes to the amniotic fluid.
- By the second trimester, the fetal kidneys begin to excrete urine, accounting for about 70–80% of the amniotic fluid.
- The renal control system for the regulation of blood pressure and other functions of the kidney are almost nonexistent until late fetal life and do not reach full development until a few months after birth.

3 fetal Metabolism

The fetus uses mainly glucose for energy and for synthesising fat.

- Metabolism of calcium and phosphate: 22.5 g and 13.5 g of calcium and phosphorus, respectively, are accumulated in the fetus during gestation, which represents only about 2% of the quantities of these substances in the mother's bones. Therefore, this is a minimal drain from the mother. Much greater drain occurs after birth during lactation.
- Accumulation of iron: iron, mainly in haemoglobin form, accumulates in the fetus even more rapidly than calcium and phosphate. About one-third of the iron in a fully developed fetus is normally stored in the liver. This iron can then be used for several months after birth by the neonate for formation of additional haemoglobin.
- Utilisation and storage of vitamins: in general, the role of vitamins is the same in the fetus as in the adult. Vitamin B_{12} and folic acid are necessary for the formation of red blood cells and nervous tissue, as well as for overall growth of the fetus. Vitamin C is necessary for appropriate formation of the bone matrix and fibres of connective tissue. Vitamin D is necessary for normal bone growth in the fetus. Vitamin E is necessary for normal development of the early embryo. Vitamin K is used by the fetal liver for formation of factor VII, prothrombin and several other blood coagulation factors. Many of these vitamins are taken up from the mother and stored in the fetal liver to be used in postnatal life.

4 Infant Adjustments to Extrauterine Life

4.1 Respiratory Readjustments at Birth

One of the most important immediate adjustments required of the infant is to begin breathing as there is a loss of the placental connection with the mother, which is the main source of metabolic support for the fetus.

- Cause of breathing at birth: the neonate generally begins to breathe within seconds and has a normal respiratory rhythm within less than one minute after birth. Initiation of breathing probably results from the following:
  1. Transient asphyxia, which develops immediately at the time of birth
  2. Sensory impulses on the skin, which are triggered with the drop in temperature at birth
  3. In a baby who does not breathe immediately at birth, hypoxia and hypercapnia provide

additional stimulus to the respiratory centre and usually cause breathing within a minute after birth

- Delayed or abnormal breathing at birth can lead to hypoxia: onset of breathing is likely to be delayed in babies (1) when mothers have been given general anaesthesia during delivery, (2) babies with birth trauma or following prolonged labour/ delivery.
- Degree of hypoxia that an infant can tolerate: in an adult, failure to breathe for just 4 minutes often causes death, but a neonate can survive a hypoxia of almost 10 minutes. Permanent and serious brain impairment often ensues if breathing is delayed more than 8 to 10 minutes.
- Expansion of the lungs at birth: at birth, the walls of the alveoli are at first collapsed because of the surface tension of the viscid fluid that fills them. More than 25 mmHg of negative inspiratory pressure in the lungs is usually required to oppose the effects of this surface tension and to open the alveoli for the first time. Fortunately, the first inspirations of the normal neonate are extremely powerful, usually capable of creating as much as 60 mmHg negative pressure in the intrapleural space. But once the alveoli do open, further respiration can be affected with relatively weak respiratory movements, and surfactant keeps them from collapsing again.
- Respiratory distress syndrome (RDS) of the newborn, or infant respiratory distress syndrome (IRDS), is caused when surfactant secretion is deficient: surfactant deficiency is an important cause of IRDS; also known as hyaline membrane disease. It is the serious pulmonary disease that develops in newborns born before their surfactant system is functional. Surface tension in the lungs is high, and the alveoli are collapsed in many areas (atelectasis). An additional factor in IRDS is retention of fluid in the lungs.
- Surfactant, a phospholipid-protein complex, which is produced by type II pneumocytes and is deposited along the alveolar surfaces, also helps counteract alveolar surface tension and promote alveolar stability. As a result of the increasing effect of surfactant, less transpulmonary pressure is needed for subsequent breaths, and functional residual capacity is soon established.
- Pulmonary blood flow increases as the lungs expand, and pulmonary vascular resistance declines under the influence of oxygen-mediated relaxation of the pulmonary arterioles. This increase in pulmonary blood flow in turn allows the patent foramen ovale and the patent ductus arteriosus to functionally close, thereby allowing further blood flow to the lungs.
- The postnatal circulation is then that of a low-resistance pulmonary circuit and high-resistance systemic circuit, and the lungs assume the responsibility of gas exchange and oxygenation.

4.2 Circulatory Readjustments at Birth

Circulatory adjustments are essential at birth as they allow for adequate blood flow through the lungs and liver, which up to this point has had little blood flow. To describe these readjustments, it is important to consider the anatomical structure of the fetal circulation.

- Specific anatomical structure of the fetal circulation: 55% of the fetal cardiac output goes through the placenta. The ductus venosus diverts some of this blood directly to the inferior vena cava (mainly bypassing the liver), and the remainder mixes with the portal blood of the fetus.
- Most of the blood entering the heart through the inferior vena cava is diverted directly to the left atrium via the patent foramen ovale. Most of the blood from the superior vena cava enters the right ventricle and is expelled into the pulmonary artery.
- The resistance of the collapsed lungs is high, and the pressure in the pulmonary artery is several mmHg higher than it is in the aorta, so that most of the blood in the pulmonary artery passes through the ductus arteriosus to the aorta. Hence, the relatively unsaturated blood from the right ventricle is diverted to the trunk and lower body of the fetus, while the head of the fetus receives the better-oxygenated blood from the left ventricle.
- From the aorta, some of the blood is pumped into the umbilical arteries and back to the placenta where the deoxygenated blood becomes oxygenated.
- Changes in fetal circulation at birth: at birth, the placental circulation is cut off and the peripheral resistance suddenly rises. The pressure in the aorta rises until it exceeds that in the pulmonary artery.
- Meanwhile, because the placental circulation has been cut off, the newborn baby becomes increasingly asphyxial. Finally, the newborn baby

gasps several times, and the lungs expand. The markedly negative intrapleural pressure (−30 to −50 mmHg) during the gasps contributes to the expansion of the lungs.

- Once the lungs are expanded, the pulmonary vascular resistance falls to less than 20% of the value in utero, and pulmonary blood flow increases markedly.
- Blood returning from the lungs raises the pressure in the left atrium, closing the foramen ovale by pushing the valve that guards it against the interatrial septum.
- The ductus arteriosus constricts within a few hours after birth, producing functional closure and permanent anatomic closure follows in the next 24–48 hours. The mechanism producing the initial constriction is not completely understood, but the increase in arterial oxygen tension plays an important role. Relatively high concentrations of vasodilators are present in the ductus in utero, especially prostaglandin $F_{2\alpha}$, and synthesis of these prostaglandins is blocked by inhibition of cyclooxygenase at birth.
- In many premature infants, the ductus fails to close spontaneously, but closure can be produced by infusion of drugs that inhibit cyclooxygenase.
- Immediately after birth, blood flow through the umbilical vein ceases, but most of the portal blood still flows through the ductus venosus, with only a small amount passing through the channels of the liver. However, within one to three hours, the muscle wall of the ductus venosus contracts strongly and closes this avenue of flow. Consequently, the portal venous pressure rises from near 0 mmHg to 6–10 mmHg, which is enough to force portal venous blood flow through the liver sinuses.

4.3 Maternofetal Oxygenation

- The uteroplacental circulation starts with the maternal blood flow into the intervillous space through decidual spiral arteries. Exchange of oxygen and nutrients take place as the maternal blood flows around terminal villi in the intervillous space.
- Maternal arterial blood pushes deoxygenated blood into the endometrial and then uterine veins back to the maternal circulation.
- The fetal–placental circulation allows the umbilical arteries to carry deoxygenated and nutrient-depleted fetal blood from the fetus to the villous core fetal vessels. After the exchange of oxygen and nutrients, the umbilical vein carries fresh oxygenated and nutrient-rich blood circulating back to the fetal systemic circulation.
- At term, maternal blood flow to the placenta is approximately 600–700 ml/min.

5 The Umbilical Cord

- At full term, the average length of the umbilical cord is 50–70 cm (20 inches) and 2 cm (0.75 inches) in diameter.
- It extends from the fetal umbilicus to the fetal surface of the placenta or chorionic plates.
- The umbilical cord contains one vein (the umbilical vein) and two arteries (the umbilical arteries).
- There are about 30–60 branches in each cotyledon, with calibres of 0.1–0.6 mm and lengths of 15–25 mm.
- There are about 15–28 cotyledons per placenta.

5.1 Abnormal Insertion of Umbilical Cord

- In >90% of placentas, the umbilical cord inserts on the fetal surface (chorionic plate) of the placenta more than 3 cm from the margin.
- In <10%, the umbilical cord inserts at or near the margin.
- In 1%, the umbilical cord inserts in the placental membranes.
- Chorionic plate arteries and veins branch from the umbilical cord insertion. Arteries always cross veins.
- Peripheral cord insertion (velamentous and marginal) is associated with increased frequency of miscarriages, preterm labour and intrauterine fetal growth restriction.
- Velamentous cord insertion is considered a marker of poor placentation and blood flow patterns.

6 Oxygen Dissociation Curve

$H^+ + HbO_2 \longleftrightarrow Hb\,H^+ + O_2$(Bohr effect)

The above equation means that oxygenation of haemoglobin (Hb) promotes dissociation of hydrogen ion (H^+) from haemoglobin, which shifts the bicarbonate buffer equilibrium towards carbon dioxide (CO_2) formation; thereby releasing carbon dioxide from the red blood cells.

7 The Haldane Effect

- The Haldane effect describes the increased ability of deoxygenated blood to carry more carbon dioxide.
- Oxygenation of blood in the lungs displaces carbon dioxide from haemoglobin, which helps to get rid of the carbon dioxide. This property is the Haldane effect. Conversely, oxygenated blood has a reduced affinity for carbon dioxide.
- Carbon dioxide binds to amino groups at the N-terminals and side chains of arginine and lysine residues in haemoglobin forming carbaminohaemoglobin.
- Carbaminohaemoglobin is the major contributor to the Haldane effect.

8 The Bohr Effect

- This is a physiological phenomenon first described in 1904 by the Danish physiologist, Christian Bohr. This phenomenon relates to the oxygen-binding affinity of red blood cells.
- The Bohr effect describes the shift of the haemoglobin dissociation curve to the right by hydrogen ions, which reduces the affinity of haemoglobin for oxygen.
- The oxygen dissociation curve is inversely related both to acidity and to the concentration of carbon dioxide.
- Carbon dioxide reacts with water to form carbonic acid; this reduces the pH of blood and the haemoglobin proteins release the oxygen to the tissues.
- Conversely, a decrease in carbon dioxide provokes an increase in pH, which results in haemoglobin picking up more oxygen.

8.1 Double Bohr and Double Haldane Effect

- Both the Bohr and Haldane effects enhance the exchange of oxygen and carbon dioxide across the placenta.
- The carbon dioxide from the fetal side diffuses into the maternal blood, causing an increase in maternal intervillous hydrogen ions, which reduces the affinity of maternal haemoglobin for oxygen, increasing oxygen transfer to the fetus.
- At the same time, the relative decrease in carbon dioxide on the fetal side causes the fetal blood to become slightly more alkaline, increasing the fetal haemoglobin uptake of oxygen.
- Both the Bohr and Haldane effect occurs on both sides of oxygen delivery/uptake: it has been called the double Bohr and double Haldane respectively.

8.2 Factors That Affect the Oxygen Dissociation Curve

- Many factors can change the shape of the oxygen dissociation curve such as exercise, increasing temperature, and 2,3 DPG. See Table 15.1.
- A rightward shift indicates that the haemoglobin under study has a decreased affinity for oxygen. This makes it more difficult for haemoglobin to bind to oxygen (requiring a higher pO_2 to achieve the same oxygen saturation), but it makes it easier for the haemoglobin to release oxygen bound to it.
- Left shift of the curve is a sign of haemoglobin's increased affinity for oxygen (e.g., at the lungs). This leftward shift indicates that the haemoglobin under study has an increased affinity for oxygen so that haemoglobin binds oxygen more easily, but unloads it more reluctantly.
- Right shift shows decreased affinity, as would appear with an increase in either body temperature, hydrogen ions, 2,3 DPG and carbon dioxide concentrations.See Figure 15.1.

Table 15.1 Factors that shift the oxygen dissociation curve

Control factors	Levels	Shift
Temperature	Increases Decreases	Right Left
Exercise	Increases Decreases	Right Left
2,3 DPG	Increases Decreases	Right Left
CO_2	Increases Decreases	Right Left

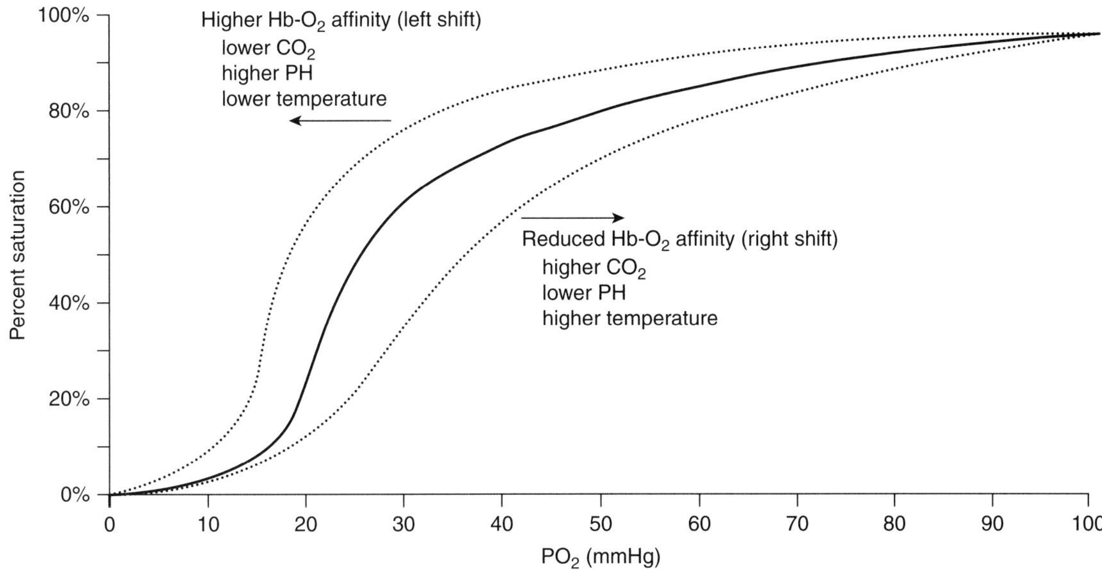

Figure 15.1 Fetal haemoglobin saturation curve. Used with permission from Lumen.

9 Fetal Haemoglobin

- Fetal haemoglobin has higher oxygen affinity than adult haemoglobin; primarily due to much-reduced affinity to 2,3 DPG.
- Mnemonic: 'CADET, face right' (CO_2, acid, 2,3 DPG, exercise, temperature).
- Fetal haemoglobin (HbF) is structurally different from normal adult haemoglobin (HbA), giving Haemoglobin F a higher affinity for oxygen than HbA.
- Haemoglobin F is composed of two alpha and two gamma chains, whereas HbA is composed of two alpha and two beta chains.
- The fetal dissociation curve is shifted to the left relative to the curve for the normal adult because of these structural differences.
- Typically, fetal arterial oxygen pressures are lower than adult arterial oxygen pressures. Hence, higher affinity to bind oxygen is required at lower levels of partial pressure in the fetus to allow diffusion of oxygen across the placenta.
- At the placenta, there is a higher concentration of 2,3 DPG formed, and 2,3 DPG binds readily to beta chains rather than to alpha chains. As a result, 2,3 DPG binds more strongly to adult haemoglobin, causing HbA to release more oxygen for uptake by the fetus, whose Haemoglobin F is unaffected by the 2,3 BDG. Haemoglobin F then delivers that bound oxygen to tissues that have even lower partial pressures where it can be released.

16 Physiology of Pregnancy and Labour

Neela Mukhopadhaya

1 The Cardiovascular System

1.1 The Conduction System of the Heart

- The electrical impulse in the heart is generated by the sinoatrial (SA) node, which is in the right atrium at the entry of the superior vena cava.
- The impulse is then transmitted across both the atria, resulting in atrial contraction.
- Once the impulse arrives at the atrioventricular node, it is stored for a few seconds to allow ventricular filling.
- The His-Purkinje system is a specialised conduction tissue, which divides into a left and right branch to innervate both the ventricles.
- The right bundle is narrow while the left bundle is wide and innervates the muscles of the larger left ventricle. The left bundle block leads to abnormal left ventricular function.
- Aberrant pathways of conduction can develop, which causes arrhythmias: an example is the Wolff–Parkinson–White (WPW) syndrome.
- Neurogenic control of the SA node is via sympathetic and parasympathetic nervous system.
- At rest, the dominant tone is parasympathetic/vagal.
- There are several factors that affect the heart rate. See Table 16.1.
- In pregnancy, the two atriums enlarge most: the left atrium increases by 5 mm and the right atrium by 7 mm.

Table 16.1 Factors that stimulate and inhibit SA node function

Factors that increase SA node discharge and heart rate	Factors that decrease SA node discharge and heart rate
Thyroxine	Hypothyroidism
High temperature	Hypothermia
Beta-adrenergic activity	Beta-adrenergic blockers
Atropine	Ischaemia (pacemakers are used)

1.2 Electrocardiogram Changes

In a normal electrocardiogram (ECG):

- P wave = atrial depolarisation = atrial contraction
- QRS complex = ventricular depolarisation = ventricular contraction
- T wave = ventricular repolarisation
- atrial repolarisation coincides with ventricular depolarisation; hence, is not detected on ECG
- the speed of the ECG paper is 25 mm/s, so each small square is 0.04 s and each large square represents 0.2 s
- in the vertical axis, each cm equals 1 Mv
- the normal PR interval is 0.12–0.20 ms
- prolongation of the PR interval occurs in first-degree blocks when the conduction of electrical impulse between the atrium and ventricle is delayed
- the PR interval is reduced in faster pathways and in aberrant conduction; a typical example is WPW syndrome where a delta wave occurs
- normal QRS width is 0.12 s:
    - any longer QRS width is suggestive of a delay in travel in the His-Purkinje system; a typical example is a bundle branch block
- the QT interval is usually 0.30–0.45 s and depends on the heart rate
- the QT interval is increased in hypocalcaemia, hypokalaemia and rheumatic carditis and with many drugs.
- the QT interval is decreased in hypercalcaemia, hyperkalaemia and digoxin.

Changes in ECG during pregnancy include:

- left ventricular hypertrophy and dilatation
- upwards displacement of the diaphragm

- the apex is shifted anterior and left
- heart rate increases by 10–15%
- left axis deviates by 15 degrees
- inverted T wave in lead III
- Q wave in lead III and augmented vector foot (AVF)
- nonspecific ST changes

  There is no change in the contractility.

1.3 Haemodynamic and Cardiac Events in Pregnancy

See Table 16.2 and Table 16.3.

- Plasma volume increases from 2600 ml to 3800 ml. This occurs early in pregnancy (6–8 weeks). No further increase occurs after 32 weeks.
- Red cell mass increases from 1400 ml to 1800 ml with a steady increase until term. This is proportionately lower than the plasma volume increase; hence, the haematocrit and haemoglobin concentration falls.
- Cardiac output increases by more than 40% (4.5–6 L/min); this occurs early in pregnancy and plateaus at 24–30 weeks. It falls to prepregnancy level after delivery (variable times).
- Heart rate increases by 10% from 80 beats per minute (BPM) to 90 BPM (late in pregnancy).
- Stroke volume increases early in pregnancy.
- Supine hypotension syndrome: this occurs due to pressure of the gravid uterus on the inferior vena cava reducing the cardiac output.
- Oxygen consumption increases by an extra 30–50 ml/min.
- Alteration in regional flow occurs with preferential redistribution of blood to the:
  - uterus
  - kidney
  - skin
  - breasts
  - skeletal muscle
- The arteriovenous oxygen gradient falls.
- At term, the distribution of the 1.5 L of extra blood is as follows:
  - uterus 400 ml/min
  - kidney 300 ml/min
  - skin 500 ml/min
  - gastrointestinal system, breasts and others: 300 ml/min
- Early in pregnancy, extra blood supply is to the skin and breasts.
- Blood pressure (BP) changes in pregnancy: peripheral vascular resistance falls from 8 to 36 weeks
  - systolic BP falls by 5 mmHg
  - diastolic BP falls by 10 mmHg
- Other factors like position, uterine contractions and drugs affect blood pressure.
- Blood enters the right heart via the superior and inferior vena cava.
- Blood from the head via the superior vena cava has less oxygen as the oxygen consumption of the brain is high.
- The blood that reaches the right atrium is mixed and the mixed venous oxygen concentration in the right atrium is around 60%.
- The oxygen concentration in the left atrium is about 96%.
- The left atrium and ventricle have a similar oxygen concentration.
- True mixed venous blood is best sampled from the pulmonary artery.
- The fixed reference point for the pressures in the heart is the level of the right atrium. See Table 16.4.

Table 16.2 Changes in the cardiovascular parameters

Stroke volume	**+30%**
Heart rate	+10–15%
Systemic vascular resistance	–5%
Systolic blood pressure	–10 mmHg
Diastolic blood pressure	–15 mmHg
Mean blood pressure	–15 mmHg
Oxygen consumption	+20%

Table 16.3 Percentage changes in cardiovascular function during pregnancy

Blood volume	+30%
Plasma volume	+40%
Red blood cell volume	+20%
Cardiac output Early phase Late phase	+40% +50% +70%

Table 16.4 Pressures in the four heart chambers

Right atrium: 1–7 mmHg (average: 4 mmHg)	Left atrium: 10–15 mmHg
Right ventricle: Systolic 15–25 mmHg Diastolic 0–8 mmHg	Left ventricle: End diastolic pressure <12 mmHg

Table 16.5 Vasodilators and vasoconstrictors

Substances causing vasodilatation	Substances causing vasoconstriction
Endothelium derived relaxing factor	Angiotensin II
Prostacyclin	Thromboxane
Prostaglandin A and E	Prostaglandin F2-alpha

1.4 Blood Pressure Control in Pregnancy

- Blood pressure = cardiac output x peripheral resistance.
- Cardiac output = stroke volume x heart rate.
- Peripheral resistance is controlled by the autonomic nervous system.
- Peripheral resistance is also affected by drugs and chemical substances like angiotensin II, serotonin, kinins, catecholamines, adenosine, potassium, hydrogen ion, partial pressure of carbon dioxide (pCO_2), partial pressure of oxygen (pO_2) and prostaglandins.
- Blood viscosity will rise hugely when the haematocrit rises above 45%.
- The receptors involved in blood-pressure control are cholinergic, alpha and beta-adrenergic receptors.
- Adrenergic stimulation causes vasoconstriction, and vasodilatation is mainly due to a reduction in vasoconstrictor tone.
- The autonomic system controls blood pressure mainly by the cardioinhibitory and the vasomotor centres.
- The cardioinhibitory centre is the dorsal motor nucleus of the vagus nerve.
- The baroreceptors send impulses to the cardioinhibitory centre and cause slowing of the heart rate and a drop in blood pressure.
- Sympathetic output to the heart and blood vessels is controlled by the vasomotor centre. Input impulses are from baroreceptors and chemoreceptors.
- Fall in pO_2 and pH, or rise in pCO_2 stimulates vasomotor centre and increases blood pressure.
- Rise in cerebrospinal fluid (CSF) pressure will also stimulate vasomotor centre causing a rise in blood pressure (Cushing reflex).
- Tissue metabolites accumulated following anaerobic metabolism can cause vasodilatation.
- Autoregulation takes place at a local level with vasodilatation and improved blood flow.
- Prostaglandins can cause blood vessels to constrict or dilate.
- Prostaglandin A and prostaglandin E cause a fall in blood pressure by reducing splanchnic vascular resistance, while prostaglandin F causes uterine contraction and bronchial constriction.
- Prostacyclin causes vasodilatation while thromboxane causes vasoconstriction. See Table 16.5.

2 The Respiratory system

2.1 Respiratory Changes in Pregnancy

2.1.1 Lung Volumes

- Tidal volume: the lung volume that represents the normal volume of air displaced between normal inhalation and exhalation when extra effort is not applied. In a healthy, young human adult, tidal volume is approximately 500 mL per inspiration or 7 ml/kg of body mass.
- Total lung capacity is 5 L. Of this, 1.5 L remains at the end of a forced expiration called residual volume (RV).
- Vital capacity: the air that can be inhaled after a forced expiration to a forced inspiration. This is the total of tidal volume, inspiratory reserve volume and expiratory reserve volume.
- Functional residual capacity (FRC): the volume of air present in the lungs at the end of passive expiration. At the end of a normal expiration, there are opposing effects of the elastic recoil forces of the lung and chest wall, which balance it, and there is no exertion on the diaphragm. However, in chronic obstructive pulmonary disease (COPD), there is a loss of elastic recoil and an increased FRC. Additionally, in chronic emphysema or other airway obstructions, the FRC increases.

- In pregnancy, due to the pressure of the gravid uterus which moves the diaphragm up, there is reduced FRC and reduced expiratory residual capacity (ERV).
- ERV: the additional amount of air that can be expired from the lungs by determined effort after normal expiration: FRC = RV + ERV.

The main changes in pregnancy are as follows (see Figure 16.1):

- Elevation of the diaphragm and altered chest configuration: there is a 5 cm upwards displacement in the resting position of the diaphragm. The chest height reduces, but the rib cage expands outwards hence the total lung capacity remains the same or decreases by 200 ml. Chest compliance reduces, especially in lithotomy. Lung compliance is unaffected.
- Negative pleural pressure increases, and earlier closure of the small airways causes the reduction in FRC and ERV. This progressively decreases by 20% at term.
  - Inspiratory reserve volume increases early and decreases late in pregnancy.
  - Progesterone alters the smooth muscle tone of the airways, resulting in a bronchodilator effect. It also mediates hyperaemia and oedema of mucosal surfaces, causing nasal congestion.
- Increased progesterone directly stimulates the central respiratory centre and causes increased minute ventilation. Ventilation increases by 40% (from the first trimester). This is thought to be due to progesterone, which stimulates the respiratory centre both directly and indirectly. A similar increase in ventilation is also seen in women on progesterone-only pills and in the luteal phase of the menstrual cycle.
- Breathing is more diaphragmatic than thoracic.
- Seventy percent of pregnant women experience subjective dyspnoea.
- Increased risk of pulmonary embolism.
- Respiratory rate does not change.
- Increase in tidal volume.
- Oxygen consumption and carbon dioxide production increases by 20–30% by the third trimester and up to 100% during labour, necessitating increased minute ventilation to maintain normal acid-base status. Oxygen consumption increases (50 ml/min at term):
  - fetus 20 ml/min
  - cardiac output 6 ml/min
  - renal system 6 ml/min
  - overall metabolic rate 18 ml/min
- Respiratory resistance increases: this is measured clinically by the forced expiratory volume in 1 second (FEV_1). This is directly dependent on the vital capacity and is expressed as FEV_1/forced vital capacity (FVC). The normal ratio is >75%. This ratio falls with age, asthma and lung disease. The resistance is also measured by peak flow rate, which normally is >600 L/min. There is no change in FEV_1, or peak flow rate during pregnancy.
  - Total pulmonary and airways resistance decrease in late pregnancy.
  - Respiratory changes in pregnancy are the same in singleton and twin pregnancies.
  - Basal metabolic rate increases by 14%.

2.1.2 Acid-base Balance in Pregnancy

- The increase in ventilation is greater than the increase in oxygen consumption.
- Partial pressure of oxygen (pCO_2) decreases to 31 mmHg (due to hyperventilation).
- pO_2 increases to 14 kPa during the third trimester and then falls to <13.5 kPa at term (increased cardiac output (CO) is unable to compensate for increased oxygen consumption).
- Bicarbonate (HCO_3) decreases to maintain a normal pH.
- Sodium (Na) decreases.
- Osmolarity decreases by 10 mmol/L.
- The net effect is a mild chronic respiratory alkalosis with a decrease in the arterial pCO2, a slight increase in the pO_2 (alveolar gas equation), a slightly elevated pH and a slightly decreased HCO_3 (renal compensation).

2.1.3 Summary of Changes in the Respiratory System During Pregnancy

- tidal volume increases, but not the respiratory rate
- no change in vital capacity
- residual volume decreases by 200 ml
- expiratory reserve volume decreases
- inspiratory reserve volume decreases early and increases late in pregnancy
- mild chronic respiratory alkalosis

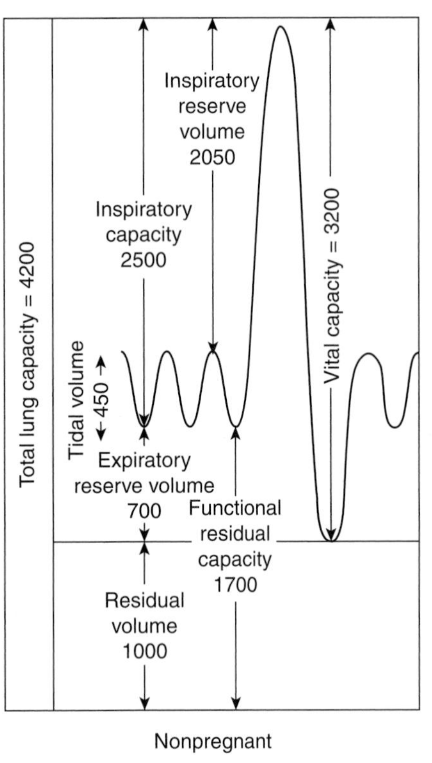

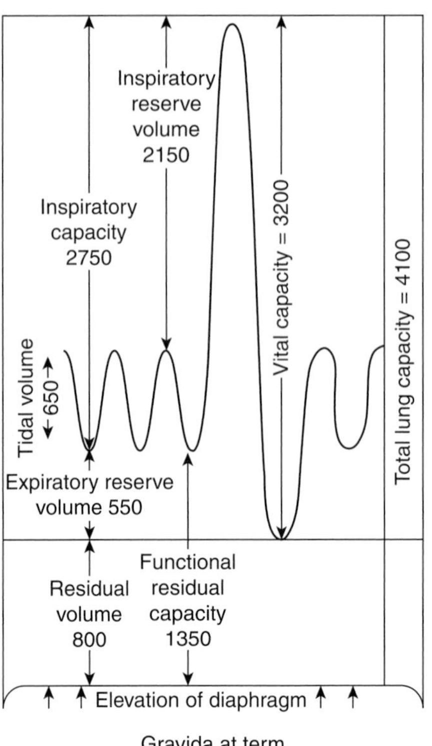

Figure 16.1 Lung volume changes in pregnancy (units in mL). Used with permission from Gardner, M. O., Doyle, N. M. (2004). Asthma in pregnancy. *Obstet Gynecol Clin*, 31, 390.

2.1.4 Composition of Inhaled and Exhaled Air

- The partial pressures and the composition of dry air, inspired air, alveolar air and expired air differ.
- In all cases, the relative concentration of gases is nitrogen > oxygen > water vapour > carbon dioxide. The amount of water vapour present in alveolar air (47 mmHg) is greater than that in atmospheric air (5.7 mmHg).
- Total volume of alveolar air is 2 L. Alveolar ventilation is 350 ml for each breath.
- Gas exchange occurs at two sites in the body: in the lungs, where oxygen is picked up and carbon dioxide is released at the respiratory membrane, and at the tissues, where oxygen is released and carbon dioxide is picked up.
- External respiration is the exchange of gases with the external environment, and occurs in the alveoli of the lungs. Internal respiration is the exchange of gases with the internal environment, and occurs in the tissues. The actual exchange of gases occurs due to simple diffusion.
- Ventilation is the process that moves air into and out of the alveoli. Perfusion affects the flow of blood in the capillaries. Both are important in gas exchange, as ventilation must be sufficient to create a high pO_2 in the alveoli. If ventilation is insufficient and the pO_2 drops in the alveolar air, the capillary is constricted and blood flow is redirected to alveoli with sufficient ventilation.

2.1.5 Control of Respiration

- The respiratory centre is responsible for controlling the depth and rhythmicity of the respiration.
- The respiratory centre is under the influence of chemoreceptors:
  - central chemoreceptors
  - peripheral chemoreceptors around the aortic arch and in the carotid body
- The aortic arch chemoreceptors are innervated by the vagus nerve and the carotid body chemoreceptors by the glossopharyngeal nerve.
- Carotid body receptors are sensitive to pO_2.
- Both carotid and aortic body receptors are sensitive to changes of pH and pCO_2.

2.2 Applied Respiratory Physiology

- In pregnancy, spirometry remains normal. This includes FVC, FEV_1 and peak expiratory flow rate, which remain unaltered. However, lung volumes change.
- Asthma: corticosteroids should be used promptly to prevent critical illness.
- COPD: there is a risk of hypoxia and hypercapnia in pregnancy. It leads to severely reduced vital capacity (VC).
- Pulmonary oedema: this can occur with use of tocolytics or in preeclampsia with the use of magnesium sulphate.

2.2.1 Acute Respiratory Distress Syndrome

- Nonobstetric causes of acute respiratory distress syndrome (ARDS) include sepsis, pneumonia, intracerebral haemorrhage, blood transfusion reaction and reduced gastrointestinal sphincter tone.
- Obstetric causes include amniotic fluid embolism, preeclampsia, septic miscarriages, retained placenta and tocolysis.
- Treatment includes prompt antibiotics, intravenous hydration, mechanical ventilation and extracorporeal life support in refractory ARDS.

3 Urinary changes in pregnancy

3.1 Anatomy of the Kidney and the Physiological Changes that Occur in Pregnancy

- The parts of the nephron are as follows:
  - afferent arteriole
  - glomerulus
  - proximal convoluting tubule
  - loop of Henle
  - distal convoluting tubule
  - collecting duct
  - efferent arteriole
- The functional unit of the kidney is the nephron (about a million per kidney).
- The glomerulus is an invagination of the Bowman's capsule (the end of the renal tubule).
- The afferent arteriole brings blood to the glomerulus.
- The glomerular filtrate passes from the blood, through the capillary endothelium, basal lamina and the tubular epithelium before it reaches the tubule.
- The functional diameter of the pores in the tubular epithelium is about 8 nm. Hence, particles larger than 8 nm such as red blood cells (6.2–8.2 μm), do not cross into the glomerular filtrate.
- The capillaries of the glomerulus have negatively charged proteins in the pores; hence, albumin (negatively charged molecule) cannot pass through the glomerulus in normal circumstances.

3.2 Changes During Pregnancy

- The increased blood volume and cardiac output during pregnancy cause a 50–60% increase in renal blood flow and glomerular filtration rate (GFR). This causes an increased excretion and reduced blood levels of urea, creatinine, urate and bicarbonate. See Table 16.6.
- Mild glycosuria and/or proteinuria may occur because the increase in GFR may exceed the ability of the renal tubules to reabsorb glucose and protein.
- Increased water retention causes a reduction of plasma osmolality.
- The smooth muscle of the renal pelvis and ureter become relaxed and dilated, kidneys increase in length and the ureters become longer, more curved and with an increase in residual urine volume.
- Increase in bladder capacity due to muscle relaxation and increased risk of urinary tract infections.
- The enlarging uterus may put pressure on the ureters.

Table 16.6 Changes in kidney function during pregnancy

Urea	Decrease from 4.3 to 3.1 mmol/L
Creatinine	Decrease to 73–47 μmol/L
Urate and HCO_3	Decreases
Glucose and protein in urine (mild glycosuria and proteinuria)	Increases
Plasma osmolarity	Decreases
Renal blood flow	Increases from 1.2 L/min to 1.5 L/min
GFR	Increases to 140–170 ml/min

- Asymptomatic bacteriuria occurs in 2–10% of women in pregnancy and, if untreated, up to 30% may develop acute pyelonephritis.
- Clearance of drugs and individual substances during pregnancy changes:
  - volume of distribution increases; hence, drug dosages should be higher
  - excretion also increases
  - dosages of some drugs may need to be increased such as antiepileptic drugs and thyroxine
  - the safety of drugs used in pregnancy should be borne in mind
- Urinary protein excretion increases during pregnancy, but never to more than 300 mg/day and, therefore, overt proteinuria is abnormal.
- Women are at increased risk of urinary tract infections because of renal tract dilatation leading to urinary stasis.
- Women with one (or more) dipstick-positive proteinuria in the absence of infection should have the level of proteinuria quantified once infection and preeclampsia have been excluded.
- Baseline quantification of proteinuria should be by 24-hour collection for urine protein and by protein/creatinine ratio (PCR). PCR alone may be used for follow-up.
- Pregnant women with persistent proteinuria above 500 mg/day diagnosed before 20 weeks of gestation should be referred promptly to a nephrologist.
- Women with a nephrotic syndrome should be given prophylactic heparin for thromboprophylaxis.
- Isolated microscopic haematuria with structurally normal kidneys does not need to be investigated during pregnancy, but should be evaluated if it is persistent following delivery.
- Asymptomatic bacteriuria is found in 2% of sexually active women, and is more common (up to 7%) during pregnancy.
- In women with recurrent pyelonephritis, 20% have an underlying renal tract abnormality and this should be investigated after 12 weeks.
- Women with more severe renal impairment are more likely to suffer hypertension, preeclampsia or premature labour and to have a small baby, miscarriage or irreversible decline in renal function long term.
- Pregnancy is extremely uncommon in women with end-stage kidney disease on dialysis, for a variety of reasons; most such women are infertile. Fertility often returns rapidly after a successful renal transplant.
- Acute kidney injury in pregnancy may be due to various causes, including:
  - septicaemia; for example, septic abortion, pyelonephritis
  - haemolysis; for example, sickling crisis, malaria
  - hypovolaemia; for example, preeclampsia, antepartum haemorrhage, intrapartum or postpartum haemorrhage, disseminated intravascular coagulation (DIC) and abortion
- Renal disease may be related to diabetes, hypertensive disorders and preexisting diseases like systemic lupus erythematosus.

4 Haematological system

4.1 Haematological Changes in Pregnancy

- Plasma volume increases in pregnancy and there is physiological anaemia (maximum at 32 weeks).
- Increased erythropoiesis occurs from early pregnancy (increased erythropoietin and placental lactogen) to the end of the second trimester.
- Mean corpuscular volume (MCV) and mean corpuscular haemoglobin concentration (MCHC) are unaffected.
- Modest leucocytosis occurs in pregnancy (increased white blood cell count (WBC)) and peaks after delivery.
- Gestational thrombocytopenia affects 7–10% of women (platelets: $<150 \times 10^6$).
- Increased iron demand occurs in pregnancy:
  - total requirement: 700–1400 mg extra
  - overall requirement: 4 mg/day (from 2.8 mg/day in nonpregnant women to 6.6 mg/day by the end of pregnancy)
  - ferritin 15–300 μg/l (iron stores)
  - increased iron absorption (erythroid hyperplasia) in the latter half of the pregnancy
  - the amount absorbed depends on iron stores
  - serum iron decreases, but transferrin and total iron binding capacity (TIBC) increases
- The most common haematological problem in pregnancy is anaemia.

- Symptoms: dyspnoea, tiredness and faintness (common in pregnancy).
- Serum iron <12 μmol/L.
- TIBC saturation <15%.
- Hypercoagulable state (increase in factors VII, VIII, IX, X and fibrinogen).
- Increased coagulation factors in all except XI and XIII (from the third month).
- Fibrinolysis decreases, especially to protect against a haemorrhage in labour:
  - remains low in labour
  - returns to normal within one hour of delivery of placenta
  - increased erythrocyte sedimentation rate (ESR)
  - increased platelet count, but decreases due to dilution
  - platelet function remains same
  - routine coagulation screening is normal
  - evidence that the inhibition of fibrinolysis is mediated through the placenta (plasminogen activator inhibitor 2). See Table 16.7.

4.2 Conditions That Cause Haematological Impairment

4.2.1 Preeclampsia

- During the last few months of pregnancy, about 5% of pregnant women have a rapid rise in arterial blood pressure along with appearance of large amounts of protein in the urine. This condition is called preeclampsia or toxaemia of pregnancy.
- It is characterised by excess salt and water retention by the mother's kidneys and by weight gain and development of oedema and hypertension in the mother.
- In addition, there is impaired function of the vascular endothelium and arterial spasm occurs in many parts of the mother's body, most significantly in the kidneys, brain and liver.
- The renal blood flow and the GFR are decreased, which is exactly opposite to the changes that occur in the normal pregnant woman.

4.2.1.1 Pathophysiology of Preeclampsia

- Although various attempts have been made to prove that preeclampsia is caused by excessive secretion of placental or adrenal hormones, proof of a hormonal basis is still controversial.
- Presence of a fetus leading to autoimmunity or allergy has also been suggested as a causative theory for this condition as the acute symptoms usually disappear within a few days after birth of the baby.
- There are some studies suggesting that preeclampsia is initiated by insufficient blood supply to the placenta, resulting in the placenta's release of substances, which cause widespread dysfunction of the maternal vascular endothelium.

Table 16.7 Clotting changes during pregnancy

Condition	PT	PTT	BT	Platelets
Aspirin			↑	
Congenital afibrinogenaemia	↑	↑	↑	
DIC	↑	↑	↑	↓
Early liver failure	↑			
Late liver failure	↑	↑	↑	↓
Factor V deficiency	↑	↑		
Factor X deficiency				
Haemophilia		↑		
Thrombocytopenia			↑	↓
Uraemia			↑	
Vitamin K deficiency	↑	↑		
Von Willebrand's disease		↑	↑	

PT: prothrombin time; PTT: partial thromboplastin time; BT: bleeding time; ↑: increased; ↓: decreased

- The role of various increased levels of inflammatory cytokines has also been suggested.
- However, the precise role of the various factors released from the ischaemic placenta in causing the multiple cardiovascular and renal abnormalities in women with preeclampsia is still uncertain.

4.2.2 Eclampsia

- Eclampsia is characterised by vascular spasm throughout the body: it causes clonic seizures in the mother, sometimes followed by coma, greatly decreased renal output, liver dysfunction, often extreme hypertension and a generalised toxic condition of the body.
- It usually occurs shortly before birth of the baby and is associated with high morbidity and mortality.
- However, with optimal and immediate use of rapidly acting vasodilating drugs to reduce the arterial pressure to normal, followed by immediate delivery of the baby by caesarean section, morbidity can be reduced.

4.2.3 HELLP Syndrome

- HELLP syndrome is a variant of preeclampsia with haemolysis (H), elevated liver enzymes (EL) and low platelets (LP).
- It causes severe epigastric pain and upper abdominal pain.
- Other symptoms include nausea, vomiting, backache, anaemia, hypertension, headache and visual disturbances.
- Spontaneous haematoma can occur, especially rupture of the liver capsule in the right lobe.

4.2.3.1 Risk Factors for HELLP

- increased body mass index (BMI)
- metabolic disorders such as antiphospholipid syndrome
- previous HELLP

4.2.3.2 Pathophysiology of HELLP

HELLP is mainly an endothelial cell injury, leading to:

- acute renal failure
- thrombotic thrombocytopenic purpura
- decreased endothelium derived relaxing factors
- increased von Willebrand factor (vWF), leading to a coagulation cascade
- placental component causing inflammation, and increased cytokines, leucocytes, interleukins and complement

4.2.4 Thalassaemia

- Thalassaemia is an inherited disorder, which impairs the body's ability to make clots.
- Bleeding is longer than usual, with easy bruising and with bleeding in the joints and the brain.
- There are two types of thalassaemia: alpha thalassaemia occurs when a gene or genes related to the alpha globin protein are missing or changed (mutated). Beta thalassaemia occurs when similar gene defects affect production of the beta globin protein.

4.2.5 Haemophilia

- There are five types: haemophilia A, haemophilia B, haemophilia C, parahaemophilia and acquired haemophilia. See Table 16.8.

4.2.5.1 Treatment of Haemophilia

- desmopressin and tranexamic acid
- heparin and warfarin should be avoided as these can aggravate clotting deficiencies
- nonsteroidal anti-inflammatories (NSAIDs) should be avoided as these can prolong bleeding

4.2.6 Sickle Cell Disease

- single-gene autosomal recessive
- group of disorders, which affect haemoglobin chains

Table 16.8 Types and cause of haemophilias

Types	Causes	
Haemophilia A	Factor VIII deficiency	X-linked recessive, women affected
Haemophilia B	Factor IX deficiency	X-linked recessive, women affected
Haemophilia C	Factor XI deficiency	Not completely recessive – heterozygous also show increased bleeding, both sexes affected, Ashkenazi Jews
Parahaemophilia	Factor V deficiency	Usually mild, can be acquired or inherited
Acquired haemophilia	Cancers, autoimmunity, pregnancy	Acquired

Table 16.9 Sickle cell disease variants

HbAS	Trait
HbSS	Disease
HbSC	Haemoglobin C chain (variant)
HbSB	β thalassemia variant

Table 16.10 Distribution of HbA and HbS in sickle cell disease and traits

HbS 40% and HbA 60%	Sickle cell trait
HbS majority and HbF 10%, no HbA	Sickle cell disease

- higher incidence in African, Caribbean, Middle Eastern, Mediterranean and Asian people
- unusual shape of haemoglobin: rigid and fragile cells
- increased breakdown of red blood cells causing haemolytic anaemia
- this breakdown causes vaso-occlusion in small vessels and painful crisis – see Tables 16.9 and 16.10

4.2.5.1 Diagnosis

Diagnosis of sickle cell disease or a variant is usually made at the booking of the pregnancy. The booking bloods include haemoglobin electrophoresis, which will diagnose the condition.

4.2.5.2 Management of sickle cell crisis

- analgesia such as NSAIDs
- mobilisation
- hydration
- folic acid: 5 mg preconception and throughout the pregnancy
- thromboprophylaxis if admitted antenatally
- blood transfusion usually not required, but a cytomegalovirus (CMV) negative blood should be used

4.3 Blood Group and Rhesus Testing

4.3.1 Atypical Red Cell Antibodies: Serological and Cross-Matching Problems

- Samples referred for the investigation of atypical antibodies should be tested, both to confirm the specificity of the antibodies and to exclude the presence of additional alloantibodies.
- The patient's rhesus (Rh) and atypical phenotype is performed on the first sample received from that patient, plus testing for any other implicated antigens.
- Patients who may require long-term transfusion support are phenotyped for all the major blood group antigens. Patients who have received recent multiple transfusions may be genotyped for the same antigens.

4.3.2 Red Cell Genotyping

- Blood groups currently determined by this method are: Rh C, c, E, e, Cw, M, N, S, s, K, k, Jk^a, Jk^b, Fy^a, Fy^b, Do^a, Do^b.

4.3.3 Haemolytic Transfusion Reactions

- ABO typing, Rh phenotyping, direct antiglobulin test (DAT) or Coombs test and antibody screen/identification is performed on both pre- and post-transfusion samples if available. If no antibodies are detected by standard methods, a more sensitive method may be applied.
- If all reactions are negative, further investigations will be considered for nonhaemolytic transfusion reactions; for example, human leucocyte antigen (HLA) antibodies and anti-immunoglobulin A (IgA).
- ABO, Rh phenotype matched and K negative blood is used for transfusion. Pretransfusion tests will be performed using the post-transfusion sample.

4.3.4 Problems with ABO/RhD grouping

- Samples can be referred for investigation if anomalous results are obtained with routine ABO or RhD grouping; for example, to distinguish between 'D variants' and weak D antigens.
- In case of ABO grouping problems, saliva may be requested.
- It is important to include relevant clinical data.
- A blood-group card can be issued.

4.3.5 Positive Direct Antiglobulin Test

- In a high proportion of DAT-positive cases with free autoantibodies, alloantibodies are also present.
- Therefore, it is recommended that samples from patients requiring a transfusion and with a positive DAT are referred so that clinically significant alloantibodies, which may be masked, can be detected and identified.

- In recently transfused patients who develop a positive DAT, this may be caused by alloantibodies bound to donor red cells (indicating a possible delayed haemolytic reaction). In such cases, an eluate needs to be prepared, for which at least 3 ml of packed red cells are needed.
- In patients with a positive DAT and a negative antibody screen who need transfusions, samples should not routinely be referred prior to each transfusion episode. An eluate is indicated only if there is evidence of a delayed haemolytic transfusion reaction, a change in serology or if a higher frequency of transfusion than normal is required to maintain an adequate level of haemoglobin. The DAT may be positive in patients or in healthy individuals without overt haemolysis.

4.3.6 Transfusion of RhD-Positive Blood to RhD-Negative Recipients

- If RhD-positive blood has been given to a RhD-negative female recipient of childbearing potential, the case should be discussed with a National Health Service Blood and Transplant (NHSBT) medical consultant.
- The volume of RhD-positive red cells infused can be calculated and advice given on the management of the patient. The removal of these cells from the patient´s circulation can be monitored by flow cytometry.

4.3.7 Investigation of IgA Deficiency and IgA Antibodies

- In cases of anaphylactic transfusion reactions, or other indications, samples can be referred to test for IgA deficiency and the presence of antibodies to IgA.

4.3.8 Investigation of Haemolytic Disease of the fetus and Newborn

- Suspected cases of haemolytic disease of the fetus and newborn (HDFN) are investigated by the reference laboratory to detect and identify the causative red cell antibody, including immune ABO antibodies. Tests applied include direct antiglobulin test and eluate from the baby's cells.
- Coombs test: also known as antiglobulin test. There are two types: direct (DAT) or indirect Coombs test (also called indirect antiglobulin test).

4.3.8.1 Direct Coombs Test or DAT

- The DAT is used for autoimmune haemolytic anaemia. In certain diseases, there can be immunoglobulin G (IgG) antibodies in the blood, which bind to antigen in the red blood cells' membrane. The red blood cells then become coated with the IgG alloantibody or autoantibodies and complement proteins bind to them and cause destruction of the red blood cells. The DAT detects any complement proteins or antibodies that are bound to the surface of the red cells.
- Process: a blood sample is taken and washed removing the blood plasma and then incubated with antihuman globulin. If agglutination occurs, then there is evidence of antibodies and the test is positive.

4.3.8.2 Indirect Coombs Test

- used in prenatal testing in pregnant women at booking
- undertaken prior to blood transfusion
- it detects unbound antibodies in the serum
- serum from the patient is incubated with red blood cells of unknown antigenicity
- antihuman globulin is added
- indirect Coombs test is positive if agglutination occurs

5 Gastrointestinal System

5.1 Gastrointestinal Changes in Pregnancy

5.1.1 Gastric Relaxation

In a pregnant woman, under the influence of progesterone, there are some changes:

- delayed gastric emptying
- relaxation of the gastro-oesophageal sphincter
- reflux of gastric acid: 80% heart burn at term
- prone to gastric aspiration (Mendelson's syndrome)
- slower bowel peristalsis: constipation common

5.1.2 Changes Affecting the Liver

- alkaline phosphatase (ALP) increases by three times the normal level (placental production)
- cholecystokinin release decreases
- gall bladder contractility decreases
- prone to gallstones

5.1.2.1 Obstetric Cholestasis

- Obstetric cholestasis is diagnosed when otherwise unexplained pruritus occurs in pregnancy and abnormal liver function tests (LFTs) and/or raised bile acids occur in the pregnant woman and both resolve after delivery. Pruritus that involves in the palms and soles of the feet is particularly suggestive.
- Other causes of pruritus and abnormal LFTs should be sought. This may include carrying out viral screens for hepatitis A, B and C; Epstein–Barr virus and CMV; a liver autoimmune screen for chronic active hepatitis and primary biliary cirrhosis (for example, anti-smooth muscle and antimitochondrial antibodies) and liver ultrasound.
- Interaction between inherited and acquired abnormalities and bile salt transporters occurs.
- Liver enzymes and bile salts increase.
- The condition is similar to liver dysfunction with combined contraceptive pills.
- It is associated with intrauterine fetal death, fetal distress in labour.
- In obstetric cholestasis, the proposed mechanism of action of ursodeoxycholic acid is displacement of more hydrophobic endogenous bile salts from the bile acid pool. This may protect the hepatocyte membrane from the damaging toxicity of bile salts and enhance bile acid clearance across the placenta from the fetus.

5.1.2.2 Hyperemesis Gravidarum

- Hyperemesis gravidarum is the severe, protracted nausea and vomiting with the triad of more than 5% prepregnancy weight loss, dehydration and electrolyte imbalance.
- Diagnosis includes ruling out the differentials of urinary tract infections, liver diseases and gastroenteritis.
- Investigations include urea and electrolytes, liver function tests, urinalysis. The mainstay of treatment includes intravenous hydration, antiemetics, thromboprophylaxis and thiamine.
- For women with persistent or severe hyperemesis gravidarum, the parenteral or rectal route may be necessary and more effective than an oral regimen.
- Women should be asked about previous adverse reactions to antiemetic therapies.
- Drug-induced extrapyramidal symptoms and oculogyric crises can occur with the use of phenothiazines and metoclopramide. If this occurs, there should be prompt cessation of the medications.
- Metoclopramide is safe and effective, but because of the risk of extrapyramidal effects it should be used as second-line therapy.
- There is evidence that ondansetron is safe and effective, but because data are limited it should be used as second-line therapy.

6 Endocrinology

6.1 Function of the Placenta

The maternal portion of the placenta is a large blood sinus. Villi of the fetal portion, which contain small branches of the fetal umbilical arteries and vein, project into this 'lake'.

The main functions of the placenta are as follows:

- Respiratory, excretory and nutritive functions: transfer of gases, nutrients and waste products occurs between the mother and fetus.
- Endocrine function: the placenta is an endocrine gland. It produces both steroid and peptide hormones to maintain pregnancy.
- Barrier function: the placenta has long been considered as a protective barrier to the fetus against noxious agents circulating in the maternal blood, but there are exceptions like various antigens, antibodies and pharmacological drugs.
- Immunological function: the fetus and the placenta contain paternally determined antigens, which are foreign to the mother. Despite this, there is no evidence of graft rejection. Placenta probably offers immunological protection against rejection.

6.2 Hormonal Factors in Pregnancy

In pregnancy, the placenta forms especially large quantities of human chorionic gonadotropin, estrogens, progesterone, and human chorionic somatomammotropin (hCS). All are essential to a normal pregnancy.

6.2.1 Human Chorionic Gonadotropin

- Human chorionic gonadotropin (hCG) causes persistence of the corpus luteum and prevents menstruation.
- It causes the corpus luteum to secrete even larger quantities of its sex hormones progesterone and estrogen for the next few months until the placenta takes over the function.

- It exerts an interstitial cell-stimulating effect on the testes of the male fetus, resulting in the production of testosterone in male fetuses until the time of birth.

6.2.2 Estrogen

- estrogen exerts mainly a proliferative function on most reproductive and associated organs of the mother.

6.2.3 Progesterone

- Progesterone facilitates development of the decidual cells (which are responsible for nutrition of the early embryo).
- It decreases the contractility of the pregnant uterus, preventing spontaneous abortion.
- It assists estrogen in preparing the mother's breasts for lactation.

6.2.4 Human Chorionic Somatomammotropin

- A protein hormone, which is lactogenic and has a small amount of growth-stimulating activity. This hormone has been known as chorionic growth hormone-prolactin and human placental lactogen, but it is now generally called hCS.
- The structure of hCS is very similar to that of human growth hormone; hence, hCS has most of the actions of growth hormone. It functions as a 'maternal growth hormone of pregnancy' to bring about the nitrogen, potassium and calcium retention, lipolysis and decreased glucose utilisation. The last two actions divert glucose to the fetus. The amount of hCS secreted is proportionate to the size of the placenta, which normally weighs about one-sixth as much as the fetus, and low hCS levels are a sign of placental insufficiency.

6.2.5 Other Hormonal Factors in Pregnancy

- Pituitary secretion: there is an increased production of corticotropin, thyrotropin and prolactin from the anterior pituitary. Conversely, pituitary secretion of follicle stimulating hormone and luteinising hormone is almost totally suppressed as a result of the inhibitory effects of estrogens and progesterone from the placenta.
- Increased corticosteroid secretion: augmented secretion likely helps in mobilising amino acids from the mother's tissues so that these can be used for synthesis of tissues in the fetus.
- Increased thyroid gland secretion: the increased thyroxine production is caused, at least partly, by a thyrotropic effect of human chorionic gonadotropin secreted by the placenta and by small quantities of a specific thyroid stimulating hormone, human chorionic thyrotropin, also secreted by the placenta.
- Increased parathyroid gland secretion: heightened secretion causes calcium absorption from the mother's bones, thereby maintaining normal calcium ion concentration in the mother's extracellular fluid, even while the fetus removes calcium to ossify its own bones. This secretion of parathyroid hormone is even more intensified during lactation after the baby's birth because the growing baby requires many times more calcium than the fetus does.
- Secretion of 'relaxin' by the ovaries and placenta: relaxin is mainly secreted by the corpus luteum of the ovary and by placental tissues. It likely softens the cervix of the pregnant woman at the time of delivery.

6.2.6 Fetoplacental Unit

- The fetus and the placenta interact in the formation of steroid hormones.
- The placenta synthesises pregnenolone and progesterone from cholesterol. Some of the progesterone enters the fetal circulation and provides the substrate for the formation of cortisol and corticosterone in the fetal adrenal glands. Some of the pregnenolone enters the fetus and, along with pregnenolone synthesised in the fetal liver, is the substrate for the formation of dehydroepiandrosterone sulphate (DHEA-S) and 16-hydroxydehydroepiandrosterone sulphate (16-OHDHEAS) in the fetal adrenal.
- DHEA-S and 16-OHDHEAS are transported back to the placenta, where DHEA-S forms estradiol and 16-OHDHEAS forms Estriol.
- fetal 16-OHDHEAS is the principal substrate for the estrogens. Hence, the urinary estriol excretion of the mother can be monitored as an index of the state of the fetus.

7 Physiology of Labour and Lactation

The duration of pregnancy in humans averages 270 days from fertilisation (284 days from the first day of the menstrual period preceding conception).

Parturition means birth of the baby. Near term, there is an increased progressive uterine excitability, which leads to the expulsion of the baby. The exact cause of the increased activity of the uterus is not known, but two major categories of effects have been postulated: (1) progressive hormonal changes, which cause increased excitability of the uterine musculature and (2) progressive mechanical changes.

7.1 Hormonal Factors That Increase Uterine Contractility

- Increased ratio of estrogens to progesterone: progesterone has an inhibitory effect on uterine contractility during pregnancy. Conversely, estrogen has a stimulatory effect. Both progesterone and estrogen are secreted in progressively greater quantities throughout most of pregnancy, but from the seventh month onward, estrogen secretion continues to increase, while progesterone secretion remains constant or perhaps even decreases slightly. This leads to increased ratio of estrogen-to-progesterone, resulting in increased contractility of the uterus.
- Oxytocin causes contraction of the uterus: oxytocin is a hormone secreted by the neurohypophysis. There are four reasons to believe that oxytocin might be important in increasing the contractility of the uterus near term: (1) the uterine muscle has heightened responsiveness to oxytocin owing to an increase in oxytocin receptors, (2) oxytocin secretion is considerably increased at the time of labour, (3) labour is prolonged in hypophysectomised animals and (4) experiments in animals indicate that irritation or stretching of the uterine cervix, as occurs during labour, can cause a neurogenic reflex, whereby there is an increased secretion of oxytocin.
- Effect of fetal hormones on the uterus: at the time of labour, the fetus's pituitary gland secretes oxytocin, its adrenal gland secretes cortisol and fetal membranes release prostaglandins in high concentration. All these have a stimulatory effect on the intensity of uterine contractions.

7.2 Mechanical Factors That Increase Uterine Contractility

- Stretch of the uterine musculature: simply stretching smooth muscle organs usually increases their contractility. The importance of mechanical stretch in eliciting uterine contractions is supported by the observation that twins are born, on average, 19 days earlier than a single child.
- Stretch or irritation of the cervix: stretching or irritating the uterine cervix is particularly important in eliciting uterine contractions. It has been postulated that stretching or irritation of nerves in the cervix initiates reflexes to the body of the uterus, but the effect could also result simply from myogenic transmission of signals from the cervix to the body of the uterus.

7.3 Onset of Labour: A Positive Feedback Mechanism for Initiation of Parturition

- Throughout the pregnancy, the uterus undergoes periodic episodes of weak and slow rhythmical contractions called Braxton-Hicks contractions.
- However, around term, these contractions become progressively stronger, which starts stretching the cervix and later forces the baby through the birth canal, thereby causing parturition. This process is called labour, and the strong contractions that result in final parturition are called labour contractions.
- Mechanism of onset of labour: the positive feedback theory suggests that stretching of the cervix by the fetus's head finally becomes great enough to elicit a strong reflex increase in contractility of the uterine body. This pushes the baby forwards, which stretches the cervix more and initiates more positive feedback to the uterine body. Thus, the process repeats until the baby is expelled.
- During labour, spinal reflexes and voluntary contractions of the abdominal muscles ('bearing down') also aid in delivery. However, delivery can occur without bearing down and without a reflex increase in secretion of oxytocin, since paraplegic women can go into labour and deliver.
- Mechanics of parturition: during labour, stronger uterine contraction initiates mainly at the top of the uterine fundus and spreads downwards over the uterine body. Each uterine contraction tends to force the baby downwards towards the cervix. The frequency and intensity of uterine contraction increases with progression of labour with subsequent decrease in relaxation periods.
- In more than 95% of births, the head is the first part of the baby to be expelled and, in most of the

remaining instances, the buttocks are presented first. When the baby enters the birth canal with the buttocks or feet first, this is called a breech presentation.

- The first major obstruction to expulsion of the fetus is the uterine cervix. Towards the end of pregnancy, the cervix becomes soft, which allows it to stretch when labour contractions begin in the uterus. The so-called first stage of labour is a period of progressive cervical dilation, lasting until the cervical opening is as large as the head of the fetus.
- Once the cervix has dilated fully, the fetal membranes usually rupture and the amniotic fluid is lost suddenly through the vagina followed by rapid movement of the fetus's head into the birth canal until delivery is effected.
- Separation and delivery of the placenta: after the birth of the baby, the uterus continues to contract to a smaller and smaller size, which causes a shearing effect between the walls of the uterus and the placenta; thus, separating the placenta from its implantation site. Separation of the placenta opens the placental sinuses and causes bleeding. However, bleeding is limited to an average of 350 ml only as the smooth muscle fibres of the uterine musculature are arranged in figures of eight around the blood vessels. As a result, contraction of the uterus after delivery of the baby constricts the vessels, minimising the blood loss. In addition, vasoconstrictor prostaglandins formed at the placental separation site causes additional blood vessel spasm.
- Involution of the uterus after parturition: during the first four to five weeks after parturition, the uterus involutes. The process is aided by lactation, which causes suppression of pituitary gonadotropin and ovarian hormone secretion during the first few months of lactation.

7.4 Lactation

- Development of the breasts: many hormones are necessary for full mammary development. In general, estrogens are primarily responsible for proliferation of the mammary ducts and progesterone for the development of the lobules. The role of prolactin, although documented in rats, is controversial in humans. During pregnancy, prolactin levels increase steadily until term, and levels of estrogens and progesterone are elevated as well, producing full lobuloalveolar development.
- Initiation of lactation after delivery: in response to increased levels of estrogens, progesterone, prolactin and possibly hCG, breasts enlarge during pregnancy. A very small amount of milk is secreted into the ducts as early as the fifth month.
- Expulsion of placenta leads to abrupt decline in levels of estrogens and progesterone and this initiates lactation. Prolactin and estrogen synergise in producing breast growth, but estrogen antagonises the milk-producing effect of prolactin on the breast.
- In women who do not wish to nurse their babies, estrogens may be administered to stop lactation.
- Milk ejection reflex: oxytocin causes contraction of the myoepithelial cells (smooth-muscle-like cells that line the ducts of the breast). This squeezes the milk out of the alveoli of the lactating breast into the large ducts (sinuses) and thence out of the nipple (milk ejection).
- Ejection of milk is mainly initiated by a neuroendocrine reflex. The touch receptors around the nipples of the breasts are mainly involved in this reflex. Impulses generated are relayed from the somatic touch pathways to the supraoptic and paraventricular nuclei of the hypothalamus. Subsequently, oxytocin-containing neurons cause secretion of oxytocin from the posterior pituitary into the bloodstream.
- The baby suckling at the breast stimulates the touch receptors, the hypothalamic nuclei are stimulated, oxytocin is released and the milk is expressed into the sinuses, ready to flow into the mouth of the waiting baby.
- In lactating women, genital stimulation and emotional stimuli also produce oxytocin secretion, sometimes causing milk to spurt from the breasts.
- Effect of lactation on menstrual cycles: nursing women, generally, have amenorrhea for 25 to 30 weeks. Conversely, women who do not nurse their infants usually have their first menstrual period six weeks after delivery.
- Nursing is known to stimulate prolactin secretion, which in turn inhibits gonadotropin-releasing hormone (GnRH) secretion, inhibits the action of GnRH on the pituitary and antagonises the action of gonadotropins on the ovaries.

- estrogen and progesterone output falls to low levels when ovulation is inhibited and the ovaries are inactive. Even after continuation of menses, for the first six months, cycles are anovulatory.
- Consequently, nursing has long been known to be an important, if only partly effective, method of birth control.
- Chiari–Frommel syndrome: this is a rare condition in which there is a persistence of lactation (galactorrhoea) and amenorrhea in women who do not nurse after delivery. It may be associated with some genital atrophy and is due to persistent prolactin secretion without the secretion of the follicle stimulating hormone and luteinising hormone necessary to produce maturation of new follicles and ovulation.
- Similar symptoms with high prolactin levels is also seen in nonpregnant women with chromophobe pituitary tumours and in women in whom the pituitary stalk has been cut during cancer treatment.

8 Weight Gain and Metabolic Changes in Pregnancy

8.1 Response of the Mother's Body to Pregnancy

- Increased size of the various sexual organs.
- The uterus increases from about 50 g to 1100 g
- Breasts approximately double in size.
- Hormonal changes such as development of oedema, acne and masculine or acromegalic features.

8.2 Weight Gain in the Pregnant Woman

- The usual weight gain during pregnancy is about 25–35 lb, with most of this gain occurring during the last two trimesters.
- Respective contribution:
  - fetus (8 lb)
  - amniotic fluid, placenta, and fetal membranes (4 lb)
  - uterus (3 lb)
  - breasts (2 lb)
  - extra fluid in the blood and extracellular fluid (5 lb)
  - fat accumulation (3–13 lb)

8.3 Metabolism During Pregnancy

- Basal metabolic rate of the pregnant woman increases by about 15% during the latter half of pregnancy owing to the increased secretion of many hormones like thyroxine, adrenocortical hormones and the sex hormones.

8.4 Nutrition During Pregnancy

- The greatest growth of the fetus occurs during the last trimester of pregnancy; its weight almost doubles during the last two months of pregnancy.
- The mother does not absorb sufficient protein, calcium, phosphates and iron from her diet during the last months of pregnancy to supply these extra needs of the fetus.
- If appropriate nutritional elements are not present in a pregnant woman's diet, a number of maternal deficiencies can occur, especially in calcium, phosphates, iron and the vitamins.

17 Physiology of Wound Healing

Anita Pawar

1 Phases of Wound Healing

- Coagulation (begins immediately after injury): Platelets adhere to exposed matrix via integrins that bind to collagen and laminin. Blood coagulation produces thrombin, which promotes platelet aggregation and granule release.
- Inflammation (begins shortly thereafter): the platelet granules generate an inflammatory response. Inflammatory cells (neutrophils and macrophages) are attracted to the injury site and undergo activation. Macrophages secrete various growth factors, which in turn stimulate the infiltration, proliferation and migration of fibroblasts and endothelial cells, leading to angiogenesis and generation of antioxidants.
- Within hours of injury, an epidermal covering composed predominantly of keratinocytes begins to migrate and undergo stratification and differentiation to reconstitute the barrier function of epidermis (epithelisation). It also promotes extracellular matrix production, growth factor and cytokine expression, and angiogenesis.
- Overall, the inflammatory process is a defence against infections and a bridge between tissue injury and new cell growth.
- Migratory and proliferation (begins within days): cells (mainly epithelial cells, fibroblasts, and endothelial cells) recruited undergo rapid mitosis and begin to define the ultimate structure of the scar.
- Ultimately, with the synthesis of extracellular proteins and proteoglycans and a balance of collagen lysis and collagen synthesis, the remodelling of new tissue initiates. The processes are dependent on the availability of metabolic substrates, oxygen concentration and growth factors.
- Remodelling (lasts up to a year): refers to changing patterns in the deposition of matrix components during wound healing.
- Initially, the wound matrix consists of a clot of fibrin and fibronectin, resulting from haemostasis and macrophage activation. Over time, it changes to a mixture of glycosaminoglycans, proteoglycans and other proteins, which support the deposition of future matrix components. There is proliferation and migration of fibroblasts and collagen synthesis. Collagen fibres, originally thin and randomly oriented, gradually increase in thickness and, aided by proteinases, are rearranged along the stress line of the wound.
- Remodelling contributes to the development of the tensile strength in the wound. Wounds gain 20% of their ultimate strength in three weeks and later gain more strength, but they never reach more than about 70% of the strength of normal skin.

2 Angiogenesis

- Angiogenesis refers to the reconstitution of blood supply to the wound.
- The stimulus for vessel formation and growth is provided by activated macrophages and keratinocytes.
- The direction for their growth is governed by low oxygen tension, high lactate concentration and/or oxidant signalling.
- Fibroblasts in the wound site provide the scaffolding and tensile strength for vessel growth.

3 Factors Affecting Wound Healing

Identification of various factors that affect wound healing has provided better knowledge of improving the clinical management of chronic wounds. Patients with risk factors for wound healing may be identified and treated more aggressively, or may be better managed for prevention of infection and/or nonhealing wounds.

Factors affecting wound healing fall into several categories, based on their source: local, regional or systemic.

3.1 Local Factors

1. Growth factors: during the course of wound healing, growth factors have been implicated in such activities as angiogenesis, mitogenesis, chemotaxis, migration and remodelling. However, local therapy with exogenous growth factors has been disappointing, mainly because the added growth factors are quickly destroyed by proteolysins and oxidants. In addition, fibroblasts taken from chronic wounds are often deficient in several ways, and these deficiencies prevent a constructive response to growth factors. Recent clinical trials have found a way to circumvent this problem by making the environment of human chronic wounds more hospitable and the cells made more receptive by doing radical debridement and weight offloading of the wound. Use of autologous skin grafts provide essential growth factors, which help with healing. Now it is possible to construct skin replacements so that the cells they contain release growth factors, but, in this case, they release the factors into a more receptive environment achieved by radical debridement of the surface tissue.
2. Oedema and ischaemia: oedema and/or ischaemia and associated tissue necrosis is associated with delayed healing of chronic wounds. Oedema is common in individuals with venous leg ulcers. One way to improve wound healing in these patients is by reducing oedema by leg elevation and compression. However, the mechanism by which reduction in oedema improves wound healing is not clear.
3. Low oxygen tension: low oxygen tension may result in the inhibition of collagen deposition, decreased phagocytic activity of macrophages and neutrophils, and increased growth of microorganisms due to the hypoxia-related reduction in leucocyte bacterial killing capacity. Maintaining a high oxygen tension in the arterial blood, along with manipulations to increase perfusion (e.g., keeping the wound warm), can facilitate wound healing.

3.2 Regional Factors

1. Arterial insufficiency: arterial insufficiency develops as a result of regional ischaemia and leads to tissue hypoxia. It may also lead to regional tissue necrosis, which eventually results in infection, ulceration and possible amputation.
2. Venous insufficiency: venous insufficiency may develop as a result of valvular dysfunction. It can lead to venous hypertension and capillary oedema, changes in surrounding skin (hyperpigmentation, venous dermatitis, xerosis, lipo-dermato-sclerosis), and skin ulceration.
3. Neuropathy: in some patients, comorbid conditions such as diabetes, nutritional disturbances, infectious diseases or trauma can lead to sensory, motor or autonomic neuropathy, which can result in repeated trauma and ulcerations. In such cases, offloading of pressure points and debridement are enough to allow healing.

3.3 Systemic Factors

1. Inadequate perfusion: insufficient regional circulation has the potential to delay wound healing by interfering with the delivery of oxygen and nutrients.
2. Metabolic disease: comorbid metabolic disorders have the potential to delay wound healing. In patients with diabetes, for example, the incidence of infection and the time to healing may be increased. Adequate control of diabetes is essential for wound healing to occur.

Section 4

Genetics

Jane Ding

18

Cell Structure and Function

Jane Ding

1 Prokaryotic and Eukaryotic Cells

See Table 18.1.

2 Organelles and Suborganelles

2.1 Cytoplasm

- thick solution filling the cell
- contains water, electrolytes and proteins

2.2 Nucleus

- largest organelle
- surrounded by nuclear envelope
- contains nucleolus
- contains chromosomes
- location of the majority of DNA/RNA replication and synthesis

2.3 Nuclear Envelope

- separates cytoplasm from nucleus
- protects DNA
- double layered
- outer nuclear membrane is usually continuous with the rough endoplasmic reticulum

Table 18.1 Prokaryotic and eukaryotic cells

	Prokaryotic	Eukaryotic
Definition	No defined membrane around nucleus	Has defined membrane around nucleus
Example	Bacteria	Plant, animal cells
Size	1–10 μm	10–100 μm
Internal organisation	Simple	Complex

2.4 Nucleolus

- location of RNA synthesis

2.5 Mitochondria

- cellular respiration: glucose burning to produce adenosine triphosphate (ATP)
- glucose travels across inner membrane back and forth to produce ATP
- structure:
  - smooth outer membrane
  - cristae: involuted inner membrane
  - matrix: space inside inner membrane

2.6 Endoplasmic Reticulum

- network of folded membranes in the cytoplasm
- rough and smooth types
- rough endoplasmic reticulum
- rough: due to ribosomes attached to outer surface
- ribosomes synthesise membrane, cellular and secretory proteins
- after synthesis, proteins exit within minutes to the Golgi complex via vesicles
- smooth endoplasmic reticulum
- smooth: no ribosome on outer surface
- synthesises fatty acids and phospholipids
- more abundant in liver: detoxifies chemicals

2.7 Golgi Complex

- modifies secretory and membrane proteins

2.8 Lysosomes

- contains digestive enzymes (pH 4.8), which degrade unwanted proteins, nucleic acid, polysaccharides and old organelles

- surrounded by single membrane
- endocytosis: plasma membrane invaginates to form vesicles for small materials
- phagocytosis: plasma membrane envelopes large items (bacteria)

2.9 Peroxisomes

- contains oxidases to degrade organic substances
  - produces hydrogen peroxide (H_2O_2), which converts to oxygen (O_2) + water (H_2O)
- oxidases fatty acid for synthetic pathway
- clears toxins from liver and kidney

2.10 Cytosol

- inside of cell, which contains all organelles

2.11 Cytoskeleton

- provides cell rigidity and strength
- three types:

1. microtubule: 20 nm diameter
2. microfilament: 7 nm diameter
3. intermediate filament: 10 nm diameter

19 Structure of Chromosomes and Genes

Jane Ding

1 Structure of DNA/RNA

The three parts of nucleotide are as follows:

1. Nitrogen-containing bases:
   - purine:
     - fused nitrogen-containing ring
     - include adenine and guanine
   - pyrimidine:
     - single nitrogen-containing ring
     - include cytosine, thymine and uracil
   - DNA: adenine, guanine, cytosine and thymine
   - RNA: adenine, guanine, cytosine and uracil
2. Pentose (5-carbon sugar)
   - DNA: deoxyribose
   - RNA: ribose
3. Phosphate: linked to pentose by phosphodiester bond

2 Nucleotide

- basic structural unit of DNA/RNA:
  - DNA: 100 million nucleotides; double-stranded helix
  - RNA: 100–1000 nucleotides, single stranded
- triplet nucleotide = codon = produces a single amino acid:
  - one amino acid can have several codons
  - one codon can produce only one amino acid
- two ends:
  - five-prime end: phosphate attaches to C5 of pentose
  - three-prime end: hydroxyl attaches to C3 of pentose
- base pairing:
  - A-T (two weak hydrogen bonds, DNA)
  - C-G (three weak hydrogen bonds, DNA)
  - A-U (three weak hydrogen bonds, RNA)

3 Types of RNA

- messenger RNA (mRNA): carries codon
- transfer RNA (tRNA): carries anticodon and single amino acid
- ribosomal RNA (rRNA): assembles amino acids

4 DNA Replication

1. DNA double helix unwinds as helicase breaks down hydrogen bonds and forms replication fork
2. DNA polymerase adds nucleotides to the leading strand (oriented 3-prime to 5-prime)
   - polymerase travels from 5-prime to 3-prime to form a new strand continuously
3. DNA polymerase adds nucleotides to lagging strand (oriented 5-prime to 3-prime)
   - polymerase travels from 5-prime to 3-prime to form a new strand, but in segments (called Okazaki fragments)
   - DNA ligase joins the Okazaki fragments together
4. This process is performed at many points on DNA simultaneously to save time

5 Process of DNA Synthesising Protein

1. Transcription: DNA is copied into mRNA
2. Gene splicing
3. Translation: mRNA translates into amino acids into protein
4. Protein structure formation
5. Posttranslational modification

6 Transcription

1. DNA strands unwind, and the DNA template strand opens up
2. RNA polymerase adds nucleotides from 5-prime to 3-prime onto coding strand
   - uracil replaces thymine in the process
3. DNA strands reanneal after mRNA is released
4. This process is performed at many points on DNA simultaneously

7 Gene Splicing

- removes introns (noncoding sequences) and joins exons (protein-coding sequences)
- alternative splicing: single gene translated into many proteins with different functions

8 Translation

1. tRNA carries anticodon to pair onto codon on mRNA
2. tRNA releases amino acid as anticodon attaches to codon
3. Ribosome (containing rRNA + proteins) carries the growing polypeptide and releases rRNA
4. Ribosome falls off after polypeptide completed
5. This process occurs at many points on mRNA simultaneously to save time

9 Protein Structure Formation

1. Primary structure: initial polypeptide strand
2. Secondary structure: folding into chains (alpha chain) or sheets (beta sheet) via hydrogen bonds
3. Tertiary structure: folding into final structure via hydrophobic interaction + disulphide bonds
4. Quaternary structure: multiple polypeptides combine into multimeric proteins

10 Posttranslational Modification

- acetylation (add acetyl group): affects lifespan of protein
- phosphorylation (add phosphate group): affects activity of protein
- glycosylation (add carbohydrate chain)

11 Chromosome

- cells and number of chromosomes:
  - somatic cells (most of the body): 46 chromosomes or 23 pairs (diploid); identical in body
  - germ cells or gametes (ovum and sperm only): 23 chromosomes (haploid); nonidentical due to recombination
  - autosome: first 22 pairs (numbered 1–22); numbering based on decreasing chromosome length
  - sex chromosomes: twenty-third pairs are X and Y: XX (female), XY (male)
- shape of chromosomes
  - short arm of chromosome: p arm
  - long arm of chromosome: q arm
  - metacentric chromosome: short and long arm equal length (centromere near middle of the chromosome)
  - submetacentric chromosome: one arm longer than the other (centromere closer to one side of the chromosome)
  - acrocentric chromosome: one arm much longer than the other (centromere at top of the chromosome)
  - isochromosome chromosome: unbalanced, with duplication of the arms, which are mirror images resulting in two copies of either the long arm or the short arm (simultaneous duplication and deletion of genetic material)
  - chromatid: single strand of a chromosome (chromosomes in somatic cells come in pairs)
  - centromere: special DNA sequence where the two sister chromatids link
  - telomere: repetitive nucleotides at the end of chromosomes; protects end of chromosome (like plastic tips on shoelaces)
  - histone: protein that DNA wraps around to condense into chromosomes (like spools for thread)

12 Genes

- definition: stretch of DNA sequence, which codes for a specific protein
- human genome: 20 000 genes

Table 19.1 Cell division

Stage	Description
Interphase	Gap 0 (G0): quiescent phase Gap 1 (G1): cell growth, protein production S phase: DNA replication Gap 2 (G2): cell growth, protein production
Prophase	Chromosomes condense
Metaphase	Mitotic spindles captures all chromosomes aligned at centre of cell
Anaphase	Sister chromatids separate from each other to opposite poles
Telophase	Nuclear envelop breaks down and reforms around daughter chromosomes Cytokinesis occurs: cytoplasm division to form daughter cells

13 Mitosis

- occurs in somatic cells
- the aim is to produce identical diploid cells for cell reproduction
- cytokinesis: the process of division into two cells; occurs in anaphase and telophase (see Table 19.1)

1 parent cell (23 pairs of chromosomes) [2 n] → 1 parent cell duplication → each paired chromatid separates to each daughter cell → 2 identical daughter cells (each with 23 pairs of chromosomes) [2 n + 2 n]

14 Meiosis

- occurs in germ cells (gametes) only
- the aim is to produce haploid cells, so that after fertilisation there will be 46 chromosomes (instead of 92 chromosomes)
- meiosis I and meiosis II

14.1 Meiosis I

[n = haploid, 2 n = diploid]

1 parent cell (23 chromosomes) [n] → 1 parent cell duplication + recombination [2 n] → each paired chromatid moves into each daughter cell → 2 nonidentical daughter cells (each with 23 chromosomes) [n + n]

14.2 Meiosis II

2 nonidentical daughter cells (each with 23 chromosomes) [n + n] → splitting of paired chromatids into single chromatids, which moves into each final daughter cell → 4 nonidentical final daughter cells (each with 23 chromosomes) [n + n + n + n]

15 Spermatogenesis

- produces four spermatozoa

Spermatogonium [n] → primary spermatocyte [2 n] → secondary spermatocyte (end of meiosis I) [n + n] → spermatids (end of meiosis II) [n + n + n + n] → spermatozoa (after differentiation) [n + n + n + n]

16 Oogenesis

- produces one ovum and three polar bodies
- polar bodies cannot fertilise (see Table 19.2)

Oogonium [n] → primary oocyte [2 n] → secondary oocyte + 1 polar body (end of meiosis I) [n + 1 polar body] → secondary oocyte + 3 polar bodies (end of meiosis II) [n + 3 polar bodies] → ovum + 3 polar bodies (after differentiation) [n + 3 polar bodies]

Table 19.2 Stages in oogenesis

Oogenesis	Arresting stage
Primary oocyte	Prophase I (until puberty)
Secondary oocyte	Metaphase II (until fertilisation)

17 Chromosome and Gene Abnormalities

See Table 19.3.

Table 19.3 Chromosomal and gene abnormalities

Chromosomal abnormalities	Gene abnormalities

• Nondisjunction
• Translocation
  ○ Reciprocal
  ○ Robertsonian
• Microdeletion
	• Missense mutation
	• Truncating mutation: frameshift, nonsense
	• Splice site mutation
	• Whole gene deletion
	• Partial gene deletion: exon deletion
	• Triplet repeat expansion

Table 19.4 Nondisjunction

	Meiosis I	Meiosis II
Mistake	Uneven spreading of homologous chromosomes	One pair of homologous chromosomes did not split
End of meiosis I	Daughter cell 1: 3 homologous split pairs Daughter cell 2: 1 homologous split pair	Daughter cell 1: 1 homologous unsplit pair, 1 homologous split pair Daughter cell 2: 1 homologous split pair
End of meiosis II	Final daughter cell 1: 3 chromosomes Final daughter cell 2: 3 chromosomes Final daughter cell 3: 1 chromosome Final daughter cell 4: 1 chromosome	Final daughter cell 1: 3 chromosomes Final daughter cell 2: 1 chromosome Final daughter cell 3: 2 chromosomes Final daughter cell 4: 2 chromosomes

18 Nondisjunction

See Tables 19.4, 19.5 and 19.6.

- due to mistake in meiosis I or meiosis II
- leads to trisomy and monosomy
- risk increases with maternal age

Table 19.5 Age and risk of nondisjunction

Age	Risk
20	1/1500
30	1/900
34	1/500
36	1/300
40	1/100
42	1/60
45	1/30

19 Reciprocal Translocation

- rearrangement and transfer of genetic material between two nonhomologous chromosomes
- leads to:

Table 19.6 Common nondisjunction conditions

Syndrome	Chromosomal error	Clinical features
Down	**Trisomy 21** Nondisjunction: 95% Rob (14q; 21q) translocation	• Learning difficulty (most moderate, some severe): 100% • Cardiac (VSD, ASD, AVSD 1000 x risk): 40–50% • Hypothyroidism: 20–40% • Dementia: 10–15% • Acute lymphoblastic leukaemia: less common • Facial: epicanthic folds, upslanting palpebral fissures, flat midface, brachycephaly
Edwards	**Trisomy 18** Nondisjunction: most Translocation + other	• Poor prenatal and postnatal outcome: rarely survive to age one • Learning difficulty (severe): 100% • Cardiac (VSD common): 90% • Spina bifida • Facial: clefts • Body: clenched hands, rocker-bottom feet

Patau	**Trisomy 13**
	Nondisjunction: 90%
	Rob (13q; 14q) translocation
		• Mostly spontaneous pregnancy loss
		• Poor postnatal outcome
		• Learning difficulty (severe): 100%
		• Cardiac (VSD, ASD): 80%
		• Renal anomalies
		• Omphalocele
		• Facial:
		  ◦ holoprosencephaly: 60–70%
		  ◦ microphthalmia / anophthalmia: 60–70%
		  ◦ cleft: 60–70%
		• Body: postaxial polydactyly (60–70%)

Table 19.6 (cont.)

Syndrome	Chromosomal error	Clinical features
Klinefelter	**XXY** (in XY individual)	• IQ: lower end of normal range • Tall stature • Gynaecomastia • Infertility
Triple X	**XXX** (in XX individual)	• IQ: lower end of normal range • Tall stature • Fertility: normal
XYY	**XYY** (in XY individual)	• IQ: lower end of normal range • Tall stature after puberty • Behavioural problems
Turner	**45,X** (in XX individual)	• Many do not survive to term due to hydrops • IQ: 10–15% less • Raised nuchal translucency

VSD: ventricular septal defect; ASD: atrial septal defect; AVSD: atrioventricular septal defect

- balanced reciprocal translocation: balanced exchange of material and overall normal amount of genetic material; phenotype normal
- unbalanced reciprocal translocation: one chromosome with more genetic material (trisomy) and the other with less genetic material (monosomy); phenotype abnormal

• commonest type: t(11; 22)(q23; q11) [chromosome 11 and 22 translocation]

1 parent with balanced reciprocal translocation + 1 parent normal → leads to 4 possible outcomes:

1. Normal pregnancy + normal karyotype
2. Normal pregnancy + balanced reciprocal translocation
3. Spontaneous miscarriage: due to unbalanced reciprocal translocation
4. Pregnancy to term + high risk of learning difficulties and congenital anomalies: due to unbalanced reciprocal translocation

• prenatal diagnosis of translocation:
  - if unbalanced reciprocal translocation in embryo → prenatal counselling
  - if balanced reciprocal translocation in embryo → parental karyotyping needed
    - if balanced reciprocal translocation in parent → likely no concern in child
    - if no balanced reciprocal translocation in parent → may lead to problem in child → recommend microarray comparative genomic hybridisation (array-CGH) to test for microdeletion

20 Robertsonian Translocation

• can only occur on acrocentric chromosomes: 13, 14, 15, 21, 22
• due to two long arms of acrocentric chromosomes fusing + short arms lost
• genes on the short arm are attached elsewhere: phenotype normal
• commonest types:
  - rob (13q; 14q): fusion of chromosome 13 to 14
  - rob (14q; 21q): fusion of chromosome 14 to 21
• imprinting:
  - one parental allele silenced
  - imprinting genes only on chromosomes 14 + 15
• trisomy rescue:
  - trisomy error rescued through reduction from three copies of chromosome to two copies of chromosome, leading to a balanced translocation
  - if the resultant two copies of chromosome are from the same parental origin (uniparental disomy) + contains imprinted genes → can be phenotypically abnormal (see Tables 19.7 and 19.8)

Table 19.7 Uniparental disomy 14 (UPD14)

	Wang syndrome	Temple syndrome
Chromosome abnormality	Paternal uniparental disomy of chromosome 14	Maternal uniparental disomy of chromosome 14
Trisomy rescue	47,XY + 14 OR 47,XX + 14	47,XY + 14 OR 47,XX + 14
After imprinting	46,XX OR 46,XY + 2 paternal chromosome 14	46,XX OR 46,XY + 2 maternal chromosome 14
Features	• Mostly spontaneous miscarriage • Severe learning difficulties • Feeding difficulties • Joint contractures	• Mostly survive to term • Small for gestational age • Learning difficulties • Hypotonia • Macrocephaly

Table 19.8 Uniparental disomy 15 (UPD15)

	Angelman syndrome	Prader–Willi syndrome
Chromosome abnormality	Paternal uniparental disomy of chromosome 15	Maternal uniparental disomy of chromosome 15
Trisomy rescue	47,XY + 15 OR 47,XX + 15	47,XY + 15 OR 47,XX + 15
After imprinting	46,XX OR 46,XY + 2 paternal chromosome 15	46,XX OR 46,XY + 2 maternal chromosome 15
Features	• Severe learning difficulties • Ataxic gait • Characteristic facial features	• Severe learning difficulties • Poor feeder as neonates • Insatiable appetite from childhood • Hypotonic • Short stature

1 parent with balanced Robertsonian translocation + 1 parent normal → leads to 6 possible outcomes:

1. Normal pregnancy + normal karyotype
2. Normal pregnancy + balanced Robertsonian translocation
3. Spontaneous miscarriage: due to unbalanced Robertsonian translocation (fetus trisomic or monosomic)
4. Spontaneous miscarriage: due to imprinting effect
5. Child with abnormalities: due to trisomy (monosomy will miscarry)
    - if mother carried balanced Robertsonian translocation: risk 10–15%
    - if father carried balanced Robertsonian translocation: risk <1%
6. Child with abnormalities: due to imprinting effect (risk <0.5%)

21 Chromosome Deletions

- microarray CGH: technique to detect microdeletions + microduplications
- not all are pathogenic (see Tables 19.9 and 19.10)

22 Modes of Inheritance

22.1 Types

1. Autosomal dominant
2. Autosomal recessive
3. X-linked dominant
4. X-linked recessive

22.2 Autosomal Dominant

- affected parent + unaffected parent → 50% children affected + 50% children not affected
- pedigree:
    - every generation is affected
    - male = women
    - both man + woman can have affected children

22.3 Autosomal Recessive

- pedigree:
    - only one generation affected
    - parents of affected children may be consanguineous (see Tables 19.12, 19.13, 19.14, 19.15 and 19.20)

Table 19.9 Chromosome microdeletion syndromes

Microdeletion	Syndrome	Clinical features
1p36		• Learning difficulty (severe) • Seizures • Hypotonia • Feeding difficulties • Facial: low-set horizontal eyebrows, deep-set eyes
4p15	Wolf–Hirschhorn	• Learning difficulty (severe) • Low birthweight, failure to thrive • Facial: 'Greek helmet' profile
5p15	Cri du chat	• Learning difficulty (severe) • Cat-like cry • Facial: bitemporal narrowing, hypertelorism, downslanted palpebral fissures
7q11	Williams	• Learning difficulty (mild–moderate) • Cardiac (supravalvular aortic/pulmonary stenosis) • Renal artery stenosis • Facial: short upturned nose, long philtrum, wide mouth, periorbital fullness • Personality: 'cocktail party' (outgoing)
8q24	Langer–Giedion	• Contiguous gene deletion • Learning disability (mild–moderate) • Facial: fine sparse hair, bulbous nose • Body: brittle nails, cone-shaped epiphyses (TRPS1 gene deletion), exostoses
17p11	Smith–Magenis	• Learning difficulty (severe) • Behavioural problems (self-harm) • Sleep problems • Facial: square-shaped face, heavy eyebrows
17p13	Miller–Dieker	• Lissencephaly • Facial: vertical furrowing on forehead, hypertelorism, short nose, anteverted nares
22q11	DiGeorge	• Learning difficulty (mild–moderate) • Cardiac (tetralogy of Fallot, VSD, interrupted aortic arch) • Psychiatric disorder • Renal anomaly • Hypocalcaemia • T cell immune disorder • Facial: cleft palate, velopharyngeal insufficiency, tubular nose, narrow palpebral fissures, simple ears • Body: short stature

Table 19.10 Gene abnormalities

Abnormality	Description	Example
Missense mutation	• Single base substitution	T**C**C → T**G**C
Frameshift mutation	• 1–2 base (not multiple of 3) insertion or deletion	CAG CCG ACT → CAG **T**CC GAC T
Nonsense mutation	• Single base substitution leading to stop codon	ACG GAA → ACG **T**AA (TAA is stop codon)
Splice site mutation	• Mutation at splice site (junction between introns and exons) • Leads to introns removed + 2 exons joined together	EXON1 **INTRON** EXON2 → EXON1 EXON2
Exon deletion (partial gene)	• ≥1 exon deleted	Duchenne muscular dystrophy

Table 19.10 (cont.)

Abnormality	Description	Example
Triplet repeat expansion	• Excessive duplication of single codon • Anticipation: progression of repeat size and severity in next generation • Parent-of-origin effect: more repeat size in mother rather than father + vice versa	Fragile X, Huntington's

Bold text denotes affected allele

Table 19.11 Autosomal dominant

		Affected parent	
		A	A
Unaffected parent	a	**A**a (**affected**)	aa (not affected)
	a	**A**a (**affected**)	aa (not affected)
		50% offspring affected **50% offspring not affected**	

Bold text denotes affected allele

Table 19.12 Autosomal recessive

		Affected parent	
		A	**A**
Unaffected parent	a	**A**a (**carrier**)	**A**a (**carrier**)
	a	**A**a (**carrier**)	**A**a (**carrier**)
		100% offspring carriers	

Bold text denotes affected allele

Table 19.13 Autosomal recessive

		Carrier parent	
		A	**a**
Unaffected parent	a	Aa (not affected)	**A**a (**carrier**)
	a	Aa (not affected)	**A**a (**carrier**)
		50% offspring carriers **50% offspring not affected**	

Bold text denotes affected allele

Table 19.14 Autosomal recessive

		Affected parent	
		A	**a**
Carrier parent	a	**A**a (**carrier**)	**A**a (**carrier**)
	a	**Aa** (**affected**)	A**a** (**affected**)
		50% offspring affected **50% offspring carriers**	

Bold text denotes affected allele

Table 19.15 Autosomal recessive

		Carrier parent	
		A	**A**
Carrier parent	a	Aa (not affected)	**A**a (**carrier**)
	a	A**a** (**carrier**)	**aa** (**affected**)
		25% offspring affected **50% offspring carrier** **25% offspring not affected**	

Bold text denotes affected allele

Table 19.16 X-linked recessive

		Affected father	
		X	Y
Unaffected mother	X	**X**X (**carrier**)	XY (not affected)
	X	**X**X (**carrier**)	XY (not affected)
		50% female offspring carrier **100% male offspring not affected**	

Bold text denotes affected allele

22.4 X-linked Dominant

- mostly restricted to women (males usually lead to miscarriage or neonatal death) (See Table 19.21)

22.5 X-linked Recessive

- males affected: only one X chromosome
- women not usually affected: two X chromosomes
- pedigree:
  - only males affected (women may be milder form)
  - no male-to-male transmission
  - skips generations (see Tables 19.16, 19.17, 19.18 and 19.22)

Table 19.17 X-linked recessive

		Unaffected father	
		X	Y
Carrier mother	**X**	**X**X (**carrier**)	**X**Y (**affected**)
	X	XX (not affected)	XY (not affected)
		50% female offspring carrier 50% female offspring not affected 50% male offspring affected 50% male offspring not affected	

Bold text denotes affected allele

Table 19.18 X-linked recessive

		Affected father	
		X	Y
Carrier mother	**X**	**XX** (**affected**)	**X**Y (**affected**)
	X	**X**X (**carrier**)	XY (not affected)
		50% female offspring affected 50% female offspring carrier 50% male offspring affected 50% male offspring not affected	

Bold text denotes affected allele

Table 19.19 Autosomal dominant diseases

Disease	Gene	Clinical features
Tuberous sclerosis	TSC1, TSC2	• Suspect prenatally if cardiac rhabdomyosarcomas seen • Skin: angiofibromata, hypomelanotic macules, shagreen patches • Neurological: brain hamartoma (seizure) • Renal: angiomyolipomata
Marfan	Fibrillin 1	• Cardiac: aortic dilatation • Body: tall stature, arm-height ratio >1.05, long fingers, dolichocephaly
Neurofibromatosis type 1	NF1	• Eye: optic glioma • Skin: café au lait spots, neurofibromata, axillary/inguinal freckling
Breast/ovarian cancer	BRCA1, BRCA2	• Breast cancer: 80% lifetime risk • Ovarian cancer: 20–40% lifetime risk
Hereditary nonpolyposis colon cancer	MLH	• Colon, endometrial, gastric, ovarian cancers
Huntington's	Huntingtin	• Movement disorder • Dementia • Psychiatric disorder
Polycystic kidney disease	PKD1, PKD2	• Cysts: kidney, liver, pancreas, spleen • Cardiac: mitral valve prolapse • Brain: intracranial aneurysm
Achondroplasia	FGFR3	• Short stature with proximal shortening • Relative macrocephaly

Table 19.20 Autosomal recessive diseases

Disease	Gene	Clinical features
Cystic fibrosis	CFTR	• Lung + pancreatic dysfunction
Spinal muscular atrophy	SMN	• Symmetrical proximal muscle weakness • Type of disease determines life expectancy
Tay-Sachs	HEXA	• GM_2 gangliosidosis • Cherry-red spot on retina • Motor + cognitive worsening
Haemochromatosis	HFE	• Excessive iron absorption • Iron deposits: liver (cirrhosis), pancreas (diabetes), skin (bronze skin)
α1-Antitrypsin deficiency	SERPINA1	• Lung: emphysema • Liver: cirrhosis
Congenital adrenal hyperplasia (21-hydroxylase deficiency)	CYP21A2	• Cannot synthesise cortisol • Female virilisation • Abnormal puberty: precocious in boys • Salt wasting
Connexin 26 mutation	GJB2	• Deafness

Table 19.21 X-linked dominant diseases

Disease	Gene	Clinical features
Incontinentia pigmenti	NEMO	• Blister → Blaschko's lines → hyperpigment → atrophic streaks
Rett	MECP2	• Learning difficult (severe), cognitive regression • Movement: hand wringing

Table 19.22 X-linked recessive diseases

Disease	Gene	Clinical features
Duchenne muscular dystrophy	Dystropin	• Proximal muscle myopathy • Death due to respiratory failure
Haemophilia A	Factor VIII gene	• Abnormal clotting, joint/muscle bleeding
Ocular albinism	GPR143	• Iris + retina hypopigmented, nystagmus, poor vision, abnormal decussation of optic nerves
X-linked adrenoleukodystrophy	ACBD1	• Very long-chain fatty acids in adrenal gland (adrenal failure) + brain (cognitive deterioration)
Fragile X	FMR1	• Triplet expansion of CGG • Learning difficulty

20 Genomics and Gene Regulation

Jane Ding

1 Laboratory Techniques

1.1 Blotting

See Table 20.1.

1.2 Polymerase Chain Reaction (PCR)

- aim: amplify specific DNA/RNA sequences in a sample with many DNA/RNA fragments
- if RNA is being amplified, it must first be transcribed into complementary DNA
- steps:
  1. Attach primer onto target DNA
  2. Taq polymerase adds nucleotides onto new DNA strand
  3. Process repeated to produce many DNA copies

1.3 DNA Microarrays

- aim: allows simultaneous analysis of thousands of gene expressions
- microarray is a commercially produced collection of fluorescently labelled DNA short oligonucleotides
- steps:
  1. Isolate RNA from cells
  2. Translate RNA into complementary DNA
  3. Hybridise cDNA onto microarray oligonucleotides

1.4 Bioinformatics

- definition: computing method to store, distribute and analyse large reported DNA information
- researchers report DNA fragment information into databanks
- databanks are accessible via the Internet

1.5 Proteomics

- definition: the study of the structure and function of proteins

2 Cell Cycle Control: Cancer Development, Growth, Spread

2.1 Cancer

- most cancers are caused by mutations in somatic cells (rather than germ cells)
- it takes many years to accumulate the mutations (mutations need at least 20 years to cause cancer)

Table 20.1 Blotting

Type	Aim	Process
Southern	To detect the presence and amount of a particular DNA sequence in a sample with many DNA sequences	1. Electrophoresis: separates DNA fragments by size 2. DNA fragments blotted onto nitrocellulose membrane 3. DNA fragments fixed onto membrane 4. Membrane exposed to probe containing target DNA sequence 5. Target DNA sequence detection on X-ray
Northern	To detect the presence and amount of a particular RNA sequence in a sample with many RNA sequences	Similar to Southern blotting
Western	To detect the presence and amount of a particular protein in a tissue sample	1. Electrophoresis: separates denatured proteins 2. Proteins fixed to membrane 3. Antibody (with radioactive tag) against target protein applied 4. Target protein detected on X-ray

2.2 Cell Cycle Control Checkpoints

- DNA damage checkpoints:
  - where: S phase, G1, G2
  - damage detected → cyclin-dependent kinase 2 (CDK2) inhibited → cell cycle progression stopped
  - damage not repairable → apoptosis
- spindle checkpoint:
  - where: metaphase
  - spindle fibres fail to attach to kinetochores → apoptosis

2.3 Signalling Proteins

- signalling proteins include growth factors (+ receptors), signal transduction proteins and transcription factors
- gain-of-function in these proteins can lead to cancer
- mutated alleles usually dominant

2.4 Cell Cycle Control Proteins

- cell cycle control proteins are usually tumour-suppressor proteins
- loss of function in these proteins can lead to cancer
- mutated alleles are usually recessive
- adenomatous polyposis coli (APC):
  - function:
    - activates transcription factor Myc → transcribes genes pushing movement from G1 to S phase
  - mutation:
    - if APC mutated → inappropriately activates Myc → uncontrolled cell proliferation
    - requires both APC alleles to be mutated for the protein to fail
- p53:
  - functions:
    - detects DNA damage
    - blocks CDK2
    - activates apoptosis
  - mutation:
    - requires both p53 alleles to be mutated for the protein to fail
    - fifty percent of cancers have mutations in p53
- ataxia telangiectasia mutated:
  - detects DNA damage
  - stops cell cycle
  - maintains normal telomere length: prevents chromosome shortening with DNA replication

2.5 Oncogenic Viruses

- some viruses contain proto-oncogenes and oncogenes
- DNA viruses:
  - need oncogenes for their own viral survival
  - example: human papillomavirus family
- RNA viruses:
  - retrovirus enters host → makes DNA copies from viral RNA → DNA copies inserted into host's DNA for viral replication → oncogenes produced
  - examples:
    - — Harvey sarcoma virus:
      - contains Ha-ras gene (differs from the human ras gene by a single-point mutation)
      - Ha-ras overexpression → bladder cancer
    - — Rous sarcoma virus
      - produces v-Src protein, which is a constitutively active mutant of human c-Src protein
      - leads to continuous phosphorylation of proteins

2.6 Cancer Cells

- characteristics:
  - less well differentiated
  - lose their specific function
  - become rapidly growing
- can be in one of three states:
  1. Constantly going through the cell cycle
  2. In Gap 0 (G0) state, but can enter the cell cycle any time
  3. Can no longer divide, but still contribute to tumour size

- cisplatin:
  - platinum anti-cancer drug
  - only affects dividing cells (in some tumours, only 5% are in this stage)
  - cannot discriminate between normal cells and cancer cells

2.7 Metastasis

- benign tumours: do not metastasise
- malignant tumours: metastasise (spread to secondary sites)
- steps of tumour cell spread:
  1. Breaks down adhesive contact with other cells
  2. Secretes plasminogen activator, which makes plasmin
  3. Plasmin breaks down basal lamina (basement membrane)
  4. Cells spread into bloodstream (<1 in 10 000 cancer cells survive through the bloodstream)
  5. Attaches to the endometrium of target site

Table 20.2 Prenatal tests

Screening tests	Diagnostic tests
– Combined test	– Chorionic villus sampling
– Triple test	– Amniocentesis
– Quadruple test	– Cordocentesis
– Integrated test	
– Sequential test	
– Cell-free fetal DNA	

2.8 Angiogenesis

- required to grow beyond 10^6 cells (2 mm diameter)
- tumours secrete various growth factors (VEGF)

3 Prenatal Diagnosis and Testing

- screening tests provide risk of getting a disease but are *not* diagnostic:
  - cut off for high risk 1:150
- if a screening test demonstrates high risk → diagnostic test then offered – see Table 20.2 and Table 20.5

3.1 Nuchal Translucency

- definition of nuchal translucency (NT): subcutaneous fluid at the back of fetal neck between 11–14/40 – see Tables 20.3 and 20.4
- NT increased in:
  - chromosomal abnormalities: trisomy 21
  - cardiac abnormalities
  - single-gene defects: Noonan syndrome
  - skeletal dysplasia

3.2 Cell-free fetal DNA (cffDNA)

- detects cell-free fetal DNA present in the maternal bloodstream
- for trisomy 13, 18, 21, fetal sexing, rhesus blood typing

Table 20.3 Screening tests and detection rate for trisomy 21

Test	Description of test	Detection rate
NT only		70–75%
NT + nasal bone		80–85%
NT + ductus venosus		80–85%
Combined test	NT + PAPP-A + β-hCG	90%
Triple test	α-FP + β-hCG + μE_3	70%
Quadruple test	α-FP + β-hCG + μE_3 + inhibin	81%
Integrated test	NT + PAPP-A + quadruple test	86%
Sequential test	Same as integrated but quad test done only if high risk with NT + PAPP-A	95%

PAPP-A: pregnancy-associated plasma protein A; β-hCG: β-human chorionic gonadotropin; μE_3: unconjugated estriol; α-FP: alpha-fetoprotein

Table 20.4 Markers for trisomy 21

Increased	Decreased	Others
• NT • β-hCG • Inhibin	• μE_3 • PAPP-A	• α-FP: no change • Nasal bone: absent / hypoplastic • Ductus venosus: absent / reversed A-wave

α-FP: alpha-fetoprotein

Table 20.5 Prenatal diagnostic tests

	Chorionic villus sampling	Amniocentesis	Cordocentesis
Diagnosis	• Chromosomal abnormality	• Chromosomal abnormality • Prenatal infection	• Chromosomal abnormality • fetal anaemia • Prenatal infection
Timing	$11–14^{+6}/40$	$\geq 15^{+0}/40$	$\geq 18^{+0}/40$
Cells collected from	Chorionic villi: placental cells	Amniocyte: fetal cells	fetal blood from umbilical vein
Direct result	2–3 days (If direct result abnormal → wait for culture result)	None	None
Culture result	1–3 weeks	1–3 weeks	1–3 weeks
Advantage	Fast direct result	If mosaicism detected: likely from fetus	If mosaicism detected: likely from fetus
Disadvantage	Miscarriage rate 1% Confined placental mosaicism • Chromosome abnormality in placental but *not* fetal tissue • Occurs in 1.5% of pregnancies • Presence can affect placental functioning: fetal growth restriction	Miscarriage rate 1%	Miscarriage rate 1–2%

4 Prenatal Diagnosis Laboratory Techniques

See Table 20.6.

4.1 Fluorescence in Situ Hybridisation (FISH)

- for interphase chromosomes
- DNA fluorescent probe attaches to the DNA sequence of interest

4.2 Quantitative Fluorescence PCR (QF-PCR)

- primer attaches to short tandem repeats on target DNA sequence → PCR amplification of target DNA

4.3 Multiplex Ligation-dependent Probe Amplification (MLPA)

- MLPA probe contains short DNA sequence
- primer with MLPA probe attaches to target DNA sequence → PCR amplification of MLPA probe

4.4 Array-CGH

- compares DNA from test to reference for deletion or duplication
- test and reference mixed → ratios of test to reference DNA (1:1, 1.5:1, 0.5:1) elicits specific colours

Table 20.6 Prenatal diagnosis laboratory techniques

Test	Use	Features
FISH	• Aneuploidy • Unbalanced translocation • Chromosome microdeletion	• Expensive • Labour intensive
QF-PCR	• Aneuploidy: only 13, 18, 21	• Rapid (1–2 days) • Cheap
MLPA	• Aneuploidy • Unbalanced translocation	• Rapid
Array-CGH	• Aneuploidy • Chromosome microdeletion • Chromosome microduplication	• Rapid

4.5 DNA Sequencing

- detects abnormalities within specific genes by sequencing parts of DNA
- next-generation sequencing steps
  1. DNA fragmented
  2. DNA adaptor ligated to ends of DNA fragments
  3. Fluorescent DNA primer added to adaptors
  4. Bases that are added are identified by fluorescent signal

4.6 Preimplantation Genetic Diagnosis

- used to determine the risk of a specific inherited condition in an embryo
- IVF → remove 1–2 cells from embryo at the 8-cell stage for analysis → low-risk embryo transferred to uterus

5 Genetics of Gynaecological Cancers

See Table 20.7.

Table 20.7 Genetics of gynaecological cancers

Gene mutation	Cancer	Lifetime risk
BRCA1	Breast Ovarian	60–90% 40–60%
BRCA2	Breast Ovarian	45–85% 10–30%
Mismatch repair (HNPCC)	Ovarian Endometrial	4% 50%
LKB1 (Peutz–Jeghers)	Endometrial Gastrointestinal	40% 30%
PTEN (Cowden)	Endometrial, breast, thyroid	Uncertain

PTEN: phosphatase and tensin

5.1 BRCA

- contributes to <2% of breast cancers
- if found to have BRCA mutation → recommend bilateral salpingo-oophorectomy → reduces ovarian cancer risk to 1% (primary peritoneal ovarian cancer) and breast cancer by 50%

5.2 Hereditary Nonpolyposis Colon Cancer (HNPCC)

- involves colon, gastric, ovarian and endometrial cancers

Section 5

Endocrinology

Jyotsna Pundir

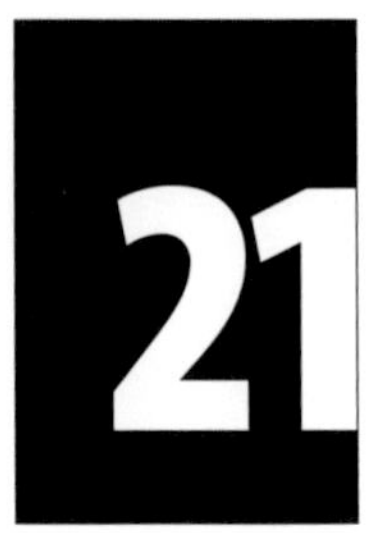

Mechanism of Action of Hormones

Jyotsna Pundir

1 Types of Hormones

1. Polypeptides:
    a. Most hypothalamic hormones
    b. Anterior and posterior pituitary hormones
    c. Pancreas and gastrointestinal (GIT) hormones
    d. Growth factors

Most hormones are peptides. Usually, these hormones are in the form of a preprohormone, which is then cleaved to form a prohormone and then the hormone. Some peptides are secreted immediately while others are stored in secretory granules.

2. Steroids:
    a. Adrenal cortex
    b. Gonadal hormones
    c. Fetoplacental unit

Steroids are the most important group of reproductive hormones. Their precursor is cholesterol derived either from circulatory low-density lipoprotein or from intracellular cholesterol esters; and all have 17-carbon atom basic ring structure with a different number of carbon atoms added.

- glucocorticoids, aldosterone and progesterone: 21 carbon atoms
- testosterone and other androgens: 19 carbon atoms
- estrogens: 18 carbon atoms

3. Amino acid hormones: some hormones such as thyroxine, catecholamines (derived from tyrosine) and melatonin (derived from tryptophan) are derived from amino acids. These are stored in granules and are regulated either by their release or by the expression of the enzymes necessary for their synthesis.
4. Prostaglandins and leukotrienes: known as eicosanoids and are derived from arachidonic acid. These are synthesised in the cell wall and release into cytoplasm or out of the cell.

2 Mechanism of action of Hormones

Hormones are the chemical messengers secreted in the bloodstream by the endocrine gland. They are target specific and bind to the specific receptor. On the basis of binding of hormone on their specific receptor, the mechanism of hormonal action is categorised into two groups:

1. Fixed membrane receptor mechanism
2. Mobile receptor mechanism

2.1 Fixed Membrane Receptor Mechanism

- Hormones that are protein or amines are water soluble and cannot pass through the lipid membrane.
- They have target receptors fixed on the cell membrane.
- The first messenger is the hormone that binds to the membrane receptor. Binding of hormone on a specific receptor on the target cell activates the enzyme adenyl cyclase in the cell membrane, which converts adenosine triphosphate to cyclic adenosine 3,5-monophosphate (cAMP).
- cAMP acts as a secondary messenger, which diffuses through the cell membrane and leads to phosphorylation of cAMP-dependent protein kinases, which results in various enzymatic reactions to cause biochemical changes.
- After the target cell responds to the changes, cAMP is deactivated by a group of enzymes called phosphodiesterases.
- A few peptide hormones activate calcium release via second messengers in the calcium signalling system.

- Neurotransmitters and peptide hormones mainly act on cell-surface receptors. Examples include polypeptide hormones: adrenocorticotropic hormone (ACTH), follicle stimulating hormone, luteinising hormone, thyroid stimulating hormone, growth hormone, parathyroid hormone, antidiuretic hormone, oxytocin, insulin, glucagon, adrenaline, biogenic amines and some prostaglandins.

2.2 Mobile Receptor Mechanism

- Lipid-soluble hormones (steroid and fatty acids hormones) can easily pass through the plasma membrane, with receptors in the cytoplasm. Binding of hormone to the specific receptor activates the enzymatic activity for biochemical changes.
- Some hormones (testosterone, progesterone, estrogen, cortisol, thyroxine and somatomedin) have receptors inside the nucleus. The hormone-receptor complex is carried inside the nucleus, which initiates transcription of the DNA to form specific mRNA.
- mRNA initiates protein (enzyme) synthesis in the cytoplasm, which results in biochemical changes in the cell. See Figure 21.1.

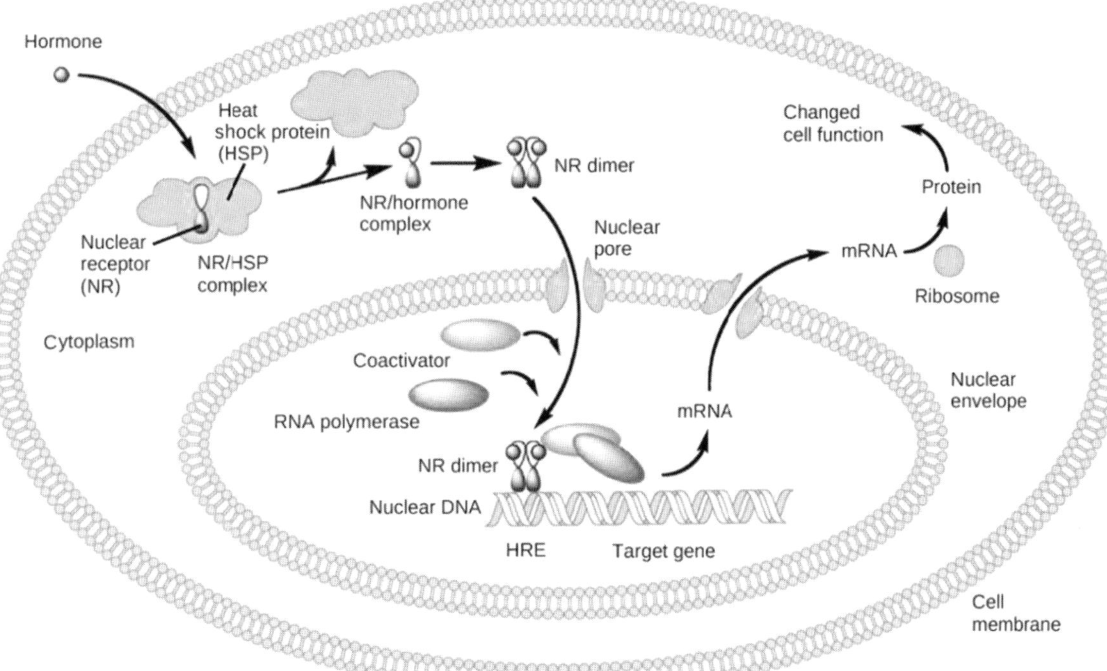

Figure 21.1 Mechanism of action of hormones. Used with permission from Lumen.

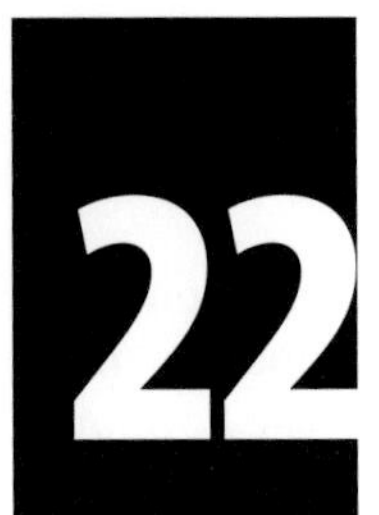

Hypothalamus and Pituitary

Jyotsna Pundir

1 Embryology

- In the early embryo, neuroectoderm of the forebrain (prosencephalon) primary brain vesicle divides to form two secondary brain vesicles: telencephalon (endbrain, cortex) and diencephalon. The thalamus and hypothalamus develop in the lateral walls of the diencephalon; the cavity that becomes the third ventricle.
- The pituitary forms two parts: the anterior adenohypophysis and the posterior neurohypophysis (hypophysis is an amalgam of two tissues). Early in gestation (4–5 weeks), a finger of ectoderm grows upwards from the roof of the mouth (oropharynx). This protrusion is called Rathke's pouch, which is eventually separated from the oral cavity by the sphenoid bone of the skull, and develops into the anterior pituitary or adenohypophysis. At the same time, another finger of ectodermal tissue evaginates ventrally from the diencephalon (floor of the third ventricle), which becomes the posterior pituitary or neurohypophysis. Ultimately, the two tissues grow into one another and become tightly apposed.
- When cells from the Rathke's pouch are left behind and form tumours, these are called craniopharyngiomas.
- The neurohypophysis (posterior pituitary) is in direct contact with the hypothalamus, while the anterior pituitary is connected to the hypothalamus via a rich vascular portal system.
- The hypothalamic-pituitary axis is established by 20 weeks of gestation.

2 Anatomy

- Hypothalamus:
    - superior: thalamus separated by hypothalamic sulcus
    - medially: third ventricle
    - inferiorly: pituitary stalk
    - anterior, lateral and posteriorly: no distinct boundaries
- Pituitary: lies within the sella turcica of the sphenoid bone at the base of the brain; it is about the size of a pea and weighs 0.5 g:
    - anteriorly: sphenoid sinus
    - inferiorly: sphenoid sinus
    - laterally: cavernous sinus with internal carotid arteries and sixth cranial nerve
    - posteriorly: clinoid processes of the sphenoid bone
    - superiorly: pituitary stalk, which merges into hypothalamus; anterior to the pituitary stalk is the optic chiasma, which may be compressed by an expanding pituitary tumour, resulting in bitemporal hemianopia
- The pituitary is connected to the hypothalamus by the infundibulum; a stalk containing nerve fibres and blood vessels.
- Blood supply: the hypothalamus, pituitary stalk and pituitary are supplied by carotid arteries via the superior and inferior hypophyseal arteries.
- Anterior pituitary:
    - chromophobes: do not stain, resting cells (chromophobe adenoma may secrete gonadotropin subunits)
    - acidophils: prolactin and growth hormone (GH)
    - basophils: gonadotropins, thyroid stimulating hormone (TSH) and adrenocorticotropic hormone (ACTH)
- The posterior pituitary is an outgrowth of the hypothalamus and its neural tissue. The axons of the paraventricular and supraoptic nuclei (hypothalamic nuclei) pass down the

Table 22.1 Hypothalamic hormones

Hormone	Role	Number of amino acids	Source
Gonadotropin-releasing hormone (GnRH)	↑ LH and FSH	10	Preoptic area
Corticotropin-releasing hormone (CRH)	↑ ACTH	41	Anterior paraventricular nucleus
Growth hormone releasing hormone (GHRH)	↑ GH	44	Arcuate nucleus
Somatostatin (SS)	↓ GH	14	Periventricular area
Thyrotropin-releasing hormone	↑ TRH	3	Medial paraventricular nucleus
Dopamine; prolactin inhibiting factor (PIF)	↓ PRL		Arcuate nucleus

LH: luteinising hormone; FSH: follicle stimulating hormone; ↑: increased; ↓: decreased; PRL: prolactin; TRH: thyroid releasing hormone; GH: growth hormone; ACTH: adrenocorticotropic hormone

infundibulum to the posterior pituitary with their terminals ending directly on capillaries. These synthesise and release oxytocin and vasopressin.

- Anterior pituitary: there are no neuronal connections with the hypothalamus; instead it is connected with hypothalamic-pituitary portal blood vessels.

3 Hypothalamic hormones

See Table 22.1.

4 Pituitary hormones

See Table 22.2.

- Antidiuretic hormone: majority is released from the supraoptic nucleus in the hypothalamus.
- Oxytocin: released from the paraventricular nucleus in the hypothalamus. Oxytocin is one of the few hormones to create a positive feedback loop. For example, uterine contractions stimulate the release of oxytocin from the posterior pituitary, which, in turn, increases uterine contractions, which continues throughout labour.
- During lactation, PRL exerts a secondary role to inhibit gonadotropin secretion, thereby reducing fertility.
- The hypothalamic-pituitary-hormonal axis:
  - Long-loop negative feedback: the hormone secreted by the third endocrine gland in a sequence exerts a negative feedback effect on the hypothalamus/pituitary (e.g., GnRH, TRH and CRH).
  - Short-loop negative feedback: the anterior pituitary hormones may exert a short-loop negative feedback inhibition on the hypothalamus. PRL acts on the hypothalamus to stimulate secretion of dopamine, which then inhibits secretion of PRL (e.g., PRL and GH).
  - Hormones not in a particular sequence can also influence secretion of the hypothalamus and/or anterior pituitary hormones. estrogen enhances secretion of PRL by the anterior pituitary.

5 Growth Hormone

- GH is produced by the pituitary somatotroph cells. Its production begins early in fetal life and continues throughout childhood and adult life, although at a progressively lower rate in the latter. GH production falls by approximately 50% every seven years. It declines from a peak during puberty to approximately one-sixth by 55 years of age.
- Its secretion is pulsatile.
- The half-life of GH in circulation is about 20 minutes.
- It stimulates hepatic synthesis and secretion of insulin-like growth factor 1, a potent growth and differentiation factor and is likely responsible for most of the growth-promoting activities of GH. Insulin-like growth factor 1 mediates most of the peripheral actions of GH.
- GH stimulates linear growth in children by acting directly and indirectly (via the synthesis of insulin-like growth factor 1) on the epiphyseal plates of long bones.
- Metabolic actions:
  - increased lipolysis, leading to mobilisation of stored triglyceride
  - stimulates protein synthesis
  - helps to maintain blood glucose levels

Table 22.2 Pituitary hormones

Hormone	Target	Role	Type	Amino acid size and weight (Da)
		Anterior pituitary		
GH	• Liver and other cells • Many organs and tissues	• Secretes insulin-like growth factor 1 (Insulin-like growth factor 1) • Stimulates growth by protein synthesis, carbohydrate and lipid metabolism	Protein	191 21 500
ACTH	Adrenal cortex	Stimulates release of cortisol	Protein	39 4500
TSH	Thyroid	Stimulates release of thyroxine	Glycoprotein	201 28 000
FSH	Female ovaries Male testes	• Stimulates follicle to mature an egg • Secretes estrogen • Stimulates sperm production	Glycoprotein	204 30 000
LH	Female ovaries Male testes	• Stimulates ovulation and progesterone production Stimulates testosterone production	Glycoprotein	204 30 000
PRL	Breast	Breast development and milk production	Protein	198 22 000
		Posterior pituitary: stores and secretes (but does not synthesise)		
Antidiuretic hormone (ADH)/vasopressin	Kidney	Stimulates retention of water	Protein	9
Oxytocin	Uterus Breast	• Stimulates contraction during labour • Stimulates contraction to express milk	Protein	9

- insulin antagonist: may lead to glucose intolerance, diabetes and features of the metabolic syndrome in GH excess
- leads to phosphate, water and sodium retention

5.1 Excess of Growth Hormone: Acromegaly and Gigantism

- Incidence of excess growth hormone: 3–8 million people.
- Mean age at diagnosis: 40 to 45 years.
- GH excess before fusion of the epiphyseal growth plates in a child or adolescent leads to pituitary gigantism. After epiphyseal fusion, it leads to acromegaly.
- The most common cause of acromegaly is a somatotroph (GH-secreting) adenoma of the anterior pituitary.
- Onset is insidious, with usually very slow progression.
- Clinical features are attributable to high serum concentrations of both GH and insulin-like growth factor 1, which is GH dependent. They have both somatic and metabolic effects.
- Pressure effect: Some patients with acromegaly and large tumours have symptoms due to direct compressive effects of the tumour mass:

  - headache, visual field defects (bitemporal hemianopsia) and cranial nerve palsies
  - it can decrease secretion of other pituitary hormones, most commonly gonadotropins, resulting in hypogonadism
  - hyperprolactinaemia occurs in approximately 30% of patients
- Somatic effects: long-term GH and insulin-like growth factor 1 excess results in overgrowth of many tissues, including connective tissue, cartilage, bone, skin and visceral organs such as characteristic findings of enlarged jaw (macrognathia) and enlarged, swollen hands and feet, macroglossia and deepening of the voice.
- Visceral organs are enlarged in acromegaly, including the thyroid, heart, liver, lungs and kidneys.
- Metabolic effects include nitrogen retention, hyperinsulinaemia, insulin resistance, overt diabetes (10–15%), impaired glucose tolerance (50%) and lipolysis.
- Systemic complications: cardiovascular disease, sleep apnoea, metabolic disorders and colon neoplasia (polyps and cancer).
- Cardiovascular: hypertension, left ventricular hypertrophy and cardiomyopathy.
- The mortality rate of patients with acromegaly appears to be increased; death is primarily from cardiovascular disease.

5.1.1 Diagnosis

- Serum insulin-like growth factor 1 concentration: a normal serum insulin-like growth factor 1 concentration is strong evidence that the patient does not have acromegaly. If the serum Insulin-like growth factor 1 concentration is high (or equivocal), serum GH should be measured after oral glucose administration. Inadequate suppression of serum GH after a glucose load confirms the diagnosis of acromegaly.
- Pituitary MRI: a pituitary adenoma is found in most cases. If the MRI is normal, then studies to identify a GHRH or GH-secreting tumour should be undertaken.

5.1.2 Treatment

- Transsphenoidal surgery is undertaken for macroadenoma that appears to be fully resectable, or a macroadenoma threatening or impairing vision.
- Long-acting somatostatin analogues for:
  - adenoma that does not appear to be fully resectable
  - patients whose risk of surgery is great
  - patients who choose not to have surgery
- Medical therapy: long-acting somatostatin analogues, GH-receptor antagonists, dopamine agonists (cabergoline) for mild disease.
- If adenoma size increases or GH/insulin-like growth factor 1 hypersecretion persists despite medical therapy, radiation therapy or repeat surgery is required.

5.1.3 Women Who Want to Become Pregnant

- Rare in pregnancy, as many women are infertile because it is often associated with hyperprolactinaemia.
- Pregnancy should be postponed until GH and insulin-like growth factor 1 levels are controlled and no residual tumour mass is seen to minimise the risk of gestational diabetes mellitus (GDM) and pregnancy-induced hypertension (PIH).
- Medical therapy should be stopped once pregnancy is confirmed. Most adenomas do not grow during pregnancy.
- Bromocriptine and cabergoline may work in 50% of cases.
- Short-acting octreotide (somatostatin analogues) can be used during pregnancy, but only for control of headache and adenoma size, and only if the potential benefits outweigh risks.
- Monitor visual fields during pregnancy in women with macroadenomas starting at the end of the first trimester and every six weeks thereafter.

6 Hypogonadotropic Hypogonadism

Hypogonadotropic hypogonadism results from a defect at hypothalamic or pituitary level. It is characterised by low FSH and LH levels.

6.1 Causes

1. Functional hypothalamic amenorrhea (FHA):
   - Excludes organic disease.
   - It can occur from severe energy restriction, increased energy expenditure or stress, or combinations of the three.
   - Female athlete triad: young exercising women with restrictive eating and amenorrhea suffer with a triad of low energy availability,

menstrual dysfunction and low bone mineral density. Associated with amenorrhea, low serum gonadotropins and estradiol and, usually, evidence of a precipitating factor (exercise, low weight, stress).
- For restoration of menses and improvement in bone density, caloric intake should be increased and exercise decreased, or both.
- Behavioural therapy should be undertaken if there is a history of irregular eating behaviour or distorted body image, and resistance to decreasing exercise and/or weight gain to manage stress and improve coping strategies.
- Hormone replacement therapy (HRT) or combined contraceptive pills replace estradiol and progesterone.
- Fertility: ovulation induction should be undertaken once the woman has achieved a healthy weight.

2. Isolated GnRH deficiency (idiopathic hypogonadotropic hypogonadism (IHH)):
   - There is a functional absence of GnRH secretion from the hypothalamus or a defect in its action at the level of the gonadotrope (mutations in the GnRH receptor).
   - IHH (with or without anosmia) can be inherited.
   - It is characterised by low serum concentrations of LH and FSH, with normal anterior pituitary function, and normal MRI of the hypothalamic-pituitary region. Anti-müllerian hormone (AMH) levels are low to normal.
   - The main differential diagnosis is constitutional delay of growth and puberty. A definitive diagnosis of IHH in the absence of a family history or prior genetic testing is difficult to make until the patient reaches at least 18 years of age, unless other suggestive features are present.
   - Management: sex steroids should be replaced to develop secondary sex characteristics and to build and sustain normal bone and muscle mass. Gonadotropin (FSH^{+}/–LH) or pulsatile GnRH therapy are used for ovulation induction in women and for induction of spermatogenesis in men.
3. Severe systemic illnesses; for example, coeliac disease, inflammatory bowel disease.
4. Infiltrative diseases and tumours such as craniopharyngioma and germinoma: MRI is indicated if associated visual field defects, headaches, other evidence of hypothalamic or pituitary dysfunction, or symptoms are suggestive of other diseases.
5. Sheehan's syndrome (pituitary infarction after major obstetric haemorrhage):
   - Infarction of the pituitary gland after postpartum haemorrhage (PPH).
   - It can be associated with panhypopituitarism or partial hypopituitarism.
   - Associated with history of severe PPH, requiring transfusion of multiple units of blood.
   - It is characterised by the loss of anterior pituitary hormones: GH, prolactin, and gonadotropin deficiency, and, less commonly, TSH and ACTH. Rarely, overt diabetes insipidus develops (subclinical vasopressin deficiency is common).
   - Severe hypopituitarism: symptoms include lethargy, anorexia, weight loss and the inability to lactate during the first days or weeks after delivery. Features of hypothyroidism and adrenocortical insufficiency may be present.
   - Less severe hypopituitarism: symptoms include failure of postpartum lactation, resume menses in the weeks and months after delivery/or persistent amenorrhoea, loss of axillary and pubic hair, milder degrees of fatigue, anorexia and weight loss.
   - Eventual development of a small pituitary within a sella of normal size: as an 'empty sella' on MRI.

6.2 Diagnosis

- Blood tests: reduced levels of gonadotropins.
- Rule out hypopituitarism: measure thyroxine (T4), TSH, cortisol and insulin-like growth factor 1. Any patient with hypopituitarism should undergo an MRI of the pituitary to exclude a pituitary tumour.

6.3 Treatment

- May resolve spontaneously.
- Pregnancy is achieved with gonadotropin stimulation for ovulation induction. Once pregnancy is achieved, the fetoplacental unit

produces enough gonadotropins, E2 and progesterone to sustain the pregnancy; hence, there is no need for any additional adjuvant treatment.

- Women who do not desire pregnancy: estrogen replacement is prescribed in the form of HRT or combined pills.
- Replacement of pituitary hormones is the treatment. Prolactin deficiency results in inability to breastfeed, but no treatment is available.

7 Hyperprolactinaemia

- Prolactinomas: pituitary adenomas that secrete PRL.
- They are invariably benign. Over 90% are small, intrasellar tumours, which rarely increase in size:
  - microadenomas (<10 mm in diameter)
  - macroadenomas (>10 mm in diameter)
- PRL secretion is enhanced by estrogen and inhibited by dopamine.
- PRL stimulates milk production and also has secondary effects on gonadal function.
- PRL-secreting adenomas may also produce TSH or ACTH: this is uncommon.
- Age: 2 to 80 years. More common in women, with a peak incidence during the childbearing years.
- Other causes of hyperprolactinaemia:
  - drugs or situations that inhibit hypothalamic production of dopamine, its transport to the pituitary due to the compression of the pituitary stalk or its effectiveness at dopaminergic receptors
  - craniopharyngioma and other sellar or parasellar masses, granulomatous infiltration of the hypothalamus, head trauma and large pituitary adenomas
  - a large nonfunctional tumour in the hypothalamus or pituitary
  - mixed GH- and PRL-secreting tumours: acromegaly in association with hyperprolactinaemia
  - chronic renal or hepatic failure: due to decreased clearance of PRL
  - polycystic ovarian syndrome (PCOS) is commonly associated with mildly elevated PRL levels
  - primary hypothyroidism: some cases have mild hyperprolactinaemia; this is due to increased synthesis of, or sensitivity to, hypothalamic TRH, which is able to stimulate pituitary lactotroph cells, but the true cause is unknown
  - during pregnancy, there is a progressive increase in prolactin levels (as high as 10 times normal) because of pituitary lactotroph hyperplasia induced by the high estrogen levels secreted by the placenta
  - PRL levels can also rise modestly after exercise, meals, chest wall/breast stimulation, stress or sexual intercourse
  - idiopathic hyperprolactinaemia
  - drugs that reduce dopamine secretion or action: metoclopramide, phenothiazines, butyrophenones, risperidone, serotonin reuptake inhibitors (rare), sulpiride, domperidone and verapamil

7.1 Symptoms

- Premenopausal women present with oligo/amenorrhoea (90%), galactorrhoea (80%) and anovulatory infertility. Women with amenorrhea present with symptoms of estrogen deficiency.
- Postmenopausal women: usually pressure effects due to large adenoma.
- Children: delayed puberty, primary amenorrhoea and galactorrhoea. Because of the increased prevalence of macroadenomas, prolactinomas in children are more frequently accompanied by neurological symptoms.

7.2 Risks or Complications

- Hyperprolactinaemia interrupts the pulsatile secretion of GnRH, inhibits the release of LH and FSH, and directly impairs gonadal steroidogenesis, leading to primary or secondary amenorrhoea.
- Chronic hyperprolactinaemia-induced hypogonadism reduces bone mineral density (BMD). After PRL normalisation, BMD increases, but does not always return to normal.
- Pressure symptoms: very large tumours result in compression of other pituitary cells or of the hypothalamic-pituitary stalk, leading to hypopituitarism.
- Neurological manifestations are common with macroadenomas or giant adenomas because they

are space-occupying lesions with possible compression of the optic chiasma. These include headaches, visual impairment ranging from quadrantanopia to classical bitemporal hemianopia, or scotomas.

- Visual field defects are seen in up to 5% of cases.
- Blindness due to an expanding prolactinoma may occur in pituitary apoplexy.

7.3 Investigations

- PRL values are not absolute; prolactinomas can present with variable elevation in PRL, and there may be dissociation between tumour mass and hormonal secretion.
- Normal levels in women are <500 mIU/L (1 µg/L = 21.2 mIU/L):
  - microadenoma: moderately elevated PRL levels >1000 mIU/L
  - macroadenoma: levels of >5000 mIU/L
  - large nonfunctional tumours: PRL levels <3000 mIU/L
  - PRL values between the upper limits of normal and 2000 mIU/L may be due to psychoactive drugs, estrogen or idiopathic causes, but can also be caused by microprolactinomas.
- Repeat PRL measurement if PRL level is >1000 mIU/L and, if still elevated, investigate further with MRI.
- Formal visual field examination should be undertaken for patients with macroadenomas that abut the optic chiasma.
- Imaging:
  - gadolinium-enhanced MRI: to assess the extent of tumour, suprasellar extension and compression of optic chiasma or invasion of the cavernous sinus
  - a normal MRI does not necessarily exclude a microadenoma
- The empirical confirmation of the diagnosis can be obtained by medical treatment with dopamine with serial assessment of serum PRL levels and adenoma size.

7.4 Management

1. Expectant: may be self-limiting in up to one-third of women.
2. Medical: all patients with macroadenomas and most patients with microprolactinomas require treatment.
   - indications for treatment:
     - infertility
     - neurological effects (particularly visual defects)
     - bothersome galactorrhoea
     - longstanding hypogonadism
     - alterations in pubertal development
     - prevention of bone loss in women because of hypogonadism
   - dopaminergic agonists: bromocriptine and cabergoline; pergolide and quinagolide are less commonly used
   - bromocriptine is less expensive; it restores ovulation in 80–90% of patients, and reduces the size of prolactinomas in 70% of cases
   - cabergoline is longer acting, and significantly better than bromocriptine in terms of patient tolerability and convenience; it causes a reduction in prolactin secretion, restoration of gonadal function and decrease in tumour volume
3. Surgical:
   - indications:
     - up to 10% of patients who do not respond to dopaminergic agonists
     - if visual field deficits do not improve
     - apoplexy with neurological signs in macroadenomas
     - cystic macroprolactinomas causing neurological symptoms
     - intolerance to dopaminergic agonists
     - nonfunctional tumours
     - suprasellar extension of a tumour, which has not regressed with medical treatment and a pregnancy is desired
   - transsphenoidal adenectomy: does not reliably lead to a long-term cure, and recurrence of hyperprolactinaemia is frequent:
     - microadenomas: the success rate is about 75%
     - macroprolactinomas: the success rate is much lower; recurrence occurs in about 20%

4. Radiotherapy: significant side effects, including hypopituitarism, damage to the optic nerve, neurological dysfunction and increased risks of stroke and secondary brain tumours. Therefore, radiotherapy is reserved for patients who do not respond to dopaminergic agonists, who are not cured by surgery or for very rare cases of malignant prolactinoma.

7.5 Hyperprolactinaemia and Fertility

- If regular menstrual cycles, no treatment is necessary. Treat only if anovulatory and fertility is desired. In anovulatory women, dopaminergic agonists restores ovulation in approximately 90% of cases, and result in a pregnancy in 80–85% of women. Treatment should be given to correct amenorrhoea and its sequelae, rather than just for normalisation of serum levels of PRL.
- The association between hyperprolactinaemia and infertility in the presence of ovulation and regular menstrual cycles is controversial. There is no evidence to support an association between prolactin and conception rates in ovulatory women. PRL levels should be measured in anovulatory women or those with symptoms of galactorrhoea or a pituitary tumour.
- When a patient with a macroprolactinoma wishes to become pregnant, pregnancy should be planned once serum PRL is normalised and the tumour volume significantly reduced to avoid or reduce the risk of compression of the optic chiasma during pregnancy.
- Surgery before pregnancy in women with macroprolactinomas to reduce the likelihood of major tumour expansion is a less preferable option, since medical therapy during pregnancy is probably less harmful than surgery.
- Transsphenoidal surgery is an option in an infertile patient with a prolactinoma who cannot tolerate or is resistant to dopaminergic drugs.

7.6 Hyperprolactinaemia and Pregnancy

- Serum PRL in pregnancy does not reliably reflect an increase in the size of prolactinomas.
- Microprolactinomas: the risk of clinically relevant tumour expansion is <2% during pregnancy. Therefore, dopaminergic agonists should be stopped as soon as pregnancy is confirmed. The patient should be advised to report for urgent assessment in the event of a severe headache or visual disturbance. Serial PRL determinations are not necessary.
- Macroadenomas: symptomatic tumour expansion occurs in 20–30% of women. Options include stopping the dopaminergic agonists when pregnancy is confirmed with close surveillance, or continuing the dopaminergic agonists through the pregnancy.
- If visual field defects or progressive headaches develop, an MRI should be performed without gadolinium and dopaminergic agonists restarted if the tumour has grown significantly. Visual fields should be monitored every two to three months.
- If the enlarged tumour does not respond to dopaminergic agonists therapy, alternatives include delivery if the pregnancy is far enough advanced or transsphenoidal surgery.

7.7 Safety of Dopamine Agonists in Pregnancy and Lactation

- Bromocriptine: the incidence of miscarriage or congenital malformations is no higher than that in the general population.
- Cabergoline: similar to bromocriptine, but data are limited.
- Pergolide and quinagolide: limited experience; these two drugs should not be used in this setting.
- Bromocriptine and cabergoline: the exposure of the embryo to such drugs should be limited as much as possible. Teratogenicity most often occurs during the first trimester, and the first trimester is associated with the period of lowest growth of a macroadenoma in pregnant women who have stopped therapy. Therefore, bromocriptine or cabergoline should be stopped once a pregnancy test is positive.
- Lactation: dopaminergic agonists should not be prescribed in women wishing to breastfeed because the resulting decrease in serum PRL levels will impair lactation. There are no data to suggest that breastfeeding leads to an increase in tumour size.

8 Amenorrhea

8.1 Primary Amenorrhoea

- Failure to establish menstruation by 16 years of age in girls with normal secondary sexual characteristics (SSC), or by 14 years of age in girls

Table 22.3 Tanner stages of pubertal development

Tanner stages	Breast development	Pubic hair growth
Stage I	Prepubertal	Prepubertal
Stage II	Breast buds form	Few long, downy hairs at the labia majora
Stage III	Breast buds larger	Pubic hair growth continues, but mainly central
Stage IV	Breasts in a 'mound' form	Pubic hair in the triangular adult shape, but smaller
Stage V	Breasts fully formed	Pubic hair adult in shape, quantity and type and spread to the inner thighs

with no secondary sexual characteristics. See Table 22.3 for the Tanner stages of pubertal development.

8.2 Concerns

- estrogen deficiency: risk of osteoporosis; may be increased risk of cardiovascular disease.
- estrogen deficiency in adolescents: desirable peak bone mass may not be attained.
- Infertility.
- Unpredictable spontaneous ovulation may occur, so contraception is needed.
- Women with a Y chromosome: increased risk of gonadal tumours. Gonads (residual testes) need removal either at diagnosis or, in women with androgen insensitivity, after puberty.

8.3 Causes of Primary Amenorrhoea

See Figure 22.1.

Outflow tract obstructions

- Imperforate hymen:
  - normal SSC
  - cyclical lower abdominal pain
  - visible haematocolpos with a bulging purple/blue, stretching thin hymen at introitus
  - ultrasound scan (USS): may show haematometra
  - treatment: surgery; simple cruciate incision on the hymen
- Transverse vaginal septum: due to failure of fusion or canalisation between the müllerian tubercle and sinovaginal bulb:
  - normal SSC
  - cyclical lower abdominal pain
  - pink bulge at introitus as the septum is thicker than hymen
  - treatment: surgery; risk of annular constriction
- Mayer–Rokitansky–Küster–Hauser syndrome:
  - 46,XX, normal female phenotype
  - incidence: 1:5000 female births
  - ovarian tissue: functioning normally: therefore, normal SSC
  - müllerian ducts fail to fuse: uterine development is rudimentary or absent with uterine remnants; vaginal agenesis with short and blind ending vagina
  - external genitalia: normal appearance
  - may be associated with renal tract (15–40%) and skeletal anomalies (10–20%)
  - investigations: USS, laparoscopy
  - treatment: sexual function: gradual dilation of vagina (Vecchietti procedure)
  - surgery to create neovagina: McIndoe vaginoplasty, tissue expansion vaginoplasty, Williams vaginoplasty
  - fertility: oocytes retrieval and surrogacy
- Androgen insensitivity syndrome:
  - 46,XY, 1:60 000 male births
  - inherited as an X-linked trait
  - testes are present, but end organs are insensitive to androgens
  - phenotypically female, lack pubic and axillary hair (androgen dependent), presence of breast development, but reduced
  - anti-müllerian factor: prevents development of internal müllerian structures
  - müllerian structures fail to develop due to insensitivity to androgens; external genitalia develop into default female organs
  - treatment: gonadal tissue is removed after puberty due to the risk of malignancy, followed by exogenous estrogens
- Turner's syndrome
  - most common cause of gonadal dysgenesis
  - pubertal delay

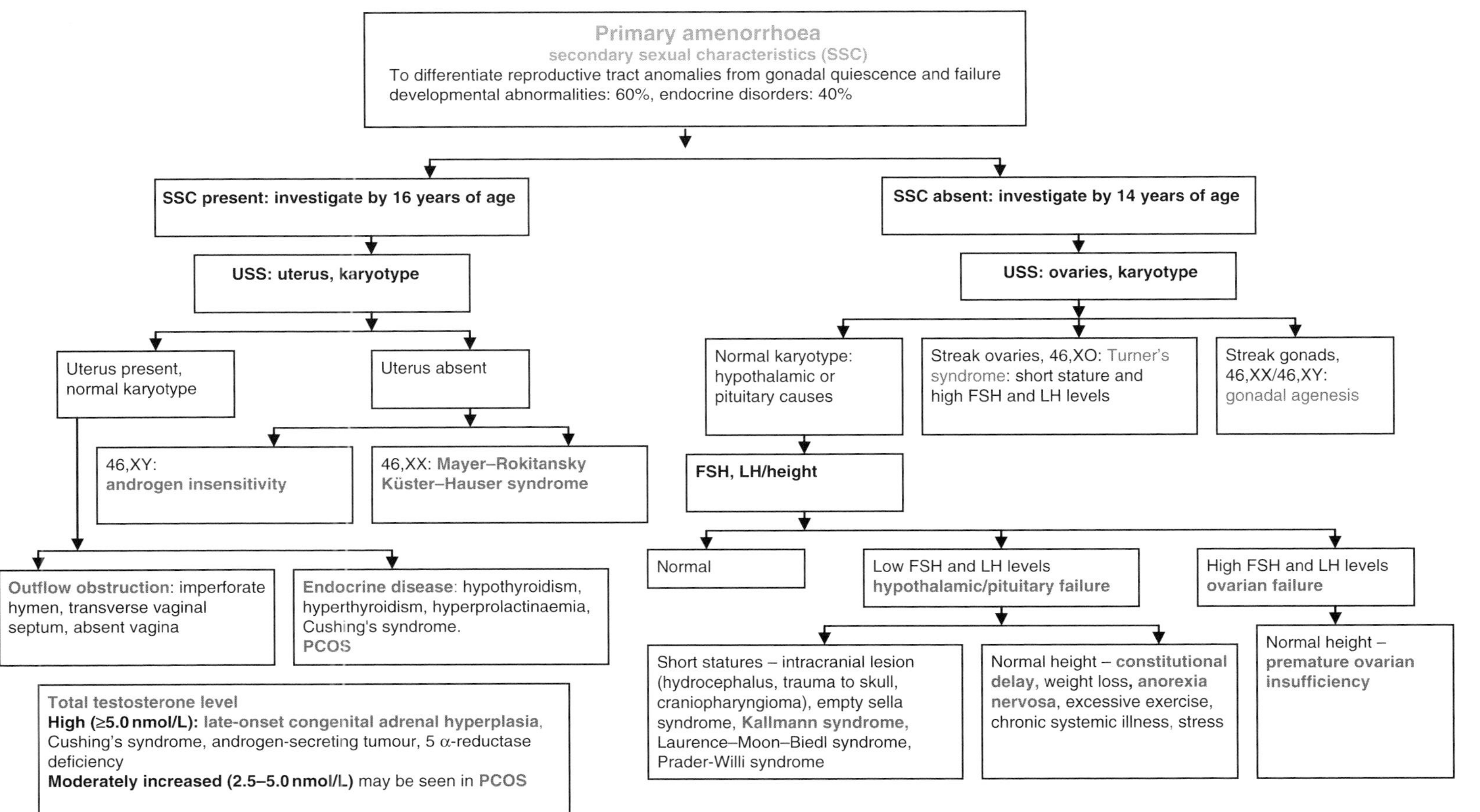

Figure 22.1 Primary amenorrhoea.
SSC: Secondary sexual characteristics

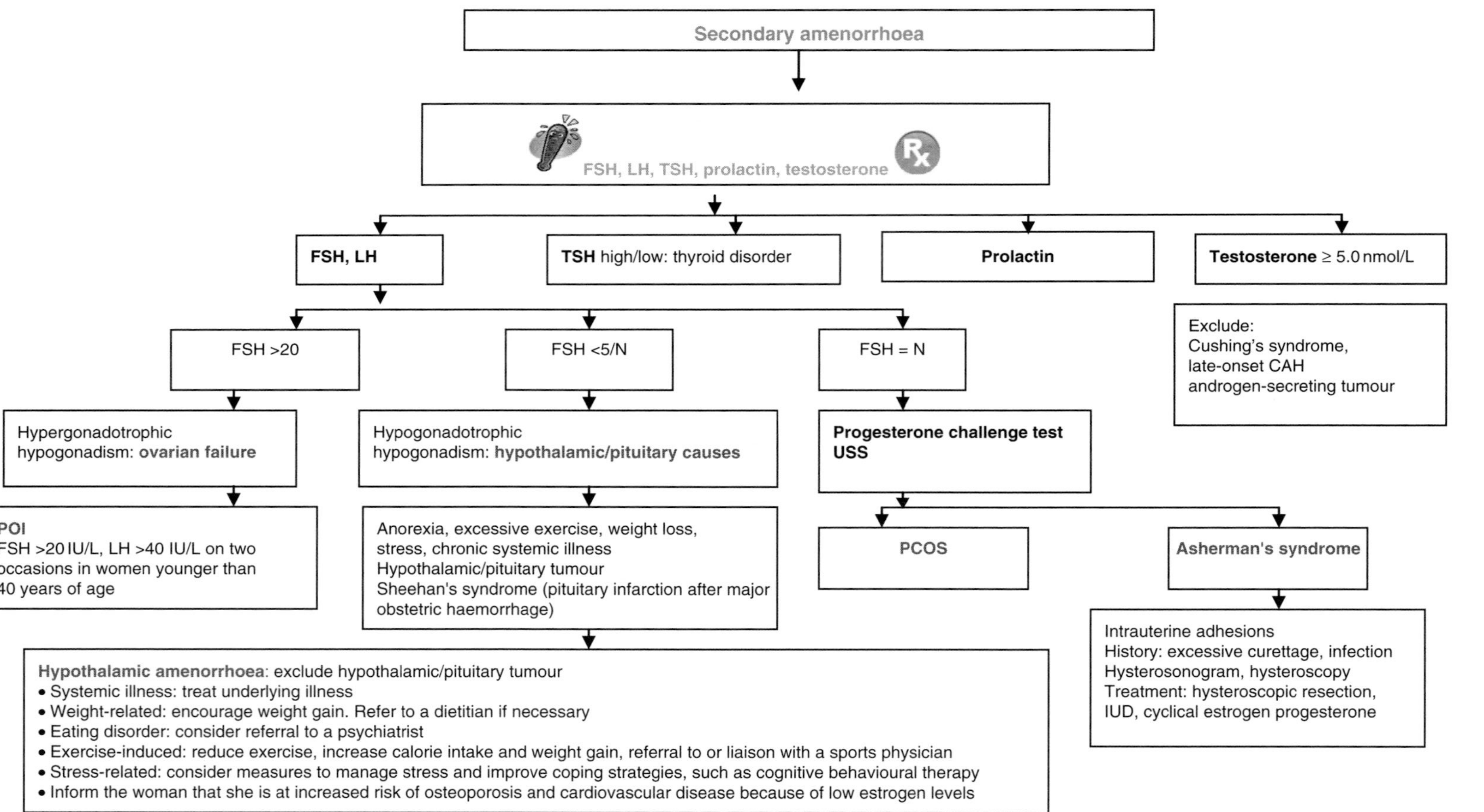

Figure 22.2 Secondary ammenorrhoea.
N: normal
CAH: congenital adrenal hyperplasia
POI: premature ovarian insufficiency
IUD: intrauterine device

- 45,XO: classical features: short stature, webbing of the neck, coitus valgus, widely spaced nipples, cardiac and renal abnormality, autoimmune hypothyroidism
  - mosaicism: spontaneous menstruation may occur, but leads to premature ovarian insufficiency (POI)
  - streak gonads
  - treatment: low-dose estrogen to promote breast development without affecting linear growth; cyclical estrogen and progesterone treatment for maintenance
  - fertility: egg donation
- Constitutional delay (physiologically delayed puberty):
  - there is no anatomical abnormality, and maturation usually occurs spontaneously by 18 years of age
  - familial
  - diagnosis is by exclusion of pathological causes
- Anorexia:
  - weight: 10–12% less than ideal body weight
  - the growth spurt usually occurs, but SSC are absent
  - associated features: constipation, hypothermia, cold intolerance, bradycardia, hypotension, lanugo-type hair
  - low LH, FSH and E2; anaemia, ECG abnormality in 52.2%, abnormal glucose tolerance test (GTT) in 37.5%
  - dietary therapy, psychotherapy and antidepressants
  - estrogen replacement
- Kallman syndrome: congenital gonadotropin deficiency characterised by anosmia and other cranial anomalies.

9 Secondary Amenorrhoea

- Absence of menstruation for at least six consecutive months in women with previously normal and regular menses, or for 12 months in women with prior oligomenorrhoea.
- The woman should be evaluated if amenorrhoea has persisted for 3–6 months. This also applies to women with amenorrhoea after stopping combined oral contraceptives.
- Investigations should begin by six months after the end of the last period; or earlier if it is clinically indicated (e.g., for hirsutism).
- Women who are amenorrhoeic after cessation of an injectable progestogen should be investigated nine months after the last injection.
- Pregnancy should be excluded (see Figure 22.2).

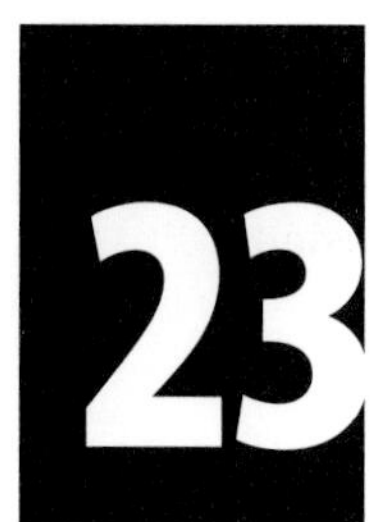

Puberty

Jyotsna Pundir

- Puberty is the transition from sexual immaturity to sexual maturity. There are two main physiological events in puberty:
  - gonadarche is the activation of the gonads by the pituitary and follicle stimulating hormone (FSH) and luteinising hormone (LH)
  - adrenarche is the increase in production of androgens by the adrenal cortex
- Thelarche: the appearance of breast tissue, which is primarily due to the action of estradiol from the ovaries.
- Menarche: the time of the first menstrual bleed. Initial bleeds are caused by the effects of estradiol on the endometrial lining. Menstrual bleeding in regular menstrual cycles after maturity follows regular ovulation and interplay of estradiol and progesterone.
- Spermarche: the time of the first sperm production (heralded by nocturnal sperm emissions and appearance of sperm in the urine), which is due to the effects of FSH and LH, via testosterone.
- Pubarche: the appearance of pubic hair, axillary hair, apocrine body odour and acne, which is primarily due to the effects of androgens from the adrenal gland.
- The critical hormonal event in puberty is an increase in the pulsatile secretion of gonadotropin-releasing hormone (GnRH) from the hypothalamus, resulting in increases in both frequency and amplitude of pulses of LH secretion and FSH, which in turn stimulate sex-steroidogenesis and, eventually, gametogenesis.
- FSH stimulates the growth of ovarian follicles and, in conjunction with LH, stimulates production of estradiol by the ovaries. estradiol stimulates breast development and growth of the skeleton, leading to pubertal growth acceleration. estradiol also induces maturation of the skeleton, eventually resulting in fusion of the growth plates and cessation of linear growth.
- Gonadarche and adrenarche are physiologically distinct events. Individuals with defects in the hypothalamic-pituitary-gonadal axis can still undergo adrenarche.
- Adrenarche begins when the zona reticularis of the adrenal gland begins to synthesise the adrenal androgens dehydroepiandrosterone and androstenedione. Although less potent than testosterone, these induce androgenic changes, including growth of pubic and axillary hair and maturation of the apocrine sweat glands.
- The earliest detectable secondary sexual characteristic (SSC) is breast/areolar development (thelarche). Growth acceleration typically precedes breast development. Menarche occurs on average 2–2.5 years after the onset of puberty.

1 Precocious Puberty

- Precocious puberty is puberty that occurs younger than two standard deviations before the average age.
- The normal age of pubertal onset is 8–13 years of age in girls.
- Prevalence of precocious puberty: girls: 0.2%, boys: < 0.05%.

1.1 Causes

1.1.1 Central or gonadotropin-Dependent Precocious Puberty

- premature activation of the hypothalamic-pituitary-gonadal axis: serum gonadotropins are elevated with the same pattern of endocrine change as in normal puberty (consonant)
- breast with or without pubic hair development
- increased growth velocity, possible acne, oily skin, hair and emotional changes

- variable serum estradiol
- peak LH level after GnRH agonist (GnRHa) stimulation: in pubertal range
- advanced bone age
- developed uterus on ultrasound scan (USS)

1.1.2 Peripheral or gonadotropin-Independent Precocious Puberty

- premature activation of the ovaries or adrenal glands independent of gonadotropin secretion
- secretion of sex steroids is autonomous with loss of normal feedback regulation: sex steroid concentrations are elevated with low gonadotropins
- pubertal development does not follow the pattern of normal puberty (disconsonant)
- varied pubertal symptoms depending on the nature of sex steroid produced
- high/markedly elevated serum estradiol in girls
- low peak serum LH after GnRHa stimulation
- advanced bone age
- developed uterus on USS
- may have advanced pubic and axillary hair growth prior to breast development, or menstruation with minimal breast development

1.1.3 Benign Variants of Precocious Pubertal Development

- usually isolated SSC
- no/slightly increased growth velocity
- bone age within normal range
- low serum levels of sex steroids
- peak LH levels after GnRHa stimulation: prepubertal range
- normal pelvic USS

1.1.4 CNS Lesions

- Hypothalamic tumour (glioma involving the hypothalamus or optic chiasma, germ-cell tumour).
- Hypothalamic hamartoma.
- Injury: cranial irradiation, head injury, infection such as meningitis or encephalitis, perinatal insult.

1.1.5 Autonomous Gonadal Activation

McCune–Albright syndrome: the classic triad is precocious puberty, café-au-lait spots and fibrous dysplasias of bone. There is rapid progression of breast development and early vaginal bleeding. Autonomous hyperfunctioning most commonly involves the ovary, but other endocrine involvement includes the thyroid (thyrotoxicosis), adrenals (Cushing's syndrome), pituitary (gigantism/acromegaly or hyperprolactinaemia) and parathyroid glands (hyperparathyroidism). Large ovarian cysts are seen on USS.

1.1.6 Ovarian Tumours

- Granulosa cell tumour: rapid progression of breast development and possible abdominal pain.
- Androgen-producing tumour: Leydig cell tumours, and gonadoblastoma. Progressive virilisation.
- Adrenal disorders: increased androgen production, leading to virilisation.

1.2 Management

- The aim is to prevent the progression of SSC and onset of menarche, and to maximise the growth potential and psychosocial wellbeing. Any underlying cause should be treated.
- Central precocious puberty: GnRHa provides continuous stimulation of the pituitary gonadotrophs, leading to desensitisation and a decrease in the release of LH and FSH. This results in the regression or stabilisation of pubertal symptoms as it is only the pulsatile exposure that triggers pubertal progression.
- Peripheral precocious puberty: the underlying cause should be managed. Agents are used to inhibit steroidogenesis, so as to reduce estrogen formation, which is a prime driver of bone maturation acceleration.
- Central lesion: any brain neoplasms should be managed. Managing the causal lesion generally has no effect on the course of pubertal development. Treatment with GnRH agonists can lead to a reduction in the growth rate due to a reduction in growth hormone (GH) and insulin-like growth factor 1 levels. Addition of GH may lead to a better growth velocity, although data is limited.

2 Delayed Puberty

- The absence of signs of puberty by an age 2-to-3 standard deviation (SD) above the mean age of onset of puberty of that sex and culture have initiated sexual maturation.
- See section on primary amenorrhea in Chapter 22.

24 Premature Ovarian Insufficiency

Jyotsna Pundir

1 Background and Prevalence

- menopause before the age of 40 years
- diagnosis: follicle stimulating hormone (FSH) levels >40 IU/mL and estradiol level <50 pmol/L
- prevalence: 1% under the age of 40 and 0.1% under the age of 30
- two main mechanisms:
  - dysfunction of follicular maturation
  - depletion in the follicular pool
- risks or complications: premature morbidity and mortality; increased risk of osteoporosis, cardiovascular disease, dementia, depression and cognitive decline

2 Causes

- Autoimmune oophoritis: premature ovarian insufficiency (POI) is frequently associated with autoimmune disorders, including hypothyroidism, insulin-dependent diabetes mellitus (IDDM) and antibodies including parietal cell antibodies and the acetylcholine esterase antibodies seen in myasthenia gravis.
- Turner syndrome: due to accelerated atresia of the primordial follicles during later fetal life, the ovarian follicle pool is depleted by puberty, resulting in primary amenorrhoea.
- Mosaic genotype (45,XO/46,XX): the rate of atresia, although accelerated, is relatively slower and patients present with secondary amenorrhoea.
- 46,XY gonadal dysgenesis.
- Fragile X syndrome permutation: the individual is phenotypically normal.
- Iatrogenic: secondary to cancer treatment: surgical, radiotherapy or chemotherapy. The likelihood of POI depends on the woman's age and the dose of radiation or chemotherapeutic agents used. Of all survivors of childhood cancers, 8% experience POI and this increases to 30–40% among those who receive a combination of radiotherapy and chemotherapy.
- Accumulation of toxic metabolites or immune mediated: galactosaemia is the direct toxicity from galactose-1-phosphate and galactitol, caused by the aberrant glycosylation of glycoproteins and glycolipids involved in ovarian function, and the activation of apoptosis of oocytes and ovarian stromal cells.
- Primary: idiopathic, most common, seen in 88%.

3 Presenting Features

- The most common presentation is secondary amenorrhoea with normal pubertal development. In 20% of cases, there is primary amenorrhoea with pubertal development delay.
- Symptoms of estrogen deficiency: vasomotor symptoms (VMS) of hot flushes, night sweats and loss of libido.
- History of chemotherapy, radiotherapy or pelvic surgery; autoimmune disorders, including hypothyroidism or adrenal insufficiency.
- Family history of POI (14–31%). Familial disorder can be identified; for example, Perrault syndrome (XX gonadal dysgenesis with sensorineural deafness), FSH receptor mutations and fragile X permutations.

4 Differential Diagnosis

- Differential diagnosis is made by excluding other common causes of primary and secondary amenorrhoea. Pregnancy should be ruled out.

5 Investigations

- to confirm the diagnosis, the following should be carried out:

  - serum FSH, LH and estradiol, repeated after 4–6 weeks to confirm the diagnosis
  - endocrine screen: serum prolactin and thyroxine levels
  - if there are signs of hyperandrogenism, serum dehydroepiandrosterone sulphate (DHEA-S) and testosterone
  - ultrasound scan (USS) to assess endometrial thickness and antral follicle count
- once the diagnosis of POI is confirmed, the following second-line investigations should be carried out:
  - karyotyping and fragile X premutation analysis
  - screening for autoimmune diseases (anti-adrenal, anti-21-hydroxylase, antithyroid peroxidase and antithyroglobulin antibodies)
  - dual-emission X-ray absorptiometry scan for baseline assessment due to the risk of osteopenia

6 Management

- general measures to avoid bone loss include physical activity, a calcium-rich diet, vitamin D supplementation and advice to avoid smoking and alcohol
- there is no evidence that estrogen replacement up to the natural age of menopause (51 years) increases the risk of breast cancer or ovarian cancer
- for estrogen deficiency symptoms:
  - hormone replacement therapy (HRT), unless contraindicated, until the age of menopause; women may need a higher dose of estrogen to control VMS
  - HRT has beneficial effects on cardiovascular status and bone mineral density; early treatment provides more long-term benefits
  - for women with a uterus, add a progestogen to avoid unopposed effects of estrogen on the endometrium
  - the regimen can be sequential or continuous: sequential administration has the advantage of simulating monthly menstrual cycles; whereas continuous regimens avoid menstrual flow, but can lead to breakthrough bleeding
  - combined oral contraceptive pills may be more acceptable in younger women
  - consider androgen replacement even with normal adrenal function, as the loss of ovarian activity can reduce androgen production by 50%, which can have profound effects on general and sexual wellbeing
  - there is no need to start earlier mammographic screens in women with POI on HRT
- fertility:
  - intermittent unpredictable ovarian function with a 5–10% chance of spontaneous pregnancy
  - fertility options: adoption, oocyte or embryo donation
  - fertility preservation in women requiring chemotherapy or radiotherapy: gonadal shielding, ovarian transposition, ovarian suppression by gonadotropin-releasing hormone agonist (GnRHa) or cryopreservation of oocyte, embryo or ovarian tissue
- contraception:
  - HRT is not a contraceptive: contraception is advised if the woman wants to avoid pregnancy
- nonhormonal treatment for women with contraindications to estrogen and HRT

25 Polycystic Ovarian Syndrome

Jyotsna Pundir

- A complex disorder, with clinical manifestation of oligomenorrhoea, hirsutism and acne, often complicated by chronic anovulatory infertility and hyperandrogenism. See Figure 25.1.
- Prevalence: 6–7%.
- Polycystic ovarian syndrome (PCOS) presents at a younger age, has more severe symptoms and a higher prevalence in women of South Asian origin.

1 Presenting Features

- Symptoms vary widely with symptoms of hyperandrogenism and severe menstrual disturbances at one end of the spectrum and mild symptoms at the other:
  - infrequent or no ovulation
  - infertility
  - hirsutism or acne
  - alopecia
- Family history of PCOS.
- Women may have indirect evidence of insulin resistance.
- Acanthosis nigricans: the skin is dry and rough, with grey-brown pigmentation, palpably thickened and covered by a papillomatous elevation, giving it a velvety texture. The condition commonly affects the axillae, perineum or extensor surfaces of the elbows and knuckles.
- Obesity: especially central obesity.

2 Diagnosis

See Figure 25.2.

- The Rotterdam criteria: two of the three following criteria are diagnostic:
  - polycystic ovaries (≥12 peripheral follicles or increased ovarian volume (>10 cm^3))
  - oligo- or anovulation
  - clinical and/or biochemical signs of hyperandrogenism
- a raised luteinising hormone (LH)/follicle stimulating hormone (FSH) ratio is no longer a diagnostic criterion for PCOS

3 Health Issues

1. Irregular menstrual cycles: risks of cancer:
   - oligo- or amenorrhoea may predispose to endometrial hyperplasia and later carcinoma
   - treatment is with progestogens to induce a withdrawal bleed at least every 3–4 months
   - options: combined oral contraceptives (COCs), cyclical progestogen for 14 days every 1–3 months, levonorgestrel-releasing intrauterine system (LNG-IUS); if the woman is unwilling to take cyclical hormone treatment or use a LNG-IUS, regular ultrasound scans are undertaken (every 6–12 months) to assess endometrial thickness and morphology
2. Hirsutism and acne
3. Subfertility/anovulation: management of anovulation is with ovulation induction:
   - first line: lifestyle changes and weight loss
   - second line: clomiphene citrate, letrozole or metformin; or a combination
   - third line: gonadotropins or laparoscopic ovarian drilling; clomiphene citrate plus metformin
   - fourth line: assisted reproduction

4 Long-term Health Issues

- The metabolic consequences of PCOS include insulin resistance, and later the development of impaired glucose tolerance and type 2 diabetes mellitus (DM). Type 2 DM is increased even in

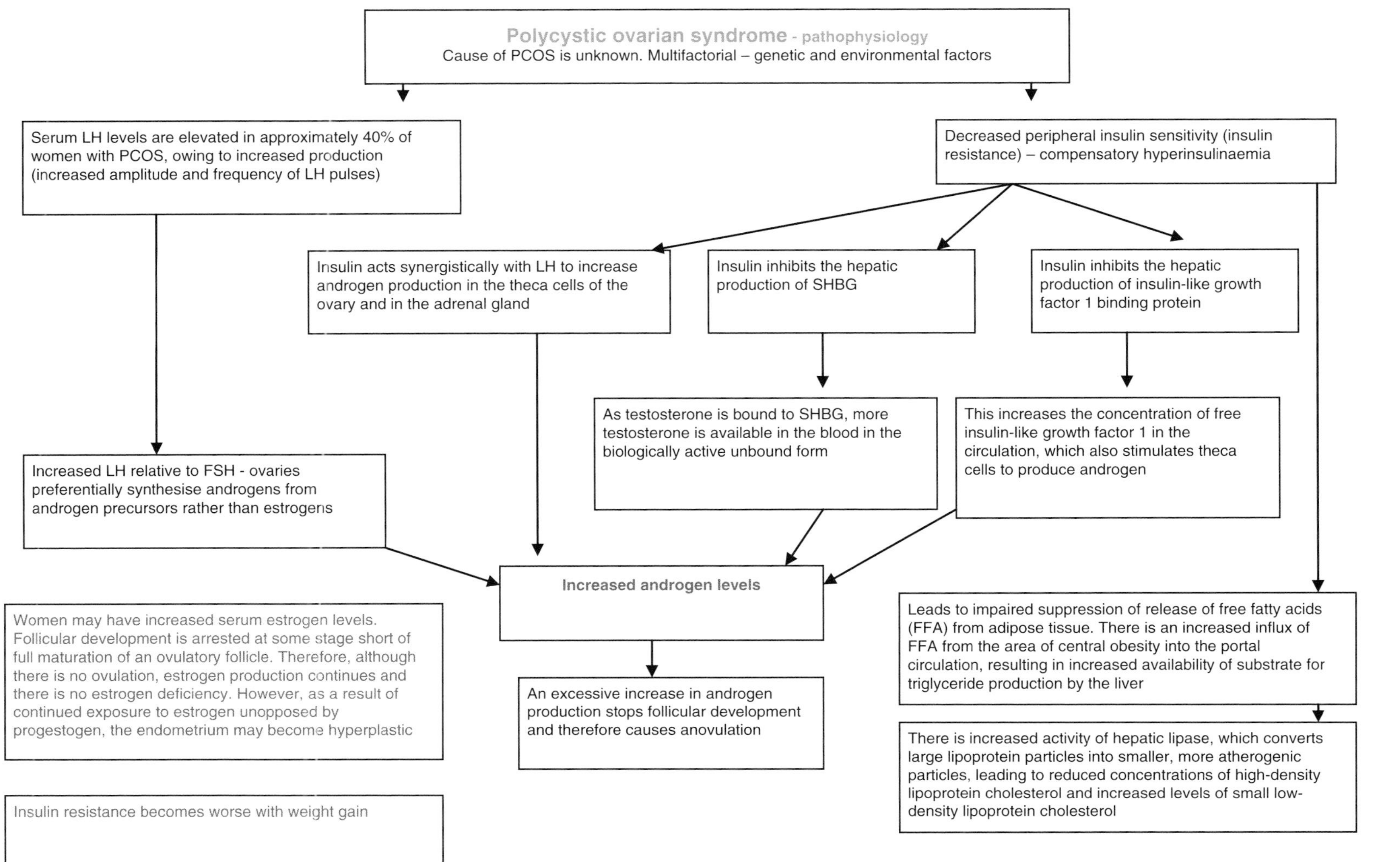

Figure 25.1 Polycystic ovarian syndrome.
SHBG – Serum hormone binding globulin

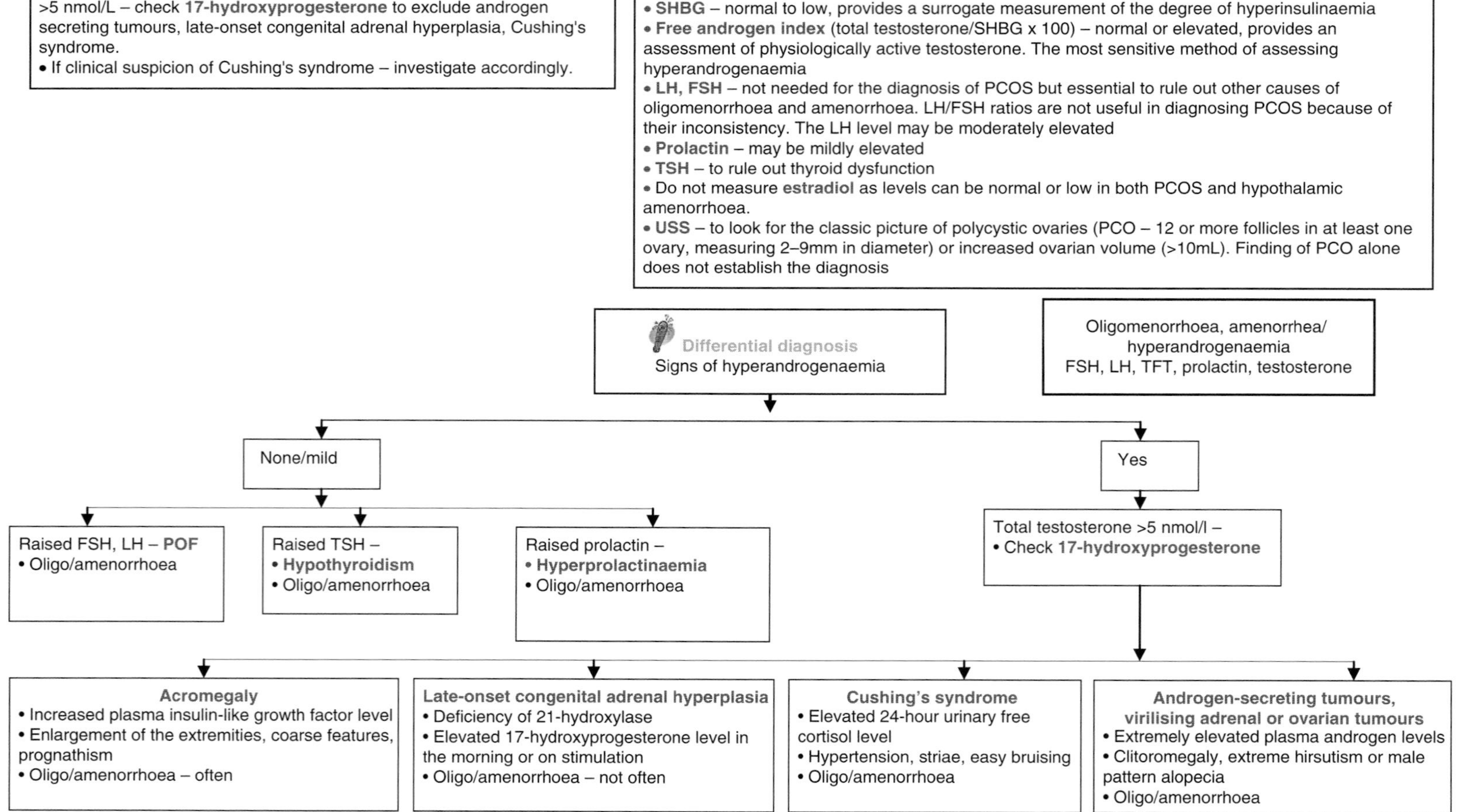

Figure 25.2 Investigations.
TFT – Thyroid function test

women with PCOS who are not obese. Women with raised fasting blood glucose (FBG) should be screened annually.

- Higher cardiovascular risk: these women have increased cardiovascular risk factors such as obesity, hyperandrogenism, hyperlipidaemia and hyperinsulinaemia. They can also have abnormal lipid profiles: raised triglycerides, total and low-density lipoprotein cholesterol. Evidence on hypertension is less consistent. Morbidity and mortality from coronary heart disease has not been shown to be as high as predicted.
- Obstructive sleep apnoea, even after controlled for body mass index (BMI): the strongest predictors for sleep apnoea are fasting plasma insulin levels and glucose-to-insulin ratio.
- In pregnancy, there can be a higher risk of gestational diabetes mellitus (GDM). Screening for GDM should be undertaken before 20 weeks of gestation.

5 Management

- Lifestyle:
  - diet and exercise: weight loss results in spontaneous resumption of ovulation, improvement in fertility, increased sex hormone-binding globulin and reduced basal level of insulin accompanied by a normalisation in glucose metabolism
  - lifestyle alteration reduces the likelihood of developing type 2 DM later in life
- Medical management:
  - insulin-sensitising agents: metformin and the thiazolidinediones reduce insulin resistance and reduce the risk of developing DM and other metabolic sequelae
  - weight-reduction drugs may be helpful in reducing insulin resistance through weight loss; orlistat and sibutramine significantly reduce body weight and hyperandrogenism in women with PCOS
- Surgical management:
  - bariatric surgery may be indicated in selected women with morbid obesity
  - ovarian diathermy should be reserved for selected anovulatory women with a normal BMI or where a laparoscopy is required for other indications

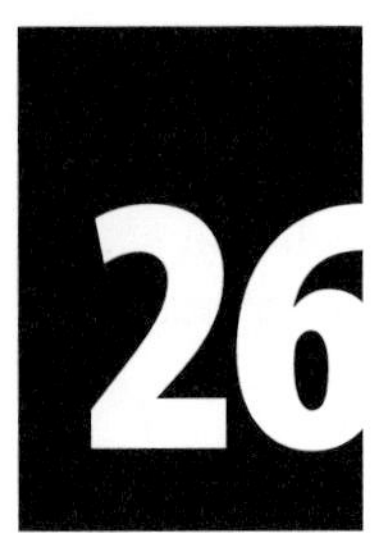

Menopause

Jyotsna Pundir

1 Background and Prevalence

- A woman is defined as postmenopausal from one year after her last menstrual period.
- In the UK, the mean age of the natural menopause is 51 years of age, although this can vary between groups of different family origin.
- The perimenopause, also called the menopausal transition or climacteric, is the interval in which a woman has irregular cycles of ovulation and menstruation before the menopause. It is the period before the menopause when the endocrinological, biological and clinical features of approaching menopause commence due to decreasing estrogen levels.
- Many women experience a range of symptoms, which are often short lived and lessen or disappear over time. The most common include vasomotor symptoms (VMSs), effects on mood and urogenital symptoms.
- Postmenopausal women are at increased risk of long-term conditions, such as osteoporosis, cardiovascular disease and changes in the vagina and bladder. These occur because of natural ageing as well as estrogen depletion.
- About 80% of women in the UK experience menopausal symptoms and 45% find the symptoms distressing. VMSs occur in 70–80% of perimenopausal women. They are most common in the first year after the final menstrual period. Vaginal symptoms occur in about 30% of women during the early postmenopausal period and in up to 47% of women during the later postmenopausal period. Only 10% seek medical advice. Racial, cultural, religious, sociological and nutritional factors modify the quality and incidence of menopausal symptoms.

2 History: Symptoms

- The menstrual cycle length may shorten to 2–3 weeks or lengthen to many months.
- VMSs: hot flushes and night sweats. Hot flushes arise as a sudden feeling of heat in the upper body (face, neck and chest) and spread upwards and downwards. Diffuse or patchy flushing of the skin is followed by sweating and tachycardia/palpitations. Hot flushes generally last only a few minutes.
- Sleep disturbance is often due to night sweats, but may also be due to mood disorders or primary sleep disorders. Chronically disturbed sleep can lead to irritability and to difficulties with short-term memory and concentration.
- Urinary and vaginal symptoms, such as vaginal discomfort and dryness, dyspareunia and recurrent lower urinary tract infection, are common.

3 Diagnosis

- The following are diagnosed without laboratory tests in otherwise healthy women aged over 45 years with menopausal symptoms:
  - perimenopause based on VMSs and irregular periods
  - menopause in women who have not had a period for at least 12 months and are not using hormonal contraception
  - menopause based on symptoms in women without a uterus
- Use of follicle stimulating hormone (FSH) test: a serum FSH test should not be used to diagnose menopause in women using combined estrogen and progestogen contraception or high-dose progestogen. An FSH test to diagnose menopause can be considered in:

- women aged 40 to 45 years with menopausal symptoms, including a change in their menstrual cycle
- women aged under 40 years in whom menopause is suspected

4 Initial Assessment

- the stage of menopause is assessed, whether perimenopausal or postmenopausal
- symptoms that are likely to respond to hormone replacement therapy (HRT) include VMSs and vaginal dryness
- the severity of symptoms and the extent to which they are affecting the woman's quality of life is determined
- the risk of cardiovascular disease is assessed, along with the risk of osteoporosis
- any contraindications are ruled out (e.g., history of breast cancer, venous thromboembolism (VTE))
- the risks and benefits of HRT are discussed
- body mass index (BMI) and blood pressure are recorded
- breast examination and pelvic examination is not routinely necessary
- investigations are not routinely indicated

5 Contraindications to Starting Hormone Replacement Therapy

- hormone-dependent cancers (current or past breast cancer)
- active or recent arterial thromboembolic disease (angina or myocardial infarction)
- VTE and pulmonary embolism (PE)
- severe active liver disease
- undiagnosed breast mass
- uninvestigated abnormal vaginal bleeding

6 Investigations

- FSH levels should not be routinely measured for diagnosing the menopause.
- Measurement of FSH is of limited value as:
  - FSH levels fluctuate during the perimenopause
  - normal results do not exclude the menopause
- Women using hormonal contraception: as combined oral contraceptives (COCs)suppress gonadotropins, a low level may be impossible to interpret. FSH should be measured when the woman is not taking estrogen-based contraception, either by stopping the COC or by changing to a progesterone only preparation. Six weeks should be allowed between terminating therapy and measuring FSH.
- Routine investigations should not be offered before starting HRT, unless there is:
  - a change in menstrual pattern, intermenstrual bleeding (IMB), postcoital bleeding (PCB) or postmenopausal bleeding (PMB): an endometrial assessment should be considered
  - a personal or family history of VTE: a thrombophilia screen should be considered
  - a high risk of breast cancer: mammography or MRI scan as appropriate for the woman's age should be undertaken
  - arterial disease or other risk markers for arterial disease: a lipid profile may be useful

7 Routes and Regimens

- estrogen: the transdermal (gels or patches) route avoids the first-pass effect through the liver and is not associated with an increased risk of VTE.
- Progestogen: nonhysterectomised women require 12–14 days of progestogen to avoid endometrial hyperplasia and minimise the risk of endometrial cancer with unopposed estrogen. The levonorgestrel-releasing intrauterine system (LNG-IUS) provides adequate endometrial protection with reduced systemic side effects.
- Continuous combined regimens avoid the need for regular withdrawal bleeds, but may be associated with continuous low-grade progestogenic side effects.
- Low-dose vaginal estrogenic creams, rings, tablets and pessaries should be considered for all women with symptoms of urogenital atrophy. Local estrogenic preparations may be more effective than systemic therapy and can be used in conjunction with oral/transdermal HRT. Progestogenic opposition is not required as systemic absorption is minimal with estradiol and estriol preparations.
- Drospirenone, a spironolactone analogue, has antiandrogenic and antimineralocorticoid properties. It has been incorporated with low-dose estrogen in a continuous combined formulation.

- With both cyclical and continuous regimens, there may be some erratic bleeding to begin with, but 90% of these women will eventually be completely bleed free.

8 Benefits of Hormone Replacement Therapy

8.1 Short-term Menopausal Symptoms

- VMSs: estrogen remains the most effective treatment. Do not routinely offer selective serotonin reuptake inhibitors (SSRIs), serotonin and norepinephrine reuptake inhibitors (SNRIs) or clonidine as first-line treatment for VMSs alone. There is some evidence that isoflavones or black cohosh may relieve VMSs. However, multiple preparations are available and their safety is uncertain; different preparations may vary and interactions with other medicines have been reported.
- Psychological symptoms: consider HRT and cognitive behavioural therapy to alleviate low mood or anxiety that arises as a result of the menopause. There is no clear evidence for SSRIs or SNRIs to ease low mood in menopausal women who have not been diagnosed with depression.
- Altered sexual function: HRT – systemic or topical – may improve sexual function in women with dyspareunia secondary to vaginal atrophy, through its proliferative effect on the vulval and vaginal epithelium and by improving vaginal lubrication. Systemic testosterones result in significant improvement in sexual function, including sexual desire and orgasm. Testosterone supplementation should be considered for menopausal women with low sexual desire if HRT alone is not effective.
- Urogenital atrophy: vaginal estrogen is offered to women with urogenital atrophy (including those on systemic HRT) and treatment continued for as long as needed to relieve symptoms. Vaginal estrogen should be considered for women with urogenital atrophy in whom systemic HRT is contraindicated. Symptoms often return when treatment is stopped. Adverse effects from vaginal estrogen are very rare. Advise women to report any unscheduled vaginal bleeding. Moisturisers and lubricants can be used alone or in addition to vaginal estrogen. There is no need to routinely monitor endometrial thickness during treatment for urogenital atrophy. estrogen has a proliferative effect on the bladder and urethral epithelium, and may help relieve symptoms of urinary frequency and urgency, and possibly reduce the risk of recurrent urinary tract infections in women with urogenital atrophy.
- Musculoskeletal effects: estrogen therapy has a protective effect against connective tissue loss. There is limited evidence suggesting that HRT may improve muscle mass and strength.
- Colorectal cancer: oral HRT reduces risk of colorectal cancer.

8.2 Long-term Benefits and Risks of Hormone Replacement Therapy

- Osteoporosis: the baseline population risk of fragility fracture for women around menopausal age in the UK is low and varies from one woman to another. HRT is effective in preserving bone density and preventing osteoporosis in both the spine and hip, as well as reducing the risk of osteoporosis-related fractures. The bone-protective effect of estrogen is dose related. The bone-preserving effect of HRT on bone mass density (BMD) declines after discontinuation of treatment. Bisphosphonates and other pharmacological agents can be used as an alternative to HRT to preserve bone density, but there can be side effects.
- Cardiovascular:
    - HRT does not increase cardiovascular disease risk when started in women aged under 60 years, and does not affect the risk of dying from cardiovascular disease. The presence of cardiovascular risk factors is not a contraindication to HRT if they are optimally managed. The baseline risk of coronary heart disease and stroke for women around menopausal age varies from one woman to another according to the presence of cardiovascular risk factors. HRT with estrogen alone is associated with no, or reduced, risk of coronary heart disease (CHD). HRT with estrogen and progestogen is associated with little or no increase in the risk of CHD.
    - Early cohort studies suggested that HRT is associated with a significant reduction in the incidence of heart disease, whether estrogen

alone or combined with progestogen, when commenced within 10 years of the menopause: this is referred to as the 'window of opportunity' for primary prevention. 'Early harm' can occur when therapy is commenced in women aged over 60 years old with relative overdoses of oral estrogen.
  - Oral (but not transdermal) estrogen is associated with a small increase in the risk of stroke. The baseline population risk of stroke in women aged under 60 years is very low.

- VTE: risk is increased by oral HRT compared with baseline population risk. The risk associated with transdermal HRT given at standard therapeutic doses is no greater than baseline population risk. Transdermal HRT is prescribed for menopausal women who are at increased risk of VTE, including those with a BMI over 30 kg/m^2. Refer women at high risk of VTE (e.g., those with a strong family history of VTE or a hereditary thrombophilia) to a haematologist for assessment before considering HRT.
- Type 2 diabetes: HRT (either orally or transdermally) is not associated with an increased risk of developing type 2 diabetes. HRT is not generally associated with an adverse effect on blood glucose control. HRT is considered for menopausal symptoms in women with type 2 diabetes after taking comorbidities into account.
- Dementia: the likelihood of HRT affecting a woman's risk of dementia is unknown.
- Breast cancer: the baseline risk of breast cancer for women around menopausal age varies from one woman to another according to the presence of underlying risk factors. HRT with estrogen alone is associated with little or no change in the risk of breast cancer. HRT with estrogen and progestogen can be associated with an increase in the risk of breast cancer. Any increase in the risk of breast cancer is related to treatment duration and reduces after stopping HRT. See Table 26.1.

9 Management

- HRT dosage, regimen and duration should be individualised, with annual evaluation of advantages and disadvantages.
- Transdermal estradiol is unlikely to increase the risk of VTE or stroke above that of nonusers and is associated with lower risk compared with oral estradiol.
- Limited evidence suggests that micronised progesterone and dydrogesterone may be associated with a lower risk of breast cancer and VTE compared to other progestogens.
- Arbitrary limits should not be placed on the duration of use of HRT; if symptoms persist, the benefits usually outweigh the risks.
- HRT prescribed before the age of 60 or within 10 years of the menopause has a favourable benefit/risk profile and is likely to be associated with a reduction in CHD and cardiovascular mortality.
- If HRT is used in women over 60 years of age, low doses should be started, preferably with a transdermal estradiol preparation.

9.1 Women With Intact Uteruses

- Perimenopausal women: if the last menstrual period (LMP) was within the previous year, a sequential combined regimen should be started; that is, continuous estrogen with progestogen for 12–14 days per month. This gives predictable withdrawal bleeding, whereas continuous regimens often cause unpredictable bleeding. A switch from cyclical therapy to continuous combined therapy should be considered when the woman is considered to be postmenopausal.
- Postmenopausal women: after a minimum of one year of HRT, or one year after the LMP (two years in premature ovarian insufficiency (POI)), women who wish to avoid a monthly withdrawal bleed should be switched to a continuous combined regimen. If breakthrough bleeding occurs following the switch to continuous combined HRT, and does not settle after 3–6 months, then the woman can be switched back to a sequential regimen for at least another year. Cyclical HRT may be used, but continuous combined preparations are generally preferred because they do not induce bleeding.
- If the woman requires treatment for decreased libido, tibolone (licensed use) or testosterone replacement (unlicensed) can be considered.

9.2 Women Who Have Had a Hysterectomy

- Oral or transdermal estrogen replacement should be used.

Table 26.1 Incidence per 1000 menopausal women over 7.5 years, NICE Guidelines 2015

	Baseline population risk in the UK/1000 postmenopausal women			Current HRT users	Treatment duration <5 years	Treatment duration 5–10 years	>5 years since stopping treatment
CHD	26.3	estrogen alone	RCT	6 fewer (−10 to 1)	–	–	6 fewer (−9 to −2)
			Obs	6 fewer (−9 to −3)	–	–	-
		EP	RCT	5 more (−3 to 18)	–	–	4 more (−1 to 11)
			Obs	-	–	–	-
Stroke	11.3	estrogen alone	RCT	0 (−5 to 10)	–	–	1 more (−4 to 9)
			Obs	3 more (−1 to 8)	–	–	-
		estrogen/ progesterone	RCT	6 more (−2 to 21)	–	–	4 more (−1 to 13)
			Obs	4 more (1 to 7)	–	–	-
Breast cancer	22.48	estrogen alone	RCT	4 fewer (−11 to 8)	–	–	5 fewer (−11 to 2)
			Obs	6 more (1 to 12)	4 more (1 to 9)	5 more (−1 to 14)	5 fewer (−9 to −1)
		estrogen/ progesterone	RCT	5 more (−4 to 36)	-	-	8 more (1 to 17)
			Obs	17 more (14 to 20)	12 more (6 to 19)	21 more (9 to 37)	9 fewer (−16 to 13)
Fragility fracture	106 (follow-up: 5 years)	Any HRT	RCT	23 fewer (−10 to −33)	25 fewer (−9 to −37)	-	-
			Obs	16 fewer (−15 to −18)	15 fewer (−11 to −17)	18 fewer (−15 to −20)	2 more (−19 to 27)

RCT: randomized controlled trial; Obs: observational; HRT: hormone replacement therapy; EP – Estrogen + progesterone

9.3 Urogenital Symptoms Alone

- Low-dose vaginal estrogen (cream, pessary, tablet or ring).

10 Follow-up

- Unscheduled vaginal bleeding is a common side effect of HRT within the first three months of treatment, but should be reported at the three-month review appointment, or promptly if it occurs after the first three months.
- If bleeding is heavy or erratic on a sequential regimen, the dose of progestogen can be doubled or the duration increased to 21 days. Persistent bleeding problems of over six months warrant investigation with ultrasound scan and/or endometrial biopsy.
- Review should be at three months and once each year thereafter. The initial review is at three months as most menopausal symptoms respond by then: VMS improvement is usually noted within four weeks. At the initial three-month review:
    - the effectiveness of treatment is assessed and adjusted to achieve symptom relief
    - any bleeding patterns and adverse effects are discussed
    - blood pressure and body weight are checked
- An annual review is undertaken because the risks and benefits of HRT change over time and need to be discussed regularly:
    - the effectiveness of treatment is checked and any adverse effects discussed
    - the need for continued use is reassessed
    - breast awareness is encouraged
    - blood pressure and BMI are checked
- Women can stop HRT by gradually reducing or immediately. Gradually reducing HRT may limit the recurrence of symptoms in the short term. Gradually reducing or immediately stopping HRT makes no difference to their symptoms in the longer term.

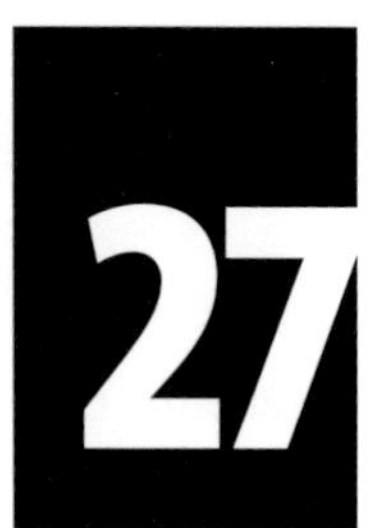

Thyroid and Parathyroid

Jyotsna Pundir

- The thyroid gland weighs 10–20 g in normal adults.
- There are two biologically active thyroid hormones: thyroxine (T4) and 3,5,3'-triiodothyronine (T3). T4 is solely produced in the thyroid gland, whereas T3 is produced both in the thyroid gland and in many other tissues by deiodination of T4.
- Approximately 80% of T3 produced is formed by 5'-deiodination of T4 in extrathyroidal tissue, leading to increased biologic activity.
- The thyroid gland contains large quantities of T4 and T3 incorporated in thyroglobulin, the protein within which the hormones are both synthesised and stored.
- T4 and T3 of thyroidal origin are synthesised by iodination, and coupling of tyrosyl residues within thyroglobulin, which is stored in the colloid space. Endocytosis of colloid and release of thyroid hormone occurs in response to thyroid stimulating hormone (TSH).
- T3 occupies specific nuclear receptors, mediating the physiologic action of thyroid hormone.
- Iodine is essential for normal thyroid function, and it can be obtained only by food. Severe iodine deficiency in fetuses and infants results in severe mental and growth retardation, and even mild deficiency is associated with thyroid enlargement and learning disabilities in children.
- More than 99.95% of the T4 and 99.5% of T3 in serum are bound to serum proteins: thyroxine-binding globulin (TBG), transthyretin (TTR/ thyroxine-binding prealbumin (TBPA)), albumin and lipoproteins.
- Because nearly all the T4 and T3 in serum is bound, changes in the serum concentrations of binding proteins, especially TBG, have a large effect on serum total T4 and T3 concentrations and the fractional metabolism of T4 and T3. They do not, however, alter free hormone concentrations or the absolute rates of metabolism of T4 and T3.
- Free T4 and T3 concentrations determine the hormones' biological activity.

1 Regulation of Thyroid Hormone

- Regulation of thyroidal biosynthesis and secretion of T4 and T3 is by TSH. The secretion of TSH is inhibited by T4 and T3 and is stimulated by thyrotropin-releasing hormone (TRH).
- The regulation of extrathyroidal conversion of T4 to T3 is by nutritional, hormonal and illness-related factors. The effect of these factors differs in different tissues.
- T4 and T3 inhibit the synthesis and release of both TSH and TRH.
- Somatostatin, dopamine and glucocorticoids may be physiologically important inhibitors of TSH secretion. Dopamine decreases serum TSH concentrations. Conversely, serum TSH concentrations rise after the administration of dopamine antagonists such as metoclopramide. The overall impact of the inhibitory actions of somatostatin, dopamine and glucocorticoids on TSH secretion is probably small.
- Thyroid hormone has important effects on neural and somatic development, both during fetal life and the first years of postnatal life. Major targets of thyroid hormone are the skeleton, the heart and the metabolic regulation.

2 Hypothyroidism

See Table 27.1.

- Hypothyroidism can result from a defect anywhere in the hypothalamic-pituitary-thyroid axis. Most commonly, it is caused by thyroid

Table 27.1 Causes of hypothyroidism

Primary hypothyroidism	Hashimoto's disease (chronic autoimmune thyroiditis; most common) Idiopathic (primary) hypothyroidism Iatrogenic: surgery, radiotherapy Drugs: lithium, amiodarone, interferon-alfa, interleukin-2, tyrosine kinase inhibitors, thionamides Infiltrative diseases: fibrous thyroiditis, haemochromatosis, sarcoidosis Congenital thyroid agenesis, gene receptor defects, dysgenesis or defects in hormone synthesis Transient: postpartum thyroiditis, subacute granulomatous thyroiditis, lymphocytic thyroiditis
Central hypothyroidism	
Secondary	TSH deficiency
Tertiary	TRH deficiency

disease (primary hypothyroidism) and less often by decreased secretion of TSH from the anterior pituitary or by decreased secretion of TRH from the hypothalamus.

- Primary hypothyroidism: high serum TSH and a low free T4.
- Subclinical hypothyroidism: normal free T4 with an elevated TSH concentration.
- Secondary (central) hypothyroidism: low serum T4 with a TSH concentration that is not appropriately elevated.
- Prevalence of overt hypothyroidism varies from 0.1% to 2%; and that of subclinical hypothyroidism is higher, ranging from 4% to 10% of adults.
- Hypothyroidism is five to eight times more common in women than men.

2.1 Causes of Hypothyroidism

2.1.1 Iodine

- Iodine deficiency (iodine intake less than 100 mcg/day) is the most common cause of hypothyroidism (and goitre) worldwide.

2.1.2 Hashimoto's Thyroiditis

- Hashimoto's thyroiditis is a chronic autoimmune thyroiditis caused by cell- and antibody-mediated destruction of thyroid tissue. The disorder has two forms: goitrous and atrophic. They differ in the extent of lymphocytic infiltration, fibrosis and thyroid follicular cell hyperplasia of the thyroid gland, but not in their pathophysiology.
- More than 90% of patients have high serum concentrations of autoantibodies to thyroglobulin and thyroid peroxidase. Many patients also have antibodies that block the action of TSH on the TSH receptor or that are cytotoxic to thyroid cells.
- The usual course is gradual loss of thyroid function. Subclinical hypothyroidism, with light increases in TSH and the presence of thyroid antibodies, leads to overt hypothyroidism and occurs at a rate of approximately 5% per year.
- It is usually, but not always, permanent.
- It is more common in women, especially older women.
- Personal or family history of other autoimmune diseases, such as adrenal insufficiency and insulin-dependent diabetes mellitus (IDDM). It is one of the components of polyglandular autoimmune syndrome 2.

2.1.3 Central Hypothyroidism

- Seen in less than 1% of patients who have hypothyroidism.
- Secondary hypothyroidism: can be caused by any of the causes of hypopituitarism; most often a pituitary tumour. Other causes include Sheehan's syndrome, trauma, hypophysitis, nonpituitary tumours such as craniopharyngiomas, infiltrative diseases and inactivating mutations in the gene for either TSH or the TSH receptor. TSH deficiency may be isolated, but, more often, it is associated with other pituitary hormone deficiencies.
- Tertiary hypothyroidism: can be caused by any disorder that damages the hypothalamus or interferes with hypothalamic-pituitary portal blood flow, mutations in the gene for the TRH receptor. TRH deficiency can be isolated or occur in combination with other hormonal deficiencies.
- TSH and TRH deficiency cannot be distinguished by biochemical tests. Any patient with findings suggestive of central hypothyroidism should have an MRI of the hypothalamus and pituitary.

2.2 Clinical Features

- The symptoms and signs vary according to the level of hormone deficiency and the acuteness with which the deficiency develops. See Table 27.2.
- Clinical features reflect one of two changes:
  - a generalised slowing of metabolic processes
  - accumulation of matrix glycosaminoglycans in the interstitial spaces of tissues
- Clinical features of central hypothyroidism are similar to those of primary hypothyroidism. When hypothyroidism is caused by hypothalamic-pituitary disease, the manifestations of associated endocrine deficiencies such as hypogonadism and adrenal insufficiency may mask the manifestations of hypothyroidism.
- Metabolic abnormalities include hyponatraemia, hyperlipidaemia, anaemia and high serum muscle enzyme concentrations.
- Clearance of drugs is decreased, such as antiepileptic, anticoagulant, hypnotic and opioid drugs.

2.3 Treatment

- Patients should be observed in transient hypothyroidism; for example, as after painless thyroiditis or subacute thyroiditis.
- The causative agent should be removed such as drugs that can be discontinued.
- All other patients with overt hypothyroidism should be treated. Goals are symptom control, normalisation of TSH secretion, reduction in size of goitre if present, and avoidance of overtreatment.
- Synthetic thyroxine should be replaced. Serum TSH should be checked six weeks after changing dose or preparations to confirm that the serum TSH is still within the therapeutic target, and the dose adjusted accordingly. Symptoms may begin to resolve after two to three weeks, but steady-state TSH concentrations are not achieved for at least six weeks. The aim is to keep TSH within the normal reference range (0.4 to 4.0 mU/L).
- T4–T3 combination is needed in selected patients, such as after thyroidectomy or ablative therapy with radioiodine. The T4:T3 ratio should be approximately 13:1 to 16:1.

Table 27.2 Clinical features of hypothroidism

Mechanism	Symptoms	Signs
Slowing of metabolic processes	Fatigue (90%) Cold intolerance (80%) Weight gain Dyspnoea on exertion Cognitive dysfunction Intellectual disability Constipation Growth failure Carpal tunnel syndrome Musculoskeletal aches and pains	Slow movement Slow speech Delayed relaxation of tendon reflexes Bradycardia Caroteneamia
Accumulation of matrix substances	Dry, scaly skin (90%) Hoarseness Oedema	Coarse skin (90%) Puffy facies (90%) Loss of eyebrows Coarse brittle thinning hair Periorbital oedema Macroglossia
Others	Decreased hearing Myalgia and paraesthesia Depression (70%) Poor concentration (65%) Psychosis Menorrhagia Arthralgia Pubertal delay	Diastolic hypertension Pleural and pericardial effusions Ascites Galactorrhea Anaemia

3 Hyperthyroidism

- Hyperthyroidism is more common in women than men (5:1 ratio).
- Prevalence: approximately 1.3%; increases to 4–5% in older women.
- Graves' disease is seen most often in younger women, while toxic nodular goitre is more common in older women.
- Two different mechanisms can be distinguished by the findings on the 24-hour radioiodine uptake:
    - A normal or high radioiodine (RI) uptake: indicates *de novo* synthesis of hormone. These disorders can be treated with a thionamides, which will interfere with hormone synthesis.
    - A near absent RI uptake indicates either inflammation and destruction of thyroid tissue with release of preformed hormone into the circulation or an extrathyroidal source of thyroid hormone. Thyroid hormone is not being actively synthesised when hyperthyroidism is due to thyroid inflammation; as a result, thionamide therapy is not useful in these disorders. See Table 27.3.

3.1 Causes

- Graves' disease: autoimmune disorder resulting from TSH receptor antibodies (thyroid stimulating immunoglobulins), which stimulate thyroid gland growth, thyroid hormone synthesis and release. Also associated with ophthalmopathy and pretibial myxoedema.

Table 27.3 Causes of hyperthyroidism

Normal/high RI uptake	Autoimmune thyroid disease: Graves' disease (most common cause); hashitoxicosis Autonomous thyroid tissue: toxic adenoma; toxic multinodular goitre TSH-mediated: TSH-producing pituitary adenoma; nonneoplastic TSH-mediated hyperthyroidism HCG mediated: hyperemesis gravidarum; trophoblastic disease
Near-absent RI uptake	Thyroiditis: subacute granulomatous (de Quervain's) thyroiditis; painless thyroiditis (silent thyroiditis, lymphocytic thyroiditis, postpartum thyroiditis); amiodarone; radiation Exogenous thyroid hormone intake Ectopic hyperthyroidism struma ovarii; metastatic follicular thyroid cancer

- Hashitoxicosis: rare; patients with autoimmune thyroid disease who initially present with hyperthyroidism and a high radioiodine uptake caused by TSH receptor antibodies similar to Graves' disease, which is followed by the development of hypothyroidism due to infiltration of the gland with lymphocytes and resultant autoimmune-mediated destruction of thyroid tissue similar to chronic lymphocytic thyroiditis (Hashimoto's thyroiditis). The initial treatment is similar to that for Graves' disease, but hypothyroidism may intervene, making further antithyroid therapy unnecessary.
- Toxic adenoma and toxic multinodular goitre: these are the result of focal and/or diffuse hyperplasia of thyroid follicular cells whose function is independent of TSH. Mutations of the TSH receptor gene are most common, which activate adenylyl cyclase in the absence of TSH.
- Trophoblastic disease and germ-cell tumours: in women with a hydatidiform mole or choriocarcinoma or in men with testicular germ-cell tumours via direct stimulation of the TSH receptor. High levels of isoforms of human chorionic gonadotropin (hCG) with more thyrotropic activity are responsible for the hyperthyroidism. Treatment is directed against the tumour.
- TSH-mediated hyperthyroidism: rare. There are two forms:
    - Neoplastic: these are usually macroadenomas by the time of diagnosis, and some are locally invasive. Almost all these patients have a goitre, 40% have a visual field defect, and one-third of women have galactorrhea. All patients have high serum thyroid hormone concentrations. Treatment is directed at the pituitary tumour.
    - Nonneoplastic: TSH-mediated hyperthyroidism is due to resistance to the feedback effect of thyroid hormone on pituitary TSH production, usually due to mutations in the nuclear T3 receptor. Treatment is rarely satisfactory.
- Thyroiditis: a group of heterogeneous disorders that result in inflammation of thyroid tissue with transient hyperthyroidism due to release of

preformed hormone from the colloid space. This initial presentation is followed by a hypothyroid phase and then recovery of thyroid function.

- Subacute thyroiditis is subacute granulomatous thyroiditis (de Quervain's thyroiditis), which is a viral or postviral syndrome characterised by fever, malaise and an exquisitely painful and tender goitre.
- Painless thyroiditis (silent thyroiditis or subacute lymphocytic thyroiditis) is part of the spectrum of autoimmune thyroid disease and occurs in the postpartum period (postpartum thyroiditis).
- radioactive (RA) uptake is less than 1%. Both RI therapy and thionamides are inappropriate, since new hormone is not being synthesised. Treatment is with beta blockers for symptomatic control and nonsteroidal anti-inflammatory drugs and, in severe cases, prednisone.

3.2 Clinical Features

See Table 27.4.

- Symptoms: the presence and size of a goitre depends on the cause of the hyperthyroidism. Exophthalmos, periorbital and conjunctival oedema, limitation of eye movement, and infiltrative dermopathy (pretibial myxoedema) occur only in patients with Graves' disease.

Table 27.4 Clinical features of hyperthyroidism

Mechanism	Symptoms	Signs
Skin	• Sweating and heat intolerance due to increased calorigenesis. • Pruritus and hives • Vitiligo • Alopecia areata • Thinning of hair	• Warm due to increased blood flow; smooth because of a decrease in the keratin layer • Onycholysis (loosening of the nails from the nail bed) and softening of nails • Hyperpigmentation in severe cases due to accelerated cortisol metabolism, leading to increased ACTH secretion • Infiltrative dermopathy in Graves' disease: skin overlying the shins is raised, hyperpigmented, violaceous, orange-peel-textured papules: 'Pretibial myxoedema'
Eyes	• Ophthalmopathy: gritty feeling or pain in eyes, diplopia due to extraocular muscle dysfunction • Severe proptosis: optic neuropathy and blindness	• Stare and lid lag due to sympathetic overactivity • Corneal ulceration due to proptosis and lid retraction • Ophthalmopathy seen only in Graves' disease: inflammation of the extraocular muscles, orbital fat and connective tissue, resulting in proptosis (exophthalmos), impairment of eye muscles and periorbital and conjunctival oedema
CVS	• Decreased hearing • Myalgia and paraesthesia • Palpitations	• Increase in cardiac output due to increased peripheral oxygen needs and increased cardiac contractility • Heart rate is increased, wide pulse pressure and peripheral vascular resistance is decreased • Systolic hypertension • High or normal output: congestive heart failure can occur in severe cases • Atrial fibrillation, mitral valve prolapse, mitral regurgitation
Metabolic		Impaired glucose tolerance
Respiratory	Dyspnoea and dyspnoea on exertion	• Oxygen consumption and carbon dioxide production increase, which stimulate ventilation • Respiratory muscle weakness and decreased lung volume • Tracheal obstruction from a large goitre • Pulmonary arterial systolic pressure is increased
GIT	Weight loss due to increased basal metabolic rate (BMR)	• Hyperphagia • Dysphagia due to goitre
Haematologic		Normochromic, normocytic anaemia: RBC mass increases but the plasma volume increases more

Table 27.4 (cont.)

Mechanism	Symptoms	Signs
Genitourinary	Urinary frequency and nocturia	Women: • Serum SHBG is high, resulting in high serum estradiol and low/normal serum free E2, high LH, reduced midcycle surge in LH, oligomenorrhea and anovulatory infertility • Amenorrhea can occur in severe cases Men: • Increase in serum SHBG results in high serum total testosterone, but serum free testosterone is normal or low • Serum LH may be slightly high • Extragonadal conversion of testosterone to estradiol is increased, resulting in high serum estradiol, which can cause gynaecomastia, reduced libido and erectile dysfunction • Spermatogenesis may be decreased or abnormal; e.g., more spermatozoa are abnormal or nonmotile
Bone	Graves' disease: thyroid acropachy: clubbing and periosteal new bone formation in the metacarpal bones or phalanges	• Stimulates bone resorption • May lead to an increase in serum calcium, inhibiting PTH secretion and the conversion of calcidiol to calcitriol: impaired calcium absorption and an increase in urinary calcium excretion, resulting in osteoporosis and an increased fracture risk
Neuropsychiatric	Anxiety, restlessness, irritability and insomnia	• Behavioural and personality changes: psychosis, agitation and depression in thyrotoxicosis • Cognitive: impaired concentration, confusion, poor orientation, amnesia

ACTH: adrenocorticotropic hormone; CVS: cardiovascular system; GIT: gastrointestinal; RBC: red blood cell; SHBG: sex hormone-binding globulin; LH: luteinising hormone; PTH: parathyroid hormone

3.3 Diagnosis

- Primary hyperthyroidism:
  - Overt: low TSH; high free T4 and T3. In some patients, only the serum T3 or T4 is elevated.
  - Subclinical: TSH is below normal and serum free T4, T3 and free T3 are normal.
- The cause of the hyperthyroidism should be determined. The diagnosis may be obvious on presentation: a patient with new-onset ophthalmopathy, a large nonnodular thyroid and moderate-to-severe hyperthyroidism has Graves' disease. If the diagnosis is not apparent based on the clinical presentation, measurement of thyrotropin receptor antibodies and radioactive iodine uptake should be undertaken.

3.4 Treatment of Grave's Hyperthyroidism

- Aim:
  - rapid amelioration of symptoms with a beta blocker
  - measures to decrease thyroid hormone synthesis: thionamide, radioiodine ablation or surgery
- Beta blocker for hyperadrenergic symptoms until euthyroidism is achieved.
- Thionamide: to achieve euthyroidism quickly. Methimazole is used (except during the first trimester of pregnancy) because of its longer duration of action, allowing for once-daily dosing, more rapid efficacy and lower incidence of side effects.
- Primary antithyroid drug therapy may be preferable for patients with mild disease and small goitres who are more likely to achieve a remission after a year of treatment.

- Definitive therapy: once patients are euthyroid on methimazole with RI or surgery:
  - in the absence of moderate-to-severe orbitopathy, RI therapy is recommended as it has a lower cost and a lower complication rate than surgery
  - for patients who are tolerating hyperthyroid symptoms and who are not at risk for complications from hyperthyroidism, RI can be used as initial therapy
  - surgery: for patients with hyperthyroidism due to a very large or obstructive goitre, patients who are allergic to thionamides and are unable to or do not want to receive radioiodine, and for patients with active orbitopathy
- Women who want to become pregnant: RI should be considered or surgery six months before a planned pregnancy to avoid the need for a thionamide during the pregnancy. However, if radioiodine or surgery is not desired, treatment is with propylthiouracil (PTU) during the first trimester of pregnancy and this may be continued throughout the pregnancy.
- Monitoring is with periodic clinical assessment and measurements of serum free T4 and total T3 levels. Measurement of serum TSH can be misleading in the early follow-up period because it can remain low for weeks, or even months, even when the patient is biochemically euthyroid.

4 The Thyroid in Pregnancy

- The major changes in thyroid function during pregnancy are:
  - an increase in serum thyroxine-binding globulin (TBG)
  - stimulation of the thyrotropin (TSH) receptor by hCG
- During pregnancy, serum TBG concentrations rise almost two-fold because of estrogen. TBG excess leads to an increase in total, but not free, T4 and T3 concentrations. Levels of total T4 and T3 rise by approximately 50% during the first half of pregnancy, plateauing at approximately 20 weeks of gestation.
- hCG (one of a family of glycoprotein hormones, including TSH) has a common alpha subunit and a unique beta subunit. However, there is considerable homology between the beta subunits of hCG and TSH. As a result, hCG has weak thyroid stimulating activity. Serum hCG concentrations increase soon after fertilisation and peak at 10 to 12 weeks. During this peak, total serum T4 and T3 concentrations increase and serum TSH concentrations are appropriately reduced. This transient, usually subclinical, hyperthyroidism should be considered a normal physiologic finding.
- Because of the changes in thyroid physiology during pregnancy, for the diagnosis and management of thyroid disease during pregnancy and postpartum, population-based, trimester-specific reference ranges are used for TSH and free T4.
- The fetus is dependent on maternal thyroid hormone until 12 weeks of gestation when autonomous fetal thyroid function begins.

4.1 Hypothyroidism During Pregnancy

- Severe hypothyroidism is associated with anovulation and subfertility.
- Untreated severe hypothyroidism in pregnancy is associated with increased rate of miscarriage, anaemia, fetal loss, preeclampsia and low birth-weight babies.
- Clinical features of hypothyroidism during pregnancy are similar to those that occur in nonpregnant patients.
- Newly diagnosed:
  - Overt hypothyroidism is treated with levothyroxine.
  - Initiate T4 replacement in pregnant women with subclinical hypothyroidism.
  - TSH should be measured every four weeks during the first half of pregnancy because dose adjustments are often required. The goal of treatment is to maintain TSH in the lower half of the trimester-specific reference range (or approximately <2.5 mU/L).
- Preexisting hypothyroidism:
  - Women who are planning to become pregnant should be optimised preconception. The goal is for serum TSH to be between the lower reference limit and 2.5 mU/L.
  - T4 dose requirements may increase during pregnancy. Serum TSH is measured as soon as pregnancy is confirmed, then again four weeks later, four weeks after any change in the dose of

T4, and at least once each trimester. The dose should be adjusted as needed every four weeks to achieve a normal TSH level, using a trimester-specific reference range.

4.2 Hyperthyroidism During Pregnancy

4.2.1 Overt Hyperthyroidism

- Occurs in 0.1 to 0.4% of all pregnancies.
- Graves' disease and hCG-mediated hyperthyroidism are the most common causes.
- Diagnosis: suppressed (<0.1 mU/L) or undetectable (<0.01 mU/L) serum TSH value and a serum free T4 and/or free T3 (or total T4 and/or total T3) exceeds the normal range during pregnancy.
- Women with symptomatic and/or moderate-to-severe, overt hyperthyroidism due to Graves' disease, toxic adenoma, toxic multinodular goitre or gestational trophoblastic disease require treatment.

4.2.2 Subclinical Hyperthyroidism

- Low TSH, normal free T4, or total T4, and T3 <1.5 times the upper limit of normal for nonpregnant adults.

4.2.3 Treatment

- Asymptomatic and/or mild, overt hyperthyroidism may be followed with no treatment. Monitoring is with TSH, free T4, and/or total T4, or total T3 every four to six weeks.
- Beta blocker for moderate-to-severe hyperthyroidism and hyperadrenergic symptoms of tachycardia, sweating and tremors. Possible side effects include fetal growth restriction, hypoglycaemia, respiratory depression and bradycardia. Beta blockers should be weaned as soon as the hyperthyroidism is controlled by thionamides (usually within three weeks).
- Women with moderate-to-severe hyperthyroidism: thionamide –carbimazole (CBZ) and PTU. Both cross the placenta; PTU less so than CBZ and in high doses may cause neonatal hypothyroidism and goitre.
- Thyroid function tests (TSH and free T4) should be given every four weeks throughout pregnancy. The thionamide dose should be adjusted based on the results of the TFTs to maintain serum free T4 at or just above the upper limit of normal. Serum TSH should be maintained below the reference range for pregnancy.
- Use PTU in newly diagnosed cases (less transfer across the placenta and breast milk). Patients taking PTU during the first trimester can either switch to methimazole after 16 weeks or continue PTU throughout the pregnancy.
- CBZ can cause a scalp defect, aplasia cutis. Rarely, it may cause neutropenia and agranulocytosis.
- For women with symptomatic, moderate-to-severe, overt hyperthyroidism who cannot tolerate thionamides because of allergy or agranulocytosis, thyroidectomy during pregnancy may be necessary.
- RI therapy for pregnant women is absolutely contraindicated.
- fetal monitoring: monitoring should be undertaken for signs of fetal thyrotoxicosis by assessment of fetal heart rate and fetal growth. If fetal thyrotoxicosis is suspected, prenatal thyroid ultrasound is performed to rule out fetal goitre.
- Given the concerns about potential PTU-associated hepatotoxicity, methimazole is used for nursing mothers.
- Women with Graves' disease who have been treated before or during pregnancy need careful monitoring during the postpartum period as they may experience an exacerbation.

5 Parathyroid Hormone

- PTH is synthesised as a 115-amino acid polypeptide called prepro-PTH, which is cleaved within parathyroid cells first to pro-PTH (90 amino acids) and then to PTH (84 amino acids).
- PTH 1–84 has a plasma half-life of two to four minutes.
- Once secreted, PTH is rapidly cleared from plasma through uptake by the liver and kidney, where it is cleaved into amino- and carboxyl-terminal fragments, which are then cleared by the kidney.
- PTH secretion is primarily regulated by extracellular calcium, along with extracellular phosphate, calcitriol, and fibroblast growth factor 23 (FGF23).
- A decrease in serum ionised calcium concentration produces a large increase in serum PTH concentration within minutes; conversely, an equally small increase in serum ionised calcium rapidly lowers the serum PTH concentration.

- PTH acts by binding to and activating one of several types of PTH receptors, which ultimately stimulate bone resorption, renal tubular calcium reabsorption, and phosphate excretion and/or hydroxylation of calcidiol to calcitriol, which enhances gastrointestinal absorption of calcium.
- The increase in PTH release in response to low calcium levels raises the serum calcium concentration towards normal via three actions:
  - increased bone resorption, which occurs within minutes
  - increased intestinal calcium absorption mediated by increased production of calcitriol, the most active form of vitamin D
  - decreased urinary calcium excretion due to stimulation of calcium reabsorption in the distal tubule, which occurs within minutes
- PTH acts on bone, the main reservoir of calcium, to release calcium in two phases:
  - the immediate effect of PTH is to mobilise calcium from skeletal stores that are readily available and in equilibrium with the extracellular fluid
  - later, PTH stimulates release of calcium (and also phosphate) by activation of bone resorption
- PTH, along with FGF23, inhibits mostly proximal, but also distal, tubular reabsorption of phosphorus.
- PTH stimulates the synthesis of 1-alpha hydroxylase in the proximal tubules and, thus, conversion of calcidiol to calcitriol. PTH also decreases the activity of a 24-hydroxylase that inactivates calcitriol. This is a particularly important action of PTH in maintaining calcium homeostasis in states of vitamin D deficiency.
- The change in calcium concentration is sensed by an exquisitely sensitive calcium-sensing receptor (CaSR) on the surface of parathyroid cells. Activating or inactivating mutations in the CaSR produce altered extracellular calcium sensing and, therefore, inappropriate PTH release.

6 Hyperparathyroidism

- Primary hyperparathyroidism is caused by parathyroid adenoma or hyperplasia; PTH secretion is inappropriately high in relation to the serum calcium concentration.
- Secondary hyperparathyroidism seen in patients with kidney failure results in reduced responsiveness to serum calcium levels, with continued secretion of PTH, despite normal or high serum calcium levels and, ultimately, in some cases, in true parathyroid autonomy; that is, secretion of PTH independent of the prevailing level of serum calcium.

6.1 Primary Hyperparathyroidism

- Asymptomatic primary hyperparathyroidism (PHPT): the serum PTH concentration is either frankly elevated or within the normal range but inappropriately elevated given the patient's hypercalcaemia as they have mild and sometimes only intermittent hypercalcaemia. They may have nonspecific symptoms, such as fatigue, weakness, anorexia, mild depression and mild cognitive or neuromuscular dysfunction. It is suspected because of the incidental finding of an elevated serum calcium concentration on biochemical screening tests or in a patient with nephrolithiasis. PHPT is diagnosed by finding a frankly elevated PTH concentration in a patient with hypercalcaemia.
- Normocalcaemic hyperparathyroidism: patients typically come to medical attention in the setting of an evaluation for low bone mineral density (BMD), during which time PTH levels are drawn and found to be elevated in the absence of hypercalcaemia. In such cases, BMD at cortical sites may be preferentially affected. To make this diagnosis, all secondary causes for hyperparathyroidism must be ruled out, and ionised calcium levels should be normal.
- Atypical presentations: include a spectrum of disturbances in calcium homeostasis, ranging from symptomatic severe hypercalcaemia (parathyroid crisis) to normocalcaemic PHPT.
- Parathyroid crisis: rare. Characterised by severe hypercalcaemia, with the serum calcium concentration >15 mg/dL and marked symptoms of hypercalcaemia: in particular, there is central nervous system dysfunction.
- Classical: for example, osteitis fibrosa cystica and nephrolithiasis. These are due to prolonged excessive PTH secretion and hypercalcaemia. The classical manifestations ('bones, stones, abdominal moans, and psychic groans') are

uncommon in the developed countries, but are still prevalent in other countries. Nephrolithiasis and bone disease are due to prolonged excess PTH and symptoms attributable to hypercalcaemia include anorexia, nausea, constipation, polydipsia and polyuria.

- Subclinical renal manifestations of PHPT include asymptomatic nephrolithiasis, hypercalciuria, nephrocalcinosis, chronic renal insufficiency, and several abnormalities in renal tubular function: in particular, decreased concentrating ability.

6.2 Management

- Symptomatic PHPT (nephrolithiasis, symptomatic hypercalcaemia): parathyroidectomy cures the disease, decreases the risk of kidney stones, improves BMD and may decrease fracture risk.
- Asymptomatic PHPT: surgical guidelines are based on risk for end-organ effects and for disease progression. In patients who meet the criteria as per the guidelines, surgical intervention is advised as opposed to observation. For asymptomatic individuals who do not meet surgical criteria, serum calcium and creatinine are monitored annually and BMD every one to two years; if disease progression occurs, surgery is then undertaken. Patients with asymptomatic PHPT who do not meet surgical intervention criteria may still choose parathyroidectomy because it is the only definitive therapy.
- In patients (symptomatic or asymptomatic) who are unable to have surgery and whose primary indication for surgery is osteoporosis and risk for fracture, bisphosphonates are the treatment of choice.
- In patients who are unable to have surgery and whose primary indication for surgery is symptomatic and/or severe hypercalcaemia (particularly those in whom bone density is normal), cinacalcet is the treatment of choice.
- If there is no need to improve BMD or to lower the serum calcium, pharmacologic therapy is not used.
- PHPT and concomitant vitamin D deficiency: vitamin D repletion and serum and urine calcium are monitored to identify worsening hypercalcaemia and/or hypercalciuria.

6.3 Pregnancy

- PHPT is uncommon during pregnancy. However, moderate-to-severe hypercalcaemia during pregnancy may carry significant maternal and fetal risks.
- Maternal presentation includes hyperemesis, nephrolithiasis, recurrent urinary tract infections and pancreatitis.
- Neonatal complications: hypocalcaemia and tetany, secondary to fetal PTH suppression, preterm delivery, low birthweight and fetal demise.
- Total serum calcium declines across gestation, likely due to plasma volume expansion. The upper limit of normal for total serum calcium is 9.5 mg/dL in pregnancy. The active, ionised calcium level does not change significantly during a normal pregnancy.
- Treatment is based on severity and symptoms, but consideration of gestational age is also important.
- If a woman with diagnosed PHPT plans a pregnancy, parathyroidectomy should be done prior to conception.
- Observation may be appropriate in some patients with asymptomatic, very mild hypercalcaemia. Neonatologists should be alerted to the possibility of hypocalcaemia in the newborn (due to possible suppression of the fetal parathyroid gland).
- Surgery during the second trimester is the preferred treatment for symptomatic patients.

7 Hypoparathyroidism

- Hypoparathyroidism can be the result of destruction of the parathyroid glands (surgical, autoimmune; most common), abnormal parathyroid gland development, altered regulation of PTH production, or impaired PTH action.

7.1 Clinical Features

- Range from few if hypocalcaemia is mild, to life-threatening seizures, refractory heart failure or laryngospasm if it is severe. In addition to severity, the rate of development of hypocalcaemia and chronicity determine the clinical manifestations:
  - mild: perioral numbness, paraesthesias of the hands and feet, muscle cramps

  - severe symptoms of neuromuscular irritability: carpopedal spasm, laryngospasm and focal or generalised seizures
  - asymptomatic patients: incidentally noted to have a low serum total calcium, particularly when there is a personal or family history of autoimmune diseases, past history of head and neck surgery, or the presence of a neck scar

7.2 Diagnosis

- Measure serum total calcium, albumin, magnesium, phosphorus and intact PTH levels. Persistent hypocalcaemia with a low or inappropriately normal PTH level and hyperphosphataemia, in the absence of hypomagnesaemia, is diagnostic.
- The combination of low or inappropriately normal intact PTH with a low corrected serum calcium may also be found in patients with hypomagnesaemia and in patients with an activating mutation of the CaSR.

7.3 Acute Hypoparathyroidism

- Acute hypoparathyroidism can occur after total or near-total thyroidectomy. Monitoring for hypocalcaemia after near-total or total thyroidectomy is necessary. Oral and/or IV calcium and oral calcitriol supplementation is given based on the results of the serum calcium corrected for albumin.
- The goals of therapy are to relieve symptoms, to raise and maintain the serum calcium concentration in the low normal range (e.g., 8.0–8.5 mg/dL), and to prevent iatrogenic development of kidney stones.
- Patients with acute hypoparathyroidism have a rapid decline in serum calcium and PTH, precipitating acute symptoms. Emergency therapy is indicated in patients with tetany, seizures or markedly prolonged QT intervals on electrocardiogram.
  - in adults: IV 10 mL ampoule of 10% calcium gluconate in 50 mL of 5% dextrose infused over 10 to 20 minutes, followed by an IV infusion of calcium gluconate
  - in children: IV calcium gluconate (90 mg elemental calcium/10 mL vial) at a slow rate while closely monitoring pulse rate (and the QT interval)
- For asymptomatic patients with an acute decrease in serum corrected calcium to ≤7.5 mg/dL (1.9 mmol/L): IV calcium therapy.
- For adults with milder degrees of symptoms (e.g., paraesthesias) and hypocalcaemia: initial treatment with oral calcium and vitamin D supplementation is sufficient.

7.4 Chronic Hypoparathyroidism

Initial management is with calcium and vitamin D supplementation. Calcitriol is the vitamin D metabolite of choice because it does not require renal activation, has a rapid onset of action (hours), and has a shorter half-life. Other acceptable vitamin D analogues include alfacalcidol or dihydrotachysterol. The addition of recombinant PTH 1–84 is an option for patients with chronic hypoparathyroidism who cannot maintain stable serum and urinary calcium levels with calcium and vitamin D supplementation.

7.5 Pregnancy

There are conflicting data as to whether calcitriol requirements fall or do not fall during pregnancy, whereas there is uniform agreement that calcitriol requirements decrease during lactation.

Serum concentrations of 1,25 D (calcitriol) double during a normal pregnancy. However, intact PTH concentrations remain low to normal, suggesting that PTH does not mediate the late partum rise in 1,25 D production. Thus, serum calcium concentrations should be measured frequently during late pregnancy and lactation in women with hypoparathyroidism, who may have a rise in serum calcium requiring a decrease in calcitriol dose. If the calcitriol dose is not reduced, the combination of elevated serum 1,25 D and PTH-related protein can lead to increases in intestinal absorption and bone resorption and hypercalcaemia. The requirement for calcitriol will return to antepartum levels with cessation of lactation.

28 Adrenals

Jyotsna Pundir

- Adrenal cortex: adrenocorticotropic hormone (ACTH) acts on the adrenal cortex to increase cortisol secretion by increasing its synthesis. The major adrenal steroid hormones are synthesised in different areas of the adrenal cortex:
    - G: zona glomerulosa – mineralocorticoids (particularly aldosterone)
    - F: zona fasciculata – glucocorticoids (particularly cortisol)
    - R: zona reticularis – androgens (mainly dehydroepiandrosterone (DHEA))
- Cholesterol is the substrate for the synthesis of all steroid hormones. See Figure 28.1.
- Four cytochrome P450 enzymes are involved in adrenal corticosteroid biosynthesis. Inherited defects in the enzymatic steps of cortisol biosynthesis result in a congenital adrenal hyperplasia (CAH).
- Adrenal medulla: catecholamine synthesis and release.
- Glucocorticoids:
    - stimulate gluconeogenesis: increases glucose levels
    - catabolic effect: reduces protein stores
    - anti-inflammatory effect
    - immunosuppressants
- Mineralocorticoids:
    - maintain fluid balance; promote sodium absorption (passive absorption of water and increase in extracellular fluid) and excretion of potassium
    - excessive hormone will result in increased extracellular fluid (ECF) and hypertension
    - lack of hormone results in sodium and water loss
- Adrenal androgens:
    - adrenals secrete DHEA, DHEA-S, androstenedione and small amounts of estrogen and progesterone
    - extra-adrenal conversion to testosterone results in androgenic effects
    - catecholamines: fight and flight hormones
    - increase heart rate, blood pressure (BP), stroke volume and respiratory rate, and results in bronchodilation and mobilises glucose and lipolysis

1 Cushing's Syndrome (Hypercortisolism)

See Table 28.1.

- The symptoms and signs of Cushing's syndrome result directly from chronic exposure to excess glucocorticoid: proximal muscle weakness, facial plethora, wasting of the extremities with increased fat in the abdomen and face, wide purplish striae, bruising with no obvious trauma, and supraclavicular fat pads. See Table 28.2.
- The severity of symptoms varies, and depends on the following:
    - The degree and duration of hypercortisolism.
    - The presence or absence of androgen excess. Signs of androgen excess in Cushing's syndrome are most common in women with adrenal carcinomas. The adrenal glands are the major source of androgens in women. In contrast, the testes are the major source of androgens in men. Thus, men with Cushing's syndrome do not have signs of androgen excess because cortisol has no androgenic activity. Adrenal carcinomas usually secrete large amounts of androgenic precursors because they are inefficient at converting cholesterol to cortisol. In comparison, signs of androgen excess are usually mild in women with

Table 28.1 Causes of hypercortisolism

ACTH dependent	Cushing's syndrome: pituitary hypersecretion of ACTH (70%) Ectopic ACTH by nonpituitary tumours (small cell lung cancer) Ectopic corticotropic-releasing hormone (CRH) nonhypothalamic tumours causing pituitary hypersecretion of ACTH
ACTH independent	Iatrogenic: administration of excessive amounts of a synthetic glucocorticoid and rarely by ACTH Adrenal adenoma/carcinoma (15–20%) Micronodular/macronodular hyperplasia
Pseudo-Cushing's syndrome	Alcoholism

ACTH-dependent Cushing's syndrome and do not occur in women with adrenal adenomas.

- The cause of the hypercortisolism:
  - hyperpigmentation is caused by increased secretion of ACTH
  - androgen excess occurs only in women with adrenal cancer or ACTH-stimulated hyperandrogenism
  - adrenal adenomas generally secrete only glucocorticoids
- Adrenal carcinoma or the ectopic ACTH syndrome can cause tumour-related symptoms such as weight loss instead of weight gain.
- Adrenal adenomas: many patients with incidentally discovered adrenal adenomas have subclinical Cushing's syndrome, but glucose intolerance and hypertension are common.

Table 28.2 Clinical features of hypercortisolism

Reproductive	Menstrual abnormalities correlated with increased serum cortisol and decreased serum estradiol levels. Since both LH and FSH levels are low, the menstrual irregularities appear to be due to suppression of secretion of GnRH.
Signs of adrenal androgen excess	• Hirsutism: mild and limited to the face. • The scalp hair often becomes thin, but temporal balding is rare. • Oily facial skin and acne on the face, neck or shoulders. • Virilisation: temporal balding, deepening voice, male body habitus and clitoral hypertrophy in women with extremely high serum concentrations of androgens due to an adrenal carcinoma. Prepubertal males may develop premature puberty.
Dermatologic	• Easy bruisability: loss of subcutaneous connective tissue due to the catabolic effects of glucocorticoid results in easy bruising. • Striae: purple striae occur as the fragile skin stretches due to the enlarging trunk, breasts and abdomen. • Skin atrophy: the skin usually atrophies, with loss of subcutaneous fat to a sufficient degree that subcutaneous blood vessels may be seen. • Fungal infections: cutaneous fungal infections, especially tinea versicolor, are often found on the trunk. • Hyperpigmentation: induced by increased ACTH, not cortisol. ACTH binds to melanocyte-stimulating hormone receptors. • Hyperpigmentation occurs most often in patients with the ectopic ACTH syndrome, less often in those with pituitary overproduction of ACTH, and not at all in patients with adrenal tumours in whom ACTH secretion is suppressed. • The hyperpigmentation is less pronounced than in patients with chronic primary adrenal insufficiency. • Acanthosis nigricans can be present in the axillae and around the neck.
Metabolic	• Glucose intolerance is primarily due to stimulation of gluconeogenesis by cortisol and peripheral insulin resistance caused by obesity, but direct suppression of insulin release also may contribute. • Progressive obesity: the most common feature of patients with Cushing's syndrome is progressive, central (centripetal) obesity usually involving the face, neck, trunk, abdomen, and, internally, spinal canal and mediastinum. The extremities are often spared and may be wasted. • Fat accumulation in the cheeks results in a 'moon' face; a 'buffalo hump' or dorsocervical fat pad. Enlarged fat pads that fill the supraclavicular fossae and obscure the clavicles are one of the most specific signs of Cushing's syndrome. Retro-orbital fat deposition may result in exophthalmos.
Cardiovascular	Increased risk of death from cardiovascular disease, including myocardial infarction, stroke and thromboembolism. Other problems include hypertension and dyslipidaemia.
Proximal muscle wasting and weakness	Induced by the catabolic effects of excess glucocorticoid on skeletal muscle. As a result, many patients cannot rise from a squatting position without assistance; patients with more severe disease may be unable to climb stairs or get up from a deep chair.

Table 28.2 (cont.)

Bone loss	Osteoporosis caused by decreased intestinal calcium absorption, decreased bone formation, increased bone resorption and decreased renal calcium reabsorption. Pathologic fractures may occur, often resulting in severe skeletal pain.
Neuropsychologic changes and cognition	• Insomnia, depression and memory loss. • Symptoms of psychiatric disease occur in over one-half of patients: emotional lability, depression, irritability, anxiety, panic attacks, mild paranoia and mania are less common.
Infection and immune function	Glucocorticoids inhibit immune function, thereby contributing to an increased frequency of infections.
Mortality	It is associated with considerable morbidity and increased mortality.

LH: luteinising hormone; FSH: follicle stimulating hormone; GnRH: gonadotropin-releasing hormone

1.1 Diagnosis

- Exclude exogenous glucocorticoid intake.
- First-line tests:
    - late-night salivary cortisol
    - 24-hour urinary free cortisol excretion
    - overnight 1 mg dexamethasone suppression test
- In patients with at least one abnormal test result, additional evaluation is needed.
- Diagnosis is made when at least two different first-line tests are unequivocally abnormal.
- Once diagnosis is established, additional evaluations are undertaken to identify the cause of the hypercortisolism.
- Plasma ACTH: to determine whether the disease is ACTH-dependent or ACTH-independent.
- A low plasma ACTH concentration of <5 pg/mL (1.1 pmol/L) indicates ACTH-independent disease: a CT scan of the adrenal glands should be arranged. Bilateral adrenal micronodular or macronodular hyperplasia require additional testing.
- Intermediate plasma ACTH concentration of 5–20 pg/mL (1.1–4.4 pmol/L): corticotropin-releasing hormone (CRH) testing is performed. The presence of an ACTH response indicates Cushing's disease.
- ACTH-dependent disease is indicated by ACTH of >20 pg/mL:
    - Pituitary MRI: if a clear pituitary lesion >6 mm and high-dose dexamethasone and CRH tests are consistent with Cushing's disease, no further tests are required.
    - Suppression of cortisol during dexamethasone administration, as well as increases in ACTH and cortisol after CRH administration, are consistent with the diagnosis of Cushing's disease.
    - Petrosal sinus sampling with CRH stimulation for patients with unclear MRI (lesions <6 mm) or nonconcordant noninvasive tests to distinguish between Cushing's disease and ectopic ACTH secretion.

1.2 Treatment

- The goal is to achieve normalisation of hypothalamic-pituitary-adrenal function and reversal of Cushingoid signs/symptoms and comorbidities.
- Surgery: the optimal treatment is localisation and removal of an ACTH-secreting pituitary or ectopic tumour or cortisol-secreting adrenal tumour. Bilateral adrenalectomy is a definitive treatment for ACTH-secreting pituitary or ectopic tumours.
- Cushing's disease is not cured by pituitary surgery: medical treatment with cabergoline or pasireotide can result in normalisation of 24-hour urinary free cortisol in 20–40% of patients.
- Pituitary irradiation is undertaken for persistent or recurrent Cushing's disease.
- Metastatic or occult ectopic ACTH-secreting tumours may respond to somatostatin analogue treatment, adrenal enzyme inhibitors or mitotane.
- Symptoms and signs of Cushing's syndrome resolve gradually over a period of two to 12 months after its effective cure. Hypertension, osteoporosis and glucose intolerance improve, but may not disappear.

1.3 Cushing's Disease

- Eighty percent of cases of Cushing's syndrome are due to pituitary adenomas.
- Cushing's disease is mostly due to a pituitary adenoma; rarely, patients have diffuse corticotroph hyperplasia. Tumours are usually microadenomas; only approximately 5–10% are macroadenomas.
- The amplitude and duration, but not the frequency, of ACTH secretory episodes are increased, and the normal ACTH circadian rhythm is usually lost.
- Increased plasma ACTH concentrations, acting alone or in concert with other growth factors, cause bilateral adrenocortical hyperplasia and hypersecretion of cortisol.
- The increased cortisol secretion is reflected by increased urinary excretion of cortisol and 17-hydroxycorticosteroid.
- Women are three to eight times more likely than men to develop Cushing's disease, approximately three times more likely to have either benign or malignant adrenal tumours, and approximately four to five times more likely to have Cushing's syndrome associated with an adrenal tumour.
- Cushing's disease occurs mainly in women aged 25 to 45 years.

1.4 Cushing's Syndrome in Pregnancy

- Up to 75% of women with Cushing's syndrome have ovulatory disorders. As a result, women with untreated Cushing's syndrome rarely become pregnant.
- Of those who do become pregnant, approximately 55% have ACTH-independent hypercortisolism (primary adrenal adenomas: 44%, or adrenal carcinoma: 11%).
- Patients may present with excessive weight gain, extensive purple striae, diabetes mellitus, hypertension (HT), easy bruising, headache, hirsutism, acne or proximal myopathy.
- Tests: combined use of urinary free cortisol (pregnancy-specific range).
- Increased cortisol level with low ACTH, which fails to suppress with a high-dose dexamethasone suppression test, suggests an adrenal cause.
- Ultrasound (USS), CT or MRI scans of the adrenals and the pituitary are undertaken for localisation.
- There is an increased risk of fetal loss, prematurity and perinatal mortality.
- There is increased incidence of severe preeclampsia, wound infection and increased maternal morbidity and mortality.
- Neonate: at risk of adrenal insufficiency as high maternal cortisol levels suppress fetal/neonatal corticosteroid synthesis.
- Surgical resection of adrenal adenomas causing Cushing's syndrome is undertaken, typically performed at 16 to 21 weeks of gestation.
- For women who do not want surgery or are diagnosed later, metyrapone is used to control maternal hypercortisolism. It is associated with severe HT.
- It may become necessary to induce early delivery of the fetus if complications of eclampsia supervene.
- Transsphenoidal surgery for Cushing's disease has been performed in the second trimester without complicating the pregnancy.

2 Adrenal Insufficiency: Adrenocortical Failure/Insufficiency

- This can be caused by diseases of the adrenal gland (primary), interference with ACTH secretion by the pituitary gland (secondary), or interference with CRH secretion by the hypothalamus (tertiary).

Secondary adrenal insufficiency

- Any process that involves the pituitary and interferes with ACTH secretion can cause secondary adrenal insufficiency. It may be isolated or occur in conjunction with other pituitary hormone deficiencies (panhypopituitarism).
- Isolated ACTH deficiency is rare. It can be secondary to autoimmune or genetic causes, familial cortisol-binding globulin deficiency, traumatic brain injury, and drugs (chronic use of high-dose progestins and opiates).

Tertiary adrenal insufficiency

- Suppression of hypothalamic-pituitary-adrenal function by chronic administration of high doses of glucocorticoids is the most common cause of tertiary adrenal insufficiency. Clinical features of

secondary and tertiary adrenal insufficiency that help distinguish them from primary adrenal insufficiency include cortisol production, which can be restored by prolonged ACTH administration, and mineralocorticoid secretion is nearly normal because this function depends mostly on the renin-angiotensin system rather than on ACTH.
- Tertiary adrenal insufficiency also occurs in patients who are cured of Cushing's syndrome by the removal of a pituitary or nonpituitary ACTH-secreting or a cortisol-secreting adrenal tumour. The chronically high serum cortisol concentrations before treatment suppress the hypothalamic-pituitary-adrenal axis in the same manner as chronic administration of high doses of glucocorticoids.

2.1 Primary Adrenal Insufficiency: Addison's Disease

- Rare disorder.
- In contrast to adrenal failure, due to pituitary disease in Addison's disease, there is a deficiency of both cortisol and aldosterone.

2.1.1 Causes

- Autoimmune adrenalitis: occurs in 70–90%:
  - Destruction of the cortex by humoral and cell-mediated immune mechanisms. Antibodies that react with several steroidogenic enzymes (most often 21-hydroxylase) and all three zones of the adrenal cortex are present in the serum in up to 86% of patients.
  - Up to 50% of patients have additional autoimmune disorders.
- Polyglandular autoimmune syndrome type 1: a rare autosomal recessive disorder caused by mutations in the autoimmune regulator gene. Hypoparathyroidism or chronic mucocutaneous candidiasis appears by the mid-twenties, followed by adrenal insufficiency and potentially by other autoimmune diseases.
- Polyglandular autoimmune syndrome type 2: more common than type 1 syndrome. Primary adrenal insufficiency is its principal manifestation, but autoimmune thyroid disease and type 1 diabetes mellitus are also common. About half of the cases are familial, with polygenic modes of inheritance. It usually presents by age 40 years.
- Infectious causes: tuberculosis, fungal infections, cytomegalovirus and *Mycobacterium avium intracellulare*, syphilis and trypanosomiasis.
- Bilateral adrenal haemorrhage can inhibit adrenal function. This usually occurs in specific settings:
  - disseminated infection: meningococcus, *Pseudomonas aeruginosa, Streptococcus pneumoniae, Neisseria gonorrhoeae, Escherichia coli, Haemophilus influenzae* and *Staphylococcus aureus*
  - clotting abnormalities: anticoagulant drug or heparin therapy or coagulopathy, thromboembolic disease, hypercoagulable states such as antiphospholipid syndrome
  - trauma, postoperative state, sepsis and severe stress
- Metastatic disease with replacement of the cortex of both adrenal glands: most commonly associated with lung, breast, stomach, colon cancer, melanoma and lymphoma.
- Drugs are an important cause of primary adrenal insufficiency in patients with limited reserves who cannot overcome their effects:
  - drugs that inhibit cortisol biosynthesis, such as etomidate, ketoconazole, fluconazole, metyrapone, mitotane and suramin
  - drugs that accelerate the metabolism of cortisol and glucocorticoids by inducing hepatic mixed-function oxygenase enzymes such as phenytoin, barbiturates, mitotane and rifampin

2.1.2 Clinical Features

- Clinical features depend on the following:
  - the rate and extent of loss of adrenal function
  - whether mineralocorticoid production is preserved
  - the degree of stress

Acute adrenal insufficiency

- The syndrome of adrenal crisis can be seen in the following:
  - in a previously undiagnosed patient with primary adrenal insufficiency who has been subjected to serious infection or other acute, major stress
  - in a patient with known primary adrenal insufficiency who does not take more

glucocorticoid during an acute infection (can occur during acute viral infections such as influenza) or other major illness or has persistent vomiting caused by viral gastroenteritis or other gastrointestinal disorders
  - after bilateral adrenal infarction or bilateral adrenal haemorrhage
  - rarely in patients with secondary or tertiary adrenal insufficiency, but is sometimes seen with acute cortisol deficiency due to pituitary apoplexy or in patients withdrawn abruptly from suppressive doses of corticosteroids
- The predominant manifestation is shock, but the patients often have nonspecific symptoms such as anorexia, nausea, vomiting, abdominal pain, weakness, fatigue, lethargy, fever, confusion or coma.

Chronic adrenal insufficiency

- Primary: most patients present with chronic malaise, lassitude, fatigue (worsened by exertion and improved with bed rest), weakness, anorexia and weight loss. Hypoglycaemia is *not* common. Other clinical manifestations are gastrointestinal symptoms, hypotension, electrolyte abnormalities and hyperpigmentation.
- Secondary or tertiary: many are the same as those for primary adrenal insufficiency and are presumably due to glucocorticoid rather than mineralocorticoid deficiency. These include weakness, fatigue, myalgias and arthralgias. The major differences from primary adrenal insufficiency are that in secondary or tertiary adrenal insufficiency:
  - hyperpigmentation is not present because ACTH secretion is not increased
  - dehydration is not present, and hypotension is less prominent
  - hyponatraemia and volume expansion may be present (reflecting increased vasopressin secretion), but hyperkalaemia is not (reflecting the presence of aldosterone)
  - gastrointestinal symptoms are less common, suggesting that electrolyte disturbances may be involved in their aetiology
  - hypoglycaemia is *more common* in secondary adrenal insufficiency

2.1.3 Diagnosis

- An appropriate level of clinical suspicion: adrenal crisis should be considered in any patient who presents with peripheral vascular collapse (vasodilatory shock).
- Isolated ACTH deficiency, although rare, should be considered in any patient who has unexplained severe hypoglycaemia or hyponatraemia.
- Prolonged administration of pharmacologic doses of synthetic glucocorticoids is the most common cause of ACTH deficiency and consequent adrenal insufficiency.
- Patients treated with glucocorticoid therapy rarely present with adrenal crisis, although sudden withdrawal of glucocorticoids can result in exacerbation of the disorder for which they were being given (e.g., asthma, inflammatory disease, or organ transplantation), symptoms of glucocorticoid deficiency or hypotension.
- Evaluation for possible adrenal insufficiency:
  - low 9 am serum cortisol; a raised ACTH level and a loss of cortisol response to synthetic ACTH stimulation test (Synacthen)
  - if adrenal insufficiency is confirmed and ACTH levels are normal or high (i.e., primary adrenal insufficiency is the diagnosis), further evaluation for mineralocorticoid deficiency should be performed (plasma renin activity, or renin concentration and serum aldosterone)
- The underlying aetiology of the adrenal insufficiency should then be determined.

2.1.4 Treatment

Adrenal crisis is a life-threatening emergency, which requires immediate treatment.

- Goal: treatment of hypotension and reversal of electrolyte abnormalities and of cortisol deficiency. Large volumes (1–3 L) of 0.9% saline solution or 5% dextrose in 0.9% saline should be infused IV to correct hypovolaemia and hyponatraemia associated with mineralocorticoid deficiency and/or syndrome of inappropriate antidiuretic hormone secretion.
- Treatment should not be delayed while diagnostic tests are performed.
- In a patient *without* a previous diagnosis of adrenal insufficiency, dexamethasone is used (which is not measured in cortisol assays), rather

than hydrocortisone while biochemical testing is performed.

- For patients *with* a previously known diagnosis of adrenal insufficiency, IV hydrocortisone or any other glucocorticoid preparation may be used.
- Mineralocorticoid administration is not necessary in the acute setting.
- Chronic primary adrenal insufficiency: hydrocortisone in two or three divided doses (total dose of 10–200 mg/m^2/day) as the glucocorticoid of choice. A daily dose of dexamethasone or prednisone may also be used. The lowest glucocorticoid dose that relieves symptoms of glucocorticoid deficiency is suggested.
- Most patients with primary adrenal insufficiency eventually require mineralocorticoid replacement with fludrocortisone.
- For minor illnesses: two to three times the usual maintenance glucocorticoid dose is given for three days (known as the 3 x 3 rule)
- For surgical procedures or severe illness: graded doses of hydrocortisone or its equivalent is given.
- All patients should wear a medical alert bracelet and have supplies for emergency glucocorticoid injections.

2.1.5 Pregnancy

- Both serum total and free cortisol levels are increased in normal pregnancy. Therefore, an abnormally low cortisol level for pregnancy may fall within the normal nonpregnant range.
- Most women adequately treated for adrenal insufficiency go through pregnancy, labour, and delivery without difficulty and babies achieve a normal birthweight.
- The usual glucocorticoid and mineralocorticoid replacement doses are continued; an occasional woman requires slightly more glucocorticoid in the third trimester.
- Glucocorticoid dose may need to be increased or need to be given by IV, if there is hyperemesis, infection, or any other stressful events (amniocentesis).
- During labour, adequate saline hydration and 25 mg hydrocortisone should be administered by IV every six hours. At the time of delivery, or if labour is prolonged, hydrocortisone should be administered by IV in a dose of 100 mg every six hours or as a continuous infusion. After delivery, the dose can be tapered rapidly to maintenance within three days.
- The regulation of plasma volume during pregnancy is complex. Secondary hyperaldosteronism is normal, associated with increased plasma renin activity and serum aldosterone concentrations. Serum concentrations of progesterone, which competes with aldosterone for binding to the type 1 corticosteroid (mineralocorticoid) receptor in the kidney and has a natriuretic effect, are increased throughout pregnancy. Plasma atrial natriuretic peptide concentrations reach their nadir late in the third trimester, when plasma renin activity and serum aldosterone concentrations reach their peak.
- There are no studies of mineralocorticoid requirement during pregnancy in women with adrenal insufficiency. Patients should be followed closely throughout pregnancy for electrolyte abnormalities and signs of volume depletion.
- Following delivery, physiological diuresis may result in profound hypotension, which can be treated with IV saline.

3 Hyperaldosteronism

- Conn's syndrome: aldosterone-producing adenoma.

3.1 Primary Aldosteronism

- Nonsuppressible (primary) hypersecretion of aldosterone is an underdiagnosed cause of HT. The classic presentation is HT and hypokalaemia.
- Renin-independent, incompletely suppressible hypersecretion of aldosterone.

3.1.1 Causes

- Bilateral idiopathic hyperaldosteronism (or idiopathic hyperplasia): 60–70%.
- Unilateral aldosterone-producing adenoma: 30–40%.
- Unilateral hyperplasia or primary adrenal hyperplasia caused by micronodular or macronodular hyperplasia of the zona glomerulosa of one adrenal gland.
- Familial.
- Pure aldosterone-producing adrenocortical carcinomas and ectopic aldosterone-secreting tumours (e.g., neoplasms in the ovary or kidney).

3.1.2 Clinical Features

- Hyperaldosteronism may be associated with resistant hypertension: failure to achieve goal blood pressure despite adherence to an appropriate, three-drug regimen including a diuretic.
- Persistent hypervolemia, which also results in marked suppression of renin release, leads to a very low plasma renin activity and plasma renin concentration.
- Although hypokalaemia is considered a 'classic' sign of primary aldosteronism, some patients with primary aldosteronism due to an adrenal adenoma and, more commonly, those with adrenal hyperplasia, are not hypokalaemic.
- Hypokalaemia is accompanied by metabolic alkalosis due to increased urinary hydrogen excretion mediated both by hypokalaemia and by the direct stimulatory effect of aldosterone on distal acidification.
- Aldosterone may raise the glomerular filtration rate and renal perfusion pressure independent of systemic hypertension. In addition, increased urinary albumin excretion is common.
- There is an increased risk of cardiovascular disease and morbidity, including left ventricular hypertrophy, atrial fibrillation, myocardial infarction and stroke.
- Mild hypernatraemia: the persistent mild volume expansion resets the osmostat, regulating antidiuretic hormone release and thirst upwards.
- Mild hypomagnesaemia due to urinary magnesium wasting.
- Muscle weakness primarily due to hypokalaemia.

3.1.3 Diagnosis

- Reduced plasma renin activity or plasma renin concentration (typically undetectable) and inappropriately high plasma aldosterone concentration.
- Aldosterone suppression test for confirmation with oral sodium loading and measurement of urine aldosterone excretion.
- The exception to the requirement for confirmatory testing is the patient with spontaneous hypokalaemia, undetectable plasma renin activity or plasma renin concentration, and a plasma aldosterone concentration ≥20 ng/dL; there is no other diagnosis except primary aldosteronism to explain these findings.
- Adrenal CT scan to distinguish between adenoma and bilateral hyperplasia. It will also exclude adrenocortical carcinoma.
- When the CT scan is normal, shows bilateral abnormalities or shows a unilateral abnormality, but the patient is over age 35 years, adrenal vein sampling is performed to confirm unilateral disease if the patient would like to pursue surgical management of their primary aldosteronism.

3.1.4 Treatment

- From a treatment perspective, the two major forms of primary aldosteronism are unilateral adrenal aldosterone hypersecretion (adenoma, unilateral hyperplasia, or carcinoma) and bilateral aldosterone hypersecretion (idiopathic adrenal hyperplasia).
- Goal: normalisation of the serum potassium in hypokalaemic patients, normalisation of BP (which often may persist after correction of the hyperaldosteronism), and reversal of the adverse cardiovascular effects of hyperaldosteronism.
- Unilateral aldosterone hypersecretion: unilateral laparoscopic adrenalectomy. Hypokalaemia should be corrected with spironolactone preoperatively. Plasma aldosterone should be measured the day after adrenal surgery to assess for cure. Serum potassium should be measured during the hospitalisation and, as an outpatient, once weekly for four weeks.
- Bilateral adrenal hyperplasia: medical treatment. BP control is often inadequate with subtotal adrenalectomy, and the risks associated with bilateral adrenalectomy (need for lifelong glucocorticoid and mineralocorticoid replacement) outweigh the potential benefits.
- Medical treatment: mineralocorticoid receptor antagonist spironolactone as the first-line drug; switched to eplerenone if the side effects are limiting. Eplerenone is a more selective mineralocorticoid receptor agonist than spironolactone, and is associated with fewer side effects, but when administered once daily and compared with spironolactone, eplerenone is a less effective antihypertensive agent. Serum potassium, creatinine and BP should be monitored frequently during the first four to six weeks of treatment.

3.1.5 Pregnancy

- Hyperaldosteronism is uncommon in pregnancy; most patients have aldosterone-producing adenomas.
- Presents with HT and hypokalaemia (serum potassium <3.0 mmol/L).
- It can lead to intrauterine growth restriction (IUGR), preterm delivery, intrauterine fetal death (IUFD), and placental abruption.
- During pregnancy, the degree of disease may be either improved or aggravated.
- Treatment depends on how difficult it is to manage the hypertension and hypokalaemia.
- In pregnant women who will be managed medically:
  - hypertension should be treated with standard antihypertensive drugs approved for use during pregnancy (methyldopa, labetalol or nifedipine)
  - hypokalaemia, if present, should be treated with oral potassium supplements and potassium sparing diuretics
- Amiloride is safe in pregnancy.
- Spironolactone crosses the placenta and results in feminisation of the newborn in animals. However, there is only one human case in the medical literature where treatment with spironolactone in pregnancy led to ambiguous genitalia in a male. (Food and Drug Administration category C).
- If hypertension and hypokalaemia are marked, then surgical and/or medical intervention is indicated.
- Unilateral laparoscopic adrenalectomy during the second trimester can be considered in those women with confirmed primary aldosteronism and a clear-cut unilateral adrenal macroadenoma (>10 mm).

4 Pheochromocytoma

- Pheochromocytoma is a rare neuroendocrine tumour with serious and potentially lethal cardiovascular complications due to the effects of secreted catecholamines. Although the clinical presentation may be quite variable, the classic triad is considered to be episodic headache, sweating and tachycardia in association with hypertension.
- Catecholamine-secreting tumours that arise from chromaffin cells of the adrenal medulla and the sympathetic ganglia are referred to as 'pheochromocytomas' and 'catecholamine-secreting paragangliomas' ('extra-adrenal pheochromocytomas'), respectively.
- Both have similar clinical presentations and are treated with similar approaches, but the distinction between the two is an important one because of implications for associated neoplasms, risk for malignancy and genetic testing.
- Pheochromocytomas may occur at any age; they are most common in the fourth to fifth decade and are equally common in men and women.
- Most catecholamine-secreting tumours are sporadic. However, approximately 40% of patients have the disease as part of a familial disorder. In these patients, the catecholamine-secreting tumours are more likely to be bilateral adrenal pheochromocytomas or paragangliomas. Hereditary catecholamine-secreting tumours typically present at a younger age than sporadic neoplasms.

4.1 Clinical Features

- Symptoms are present in approximately 50% of patients and, when present, they are typically paroxysmal.
- Symptoms are caused by tumoural hypersecretion of one or combinations of the catecholamines: norepinephrine, epinephrine, and dopamine; increased central sympathetic activity may also contribute.
- They are characterised by the classic triad of episodic headache, sweating and tachycardia. Approximately one-half of patients have paroxysmal HT; most of the rest have either primary HT or normal BP. Most patients with pheochromocytoma do *not* have the three classic symptoms.
- Sustained or paroxysmal HT is the most common sign, but 5–15% of patients present with normal BP.
- Headache, which may be mild or severe and variable in duration, is seen in up to 90% of symptomatic patients.
- Generalised sweating seen in up to 60–70% of symptomatic patients.

- Other symptoms: forceful palpitations, tremor, pallor, dyspnoea, generalised weakness and panic attack-type symptoms.
- Pheochromocytoma multisystem crisis: patients may have either hypertension or hypotension, hyperthermia (temperature >40 °C), mental status changes and other organ dysfunction.
- Orthostatic hypotension and others: orthostatic hypotension (which may reflect a low plasma volume), visual blurring, papilloedema, weight loss, polyuria, polydipsia, constipation, increased erythrocyte sedimentation rate, insulin resistance, hyperglycemia, leucocytosis, psychiatric disorders, and, rarely, secondary erythrocytosis due to overproduction of erythropoietin.
- Cardiomyopathy: rarely, pheochromocytoma is associated with cardiomyopathy attributed to catecholamine excess.
- The abnormalities in carbohydrate metabolism that occur (insulin resistance, impaired fasting glucose, apparent type 2 diabetes mellitus) are directly related to the increase in catecholamine production, which resolve after removal of the catecholamine-secreting neoplasm.

4.2 Diagnosis

- Initial biochemical testing is based on the index of suspicion that the patient has a pheochromocytoma:
  - if there is a low index of suspicion: 24-hour urinary fractionated catecholamines and metanephrines
  - if there is a high index of suspicion: fractionated metanephrines
- Examples of patients with a low index of suspicion include resistant hypertension and hyperadrenergic spells (self-limited episodes of nonexertional palpitations, diaphoresis, headache, tremor or pallor).
- Examples of patients with a high index of suspicion include a family history of pheochromocytoma, a genetic syndrome that predisposes to pheochromocytoma (MEN2), a history of resected pheochromocytoma or an incidentally discovered adrenal mass that has imaging characteristics consistent with pheochromocytoma.
- Biochemical confirmation of the diagnosis should be followed by radiological evaluation to locate the tumour. In sporadic pheochromocytoma, CT or MRI scans of the abdomen and pelvis should be undertaken. Either test detects almost all sporadic tumours because most are 3 cm or larger in diameter.
- Both CT and MRI scans are 98–100% sensitive, but are only 70% specific because of the higher prevalence of adrenal 'incidentalomas'; most of which are benign cortical adenomas.
- If CT or MRI is negative in the presence of clinical and biochemical evidence of pheochromocytoma, the diagnosis should be reconsidered. If it is still considered likely, then iodine-123 (123-I) iobenguane (also known as metaiodobenzylguanidine [MIBG]) scintigraphy may be done. An MIBG scan can detect tumours not detected by CT or MRI, or multiple tumours when CT or MRI is positive.

4.3 Treatment

- Preoperative preparation: preoperative alpha-adrenergic blockade with phenoxybenzamine is given as the first-line drug. After adequate alpha-adrenergic blockade has been achieved, beta-adrenergic blockade is begun with cautious, low-dose administration (e.g., propranolol). The dose is adjusted to control the tachycardia (goal heart rate is 60 to 80 beats per minute). The beta-adrenergic blocker should *never* be started first.
- Surgery: laparoscopic adrenalectomy.
- Familial pheochromocytoma:
  - MEN2 (a diffuse medullary disease) with evidence of bilateral disease >2 cm in diameter on imaging: complete bilateral adrenalectomy because of the risk of recurrent pheochromocytoma.
  - Von Hippel–Lindau (a less diffuse medullary disease) with evidence of bilateral disease on imaging: cortical-sparing bilateral adrenalectomy. Because of the risk of recurrent disease in these patients, long-term biochemical monitoring is needed.
- Malignant disease: resection of malignant pheochromocytoma with intent to cure, which may improve symptoms and possibly survival.

4.4 Pregnancy

- Pheochromocytomas are rare in pregnancy.

- Paroxysms of HT, palpitations, anxiety, sweating, headache, vomiting and glucose intolerance are only present in 50% of cases.
- HT with unusual symptoms such as excessive sweating, headache or palpitations should raise suspicion.
- Diagnosis is similar to nonpregnant women: raised 24-hour urinary catecholamines or raised plasma catecholamines. CT, USS or MRI is performed for localisation of the tumour.
- There is an increased maternal and fetal mortality rate.
- Medical management: alpha blockage with phenoxybenzamine or prazosin to control HT followed by beta blockers to control tachycardia.
- If pharmacological blockage is achieved before 23 weeks, surgical resection of the tumour is undertaken.
- >24 weeks of gestation: once fetal maturity is achieved, caesarean section with concurrent or delayed tumour resection can be done.

5 Congenital Adrenal Hyperplasia

5.1 Enzyme Defects

See Figure 28.1.

21-hydroxylase deficiency (90% of cases)

- Incidence: 1 in 5000 to 1 in 15 000.
- Gene: on short arm of chromosome 6.
- Results in a failure of conversion of 17α-hydroxyprogesterone to desoxycortisol and progesterone to desoxycorticosterone, leading to increased progesterone and 17α-hydroxyprogesterone (raised 50–400 times), which is therefore converted to androstenedione and subsequently to testosterone. Also results in insufficient cortisol production, stimulating increased production of corticotropin-releasing hormone and ACTH. High ACTH levels lead to adrenal hyperplasia and production of excess androgens.
- Symptoms of excessive androgens are found in varied degrees depending on the severity of the enzyme defect.
- Severe deficiency: adrenal aldosterone secretion is insufficient to stimulate sodium reabsorption by the distal renal tubules, resulting in salt wasting (seen in one-third cases) as well as cortisol deficiency, in addition to androgen excess. The child may die of wasting and vomiting within a few weeks of life due to this salt-losing syndrome.
- Prenatal treatment with daily dexamethasone may reduce the virilisation process.

11β-hydroxylase deficiency

- The second most common enzyme defect.
- Gene: on chromosome 8.
- May present with virilisation, hypertension and hypokalaemia. Hypertension is secondary to an increase in 11-deoxycortisol and deoxycorticosterone (mineralocorticoid).
- High levels of 17-OH progesterone, 11-deoxycortisol and deoxycorticosterone.

5.2 Presentation

- Newborn with ambiguous genitalia: enlarged clitoris and excessive fusion of the labioscrotal folds, which obscure the vagina and urethra, with a single opening at some point on the perineum, usually near the base of the clitoris, although sometimes along its ventral surface and rarely at the tip. Thickening and rugosity of the labia majora with some resemblance to a scrotum. The uterus, fallopian tubes and vagina are always present, and the vagina opens at some point in the urogenital sinus.
- Late onset: accounts for up to 2–20% of women presenting with hirsutism and oligomenorrhea. May mimic PCOS. 17-OH progesterone is less elevated: ACTH stimulation test with measurement of 17-OH progesterone.
- Treatment:
  - Glucocorticoids: replace glucocorticoid deficit and decrease ACTH secretion. Overtreatment should be avoided as it may cause linear growth restriction, delayed puberty and Cushingoid signs. Infants: hydrocortisone twice daily. Adults: prednisolone.
  - Mineralocorticoid replacement with fludrocortisone.
  - Clitoral reduction, vaginoplasty with correction of labial fusion, and anomalous urethral position. Timing of surgery is advised to be delayed until adolescence.
  - Women are fertile with adequate replacement therapy. There is a risk of autosomal recessive condition being passed on to next generation.

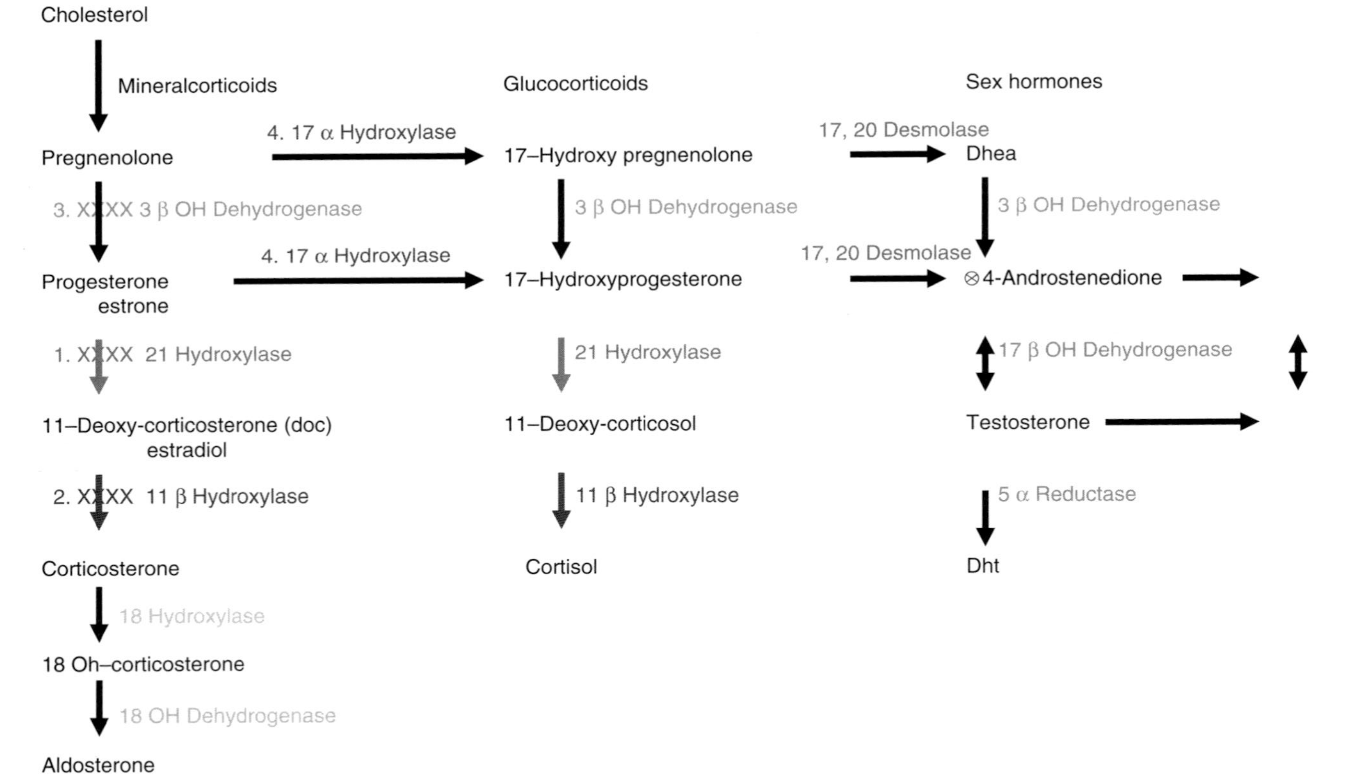

Figure 28.1 Adrenal steroid hormone synthesis steps.

5.3 Other Causes of Masculinisation in Genetic women

- Androgen-secreting tumours in pregnancy, resulting in virilisation of the fetus.
- The association between the use of progestogens and masculinisation of the fetus is extremely rare.
- Management is to exclude CAH.
- Reared in the female role.
- If no source of androgen can be identified, the possibility of the child being a 46,XX true hermaphrodite should be considered, and, if the degree of external masculinisation is considerable, gonadal biopsy considered.

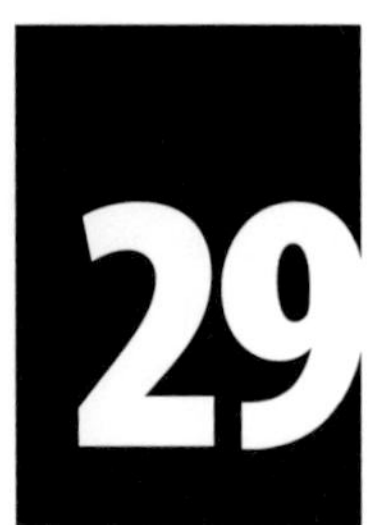

Hyperemesis Gravidarum

Jyotsna Pundir

1 Background and Prevalence

- Nausea and vomiting in pregnancy affect at least 50% of women in the first trimester of pregnancy. Symptoms usually begin at 5–6 weeks, with peak severity around week 11, and, in 90% of women, these symptoms resolve by week 16.
- Hyperemesis gravidarum (HG) is persistent vomiting in pregnancy, which leads to weight loss of >5% of prepregnancy weight with electrolyte imbalance and ketonuria. It affects 1% of pregnant woman.
- The pathogenesis is poorly understood, and the aetiology is likely to be multifactorial.

2 Risks or Complications

2.1 Maternal

- Weight loss and muscle wasting.
- Mallory–Weiss tears and haematemesis.
- Thiamine deficiency: Wernicke's encephalopathy – diplopia, abnormal ocular movements, ataxia and confusion. IV glucose may precipitate it. Thiamine replacement may improve the symptoms, but residual impairment is not uncommon.
- Korsakoff's psychosis: retrograde amnesia, impaired ability to learn and confabulation. The recovery rate is only about 50%.
- Hyponatraemia: lethargy, seizures and respiratory arrest. Both severe hyponatraemia and its rapid reversal may precipitate central pontine myelinolysis: spastic quadriparesis, pseudobulbar palsy and impaired consciousness.
- Other vitamin deficiencies (cyanocobalamin and pyridoxine) can cause anaemia and peripheral neuropathy.
- Maternal death.

2.2 Fetal

- Women with HG during pregnancy are more likely to have a baby with low birthweight and premature birth.

2.3 Psychological Impact

- affects work and quality of life
- depression
- difficulties between partners
- in some, the condition is so intolerable that the woman may elect to have a termination of pregnancy

3 Clinical Features

- severe and persistent nausea and vomiting, leading to dehydration and weight loss
- there may be ptyalism (inability to swallow saliva) and spitting
- signs of dehydration, tachycardia and postural hypotension

4 Differential Diagnoses

- urinary tract infection
- appendicitis
- hepatitis
- cholecystitis
- small bowel obstruction
- pancreatitis
- thyrotoxicosis
- gestational thyrotoxicosis
- hyperparathyroidism
- diabetic ketoacidosis
- uraemia
- Addison's disease

5 Management

- dietary and lifestyle changes: there is no evidence to prove the effectiveness of dietary changes on relieving symptoms

5.1 Nonpharmacological Therapies

- emotional support with frequent reassurance and encouragement
- psychotherapy, hypnotherapy and behavioural therapy may be helpful
- ginger and alternative therapies, such as acupuncture and acupressure, may be beneficial

5.2 Pharmacological Treatment

If no relief with conservative measures:

- Antihistamines: H1-receptor antagonists (dimenhydrinate, diphenhydramine and hydroxyzine) are considered safe in pregnancy, with no human teratogenic potential. It should be considered in the management of acute or breakthrough episodes of HG.
- Ranitidine and omeprazole: used primarily to reduce oesophageal acid reflux associated with HG. They have been shown to bring symptomatic relief, with no evidence of increased risk of congenital malformations.
- The dopamine antagonists, phenothiazines (chlorpromazine, perphenazine, prochlorperazine, promethazine, trifluoperazine) have been proven safe for use in pregnancy. Phenothiazines are safe and effective for severe HG.
- Metoclopramide: safe to be used for management of HG, although evidence for its efficacy is limited.

5.3 Admission to Hospital

- any woman unable to maintain adequate hydration should be admitted to hospital

5.3.1 Investigations

- Urea and electrolytes: hyponatraemia and hypokalaemia.
- Raised haematocrit.
- Metabolic hypochloraemic alkalosis. Severe cases: acidaemia.
- Liver function tests: raised aminotransferase and bilirubin (frank jaundice is rare).
- Urinalysis: raised specific gravity and ketonuria.
- Urine microscopy and culture: to exclude urinary tract infection (UTI).
- Ultrasound scan: to exclude molar or multiple pregnancy.
- Thyroid function tests: raised free thyroxine, reduced thyroid stimulating hormone: self-limiting. Routine thyroid function tests are questionable as clinical hyperthyroidism does not occur, and treatment is not required. They may provide an index of severity of HG, as women with abnormal thyroid function usually require longer hospitalisation to avoid readmission.

5.3.2 Rehydration

- IV rehydration with normal saline or Hartmann's solution.
- Potassium chloride with each bag of saline, particularly if there is continued vomiting.
- Fluid and electrolyte regimens must be adapted daily and titrated against daily measurements of serum sodium and potassium.
- Double-strength saline solution should be avoided, even in cases of severe hyponatraemia, as rapid correction of sodium depletion may cause central pontine myelinolysis.
- Solutions containing dextrose should be avoided because they do not contain enough sodium and may precipitate Wernicke's encephalopathy.

5.3.3 Monitoring and Others

- Weight, pulse and blood pressure should be recorded.
- Drugs that may cause nausea and vomiting (e.g., iron supplements) should be temporarily discontinued.
- Routine thiamine supplementation to prevent Wernicke's encephalopathy: oral/IV.
- Thromboprophylaxis (e.g., enoxaparin 40 mg/daily) and thromboembolic deterrent stockings.

5.3.4 Refractory: Severe Hyperemesis

- Ondansetron: the selective serotonin (5-HT$_3$) receptor antagonist. Because of its limited effectiveness, it should not be advocated for first-line use until agents with established safety and effectiveness have been tried and have failed.

- Corticosteroid therapy: may produce a dramatic and rapid improvement; may need long-term therapy. Screening for the complications of steroid treatment in pregnancy, particularly UTIs and gestational diabetes mellitus, is necessary. There is a small but significantly increased risk of oral clefting associated with first trimester exposure. The data on effectiveness is weak. It should be kept as the last line of therapy and used only when maternal benefits outweigh fetal risk.

5.3.5 Total Parenteral Nutrition

- Produces a rapid therapeutic effect.
- Recommended if optimal rehydration, antiemetic therapy and a trial of corticosteroids and/or ondansetron have failed to result in improvement.
- Risks: metabolic and infectious complications – line sepsis, bacterial endocarditis and pneumonia.

Section 6

Biochemistry

Mala Arora

30 Biochemistry in Surgical Conditions

Smita Kaushik

Following surgery, postsurgical inflammation subsequently leads to healing. Biochemical changes in the cells and the blood occur following surgery, especially with complications such as bleeding, infection, damage to the bowel or bladder, diabetic ketoacidosis or thrombosis.

The common physiological conditions that affect biochemistry in the body during the postsurgical period are:

- dehydration
- hyperventilation
- starvation/fasting
- urinary retention
- inflammation

Surgical inflammation includes five phases of inflammation either following surgery or trauma as described by the Roman scholar, Celsus, in the first century AD:

1. Calor: heat
2. Dolor: pain
3. Rubor: redness
4. Tumour: swelling
5. Functio laesa: loss of function

- The colour changes are due to traumatic and inflammatory injury.
- The acute inflammatory response to injury by mechanical energy, regardless of whether it is local or systemic, is based on the successive pathologic functional predominance of the nervous, immune and endocrine systems.
- The different blood components escape the intravascular space one by one to occupy the interstitial space, where they play the main role in the successive phases of the inflammatory response.
- The nervous or immediate functional system presents ischaemia-revascularisation and oedema, which favour nutrition by diffusion through the injured tissue. This process requires low energy and does not require oxygen (e.g., in ischaemia). If oxygen is not correctly utilised by tissues, there is subsequent excessive production of reactive oxygen and nitrogen species (ROS/RNS) that will lead to reperfusion. In this phase, with the progression of interstitial oedema in the space between the epithelial cells and the capillaries, the lymphatic circulation is activated. Thus, the injured tissues are in a state of hypoxia.
- In the ensuing immune or intermediate phase of the inflammatory response, the tissues and organs that suffered ischaemia-reperfusion are infiltrated by inflammatory cells and, sometimes, by bacteria.
- Interstitial inflammation is favoured by activation of haemostasis and complement cascades.
- In the tissues and organs that suffer oxidative stress, symbiosis of the inflammatory cells and bacteria for extracellular digestion by enzyme release (fermentation) and by intracellular digestion (phagocytosis) occurs. Furthermore, lymphatic circulation plays a major role and macrophages and dendritic cells migrate to lymph nodes where they activate lymphocytes.
- Angiogenesis characterises the last or endocrine phase of the inflammatory response, so nutrition is maintained. However, the angiogenic process becomes active early and excessive proliferation of endothelial cells takes place, which, in turn, develops a great density of endothelial sprouts. Through this initial and excessive proliferation, the endothelial cells can successively perform antioxidant and anti-enzymatic functions, leading to repair and healing.
- Inflammatory pain is caused by tissue damage generally by an upregulation of ionic channel expression in the nociceptive circuits, which causes the spontaneous neural stimulation.
- Following this is an immune phase, with cytokines, chemokines and prostaglandins derived

from glial and immune cells acting as pain mediators and modulators.

- Lastly, in an endocrine phase, neurotrophic factors, including nerve growth factor, brain-derived neurotrophic factor and neurotrophin-3 and neurotrophin-4, are associated with structural neural remodelling.
- The initial dark blue colour of the ecchymotic lesion comes from the carboxyhaemoglobin, which results from the binding of carbon monoxide to haemoglobin. Once the haemoglobin is released into the interstitial space, haemolysis results. Haemoglobin, released from red blood cells, is the major source of haem for bile pigment synthesis. Haem is converted to biliverdin (green pigment), carbon monoxide and iron by the enzyme haeme-oxygenase.
- In addition to the enzymes released by granulocytes during the process of phagocytosis and bacterial killing, the bacteria themselves produce a number of exoenzymes, which cause tissue destruction and localisation of infection. Bacteria such as *Staphylococcus aureus* strains can secrete an array of enzymes including nucleases, proteases, lipases, hyaluronidase and collagenase. Matrix metalloproteinases also collaborate in the development of enzymatic stress in the acute inflammatory tissue injury.
- Compensation of the acute phase response includes the production of positive acute phase proteins such as α_2-macroglobulin, which binds proteolytic enzymes, and α_1-antitrypsin and α_1-antichymotrypsin, which are inhibitors of leucocyte and lysosomal proteolytic enzymes. Unconjugated bilirubin is a potent inhibitor of the digestive proteases trypsin and chymotrypsin.
- In the small intestine, bilirubin glucuronides are deconjugated by beta-glucuronidase (secreted by the gut mucosa), and are also found in some strains of bacteria such as *Escherichia coli* and *Streptococcus pyogenes*.
- Cholestatic jaundice also occurs in the setting of sepsis. Liver abnormalities in sepsis include cholestasis and hyperbilirubinaemia. Gram-negative infections used to be the cause of cholestasis associated with sepsis. Hyperbilirubinaemia develops in sepsis especially with bacteraemia. Hyperbilirubinaemia precedes positive blood cultures in one-third of cases.
- Blood cells such as platelets, mast cells, neutrophils, macrophages and T-cells help with modulating inflammatory processes. As the inflammatory response progresses, certain stop signals at appropriate checkpoints prevent further oedema production and infiltration of leucocytes into tissues.
- Proinflammatory mechanisms are counterbalanced by endogenous anti-inflammatory signals, which control the severity and duration of inflammation.
- Regulatory T cells (Treg cells) have evolved to provide a complementary immunological arm to a physiological tissue-protecting mechanism driven by low oxygen tension (i.e., hypoxia) in inflamed tissues.

1 Nitric Oxide (NO): Endothelium Derived Relaxing Factor

- gaseous signalling molecule: a free radical

$$\text{Arginine} + O_2 \xrightarrow{\text{NOS, NADPH}} \text{NO} + \text{CITRULLINE}$$

1.1 Actions

- increases vasodilation
- neurotransmission
- regulates gene transcription
- mRNA translation and posttranslational modification
- causes relaxation of vascular smooth muscles, i.e. vasodilation and increases blood flow
- can diffuse freely across membranes, has paracrine effect

2 Nitric Oxide Synthase (NOS)

2.1 Isoenzymes

NOS exists in three isomers:

- eNOS: endothelial
- nNOS: neuronal
- iNOS: inducible

3 NO In Pregnancy

- contributes to maternal systemic vasodilatation
- regulates uterine and fetoplacental blood flow

- maintains uterine relaxation during antenatal period; when nearing term, NO production decreases, causing effective contractions and leading to labour
- decreased NO leads to pregnancy-induced hypertension and preeclampsia

4 NOS In Pregnancy

- uterine arteries have increased eNOS activity
- NOS is also expressed by placental syncytiotrophoblast, foetoplacental and umbilical vascular endothelium, and NO produced locally contributes to low fetoplacental vascular resistance
- the uterus also has NOS activity, but near term, exogenous NO relaxes the myometrium
- in human endometrium, iNOS activity has been found in immunocompetent endometrial cells and decidual stromal cells during menstruation, indicating that NO is involved in the initiation and maintenance of menstrual bleeding by causing tissue breakdown and vascular relaxation, and also by inhibiting platelet aggregation; eNOS has a similar role

5 The Effect of Surgery and Anaesthesia on Biochemical Parameters

- A transient rise in blood glucose, free fatty acid levels and a concomitant fall in insulin levels has been noted during surgeries. It is postulated that anxiety of surgery leads to an increase in cortisol levels, causing hyperglycaemia. Additionally, an increase in growth hormone can cause hyperglycaemia.
- Arterial blood gas values of the mother and newborn do not show any significant change during caesarean section. When mothers are supplemented with oxygen during surgery, this may lead to mild acidosis in the newborn.

31 Hormones

Smita Kaushik

1 Steroid and Nonsteroid Hormones

- Hormones may be steroid or nonsteroid.
- Steroid hormones are a group of hormones that belong to a class of compounds called steroids (see Figure 31.1). They are secreted by three steroid glands: adrenal cortex, testes and the ovaries, and during pregnancy, by the placenta.
- Nonsteroid hormones are made of amino acids. They are not fat soluble, so they cannot diffuse across the plasma membrane of target cells. Instead, a nonsteroid hormone binds to a receptor on the cell membrane. Most endocrine hormones are nonsteroid hormones, including insulin and thyroid hormones. See Table 31.1.
- All steroid hormones are derived from cholesterol. They are hydrophobic/lipophilic, and are transported in blood bound to a protein carrier to various target cells/organs, where they can enter the cell by easily passing through the plasma membrane and carry out gene transcription.
- They are often classified according to the organ that synthesises them:
  - adrenal steroids: secreted by the adrenal cortex
  - sex hormones: produced by the ovaries and testes, and the placenta during pregnancy
- There are five types of hormones based on the receptors they bind to:
  - glucocorticoids
  - mineralocorticoids
  - androgens
  - estrogens
  - progesterones
- They bind to different types of receptors. Vitamin D (also synthesised from cholesterol) is a closely related hormone system with similar receptors.
- Steroid hormones have varied functions: they help control metabolism, inflammation, immune functions, salt and water balance, and development of sexual characteristics, and are able to withstand illness and injury.
- Synthesis of steroid hormones takes place in the mitochondria of cells in the adrenal cortex and gonads (see Figure 31.2). Cholesterol is transported inside the mitochondria by a specific protein, steroidogenic acute regulatory protein (StAR). A mutation in the StAR gene leads to the severest

Table 31.1 Properties and types of steroid and nonsteroidal hormones

Nonsteroidal hormones	Steroidal hormones
Hydrophilic	Hydrophobic
Transported in blood; water soluble	Need carrier proteins
Cannot pass through the lipid layer of cells: need receptors	Can pass through cell membranes
Broken down within minutes	Persist in blood for days
Examples: • Neurotransmitters • Most hormones	Examples: • Cortisol • estrogen • Progesterone • Retinoids • Vitamin D • Thyroid hormones

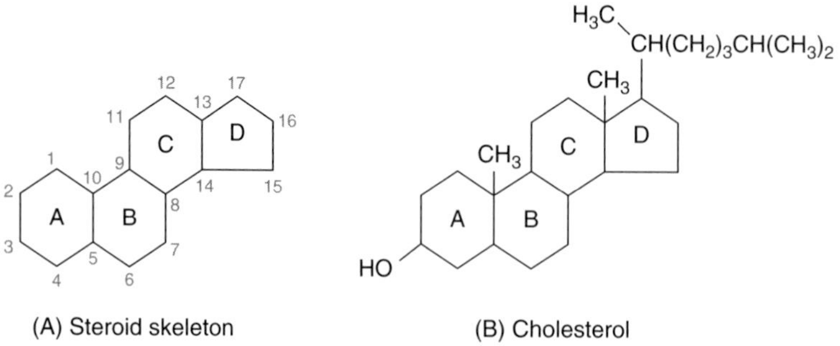

(A) Steroid skeleton

(B) Cholesterol

Figure 31.1 Structure of the steroid nucleus.

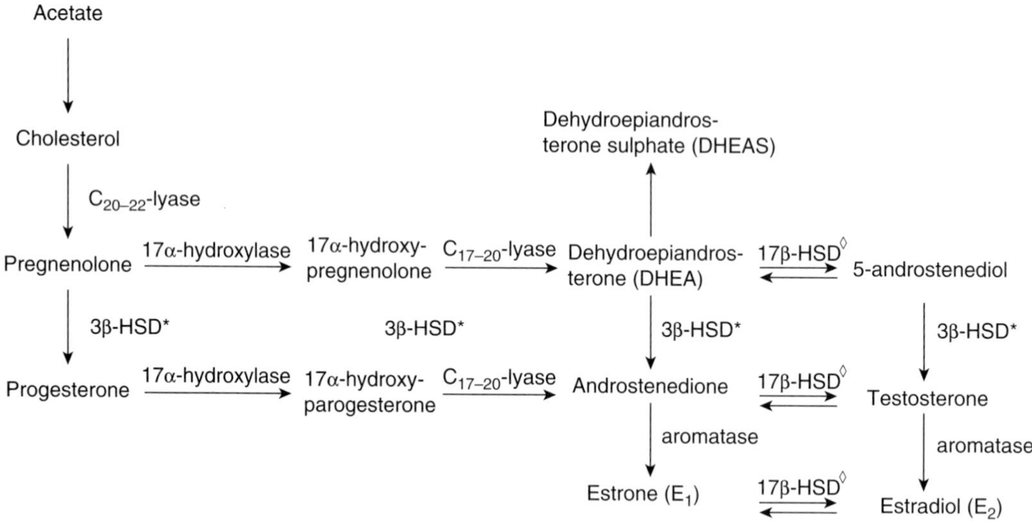

*3β-HSD = 3β-hydroxysteroid dehydrogenase-$\Delta^{5,4}$-isomerase
◊17β-HSD = 17β-hydroxysteroid dehydrogenase

Figure 31.2 Synthesis of steroid hormones in sex organs.

form of congenital adrenal hyperplasia with absence of adrenal and gonadal steroid hormones.

- The StAR gene is highly expressed in the adrenal cortex, testes and ovaries, but not in the placenta. See Figure 31.2.
- Stimulus for sex hormones synthesis: follicle stimulating hormone (FSH) and luteinising hormone (LH) (anterior pituitary).

2 Steroid Hormone Synthesis in the Adrenal Cortex

- Stimulus for steroidogenesis is ACTH secreted from the anterior pituitary. Ascorbic acid (vitamin C) and NADPH is required during synthesis.
- Cholesterol is converted to pregnenolone, which is the precursor for all the steroid hormones. See Figure 31.3.
- Steroid hormones are lipophilic and hence are transported in the blood, bound to carrier proteins such as albumin, sex hormone-binding globulin and corticosteroid-binding globulin. They reach their target organs and tissues, and enter the specific cells (without the carrier protein) across the biomembrane. Once inside the cell, they either bind to their specific cytoplasmic receptor and enter nucleus or enter the nucleus as such. They then bind to their specific hormone response element on the DNA and bring about gene transcription, leading to the synthesis of desired proteins.

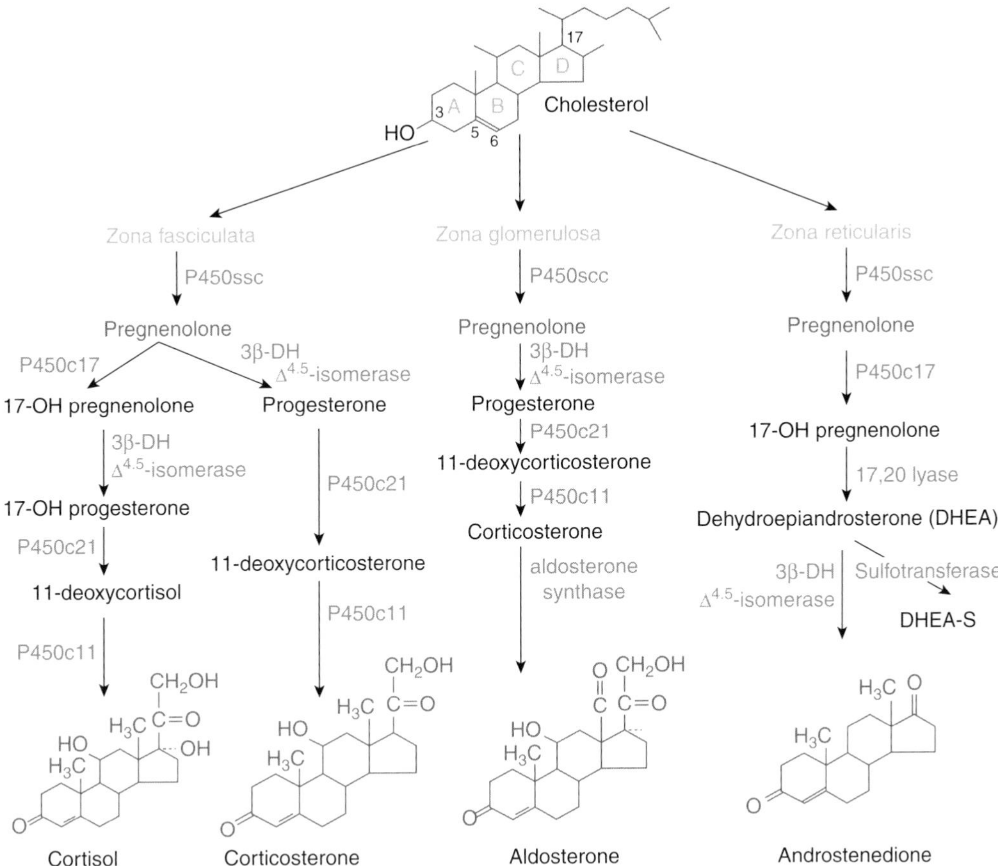

Figure 31.3 Synthesis of steroid hormones in the adrenal cortex.

3 Steroid Hormone Synthesis by the Placenta

- In humans, the placenta can acquire the ability to substitute for the ovaries during pregnancy. Trophoblast cells are responsible for steroidogenesis. Cholesterol for this purpose is taken up from maternal blood. Trophoblast cells express specific receptors (low-density lipoprotein (LDL) receptor, very low-density lipoprotein (VLDL) receptor and LDL receptor-related protein) on their surface to recognise maternal LDL, VLDL and chylomicron remnants. Also, these cells express apolipoprotein E, a ligand for all three types of lipoprotein receptors to enhance the binding of lipoproteins to their specific receptors.
- Placental cells do not express 17α-hydroxylase, which are derived from cytochrome P450, so estrogen synthesis depends on androgen secreted from fetal adrenal glands.
- There are no known cases of cytochrome P450 cholesterol side-chain cleavage enzyme ($P450_{SCC}$) deficiency, implicating that this enzyme is necessary for survival. Absence of functional $P450_{SCC}$ prevents placental progesterone and fetal adrenal and gonadal steroidogenesis, which is incompatible with life.
- Homozygous mutations (mutations in both alleles) in type I 3β-hydroxysteroid dehydrogenase gene, expressed by trophoblastic cells, are also not known; this compromises placental progesterone synthesis.

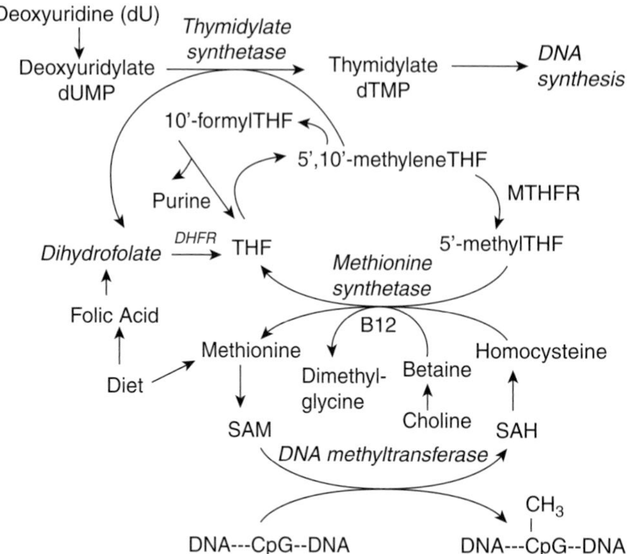

Figure 31.4 Folate metabolism.
THF: tetrahydrofolate
TMP: thymidine monophosphate
SAM: sadenosyl methionine
SAH: sadenosyl-l-homocysteine

- Placental estrogen synthesis does not occur when there is deficiency of the enzyme sulphatase (in both the fetus and the placenta), required for hydrolysis of dehydroepiandrosterone sulphate (DHEA-S) (from the fetal adrenal cortex). DHEA-S is the precursor of estrogens in the third trimester. In addition, aromatase deficiency (both fetal and placental), leads to absent or low levels of estrogens, but pregnancy does reach term, even with these enzyme deficiencies, although there is difficulty in cervical ripening due to the lack of placental estrogens. Aromatase deficiency may cause virilisation of mother and fetus.
- Regulation of placental steroidogenesis: cyclic AMP increases P450scc gene transcription in trophoblast cells. StAR protein required for cholesterol translocation into cell mitochondria for steroidogenesis is not expressed in trophoblast cells. fetal steroid hormones influence placental steroidogenesis by providing various precursors.

4 Methylenetetrahydrofolate Reductase

- Methylenetetrahydrofolate reductase (MTHFR) is the rate-limiting enzyme that catalyses the irreversible conversion of 5,10-methylenetetrahydrofolate to 5-methyltetrahydrofolate. This reaction occurs along with methylation of homocysteine to methionine (enzyme–methionine synthase), where the donor of the methyl group is 5-methyltetrahydrofolate (see Figure 31.4).
- MTHFR is a flavoprotein (closely associated with flavin adenine dinucleotide (FAD)), and utilises nicotinamide adenine dinucleotide phosphate (NADPH) as the reducing agent.
- The gene for MTHFR is present on chromosome 1.
- Certain polymorphisms and/or mutations in *MTHFR* gene have been implicated in increased susceptibility to occlusive vascular diseases due to hyperhomocysteinemia, neural tube defects, Alzheimer's disease, dementia, colon cancer and acute lymphoblastic leukaemia.
- MTHFR deficiency can lead to hyperhomocysteinaemia, which is an independent high risk factor for myocardial infarction.
- Single nucleotide polymorphisms 677C>T and 1298A>C in the *MTHFR* gene mutation results in a thermolabile enzyme variant with reduced activity. These variants in both maternal and/or fetal genes have been implicated in various pregnancy complications like miscarriage, neural tube defects, and preeclampsia, probably due to a change in DNA methylation. Miscarriage or stillbirths are probably a result of vascular disruption at the uteroplacental interface, thus preventing transport of nutrients to the fetus.

32 Minerals and Vitamins in Pregnancy

Smita Kaushik

1 Minerals

- Inorganic micronutrients are classified as (1) macroelements: calcium (Ca), phosphorus (P), sodium (Na), potassium (K), magnesium (Mg), chlorine (Cl), sulphur (S), (2) micro or trace elements: iron (Fe), zinc (Zn), fluorine (F), copper (Cu), iodine (I), selenium (Se), cobalt (Co), manganese (Mn), molybdenum (Mo).
- They are essential in the diet; deficiency may lead to certain disorders.
- The daily requirement of macroelements is >100 mg/day.
- The daily requirement of microelements is <100 mg/day.

1.1 Bulk or Macroelements

1.1.1 Calcium

- The most abundant mineral in the body; an adult contains 1.0–1.5 kg of calcium.
- Of total body calcium, 99% is in the bones and teeth as the insoluble crystalline mineral hydroxyapatite ($[Ca_3(PO_4)_2]_3.Ca(OH)_2$). The remaining 1% is in soft tissues, extracellular fluid and blood.
- Normal plasma calcium levels: 9.0–11.0 mg/100 mL (4.5–5.5 mEq/L).
- Plasma calcium exists in three forms:
  1. Ionised or diffusible: 50% of total plasma calcium (~5 mg/dL). Physiologically active form.
  2. Protein bound: 40% of total (~4 mg/dL). Bound to albumin; nondiffusible.
  3. Complexed calcium: 5–10% of total (~1 mg/dL); forms complexes with organic acids, citrate/phosphate. Diffusible form.
- All three forms remain in equilibrium with each other.
- Functions:
  1. Bone and teeth development: along with phosphate, it is deposited as hydroxyapatite
  2. Blood coagulation: clotting factor IV
  3. Muscle contraction: for excitation and contraction of muscles (smooth, skeletal and cardiac)
  4. Nerve excitability: calcium required for neurotransmitter release and impulse transmission
  5. Hormone release: insulin, parathyroid hormone (PTH) require calcium for release
  6. Enzyme activation, membrane and capillary permeability
  7. Signal transduction: as a secondary messenger
  8. Milk formation in lactating mothers
- Sources:
  - Widely distributed in plants and animals.
  - Milk and milk products: 115 mg Ca/100 mL milk.
  - Seafood.
  - Cereals, pulses, nuts, beans and leafy vegetables.
  - Recommended dietary allowance (RDA): 1000 mg/day.
  - Increased in childhood, pregnancy, lactation and postmenopause.
- Intestinal absorption: 20–40% of dietary calcium is absorbed in ionised form from the duodenum and jejunum.

1.1.1.1 Factors That Stimulate Intestinal Absorption

- presence of lactose
- acidic pH, acidic foods: calcium carbonate and phosphate soluble in acidic pH
- vitamin D (calcitriol) by inducing synthesis of calbindin in the intestinal mucosa

- calbindin increases calcium absorption from the gut
- dietary proteins favour calcium absorption such as basic amino acids like lysine and arginine

1.1.1.2 Factors That Decrease Absorption

- phytic acid (a branched fatty acid), found in plants, precipitates calcium
- alkaline pH in gut
- oxalates in green leafy vegetables (cabbage, spinach, and so on) cause the formation of calcium oxalates
- high fibre diet
- age above 60 years
- excess dietary phosphates and magnesium: precipitates as calcium phosphate; the optimal absorption of calcium and phosphorous occurs when the dietary Ca:P ratio is in the limits of 1:2 to 2:1
- diet rich in fats: formation of insoluble soaps of fatty acids
- glucocorticoids

1.1.1.3 Regulation of Calcium (and Phosphorus) Homeostasis

PTH and calcitriol act together:

- PTH: maintains normal plasma calcium levels by mobilising calcium and phosphate from bones by stimulating osteoclastic activity:
    - in the kidneys, it increases renal reabsorption of calcium and also stimulates α-1-hydroxylase enzyme, which enhances synthesis of calcitriol
- Calcitriol (active vitamin D_3): increases plasma Ca levels:
    - by increasing absorption of calcium and phosphorus by the intestine (inducing calbindin synthesis)
    - by stimulating renal reabsorption of calcium and phosphorus
- Calcitonin: tends to decrease plasma calcium levels during hypercalcaemia:
    - stimulates osteoblastic activity and inhibits osteoclastic activity
    - increases urinary excretion of calcium
- Effect of plasma protein on calcium: 40% of total plasma calcium in blood is bound to protein, mainly albumin, so total plasma calcium in patients with low or high albumin levels may not reflect the accurate free calcium concentration. The corrected calcium level is given by [0.8 x (normal albumin level – patient's albumin)] + serum Ca level.
- Inter-relationship between calcium and phosphate: a reciprocal relationship exists between calcium and phosphorus. Hypercalcaemia is accompanied by a decrease in phosphate concentration (hypophosphataemia) and hypocalcaemia is accompanied by hyperphosphataemia. The ionic product of calcium and phosphate in plasma is maintained constant at 40 (10 mg/dL Ca x 4 mg/dL P = 40) or <4 mmol^2/L^2.
- Calcium appears in urine during hypercalcaemia associated with hyperparathyroidism.
- Calcium deficiency: leads to rickets in childhood and osteomalacia in adults. Deficiency of vitamin D, calcium and phosphate may occur due to several causes. It is characterised by incomplete mineralisation of growing bones in children and demineralisation of bones in adults. It may alter the pelvic shape and diameters; thereby leading to difficulty during childbirth.
- Hypocalcaemic tetany: a plasma calcium level of <6 mg/dL causes tetany: neuromuscular hyperexcitability and convulsions. The commonest cause is hyperparathyroidism.
- A moderate decrease in calcium levels may cause muscular cramps and numbness of hands and feet.
- Blood-clotting disorders: a severe fall in calcium levels may increase the blood-clotting time.
- Osteoporosis: progressive loss of bone mineral density; loss of bone organic matrix and demineralisation. Postmenopausal women are at higher risk due to lack of estrogen. This increases the risk of fracture in Postmenopausal women.
- Hypercalcaemia: increase in plasma calcium levels beyond 12 mg/dL. Signs and symptoms are nausea and vomiting, loss of appetite and muscular weakness.
- Calcinosis (calcium deposition in kidneys, arteries, soft tissues, and so on) Commonest cause is hyperparathyroidism.

1.1.1.4 Calcium in Pregnancy

- There is an increase in calcium consumption in pregnancy and lactation as the fetus in utero and the neonate depends on maternal sources for

calcium load. Adequate calcium intake positively affects fetal bone growth. The fetus accumulates maximum calcium (almost 80%) during the third trimester when the fetal skeleton is rapidly mineralising. During pregnancy, the level of PTH remains low to normal, and vitamin D increases in early pregnancy to allow intestinal calcium absorption throughout pregnancy for normal fetal skeletal growth. Women of childbearing age should be screened for vitamin D deficiency and supplemented to allow for adequate calcium absorption during pregnancy.
- Transfer of calcium from mother to fetus is an active process, utilising energy (adenosine triphosphate [ATP]) and is regulated by parathyroid hormone related protein (PTHrP) rather than calcitriol. Syncytiotrophoblasts actively transport 80% of calcium from maternal to fetal circulation. It has high affinity to calcium ions (Ca^{2+}) and stimulates ATPase activity in the microvillus membrane, which is capable of transporting Ca^{2+} against concentration gradient. Almost 30 g of calcium is transported to the fetus in the last trimester.
- Calcium is actively secreted in milk. During lactation, a specific receptor – calcium-sensing receptor (CaSR) – is activated in mammary epithelial cells, which downregulates PTHrP levels in milk and maternal circulation and increases calcium transport into milk. CaSR is a G-protein-coupled receptor.

1.2 Phosphorus

- After calcium, phosphorus is the most abundant mineral in the body.
- Of total body phosphate, 80% is present in the bones and teeth along with calcium. The remaining 20% is in the soft tissues, extracellular fluid (ECF) and blood.
- Normal plasma levels: 2.5–4.5 mg/dL.
- Phosphorous exists in three forms:
  1. Free inorganic phosphate: approximately 40%
  2. Phosphate complexed with cations (Na^+, K^+, Ca^{2+}): approximately 50%
  3. Protein bound phosphate: approximately 10%

Biological functions

- Mineralisation of bones and teeth along with calcium as hydroxyapatite.
- Phosphorus synthesises phospholipids (the constituents of cell membrane), organic substances like nucleic acid (DNA, RNA), coenzymes (NAD, NADP, FAD, TPP, etc.), nucleotides (UTP, GTP, AMP, etc.) and second messengers (cAMP, cGMP).
- Energy metabolism in oxidative phosphorylation to generate adenosine triphosphate (ATP) and adenosine di phosphate (ADP).
- Metabolism of carbohydrate, proteins and lipids for activation of enzymes.
- RDA: adults: 700 mg/day. Pregnancy and lactation: 1200 mg/day.
- Dietary sources: phosphorous is widely distributed in animal and plant foods, milk and milk products, meat and eggs.
- Milk protein casein is a phospho-protein. Milk contains 93 mg/dl of phosphorus.
- Cereals, pulses, nuts and leafy vegetables are rich sources.
- Intestinal absorption occurs in the jejunum and only inorganic phosphate is absorbed. Vitamin D and the ratio of Ca:P in the diet influence phosphate absorption.
- Regulation of plasma phosphorus: a reciprocal relationship exists between calcium and phosphate concentrations in blood.
- PTH stimulates renal excretion of phosphorous.
- Calcitriol maintains normal levels of phosphorous during hypophosphataemia and low phosphorous levels stimulate production of calcitriol.
- Hypophosphataemia is seen in hyperparathyroidism, and vitamin D deficiency causes defective mineralisation of the bones and teeth.
- Hyperphosphataemia occurs due to hypoparathyroidism, severe renal failure and diabetes mellitus.
- Breast milk has low phosphorus, but newborns do not lose phosphate through the urine so they retain high blood levels of phosphate.

1.3 Magnesium

- Adults contain 20–25 g of magnesium: 75% in the bones and teeth in combination with calcium and phosphate; the rest is distributed in the soft tissues, ECF and blood.
- Principal cation of soft tissue: magnesium content in soft tissue is 3–5 times that of calcium.

- The plasma magnesium concentration is 2–3 mg/dL.
- Magnesium exists in three forms:
  1. Free magnesium ions (Mg^{2+}): approximately 60%: active form
  2. Complexed with anions: approximately 10%
  3. Protein bound: approximately 30%

1.3.1 The Function of Magnesium

- Magnesium is an activator of several enzymes, which have ATP as one of the substrates (e.g., kinases, glycogen phosphorylase).
- For neuromuscular transmission, hypomagnesaemia causes neuromuscular hyperirritability.
- Magnesium prevents the formation of calcium oxalate stones in the kidneys.
- Magnesium supplementation may lower blood pressure.
- RDA: 300–350 mg/day.
- Dietary sources: widely distributed in animal and plant foods, milk and milk products, meat, eggs, cereals, pulses and green leafy vegetables.
- Intestinal absorption: 50% of dietary magnesium is absorbed from the small intestine. Calcium and phosphate in large amounts reduce the absorption of magnesium.
- PTH, vitamin D and GH increase the absorption of magnesium.
- Excess alcohol, fat and phytic acids decrease the absorption of magnesium.
- Deficiency: hypomagnesaemia causes neuromuscular hyperirritability and can lead to hypomagnesaemic tetany. Deficiency can also lead to muscular weakness, cardiac arrhythmia, depression and convulsion.
- Hypermagnesaemia decreases muscle and nerve irritability. A very high concentration in the blood induces anaesthesia.

1.3.2 Magnesium in Pregnancy

- Low levels of magnesium may exaggerate morning sickness, so magnesium supplementation will reduce the symptoms. Magnesium plays a crucial role in balancing cortisol, which influences blood sugar, (hypoglycaemia is thought to be one of the main causes of morning sickness), so magnesium elevates blood sugar.
- Magnesium is a known muscle relaxant, so during pregnancy its deficiency may lead to leg cramps, especially at night.
- Magnesium is secreted in breast milk (15–64 mg/dL).

1.4 Iron

- Iron is the most essential trace element.
- An adult contains 3–5 g of iron; 70–75% of this is in the red blood cells as haem.
- Iron exists as:
  1. essential or functional iron: active form as ferrous (Fe^{2+}) in haemoproteins (haemoglobin, myoglobin (Mb), cytochromes, catalase, peroxidase, non-haem iron, etc.)
  2. storage iron: ferritin, haemosiderin and transferrin (main transport form of iron: 1%); the ionic form is ferric ion (Fe^{3+}).
- Intestinal absorption: occurs in the stomach and upper duodenum: 5–10% of dietary iron is absorbed as Fe^{2+}.

1.4.1 Factors That Stimulate Intestinal Absorption

- Vitamin C, glutathione, cysteine are reducing agents, which keep iron as Fe^{2+}, increasing the absorption of iron.
- Dietary iron exists in Fe^{3+} ionic form.
- Hydrochloric acid (HCl) favours iron absorption. It liberates non-haem iron and bound iron from food as Fe^{2+}.
- Alcohol, acidic pH and food (citrus fruits) and small weight proteins stimulate absorption of iron.
- Haem iron (animal food) is efficiently absorbed: 20–30% of haem iron is absorbed because of better bioavailability compared to non- haem iron (plant sources).
- Iron-deficient individuals absorb more iron than healthy people.

1.4.2 Factors That Inhibit Absorption

- Tea, coffee, phytic acid, oxalates and a high-fibre diet.
- Copper deficiency and achlorhydria.

1.4.3 Mechanism of Iron Absorption

- Iron absorbed as Fe^{2+} into the duodenal cells is oxidised to Fe^{3+} by ferroxidase (ceruloplasmin); which then binds with apotransferrin to form

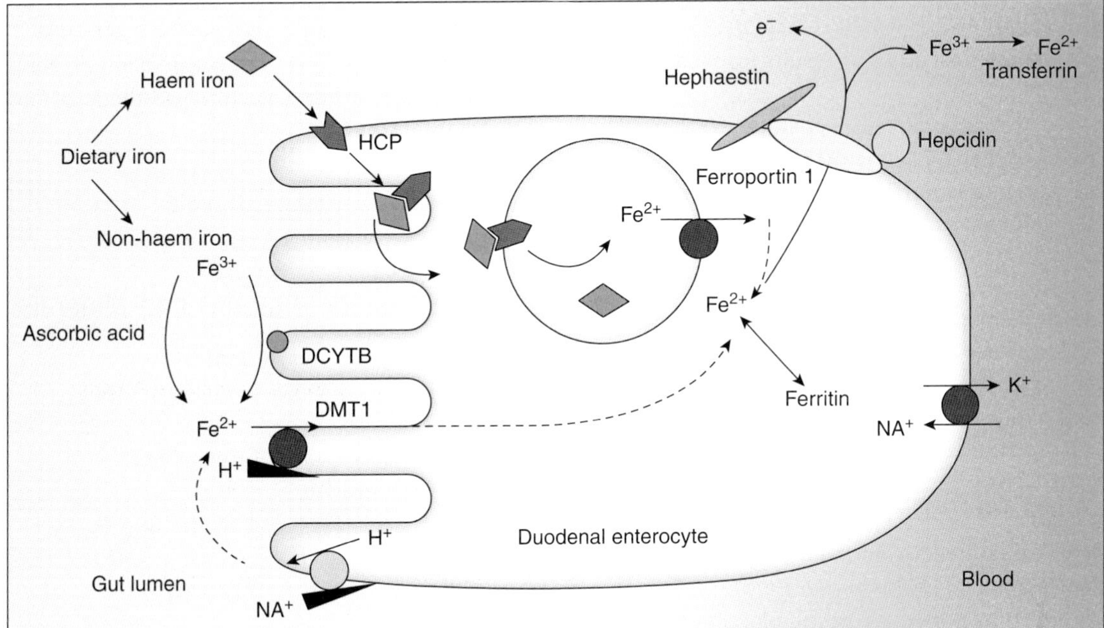

Figure 32.1 Absorption of iron in the duodenal enterocyte.
Iron transporters:
HCP: haem carrier protein
DCYTB: duodenal cytochrome b
DMT1: divalent metal transporter 1

transferrin (the transport form of iron), and with apoferritin to form ferritin (storage form). See Figure 32.1.

1.4.4 Iron Toxicity

- Haemosiderosis: excess haemosiderin deposition in tissues due to repeated blood transfusions, chronic alcoholics and excess iron absorption.
- Haemochromatosis: the deposition of haemosiderin, which causes tissue damage. It causes damage to the liver, pancreas, skin and cardiac muscle, leading to cirrhosis, pancreatic fibrosis, skin pigmentation and diabetes – together called bronze diabetes. Damage to cardiac muscle can cause cardio-myopathy.

1.4.5 Iron Transport Across Placenta

- Transplacental iron transfer involves the binding of transferrin: bound iron to the transferrin receptor, uptake into an endosome, acidification, release of iron through divalent metal transporter1 (DMT1), efflux across basolateral membrane through ferroportin.
- Iron transport across the placenta is against the concentration gradient. When the mother is iron deficient, there is increased expression of placental transferring receptor and DMT1.
- Low levels of iron are secreted into the milk.

1.5 Copper

- Copper is a trace element. The total copper in the body is 100–150 mg in the muscle (approximately 60%), bones and liver.
- Plasma concentration is 75–150 µg/dL in three forms: the majority as ceruloplasmin (ferroxidase I), albumin bound copper and ferroxidase II.
- Functions: copper is a component of many enzymes: superoxide dismutase (SOD), cytochrome c oxidase, catalase, aminolevulinic acid (ALA) synthase, ceruloplasmin, and so on.
- Copper is required for iron metabolism.
- Copper is essential for maintenance of myelin sheath, formation of bones, maturation of elastin and collagen.
- Copper synthesises haemoglobin and melanin.
- Deficiency can cause hypochromic, microcytic anaemia.
- Deficiency can cause Menkes disease (Kinky or Steel hair syndrome).

- Defective collagen and elastin cause bone demineralisation and capillary fragility.
- Hypercholesterolaemia also results from copper deficiency.
- Toxicity: excessive copper deposition can cause Wilson's disease (hepatolenticular degeneration).
- Copper accumulation in tissues is caused by low or absent ceruloplasmin, or a defect in copper binding to ceruloplasmin.
- Excessive copper deposition can cause liver cirrhosis, lenticular dysfunction, renal damage, bronze diabetes and characteristic Kayser–Fleischer ring around the cornea.
- Penicillamine is a copper chelating agent and used in treatment of copper toxicity.

1.5.1 Copper and Pregnancy

- Copper is required for normal fetal growth and organogenesis.
- Copper is transported across the placenta by a special copper receptor in the placenta, regulated by maternal estrogen and insulin. Excess copper is returned back to maternal circulation through a separate transporter.

1.6 Zinc

- Zinc is a trace element. The skin and the prostate are very rich in zinc. Red blood cells contain a higher amount of zinc than plasma. Zinc is mostly present in the enzyme, carbonic anhydrase.
- Zinc is a part of many enzymes: SOD, carbonic anhydrase, DNA and RNA, polymerase, and so on.
- Zinc is needed for proper wound healing.
- It is involved in vitamin A metabolism in the visual cycle.
- It is required for normal fetal organogenesis, placental growth and development.
- Iron transport reduces across the placenta due to zinc deficiency.
- Zinc is secreted into the breast milk through zinc transporter protein (ZIP) transporters.

2 Vitamins

2.1 Role in Pregnancy

- vitamins and minerals are essential elements of diet; they cannot be synthesised in the human body
- exceptions: vitamin D; synthesized from cholesterol
- niacin: from tryptophan (an essential amino acid)
- they act as coenzymes/cofactors/prosthetic groups of various enzymes
- vitamins:
    - water soluble (vitamins B and C)
    - fat soluble (vitamins A, D, E and K)

2.2 Erythropoietic Vitamins and Minerals

- B6: required in haem synthesis
- B12 and folic acid: DNA synthesis and cell maturation
- C: intestinal absorption of iron as $Fe2^{+}$
- A: proper cell growth
- Fe^{2+}, Zn^{2+}, Cu^{2+}: for haem synthesis

2.3 Energy-Releasing Vitamins

- thiamine
- riboflavin
- niacin
- biotin
- pantothenic acid
- lipoic acid

2.4 Fat-Soluble Vitamins

- need dietary fat and bile acids for intestinal absorption
- transported in chylomicrons from intestinal mucosa
- stored in liver and adipose tissue for a long time bound to specific binding proteins
- if taken in excess, may lead to hypervitaminosis

2.4.1 Vitamin A (Retinol)

Three forms:

- retinol (ROH)
- retinal (RCHO)
- retinoic acid (RA)

Sources

- animal: liver (polar bear liver maximum storage), milk products, eggs
- plants (contain β-carotene): spinach, mango, papaya, carrot

Storage form

- retinol and retinyl esters (bound to cytosolic retinol binding protein)

Transport form

- retinol bound to retinol binding protein
- RA to albumin

Active form

- 11-cis retinal in rhodopsin (visual purple pigment)
- retinoic acid acts as signalling molecule, binds with specific nuclear receptors and causes protein synthesis
- β-carotene converted into RA: measured in retinol equivalents (RE)
- 1RE = 6 mg β-carotene

Functions of Vitamin A

1. Maintenance of normal vision, required for synthesis of rhodopsin (rods) and iodopsin (cones), 11-cis retinal acts as the prosthetic group with OPSIN (the protein part of both pigments)
2. Retinoic acid and retinol maintain a healthy immune system and proper cell growth by regulating gene transcription and protein formation (act like steroid hormones)
3. Retinol and RA prevent keratinisation of epithelial cells and maintain healthy epithelium and mucous secretions
4. β-carotene acts as an antioxidant, quenches free radicals in high O_2 tension areas like lungs and red blood cells (RBCs)

Deficiency of vitamin A

1. Night blindness: xerophthalmia, Bitot's spots, keratomalacia
2. Squamous metaplasia of epithelium
3. Poor skull growth
4. Iron-resistant anaemia, responds to vitamin A supplements

Hypervitaminosis: toxicity

- eating polar bear liver: seen in the Inuit
- pregnant women to avoid eating liver (storage organ for many vitamins) to avoid risk of fetal damage
- signs and symptoms: nausea, vomiting, drowsiness, headache
- fatigue, insomnia, bone pain, hair loss, hepatomegaly, benign intracranial hypertension, osteoporosis.
- RDA:
  - 600–700 μg/d
  - +100 μg/d (pregnancy)
  - +350 μg/d (lactation)

Vitamin A delivery to fetus

- vitamin A is essential for maintaining pregnancy and fetal morphogenesis
- fetus obtains vitamin A from maternal circulation: retinol bound to retinol binding protein (RBP) circulates in maternal blood, retinol released from complex at maternal-fetal interface, and retinol traverses placenta bound to fetal RBP to reach fetal circulation
- fetal RBP synthesized in embryonic yolk sac
- maternal RBP does not cross placenta
- severe maternal vitamin A deficiency: early embryonic death
- moderate deficiency: fetal developmental malformations: vitamin A deficiency (VAD) syndrome

Vitamin D (calciferol)

- not a vitamin; acts like a hormone
- synthesised in the body
- has multiple target organs; just like hormones
- acts through specific nuclear receptors and regulates gene expression.

Synthesis

7-dehydrocholestrol (in skin, provitamin)
↕ UV rays (sunlight)
cholecalciferol (also called vitamin D_3, calciol)
↓
25-hydroxylase: reaches liver via blood
↓
25- hydroxycholecalciferol (calcidiol)
↓ 1,α hydroxylase (kidney)
1,25: dihydroxycholecalciferol (calcitriol –active form)

Circulating form: cholecalciferol

- storage form: cholecalciferol and ergocalciferol (vitamin D_2, plants)

- sources: sunlight, milk, egg yolk, fish oils, liver
- functions:
  - calcium homeostasis by increasing intestinal calcium absorption, increased synthesis of calbindin protein and decreased renal excretion of calcium
  - synthesis and secretion of PTH and thyroid hormone
- deficiency: rickets, osteomalacia
- PTH regulates vitamin D synthesis
- toxicity: calcinosis: hypercalcemia and calcium deposits in soft tissues

2.4.2 Vitamin D and Pregnancy

- Vitamin D deficiency causes an increased risk of preeclampsia, gestational diabetes mellitus (GDM), bacterial vaginosis, C-section.
- Human placenta can synthesize 1,25-dihydroxycholecalciferol (syncytiotrophoblast and decidual cells).
- Placental vitamin D regulates synthesis of human chorionic gonadotropin (hCG) and human palcental lactogen (hPL), estradiol, progesterone. Aids implantation and fetal growth.

2.4.3 Vitamin E (tocopherols)

- lipid-soluble chain-breaking free radical, trapping antioxidant in cell membranes
- sources: vegetable oils and nuts
- storage: adipose tissue, muscle, liver
- active form: D-α-tocopherol
- deficiency: increased haemolysis, especially in premature infants
- poor transfer of vitamin E through placenta
- colostrum and later breast milk are good sources

2.4.4 Vitamin K (hydroquinones)

- essential for blood coagulation
- three major forms:
  - phylloquinone (from diet, circulating form)
  - menaquinone (synthesised by intestinal bacteria, storage form in liver)
  - menadione (synthetic form)
- dietary sources: green vegetables, nuts, dairy products, fruits
- very little amount crosses placenta; gets secreted into milk
- premature infants prone to haemorrhagic disease of newborn (HDN)
- inhibitors: warfarin, used for treatment of thrombosis-related diseases

2.5 Water-Soluble Vitamins

2.5.1 Vitamin B Complex

- thiamine (B_1)
- riboflavin(B_2)
- nicotinamide (niacin)
- pyridoxine
- pantothenic acid
- biotin
- folic acid
- cobalamin (B_{12})

Thiamine, folate, and vitamin B12 are actively absorbed from the intestinal tract.

The rest are absorbed passively through the intestinal mucosal wall.

Not stored in the body, except B_{12}, so no toxicity.

2.5.2 Thiamine

Sources
- wheatgerm, oatmeal, yeast
- nuts, seeds, legumes.

Active form
- thiamine pyrophosphate (TPP)

Functions
- essential for carbohydrate and protein metabolism
- acts as coenzyme (TPP) for decarboxylases, transferases, dehydrogenases, transketolase, and so on
- Thiamine triphosphate (TTP) for normal nerve conduction

Deficiency
- chronic alcoholics highly prone: ethanol decreases intestinal absorption of vitamin B_1; increased intake of refined carbohydrates also causes deficiency
- eating raw fish (contains thiaminase, which breaks down thiamine)
- staple diet of white and polished rice

Deficiency diseases

- Wernicke–Korsakoff psychosis
- beriberi: dry (without fluid retention); wet (cardiac failure and oedema)
- lactic acidosis

Diagnosis of B_1 deficiency

- RBC transketolase activity measurement
- vitamin B_1 measurement by high performance liquid chromatography (HPLC)
- indirectly, by measurement of pyruvate

Thiamine and pregnancy

- required for normal metabolism of carbohydrates to provide energy
- for proper functioning of nervous system, muscles and heart
- essential for fetal brain development
- crosses placenta, secreted in milk
- excessive vomiting during pregnancy can cause depletion of vitamin
- RDA (pregnancy): 1.4 mg/d

2.5.3 Riboflavin

- an intense yellow coloured fluorescent pigment
- contains an alcohol sugar, ribitol
- heat stable but light sensitive
- used as food additive

Sources

- synthesised by plants and microorganisms
- milk and milk products
- nuts and legumes

Active forms

- flavin mononucleotide (FMN)
- flavin adenine dinucleotide (FAD)
- act as prosthetic groups of oxidoreductive enzymes; such enzymes are known as flavoproteins

Functions

- FMN and FAD act as electron(e-) carriers in oxidoreduction reactions, causing energy generation during breakdown of carbohydrate, fat and proteins
- there is generation of free radicals

Deficiency of vitamin B_2

- common but not fatal as there is very efficient conservation of tissue riboflavin
- signs and symptoms: rough, scaly skin; cheilosis; angular stomatitis; glossitis; seborrheic dermatitis
- phototherapy for neonatal jaundice may cause B_2 deficiency
- hypothyroidism may affect its conversion to active forms; also adreno-corticoptropic hormone (ACTH) and chlorpromazine

Laboratory diagnosis

- measurement of glutathione reductase activity in RBCs
- urinary levels of B_2

Riboflavin and pregnancy

- for normal growth of fetus: good vision, strong bones, muscles and nerve development
- crosses placenta; secreted into milk

2.5.4 Pantothenic Acid (B_3)

- known as anti-dermatitis factor
- widely distributed in nature
- humans cannot synthesise it
- active form: co-enzyme A (also called CoA, CoASH)
- involved in metabolism of carbohydrate, fat and proteins
- deficiency rare; causes burning feet syndrome also known as Grierson-Gopalan syndrome

2.5.5 Niacin (B_5)

- not strictly a vitamin; synthesised in the body by tryptophan (an essential, aromatic amino acid)

Generic forms

- nicotinic acid and nicotinamide

Sources

- 60 mg of tryptophan forms 1 mg of niacin in body
- yeast, meat, fish, milk, green vegetables, cereals

Functions

- NAD+ involved in energy production from glucose oxidation
- ADP+ required for reductive biosynthesis of biomolecules

- involved in DNA repair mechanism, intracellular calcium level rise in response to neurotransmitters and hormones
- mega doses of nicotinic acid inhibit fat breakdown in adipose tissue and decrease triglyceride synthesis in liver. Used in treatment of hyperlipidaemia

Deficiency

- deficiency of both niacin and tryptophan causes pellagra:
  - carcinoid syndrome
  - Hartnup's disease
  - staple diet of corn or sorghum
  - vitamin B_2, B_6 deficiency reduces niacin synthesis
  - isoniazid (INH) produces niacin deficiency
- signs and symptoms of pellagra:
  - dermatitis
  - diarrhoea
  - dementia
  - if untreated, death
- RDA: pregnancy and lactation: 30–35 mg/d
- reduces birth defects and miscarriages
- niacin crosses placenta and secreted into milk
- hypervitaminosis: vascular dilatation of skin: flushing and burning sensation

2.5.6 Pyridoxine (B_6)

- three forms:
  - pyridoxamine
  - pyridoxine
  - pyridoxal

Active form

- pyridoxal phosphate (PLP)

Sources

- plants, bacteria, yeast can synthesise
- intestinal bacterial flora also synthesises
- liver, meat, egg yolk, unrefined cereals, nuts

Functions

PLP acts as coenzyme for various enzymes:

1. Decarboxylases: causes synthesis of important biomolecules like histamine, tyramine, dopamine, gamma amino butyric acid, tryptamine, serotonin, melatonin
2. Transaminases: amino acid metabolism
3. For synthesis of haem, niacin, CoA, sphingolipids
4. Muscle glycogen breakdown

Deficiency manifestations

1. Neurological disorders: depression, nervousness, irritability, due to decreased synthesis of GABA, neurotransmitters, catecholamines and serotonin
2. Epileptic seizures in infants due to deficiency of GABA
3. Peripheral neuritis due to demyelination of nerves (decreased synthesis of sphingolipids)
4. INH treatment causes B_6 deficiency by forming an inactive hydrazone complex with pyridoxal. Leads to peripheral neuritis
5. Hyperhomocysteinaemia due to impaired cysteine catabolism; it is an independent risk factor for coronary artery disease (CAD)
6. Signs and symptoms of pellagra
7. Microcytic hypochromic anaemia due to decreased haem synthesis

RDA

- up to 2 mg/d
- requirement increases during pregnancy, lactation, antibiotic therapy, with use of oral contraceptives, INH, penicillamine

Pyridoxine and pregnancy

- Pyridoxine is given in high doses for treating nausea and vomiting in the first trimester.
- B_6 supplementation required for normal growth of developing fetus, especially for the brain and nervous system; also for normal carbohydrate and protein metabolism in the fetus
- B_6 crosses the placenta passively, also bound to placental cells
- secreted in adequate amount in breast milk
- supplements can inhibit secretion of breast milk by suppressing the elevated prolactin levels

2.5.7 Biotin (B_7)

Also known as anti-egg-white injury factor as it protects against tissue injury due to raw egg white. Raw egg white contains an antivitamin factor called avidin. Avidin binds biotin very tightly, prevents its absorption from intestine and causes B_7 deficiency.

Sources

- plants, bacteria, yeast can synthesise biotin: good sources

- intestinal bacterial flora can also synthesise
- unrefined cereals, nuts, molasses, liver, kidney, egg yolk, royal jelly
- animals cannot synthesise biotin

Functions

- biotin acts as a coenzyme (prosthetic group) for carboxylase enzymes, which bring about carboxylation (CO_2-fixation) reactions
- involved in fatty acid synthesis and gluconeogenesis

Deficiency

- very rare as it is widely distributed in food
- eating large amount of raw eggs
- broad spectrum oral antibiotics
- signs and symptoms: nausea, anorexia, glossitis, dermatitis, hyperesthesia, depression
- RDA:
  - infants: 10–15 μg/d
  - adults: 40–100 μg/d
  - dose increases during pregnancy, lactation, oral antibiotic treatment, chronic alcoholics

Biotin and pregnancy

- crucial nutrient during pregnancy: important for embryonic growth, but high doses can be dangerous to baby
- biotin is transported across placenta along with sodium ion (Na^+) and is stored in placenta against concentration gradient using ATP
- secreted in substantial amounts in breast milk
- Leiner's disease (exfoliative dermatitis), also known as erythroderma desquamativum observed in breastfed infants suffering from chronic diarrhoea due to malabsorption of biotin.

2.5.8 Folic Acid (B_9)

- folic acid from the Latin word folium meaning leaf as first isolated from spinach leaves
- contains pteridine ring, para amino benzoic acid, and 1-7 L-glutamic acid residues
- a yellow crystalline substance, soluble in water

Sources

- animals cannot synthesise B_9
- plants, bacteria, yeast, intestinal flora can synthesise
- yeast, green leafy vegetables, liver, kidney, meat, milk, eggs

Active form

- tetrahydrofolate (THF)
- folinic acid: N5-formyl THF: as therapeutic agent to provide THF
- also known as leucovorin or citrovorum factor (CF)
- folate or B_9 is a naturally occurring vitamin found in food; folic acid: a synthetic dietary supplement
- both must be converted to dihydrofolate (DHF) and then tetrahydrofolate (THF): active form, brought about by enzyme dihydrofolate reductase (DHFR); THF is then converted to methyl THF; enzyme required methylene THF reductase (MTHFR)

Functions

- act as coenzyme in reactions involving one-carbon transfers; required for DNA and RNA synthesis, and amino acid metabolism:
  1. N10-formyl THF and N5, N10-methylene: THF for *de novo* purine nucleotide and deoxythymidine monophosphate (dTMP) synthesis.
  2. Catabolism of histidine to glutamate: formiminoglutamate (FIGLU) is formed as an intermediate. It is converted to glutamate: N5-formimino-THF is required.
  3. Methylation of homocysteine to methionine: N5-methyl-THF and methylcarbylamine (B_{12}) are required as coenzymes.

Deficiency manifestations

- megaloblastic anaemia
- neural tube defects
- growth failure
- hyperhomocysteinaemia (along with B_6 and B_{12} deficiency)

Causes of deficiency

- low dietary intake
- malabsorption
- prolonged use of broad-spectrum antibiotics (sulphonamides)
- prolonged use of anticonvulsant drugs, estrogens, oral contraceptive pills (OCPs), antifolates, methotrexate, aminopterin
- chronic alcoholism

- increased demand during pregnancy
- genetic deficiency of DHFRedutase
- vitamin B_{12} deficiency causes folate trap leading to functional folate deficiency

Tests to assess folate deficiency
- blood picture showing megaloblasts
- folate levels in RBCs
- serum folate levels
- FIGLU excretion test
- hyperhomocysteinaemia

Plasma concentration of folate
- 300 ng/100 mL

RDA
- 400 μg/d
- +400 μg/d during pregnancy
- +200 μg/d during lactation
- requirement increases with oral antibiotic therapy, OCPs, estrogens, anticonvulsant drugs and chronic alcoholics
- folinic acid is used as a therapeutic agent

Folate and pregnancy
- folate helps prevent neural tube defects (NTDs) of the spinal cord (spina bifida) and brain (anencephaly)
- it also lowers the risk of other defects like cleft lip, cleft palate, some heart defects
- may reduce risk of preeclampsia
- along with B_{12}, required for proper erythropoiesis; otherwise, megaloblastic anaemia occurs (essential for production, repair and functioning of DNA: diminished synthesis of DNA prevents cells from dividing; their size increases)
- for rapid placental growth and developing fetus
- taking much higher doses than recommended during pregnancy may increase the risk of developing autism in the child, increased risk of developing insulin resistance and obesity in children later in life, increased risk of cancer in mother
- higher dose of folic acid may worsen a concomitant deficiency of vitamin B_{12} leading to damage to the nervous system
- placenta concentrates folate into fetal circulation, so fetal levels 2–4 times higher than maternal; so folate enters fetus by active transport (requires ATP), against concentration gradient
- alcohol impairs folate transport to fetus

2.5.9 Cobalamin (B_{12})

- also known as antipernicious anaemia factor and extrinsic factor of Castle
- a complex organic molecule: a corrin ring with cobalt at centre

Major forms
- cyanocobalamin: commercial form (cynide bound to Co)
- hydroxocobalamin
- methylcobalamin: physiologically active form
- 5'-deoxyadenosylcobalamin: physiologically active form

Sources
- cannot be synthesised by plants and animals
- only microorganisms (anaerobic bacteria) can synthesise
- intestinal bacterial flora synthesises
- vitamin B_{12} is found only in foods of animal origin: liver, kidney, meat, milk, milk products, fish, eggs, and so on
- liver is a very good source, as is curd (due to synthesis by lactobacilli)

Absorption of B_{12}
- absorption from ileum via a specific transport system
- requires intrinsic factor (IF) of Castle and HCl.
- IF produced in stomach (parietal cells) and binds to dietary B_{12} to form B_{12}-IF complex
- complex goes to ileum and binds to specific receptors on surface of mucosal cells, B_{12} is released from complex, enters cells through a $Ca2^{+}$-dependent process
- from cells, it enters blood where it is transported bound to:
  - transcobalamin-II
  - stored in liver bound to transcobalamin-I
  - stores are sufficient to last 3–6 years

Deficiency
- pernicious anaemia:

    - lack of IF leads to B_{12} deficiency (autoimmune destruction of gastric parietal cells)
    - gastric achylia: no secretion of HCl and pepsin: no B_{12} absorption
    - achlorhydria: no HCl secretion: no B_{12} absorption
- megaloblastic anaemia: macrocytic RBCs with anaemia; due to functional folate deficiency (folate trap)
- neurological disorders: due to progressive degeneration of myelinated nerves (due to accumulation of L-methyl malonyl CoA)
- gastrintestinal disorders: glossitis, stomatitis, mucosal atrophy

Causes of B_{12} deficiency

- dietary deficiency rare, seen in vegans
- pernicious anaemia
- chronic liver diseases
- chronic alcoholism
- gastrectomy
- malabsorption
- fish tapeworm infestation
- long-term use of OCs and estrogens

Diagnostic tests

- methylmalonic aciduria: increased levels of L-methylmalonic CoA in blood: excreted in urine
- vitamin B_{12} assay: low levels
- blood picture: megaloblastic anaemia

Normal blood levels

- 190–900 ng/mL

RDA

- 3.0 μg/d
- pregnancy and lactation: +1.0 μg/d
- vitamin B_{12} deficiency causes a functional folate deficiency (folate trap), leading to megaloblastic anaemia

Cobalamin and pregnancy

- B_{12} deficiency leads to folate deficiency: both can be fatal to fetus or may lead to severe neurological and haematological anomalies
- mild deficiency has been shown to increase risk for insulin resistance and obesity in the child
- cobalamin crosses placenta and enters fetal blood; placenta synthesises transcobalamin, to which B_{12} binds and is transported to fetus
- B_{12} also secreted into milk

3 Other essential elements in the body

3.1 Sodium (Na^+)

- principal cation of extracellular fluid (ECF): blood/plasma
- total body content: 70 g or about 3500–4000 mEq; out of which 50% is present in bones, 40% in ECF and 10% in soft tissues
- present as sodium chloride (NaCl) and sodium bicarbonate ($NaHCO_3$); concentration in blood: 135–145 mEq/L and much lower inside the cells (35 mEq/L); levels maintained by the Na^+ - K^+ ATPase pump present on the cell membrane of all cells

Sources

- common salt (NaCl) is the main dietary source
- foods rich in sodium are grains, nuts, milk, green leafy vegetables

RDA

- 1–5 g/d, but should be reduced in hypertensive patients (1 g/d)

Biochemical functions

1. Sodium is an osmotically active cation, thus maintains the osmotic pressure along with other osmotically active molecules in blood (e.g., potassium, glucose, urea). It also maintains blood pressure.
2. Helps in maintaining the acid-base balance of the body along with chloride (Cl^+) and bicarbonate (HCO_3+) ions. It is an integral part of the main extracellular and intracellular buffers respectively: the bicarbonate buffer system ($NaHCO_3$–$H2CO_3$) and the phosphate buffer system (NaH_2PO_4–Na_2HPO_4).
3. Role in neuromuscular excitability and generation of membrane potential in nerves via Na^+ - K^+ ATPase pump.
4. Role in absorption of glucose, galactose and certain amino acids in intestine.

5. Formation of bile salts (bile acids synthesised in liver from cholesterol).

Regulation of sodium levels in body

- Mainly by renin-angiotensin-aldosterone system and antidiuretic hormone.
- Ingested sodium readily absorbed in the gut. Sodium loss is through urine, stool, and sweat: about 100 mg/d; maximum through sweat, negligible through urine and stool.
- Reabsorption of sodium in kidneys is from proximal renal tubules.
- Excretion through kidneys is tightly regulated by aldosterone hormone in renal collecting ducts. Aldosterone inhibits excretion of sodium at the level of distal tubules.

Disorders

1. Hyponatraemia: a decrease in total body sodium along with low blood sodium levels. Could be seen in dehydration due to excessive loss of fluid along with obligatory Na^+ loss, or due to overhydration because of dilution. Causes:
    - prolonged severe vomiting and diarrhoea
    - diabetic ketoacidosis
    - renal failure causing reduced Na^+ reabsorption
    - diuretics causing Na^+ excretion
    - excessive loss through gastrointestinal tract
    - Addison's disease (low aldosterone leading to increased sodium excretion)
2. Hypernatraemia: an increase in blood sodium levels, along with an increase in blood volume and pressure. Severe and prolonged hypernatraemia can lead to congestive cardiac failure. Causes:
    - prolonged cortisone/steroid use: commonest cause
    - Cushing's syndrome (increased aldosterone levels due adrenocortical hyperactivity)
    - pregnancy (hormonal interplay leads to sodium and water retention during first few months)

Sodium levels during pregnancy

- A decrease in serum sodium levels is observed during normal pregnancy, possibly due to haemodilution. Multiparous pregnancies show a slight increase in sodium levels in blood.
- In preeclamptic pregnancies there is substantial reduction in serum Na^+ levels, which improves post-delivery; likely explanation may be dilutional hyponatraemia due to reduced rate of free water clearance through kidneys due to preeclampsia. Babies born to such mothers are also hyponatraemic initially. As such, it is highly recommended to monitor serum electrolytes in such mothers during pregnancy.
- Preeclampsia is therefore a common cause of hyponatraemia during pregnancy; other causes being prolonged labour, post-caesarean section, oxytocin infusion and hyperemesis gravidarum.
- Sodium is secreted in breast milk/colostrum: 11–59 mEq/L in colostrum and slightly lower amount in mature milk: 1–19 mEq/L.

3.2 Potassium (K^+)

- major intracellular cation
- total body K^+ is about 3500 mEq (150 g); 75% of this is present in muscles and the rest is distributed all over the body
- serum K^+ levels are around 3.5–5.0 mEq/L or mmol/L, whereas intracellular concentration is 150 mEq/L
- dietary sources: banana, citrus fruits, pineapple, potatoes, beans, dried apricots, chicken and meat

RDA

- 3–4 g/day

Absorption

- mainly in small intestine

Excretion

- excreted through kidneys
- aldosterone increases K^+ loss through the kidneys in exchange for Na^+ in the collecting ducts of renal tubules

Functions

1. Maintains intracellular osmotic pressure; under normal conditions, osmotic pressure of ECF is equal to that of intra cellular fluid (ICF), which are maintained mainly by Na^+ and K^+ respectively.
2. Regulation of acid base and water balance inside cells; maintain electrical neutrality inside and outside cells. Certain special channels like Na^+-K^+ATPase, and H^+-K

$^{+}$ATPase play an important role in maintaining concentration of these ions across the biomembranes.

3. Along with sodium ions, plays a significant role in nerve transmission.
4. Normal cardiac activity requires optimal K^+ concentration.
5. Protein biosynthesis in cells (cytoplasm) requires adequate levels of K^+ inside the cells.
6. Pyruvate kinase (an enzyme of glycolytic pathway) requires K^+ for optimal activity.

Disorders

- Serum/plasma K^+ levels are maintained in a narrow range (3.5–5.0 mEq/L) as a mild deviation on either side can lead to deleterious consequences.
- Hypokalaemia: plasma K^+ levels <3 mEq/L. Causes:
  - excessive loss of K^+ from the gut or kidneys, Cushing's syndrome (adrenal cortex hyperactivity) or prolonged steroid treatment promotes K^+ excretion in exchange for Na^+
  - during treatment of diabetic ketoacidosis (DKA), insulin causes K^+ entry inside the cells along with glucose leading to hypokalaemia, so potassium supplementation is necessary
  - certain diuretics (thiazides, loop diuretics tend to increase K^+ excretion through kidneys
  - seen along with metabolic alkalosis (K^+ ions moves inside the cells in exchange for H^+ ions)
  - Conn's syndrome: excess aldosterone causes K^+ loss through kidneys
  - clinical features: constipation, muscular weakness, cramps and fatigue; in severe hypokalaemia may cause respiratory failure and paralytic ileus
  - cardiac arrhythmias – may lead to cardiac arrest (ECG changes – flattening or inversion of T-wave, ST segment depression, widening of QRS complex, U-wave)
- Hyperkalaemia: plasma concentration >5.5 mEq/L. Causes:
  - renal failure with no renal loss of K^+
  - Addison's disease: aldosterone deficiency causes K^+ retention
  - diabetic ketoacidosis
  - overdose of drugs like digitalis, angiotensin converting enzyme (ACE) inhibitors, angiotensin II receptor blockers (ARBs) and beta blockers
  - dehydration
  - iatrogenic: excessive and fast supplementation of K^+
- Pseudohyperkalemia: falsely high serum K^+ levels due to haemolysis, thrombocytosis, leucocytosis, polycythaemia.
  - clinical features: increased membrane excitability may lead to ventricular arrhythmia, ventricular fibrillation, bradycardia and can cause cardiac arrest
  - ECG findings: tall T-waves, QRS complex widening, increased PR interval
  - muscular weakness may lead to flaccid paralysis

Potassium and pregnancy

- during pregnancy serum potassium levels remain normal, may rise slightly during last trimester
- deranged levels of potassium may pose a risk for complications during pregnancy
- potassium is actively secreted into milk and levels are higher than blood

3.3 Chloride (Cl-)

- mostly as a constituent of sodium chloride
- metabolism is closely related to that of sodium and potassium
- normal plasma/serum levels: 95–105 mEq/L
- normal cerebrospinal fluid (CSF) levels: 125 mEq/L, which is higher than blood

The extra- and intracellular concentrations of these macrominerals such as namely Na, K, Cl are described by the Gibbs–Donnan membrane effect, which explains the unequal distribution of diffusible ions across a semipermeable membrane in the presence of nondiffusible ions. Cells have higher concentration of K^+ and lower concentration of Cl than the plasma due to the presence of negatively charged, nondiffusible protein molecules in plasma . Similarly, CSF chloride levels are higher than plasma because CSF protein levels are lower than that of plasma.

Also, H^+ and K^+ concentrations are higher inside the RBCs than outside due to presence of haemoglobin (positively charged protein molecules). Such distribution of negatively and positively charged diffusible ions is to maintain the electrical neutrality across the semi permeable biomembranes.

- dietary sources: common salt, grains, eggs, leafy vegetables and milk
- RDA: 5–10 g as common salt
- absorbed in gastrointestinal tract
- excretion through kidneys along with Na^+
- biological functions: important constituent of gastric juice as HCl
- it plays a major role in maintaining acid-base balance in body
- chloride ions required for action of salivary amylase (ptyalin)
- amylase is required for digestion of starch

Disorders

- deranged chloride levels
- hypochloraemia:
  - prolonged severe vomiting (HCl is lost and a compensatory increase in HCO^{-3}, may lead to hypochloraemic alkalosis)
  - excessive sweating
  - Addison's disease (low levels of aldosterone increase Cl- loss)
- hyperchloraemia:
  - dehydration
  - renal tubular acidosis (RTA)
  - Cushing's syndrome (high aldosterone causes increased renal Cl^- reabsorption).
- cystic fibrosis:
  - A high sweat chloride concentration.
  - A point mutation in cystic fibrosis transmembrane regulatory protein (CFTR): CFTR is a chloride channel present in plasma membranes of tissues like lungs, pancreatic duct, intestine, sweat glands, vas deferens, and so on on their luminal side. These channels regulate Cl^+ movement across the membrane. Defective CFTR (due to the point mutation) causes excess loss of chloride ion in sweat (as NaCl) and insufficient secretion of NaCl and fluid in lungs, pancreas and intestine causing deterioration of function of these organs; also causing thick mucous, sputum, and so on, predisposing such individuals to infections and death at a young age.
- During pregnancy serum chloride levels remain within normal limits.

33 Placental Transfer

Smita Kaushik

- Fetal growth mostly depends on nutrient transport across the placenta. Changes in placental transport may directly contribute to altered fetal growth.
- Several factors influence nutrient transport across the placenta:
  1. Uteroplacental and umbilical cord blood flow
  2. Area available for exchange of nutrients/molecules
  3. Metabolism in placental cells
  4. Activity or genetic expression of various transporter pumps (proteins)
- The fetoplacental–maternal circulation is established around the tenth week of pregnancy. As the pregnancy proceeds, the cytotrophoblast layer partially disappears. Consequently, the transplacental diffusion distance decreases, increasing placental permeability. Syncytiotrophoblast is the main barrier influencing nutrient transport across the placenta. It has two polarised plasma membranes:
  1. Microvillous plasma membrane (MVM): maternal facing
  2. Basal plasma membrane (BM): fetus facing
- These express various transporters, which may be regulated by maternal, placental and fetal signals.

1 Mechanisms for Transport Across the Placenta

1. Active transport and facilitated diffusion:
   - requires energy
   - not proportional to concentration
   - similar/related molecules compete for receptor sites
   - transport depends on the membrane carrier systems
   - for example, 5-fluorouracil is transported by a system of endogenous pyrimidines and L-alpha methyldopa has an amino acid carrier system
2. Passage through membrane pores:
   - pores in lipid membranes determine permeability
   - placental pores are generally 1 nm in diameter
   - substances with molecular weight <500 Da will pass through
3. Pinocytosis/phagocytosis:
   - important mechanism of passage of small quantities of macromolecules
   - viruses and immunologically active molecules are transferred by this mechanism
   - the scale of transfer is minimal
4. Simple diffusion:
   - principal process of drug movement through cell membrane
   - no energy required
   - no competition
   - rate of transfer is proportional to the concentration gradient
   - only unionised form diffuses
   - drugs that are weak bases will equilibrate faster than strong bases
   - for example, depolarising muscle relaxants can be detected in the fetus only if hundred-fold therapeutic doses are administered to the mother
5. Other factors that influence transport:
   - Drugs with high lipid/water solubility partition ratio pass readily through the placenta.
   - Binding to plasma protein; for example, salicylate binds more strongly to maternal than fetal plasma proteins.
   - Difference in pH between maternal and fetal blood: this leads to unequal concentrations of ionisable drugs; for example, the levels of

pethidine are higher in the neonatal than the maternal blood due to lower blood pH in the neonate.

- Presence of enzymes in the placenta that destroy the drugs thereby reduces levels in the fetus. 5HT is destroyed by amine oxidase in the placenta. The placenta expresses a variety of xenobiotic-metabolising enzymes from the earlier stages of pregnancy. Drugs that have been shown to undergo significant placental metabolism include azidothymidine, dexamethasone and prednisolone. Placental enzymes catalyse phase I (drug oxidation, reduction and hydrolysis) and phase II (conjugation) reactions. Among phase I enzymes, proteins that have been identified in the placenta are cytochrome P450 (CYP) 1A1, 2E1, 3A4, 3A5, 3A7, 4B1 and 19. The most established placental phase II enzymes with regard to xenobiotic metabolism are uridine diphosphate glucuronosyltransferases .

2 Transport of Gases

- Oxygen and carbon dioxide diffuse across the placental tissue from the maternal blood due to differences in partial pressure (PP) of these gases.
- Mean PP of oxygen (pO_2) in the maternal blood is higher (26 mmHg) than in fetal blood (19 mmHg), so oxygen readily diffuses across into fetal blood. Also 2,3-bisphosphoglycerate (2,3-BPG) binds strongly to maternal haemoglobin (Hb), causing easy dissociation of oxygen from maternal Hb. Moreover, fetal Hb concentration is far higher (approximately 50% higher) than maternal Hb.
- The fetus produces a lot of carbon dioxide: the partial pressure of carbon dioxide (pCO_2) of fetal blood is higher than maternal blood, so carbon dioxide readily diffuses into maternal blood across the placenta, along with hydrogen ions (H^+). When carbon dioxide and H^+ diffuse across the placenta into maternal blood, pH decreases, causing a right-shift of oxygen-dissociation curve in the maternal blood, thus oxygen easily dissociates from the maternal Hb and diffuses across the placenta.

3 Transport of Major Nutrients

- Glucose: the major energy substrate travels across the placenta down its concentration gradient by facilitated diffusion through non-insulin-dependent glucose transporters (GLUT1 and GLUT3) present on both types of membranes (microvillus membranes (MVM) and basal membranes (BM)); more on MVM. Some glucose is oxidised to lactate in placenta, which is also utilised by the fetus for energy generation.
- Amino acids are actively transported across the placenta against their concentration gradient. Placenta expresses about 20 different types of amino acid transporters. Two main systems of amino acid transport are present on syncytiotrophoblast (MVM and BM), which bring about active transport of amino acids from the maternal blood:
  - System A: uptake of small, nonessential, neutral amino acids like glycine, alanine, serine, and so on, along with sodium ions into the cell. Alterations in activity of this system may contribute to intrauterine growth restriction (IUGR). Insulin, interleukin-6 and TNF-α stimulate activity of this system. These mediate their action through various signalling pathways; the main ones being: (a) mammalian target of rapamycin (mTOR) (regulator of fetal growth; IUGR babies show reduced activity and large babies show increased activity), (b) signal transducer and activator of transcription (STAT3) required for stimulation by leptin. Decrease in activity of System A is by glucocorticoids, hypoxia, interleukin 1 beta (IL-1β), ouabain (sodium-pump blocker), corticotropin-releasing hormone (CRH).
  - System L: sodium-independent obligatory exchanger of neutral amino acids and nonessential amino acids (taken in via System A) for essential amino acids such as leucine and phenylalanine.
  - System β or taurine transporter (TauT): TauT brings about taurine uptake against the concentration gradient along with sodium and chlorine. This pathway is more active in MVM than BM. However, activity is reduced in MVM in IUGR. Taurine is considered essential for fetal growth as the fetus is unable to synthesise taurine.
- Fatty acids: the fetus has minimal carnitine and enzymes for lipid synthesis, so maternal non-esterified fatty acids (NEFAs) and esterified

triacylglycerols (TGs) are the main sources of fatty acids. Lipoprotein lipase (LPL) on MVM cleaves TGs in lipoproteins to NEFAs. They cross lipid bilayers of placental membrane by simple diffusion, down the concentration gradient. In fetal tissues with high demand for long-chain polyunsaturated fatty acids like the brain, a specific transporter called fatty acid transport proteins enhances this transport. Facilitated diffusion is present on both MVM and BM. The placenta produces medium- and short-chain fatty acids and ketone bodies, and transports them to the fetus.

4 Transport of Antibodies

- Substantial transfer of immunoglobulin G (IgG) from maternal to fetal circulation occurs before birth. IgG transfer depends on: (a) maternal levels of IgG and specific antibodies, (b) gestational age, (c) placental integrity, (d) subclass of IgG and (e) type of antigen.
- IgG binds through its Fc base portion to its specific receptor (neonatal Fc receptor (FcRn)) on the maternal side of syncytiotrophoblasts and, after internalisation, is released on the fetal side down the concentration gradient. (An Fc receptor is a protein found on the surface of certain cells like B lymphocytes, follicular dendritic cells, natural killer cells, macrophages, neutrophils, eosinophils, basophils, human platelets and mast cells. They help with the protective functions of the immune system.) Transfer begins at about 13 weeks of gestation, but the maximum amount is transferred during the last four weeks of gestation. Thus, preterm infants tend to have lower levels of the protective immunoglobin.
- Immunoglobulin A (IgA) and immunoglobulin M (IgM) do not cross the placenta: they are generally found as polymeric forms in the blood. IgM is a pentamer and IgA is a dimer or tetramer, so they are too big to cross the placenta. If IgM antibodies are found in the newborn, it indicates an intrauterine infection.

5 Transport of Minerals

- Calcium: syncytiotrophoblast transfers about 30 g of calcium from the mother to the fetus during the last trimester, against a concentration gradient. MVM has high affinity calcium ions (Ca^{2+}) adenosine triphosphatase (ATPase) activity, capable of transferring Ca^{2+} actively. On the fetal side, there is presence of plasma membrane Ca^{2+}-ATPase (PMCA), which will extrude Ca^{2+} into fetal blood.
- Phosphate: during the latter part of gestation, phosphate transfer is against a concentration gradient. It is dependent on sodium ion as a co-transporter. It is regulated by low parathyroid hormone levels and modulated by pH, temperature, sodium and amino acid concentration.
- Magnesium: transport is also against a concentration gradient, with involvement of sodium–magnesium ion exchanger.

6 Transporters on the Placental Surface

- Na^{+}-K^{+}ATPase pump: this is involved in the active transport of sodium along with chloride and amino acids. It is present on both surfaces of the syncytiotrophoblast cells. It is not inhibited by ouabain and is more active on MVM than BM.
- Endothelial nitric oxide synthase (eNOS): NO is generated in normal placenta due to eNOS activity only. This activity is localised on syncytiotrophoblasts, and fetal vascular endothelium, in early gestation. It is involved in angiogenesis and vasculogenesis. It is also responsible for the release of human chorionic gonadotropin throughout the gestation period.
- Inducible nitric oxide synthase (iNOS): absence of iNOS activity in normal, healthy placenta. iNOS expression is induced only under

Table 33.1 Drugs that are easily transported through the placenta and can affect the fetus

Steroids
Teratogens: • Thalidomide • Alkylating agents • Antimetabolites • Barbiturates
Gaseous anaesthetics
Narcotic analgesics
Anticoagulants
Tetracyclines
Antithyroid

pathophysiological conditions (e.g., gestational diabetes mellitus). NO generation by iNOS is Ca^{2+}-independent and has cytotoxic effects and can lead to apoptosis or programmed cell death.

7 Transport of Drugs

- Drugs that are transported through the placenta are generally avoided during pregnancy and can cause undesirable effects on the fetus. Most drugs with molecular weight <500 Da cross the placenta, and most drugs with molecular weight >1000 Da do not cross the placenta (e.g., heparin, protamine and insulin). Neither succinylcholine (highly ionised) nor nondepolarising high molecular weight substances cross the placenta See Table 33.1.

34 Acid-Base Balance

Smita Kaushik

- Many biochemical compounds in the body act as weak acids or bases; that is, they can release or accept protons (hydrogen ions $[H^+]$), respectively.
- Water (H_2O) can act both as an acid and a base:

$$H_2O \leftrightarrow H^+ + OH$$

- The concentration of $[H^+]$ determine the acidity of any solution: expressed as pH.
- In solution, a weak acid dissociates reversibly:

$$HA \leftrightarrow H^+ + A^-$$

and has a dissociation constant K_a.

- The Henderson-Hasselbalch Equation describes the relationship between pH, pK_a and concentration of weak acid and its conjugate base:

$$pH = pK_a + \log\frac{[A^-]}{[HA]},$$ where pH = negative log of H^+concentration

pK_a = negative log of dissociation constant of weak acid
$[A^-]$ = molar concentration of conjugate base
$[HA]$ = molar concentration of undissociated weak acid

- Various acids are produced during metabolism in the body.
- Body fluids must be protected against minor changes in pH as all enzymes are very sensitive to pH.
- Buffers maintain pH in a range compatible with life.
- Buffers: solutions containing mixture of weak acid or weak base and its conjugate strong base or strong acid respectively.
- They resist change in pH when a small amount of acid or base is added to it. A buffer has maximal buffering capacity at its pK_a, which is the negative log of its acid dissociation constant. The buffer is strongest when the concentration of acidic and basic forms is equal; that is, $\frac{[Base]}{[Acid]} = 1$).
- A buffer is most effective at pH = $\pm$ 1 pK_a.
- Maintenance of acid-base balance involves the lungs, red blood cells (RBCs) and kidneys.
- Lungs control the exchange of gases; that is, oxygen (O_2) and carbon dioxide (CO_2) between the blood and the outside atmosphere.
- RBCs transport gases (O_2 and CO_2) between lungs and tissues.
- The kidneys are responsible for maintaining bicarbonate ion (HCO_3^-) and H^+ balance. See Figure 34.1 for reference values for arterial blood gases.

1 Physiological Buffer Systems

1.1 Extracellular Buffers

1. Bicarbonate buffer system: the most important extracellular buffer system in the body.
    - Components: weak acid: carbonic acid (H_2CO_3) [1.2 mmol/L] and conjugate base: HCO_3^- [24 mmol/L]

    $$pK_a(H_2CO_3) = 6.1$$

    - the buffering capacity of bicarbonate buffer is maximum at 7.4; the physiological pH

    $$pH = pK_a + \log\frac{[HCO2-]}{[H2CO2]}$$
    $$= 6.1 + \log\frac{[24mmol/L]}{[1.2mmol/L]} = 6.1 + 1.3 = 7.4$$

    - it is the most efficient buffer as it minimises changes in H^+ concentration when either acid or alkali is added to the blood

- changes in the acidic component of the buffer – that is, H_2CO_3 or CO_2 or partial pressure of carbon dioxide (pCO_2) – is handled by the respiratory system: the respiratory component
- changes in the basic component – that is, HCO_3^- is controlled by the kidneys and RBCs: the metabolic component
- the bicarbonate buffer system is an open system since it is connected to both the respiratory and renal systems
- RBCs and renal tubular cells are rich in an enzyme, carbonic anhydrase (CA), also called carbonic dehydratase, which causes the following reactions:

$$\underset{\text{(in tissues)}}{CO_2+H_2O} \overset{CA}{\leftrightarrow} H_2CO_3 \overset{CA}{\leftrightarrow} \underset{\text{(in kidneys)}}{H^++HCO_3^-} \overset{CA}{\leftrightarrow} \underset{\text{(in lungs)}}{CO_2+H_2O}$$

2. Plasma proteins: buffering power of plasma proteins accounts for the majority of the buffering power of blood. Albumin is a stronger buffer than globulin. The amino acid histidine, present in plasma proteins, has an imidazole group that acts as a base and an unprotonated form that can act as an acid.

1.2 Intracellular Buffers

1. Phosphate buffer: components are NaH_2PO_4 (acid) and Na_2HPO_4 (base)

   Its pK_a is 6.86
2. Proteins present in the cell
3. Haemoglobin, which is present only in erythrocytes, acts as a buffer due to histidine residues
4. Erythrocytes transport CO_2 to the lungs.
   - HCO_3^- shifts out of RBCs into the plasma, in exchange with chloride ions (Cl^-), which move into RBCs. This is known as chloride shift.
5. In the lungs, higher partial pressure of oxygen (pO_2) causes:
   - release of CO_2 from haemoglobin (Hb) = Haldane effect
   - Hb releases H^+, which react with $HCO_3^- \rightarrow H_2CO_3 \rightarrow H_2O + CO_2$ (expired)
6. Proximal tubules reabsorb HCO_3^- in the kidneys:
   - H^+ are secreted into the lumen of tubule to trap more of the HCO_3^- as H_2CO_3 to conserve HCO_3^-

Reference values of arterial blood gas (ABG) are mentioned in Table 34.1.

Table 34.1 Reference values of arterial blood gas

pH	7.35–7.45	
HCO_3^-	22–30 mmol/L	22–30 meq/L
pCO_2	4.3–6.0 kPa	32–45 mmHg
pO_2	9.6–13.8 kPa	72–104 mmHg
Anion gap	7–16 mmol/L	7–16 meq/L

pO_2: partial pressure of oxygen

2 Disorders of Acid-Base Balance

2.1 Acidosis

- Defined as pH <7.35 is more commonly seen in clinical practice. It may be:
  - respiratory acidosis (pCO_2 increase, H_2CO_3 increase):
    - chronic obstructive pulmonary disorder (COPD)
    - decrease in respiratory rate: respiratory centre depression
    - cardiac arrest
    - airway obstruction, chest deformity
  - metabolic acidosis (decreased HCO_3^-):
    - increased production of organic acids: diabetic ketoacidosis (DKA), lactic acidosis
    - impaired excretion of organic acids: renal failure
    - increased loss of HCO_3^- due to renal failure

2.2 Alkalosis

Defined as pH >7.45 is less common than acidosis. It may be:

- Respiratory
- Metabolic
  - respiratory alkalosis (pCO_2 decrease, H_2CO_3 decrease):
    - hyperventilation (anxiety, fever)
    - anaemia
    - salicylate poisoning
  - metabolic alkalosis (increased HCO_3^-):
    - excessive vomiting: resulting in loss of H^+
    - nasogastric suction
    - hypokalaemia as the kidney excretes H^+ ions to conserve potassium

Table 34.2 Compensatory mechanism of acid-base disorders

Disorder	Cause	Compensatory change	Timescale of compensatory mechanism
Respiratory acidosis	↑ in pCO_2 (↓ RR)	• ↑ in renal HCO_3^- • ↑ in bicarbonate concentration	Days
Metabolic acidosis	↓ in plasma (HCO_3^-)	↓ in pCO_2 (hyperventilation)	Minutes/hours
Respiratory alkalosis	↓ in pCO_2 (↑ RR)	• ↓ in renal HCO_3^- • ↓in bicarbonate concentration	Days
Metabolic alkalosis	↑ in (HCO_3^-)	↑in pCO_2 (hypoventilation)	Minutes/hours

↑: increase; ↓: decrease; RR: respiratory rate

3 Concept of Plasma Anion Gap

- Plasma cation concentration: [Na^+] and [K^+]: >90% of the cation concentration. Ca^{2+} and Mg^{2+} may also contribute.
- Plasma anion concentration: (Cl^-) and (HCO_3^-): >80% of the anion concentration. The remaining 20% are proteins, urates, phosphates, sulphates, lactate and organic acids (unmeasured anions).
- Anion gap (A^-) is the difference between the total concentration of measured cations ($Na^+ + K^+$) and measured anions ($Cl^- + HCO_3^-$).

Normal range: 15–20 meq/L

$$[Na^+] + [K^+] = [Cl^-] + [HCO_3^-] + [A^-]$$
$$140 + 4 = 100 + 25 + 19 \text{ mEq/L}$$

- Plasma anion gap will decrease due to:
  - increase in unmeasured cations
    - hypercalcaemia
    - hypermagnesaemia
  - ↓ in unmeasured anions
    - hypoalbuminaemia
- High anion gap acidosis: unmeasured anions increase or unmeasured cations decrease:
  - DKA
  - renal glomerular dysfunction
  - methanol poisoning
  - alcoholic acidosis
  - paracetamol poisoning
  - lactic acidosis
  - salicylate poisoning
- Normal anion gap acidosis (hyperchloraemic acidosis):
  - loss of duodenal fluid
  - increased diffusion of saline
  - acetazolamide therapy: inhibits CA
  - renal tubular acidosis

See figure 34.2 for compensatory mechanisms in acid-base balance.

4 Fetomaternal Acid-Base Homeostasis

1. During pregnancy, a chronic respiratory alkalosis prevails
   - cause: hyperventilation due to progesterone stimulating the respiratory centre
   - this is compensated by increased renal excretion of HCO_3^-
   - typical third trimester ABG values:
     - pH = 7.43
     - pCO_2 = 33 mmHg
     - pO_2 = 104 mmHg
     - [HCO_3^-] = 21 mmol/L
     - maternal 2,3-bisphosphoglycerate (2,3BPG) increases (by 30%)
     - pH is normal due to compensatory metabolic acidosis with decreased HCO_3^- from 24 to 21 mmol/L
   - The lower pCO_2 would shift the O_2 dissociation curve (ODC) to the left, but there is an increase in 2,3BPG, so there is minimal change in ODC.

Reduced maternal oxygenation
↓
Reduced placental perfusion
↓
Impeded delivery of oxygenated blood to the fetus
↓
Anaerobic metabolism in the fetus
↓
Increased production and accumulation of lactic acid
↓
fetal metabolic acidosis, fetal distress
↓
Poor Apgar score

2. Nausea and vomiting during first trimester: if severe (hyperemesis gravidarum)
   - fluid loss and electrolyte imbalance will cause metabolic alkalosis
   - with poor oral intake: ketoacidosis, which will compensate for alkalosis
3. Pregnant women are very prone to developing ketosis due to fasting.
   - ketones can cross the placenta, which are used by the fetus as an energy source and for fetal central nervous system myelination
   - in late pregnancy, insulin resistance may develop due to placental hormones
4. DKA: very severe and has adverse effects on the fetus

5 Haemoglobin

- Haemoprotein has four polypeptide chains (tetramer): 2α and 2β.
- Transports O_2 from the lungs to tissue.
- Types of Hb in normal adults:
  - HbA_1 (major form) $\alpha_2\beta_2$ (97%)
  - HbA_2 (minor form) $\alpha_2\delta_2$ (2%)
  - HbF (fetal Hb) $\alpha_2\gamma_2$ (1%): resulting in compensatory increase in sickle cell disease (SCD) and β thalassaemia
- P_{50}: partial pressure of O_2, which half saturates Hb.
- Values for P_{50}:
  - HbA_1: 26 mmHg
  - HbF: 20 mmHg
- This difference enables HbF to extract O_2 from HbA_1 from the mother's blood.
- Embryonic Hb: zeta and epsilon ($\zeta_2\varepsilon_2$); initial development (first trimester).
- By the end of the second trimester, ζ and ε are replaced by α and γ (HbF).
- Synthesis of β subunit starts only after the third trimester.
- HbF is completely replaced by HbA_1 until a few weeks postpartum.
- A compound called 2,3-diphosphoglycerate (2,3DPG) (also known as 2,3BPG) is synthesised during glycolysis in RBCs. Its synthesis is promoted by low pO_2.
- DPG binds more weakly to HbF than to HbA. Thus, HbF has higher affinity for O_2 than HbA.
- 2,3DPG shifts the ODC to the right, releasing O_2.
- Factors that shift ODC to the right:
  - increased H^+ leads to decreased pH (acidity): O_2 release: Bohr effect
  - presence of 2,3BPG
  - binding of CO_2 to Hb

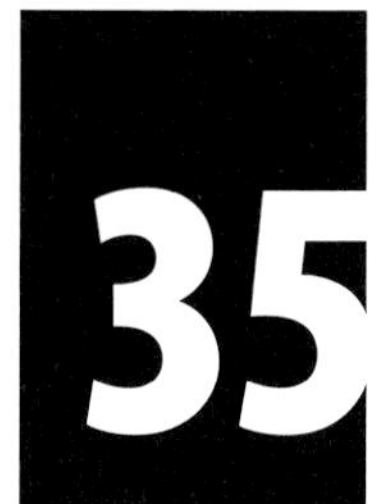

Cell Structure and Cycle

Smita Kaushik and Neela Mukhopadhaya

1 Cell Structure

Virchow in 1858 published his famous book on 'cellular pathology':

- cell theory: 'every cell derives from another existing cell like it'
- mammalian nucleated cells, 'eukaryotes', have a well-defined nucleus enclosed in a nuclear membrane
- bacteria, 'prokaryotes', lack a separate nucleus: the genomic nucleic acid is free in the protoplasm

1.1 Cell Membrane

See Figure 35.1 and Figure 35.2.

1.1.1 Structure

- the cell membrane is trilaminar in structure
- it is made of glycoprotein layers
- it contains human leucocyte antigen (HLA)
- it is attached to the centrosome

1.1.2 Function

- the cell membrane is the interface between the cell cytoplasm and interstitial tissue fluids: trilaminar
- movement of substances is by pinocytosis and phagocytosis
- cell recognition: example is antigen
- receptor: example is drugs, pathogens
- cell growth: example is proteolytic
- adhesion: example is by cadherins, integrins, HLA
- transfer: takes place by passive, active movement

1.2 Cytoplasm

- the cytoplasm is enclosed within the trilaminar cell membrane
- the mitochondria store energy
- ribosomes synthesise proteins and RNA
- the endoplasmic reticulum synthesises proteins
- centrosome: contains two centrioles
- centrioles: replicate before mitosis
- Golgi complex: forms and transports secretions
- lysosomes are the cell 'dustbins'
- phagosomes: digest unwanted substances
- microtubules give structure to cells
- microfilaments attach to desmosomes to promote adhesion

1.3 Desmosome

- desosomes are specialised cell adhesion molecules
- desmosomes help to resist shearing forces and are found in simple and stratified squamous epithelium
- the cell adhesion proteins of the desmosome, desmoglein and desmocollin, are members of the cadherin family of cell adhesion molecules

1.4 Cell Nucleus

1.4.1 Structure

- under electron microscope, the cell nucleus consists of two membranes; each 7.5 nm in width
- the perinuclear cistern is the space between the two lipid layers of the cell membrane
- the outer lamina is studded with ribosomes
- the outer layer of the nucleus is continuous with the endoplasmic reticulum
- nuclear pores are 50 nm in diameter

1.4.2 Function

- the principle component of the nucleus is DNA, which is responsible for genetic coding and inheritance
- within the nucleus is one or more mobile nucleolus, which contains RNA (involved in cell protein synthesis)

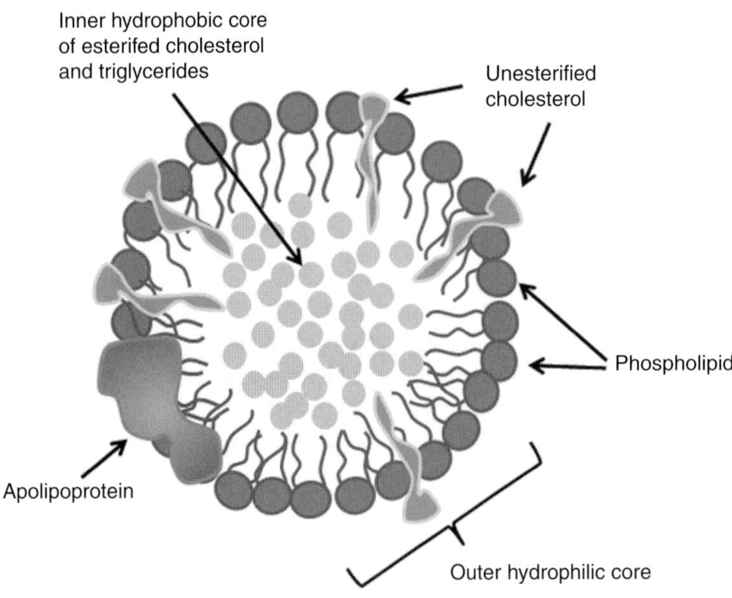

Figure 35.1 Structure of lipoproteins. Used with permission from www.researchgate.net/figure/Schematic-drawing-of-lipoprotein-structure-Information-derived-from-Champe-et-al-2005_fig2_282356824

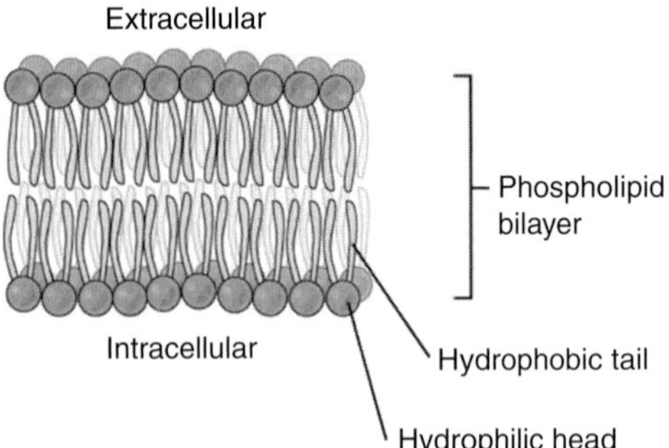

Figure 35.2 Structure of cell membrane. Used with permission from Lumen

- nuclear RNA is the precursor of cytoplasmic ribosomal RNA
- the amount of DNA is constant in all resting diploid cells and half in 'germ cells', which are haploid

1.5 Variations in the Nuclear Structure

- the sex chromatin, or Barr body, is seen in the buccal epithelial cells
- it is an inactivated X chromosome
- polyploidy occurs when there are multiple amounts of DNA: this can be normal
- it is also seen in ageing liver cells, hypertrophied muscle, irradiated fibroblasts and megaloblasts
- aneuploidy: not normal multiples; this is usually a feature of malignant cells

1.6 Mitochondria

- the mitochondria oxidise proteins, carbohydrates and fats into energy (ATP)
- they are the source of oxidative phosphorylation
- they are the site of the TCA cycle and of fatty acid oxidation
- the mitochondria contain their own genome, which is of maternal origin
- they are involved in the apoptotic pathway (final stages)

1.7 Endoplasmic Reticulum

- the smooth endoplasmic reticulum has no ribosomes
  - the site of lipid synthesis
  - responsible for drug detoxification
- the rough endoplasmic reticulum is studded with ribosomes
  - the site of protein synthesis (mRNA) translation
  - generates glycoproteins/secretory proteins

Table 35.1 Cell types

Epithelial	Connective tissue
Cover body surfaces and internal cavities	Embryonic mesoderm
Glands are derived embryologically from body surfaces	Structural support as fibrous tissue, bone, cartilage, muscle and tendon
Synthesise secretions	Body defences as leucocytes and mononuclear phagocytes

1.8 The Golgi Complex

- the Golgi complex is situated near the centrosome
- it collects, modifies, packages and transports secretions from the rough endoplasmic reticulum to the cell membrane
- it is responsible for the glycosylation of proteins

1.9 Gap Junctions

- gap junctions are specialised cell–cell junctions
- they are the mirror image of proteins
- cytoplasms are connected by narrow water-filled channels
- gap junctions allow the passage of calcium and cyclic AMP
- they increase myometrial contractility
- there are low numbers of gap junctions in pregnancy, but high numbers in labour

2 Cell Division

In human cells, replication of DNA genome occurs at a specified time during their lifespan. This period of DNA synthesis or replication is called the synthetic, or S, phase. It is separated from the mitotic, or M, phase, by nonsynthetic phases known as G1 or GAP1 and G2 or GAP2, which occur pre- and post-S phase respectively. In G1 phase, the cell prepares itself for DNA synthesis (which occurs in S phase); and in G2 for mitotic division (M phase).

1. G1 phase: growth phase and synthesis of proteins, lipids and carbohydrates occurs; longest phase of cell cycle
2. S phase: follows G1 phase; replication of genome (DNA), so the cell has double the amount of DNA
3. G2 phase: follows S phase; time for self-assessment (e.g., cell growth, DNA repair) before entering the M phase
4. M phase: mitotic cell division, forming two identical daughter cells

Cells can regulate the occurrence of each phase by expressing certain special proteins called cyclins. Cyclins are a family of proteins whose concentration increases or decreases throughout the cell cycle. They act by activating specific cyclin-dependent protein kinases (CDKs) at appropriate times during the cycle. CDKs phosphorylate specific substrates for the cycle to progress.

There are checkpoints that control progression of the cycle. These checkpoints ensure no compromised cell continues to divide to form abnormal daughter cells. A checkpoint is one of several points in the eukaryotic cell cycle at which the progression of the cell to the next stage can be halted until favourable conditions ensue.

3 Cell Cycle Checkpoints

1. G1 to S phase checkpoint: also known as restriction checkpoint or major checkpoint. At this point, the cell is committed to enter the cell cycle. During the G1 phase, depending on internal and external conditions, the cell can either: (1) delay G1 and enter G0 (quiescent phase), or (2) proceed past the checkpoint and enter S phase. See Figure 35.3.
   - Once the cell proceeds beyond the checkpoint, cyclin D levels rise and form complexes with CDK4 and CDK6, which phosphorylate certain proteins, leading to increased transcription of specific genes, followed by protein synthesis and then G1 to S transition. In addition, there is increased production of cyclin E, which binds with CDK2. The E-CDK2 complex then ensures the cell enters S phase.
   - D-CDK4/CDK6 complex in the late G1 phase binds with retinoblastoma (Rb) protein, causing its phosphorylation. Phosphorylated Rb then releases E2F transcription factor, which leads to gene activation, and transcription of crucial genes occur (e.g., dihydrofolate reductase gene). The cycle then proceeds into S phase.

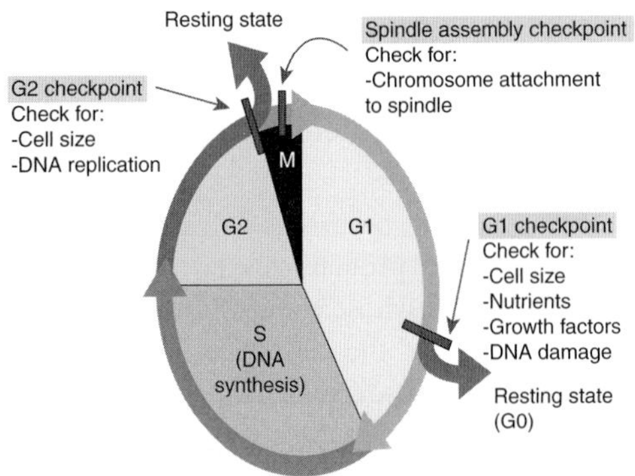

Figure 35.3 Cyclins and CDKs involved in cell cycle progression.

- If DNA damage occurs or any other defect is detected, the cell arrests in G1 phase or enters G0 phase. Ataxia-telangiectasia-mutated (ATM) brings about the phosphorylation of some specific proteins, which keeps E-CDK2 complex inactive, and the cell remains in G1 phase.
- In addition, p53 is activated by phosphorylation, which acts as an activator of many genes such as p21, which inhibits E-CDK2.

2. G2-M checkpoint: after S phase, the cell enters G2 phase, wherein further growth occurs. More proteins and other material are synthesised so that cell can enter the proliferative M phase. DNA damage or incomplete replication is identified.
3. Metaphase checkpoint: during metaphase, when all chromosomes have aligned at the mitotic plate and are under bipolar tension (attached to spindles from respective poles), mitotic spindle checkpoint occurs. See Figure 35.1.
4. Regulation of progression and initiation:
   - Progression beyond restriction checkpoint at G1/S: cyclin D and CDK 4 and 6.
   - Initiation of DNA synthesis in S phase: cyclin E and A, and CDK 2.
   - Transition from G2 to M phase: cyclin B, and CDK1.
5. Dysfunction of these checkpoints:
   - This has been linked with cancer onset.
   - Loss of ATM has been shown to precede lymphoma development.
   - BRCA1 and BRCA2 are well known tumour suppressor genes. Single mutations in these can predispose women towards breast and ovarian cancers. BRCA1 is required for S and G2/M transitions, and is involved in the cellular response to DNA damage. BRCA2 is involved in the regulation of S phase checkpoint.

3.1 Cell Cycle Regulation During Placental Growth

- Human placentation involves a high rate of trophoblast proliferation and trophoblast invasion of the uterine wall. The balance between trophoblast proliferative and invasive actions is controlled by complex interactions between cell cycle promoters and inhibitors.
- In preeclampsia and intrauterine growth restriction, promoters of the cell cycle are in low concentration (cyclin D), and inhibitors (p16, p18, etc.) of cyclin-CDK complexes increase.

Bibliography

Virchow, R. (1958). *Biological theory and modern cytology*, Bargmann, W. Dtsch Med Wochenschr. 361–4.

Carbohydrate, Protein and Lipid Metabolism

Smita Kaushik

1 Carbohydrate Metabolism

Carbohydrates are the chief components of diet (50–60% of energy per day must come from them). They include polysaccharides (starch, glycogen, cellulose, etc.), disaccharides (sucrose, lactose, maltose, etc.) and monosaccharides (glucose, fructose, galactose, etc.). After digestion, monosaccharides are absorbed from the intestine into circulation and transported to all the cells of body. Glucose is the main carbohydrate involved in cellular energy production. It is central to all of metabolism. It is the universal fuel and source of carbon for synthesis of most of the other compounds (both carbohydrate and noncarbohydrate). Other monosaccharides can be converted into glucose and have the same fate.

It reaches inside the cell through specific GLUcose Transport (GLUT) and the cholesterol is phosphorylated (addition of phosphate group) with help of an enzyme, hexokinase, to form glucose-6-phosphate. This activated glucose molecule can enter a number of pathways:

- glycolysis
- hexose monophosphate pathway (HMP) shunt
- glycogen synthesis

These three pathways are common to all cells of the body.

Different glucose transporters (GLUT 1–GLUT 5) are present on different tissues:

- GLUT 1: insulin-independent transport across cells is seen in red blood cells (RBCs), the brain, the kidneys, the colon and the placenta. It has high affinity.
- GLUT 2: insulin-independent transport is present in the liver, pancreatic β-cells, the small intestine and the kidneys. It has low affinity.
- GLUT 3: insulin-independent transport is present in neurons, the placenta, the kidneys and the testes. It has high affinity.
- GLUT 4: insulin-dependent glucose uptake is present in adipose tissue, the heart and skeletal muscle.
- GLUT 5: fructose transporter is present in the small intestine, the testes and sperm.
- SGLT 1: sodium-dependent glucose cotransporter is a symport system common to sodium and glucose, which is present in the small intestine and the kidneys. Na^+-K^+ ATPase pump maintains intracellular sodium ion concentration

1.1 Glycolysis (EMP Pathway)

EMP is an abbreviation for the names of the scientists who discovered glycolysis: Embden–Meyerhof–Parnas. It is a major pathway for glucose oxidation and provides energy as adenosine triphosphate (ATP) to the cells. It occurs in the cytoplasm of all cells. There are two types:

- Aerobic (in the presence of oxygen and the part of oxidation occurring inside the mitochondria).
- Anaerobic (in the absence of oxygen and/or mitochondria).

Aerobic glycolysis leads to the production of pyruvate, which can enter the Krebs cycle or tricarboxylic acid (TCA) cycle. Intermediates of these pathways are used for the synthesis of various amino acids and fats. The total number of ATPs formed is eight.

- Anaerobic glycolysis produces lactate. Two ATP molecules are formed.
- The main enzymes of glycolysis are:
  - hexokinase/glucokinase (only in the liver)
  - phosphofructokinase-1
  - pyruvate kinase
- These are regulatory enzymes and catalyse irreversible reactions of the pathway.
- Enolase enzyme is inhibited by fluoride ions. It is used as an anticoagulant along with potassium

oxalate during collection of blood samples for glucose estimation, and it inhibits glycolysis. It is also used in toothpaste as an anticavity agent (it inhibits glycolysis in cavity-causing bacteria).

- In RBCs, ATP production is bypassed to form an important compound, 2,3-bisphosphoglycerate (2,3-BPG), known as the Rapoport-Luebering cycle. 2,3-BPG has an important role to play in oxygen dissociation from haemoglobin (Hb) at a cellular level. 2,3-BPG levels increase at high altitude, in pulmonary hypoxia and anaemic conditions so that tissue oxygenation is improved (by increasing dissociation of oxygen from Hb in cells).
- RBCs, the lens of the eye, the retina, the renal cortex and the brain exclusively use only glucose for energy production. During prolonged starvation the brain switches over to ketone bodies as an energy source so these other tissues can use glucose.
- Regulation: insulin activates the regulatory enzymes to increase the rate of glycolysis. Glucagon inhibits glycolysis by inhibiting these enzymes.
- Lactic acidosis occurs under anaerobic or hypoxic conditions like strenuous muscular activity. Lactate accumulates in skeletal muscles, causing cramps and pain. It can also occur with deficiency of the enzyme, pyruvate kinase, or in thiamine (vitamin B_1) deficiency.
- Pyruvate synthesised in aerobic glycolysis enters the mitochondria for further oxidation via the Krebs cycle.

1.2 The Krebs Cycle (TCA Cycle)

- The Krebs cycle or tricarboxylic acid cycle occurs in the mitochondria, and is an amphibolic pathway (both oxidative and synthetic processes occur). It is the final common pathway for oxidation of carbohydrates, lipids and proteins: glucose, fatty acids and many amino acids are metabolised to acetyl-coenzyme A (CoA) or intermediates of the Krebs cycle.
- Pyruvate from glycolysis enters the Krebs cycle after conversion to acetyl-CoA with the help of the enzyme pyruvate dehydrogenase (PDH: a multienzyme complex dependent on vitamin B complex for its activity).
- Complete oxidation of acetyl-CoA to carbon dioxide and water occurs along with generation of a lot of energy as ATP (10 ATPs) for every pyruvate entering as acetyl-CoA. So, for every glucose molecule completely oxidised to carbon dioxide and water, 32 ATPs are synthesised.
- Intermediates of the Krebs cycle take part in gluconeogenesis, transamination (the conversion of one amino acid into another), fatty acid synthesis, haem synthesis, cholesterol and steroid synthesis.
- Concentration of oxaloacetate (OAA), an intermediate, is the most important limiting factor for continuation of the cycle; also concentrations of nicotinamide adenine dinucleotide hydrogen (NADH) and/or ATP in the cell.

1.3 Glycogen Metabolism

- Glycogen (homopolysaccharide) is the storage form of glucose in all cells. The liver and skeletal muscles have the maximum amount.
- Glycogen synthesis (glycogenesis) is a process requiring energy (ATP), starting with glucose-6-phosphate with more glucose units binding in a head-to-tail fashion. It is a highly branched structure. The enzyme is glycogen synthase and is a branching enzyme (introducing branch points after every 5–6 glucosyl units). The donor of glucose units is UDP-glucose.
- Glycogen breakdown (glycogenolysis) occurs in a fasting state when energy is required quickly. The enzyme glycogen phosphorylase removes one glucose unit at a time as glucose 1-phosphate from the ends of glycogen chains. A debranching enzyme removes glucose residue from each branch point.
- Liver glycogen serves as a source of blood glucose: this maintains blood glucose levels due to the liver having an enzyme called glucose-6-phosphatase, which converts into glucose.
- Muscle glycogen, on breakdown, forms lactate and provides energy to the muscle only: it cannot contribute to blood glucose. Glucose-6-phosphatase is absent in muscle, so glucose cannot be formed.
- In the liver, glycogenesis is promoted by a high insulin:glucagon ratio (fed state) and glycogenolysis is promoted by a low insulin: glucagon ratio (starvation).

- Under stress conditions, epinephrine acts on the muscle and liver to promote glycogen breakdown.
- Cyclic AMP (cAMP) integrates regulation of glycogen breakdown and synthesis in a reciprocal manner by promoting activation of phosphorylase and inhibiting glycogen synthase.
- In utero, the fetus receives a constant supply of glucose through the placenta. fetal tissues function in an environment dominated by insulin, which promotes fetal growth. This also leads to increased glycogen synthesis and storage. At birth, when the cord is clamped, maternal glucose supply cuts off abruptly and release of the counterregulatory hormones, glucagon and epinephrine, occurs to maintain the blood glucose levels of newborn.
- The inability to maintain blood glucose after birth could be due to maternal malnutrition (the fetus did not receive enough glucose in the antenatal period), inborn error of glycogen metabolism (glycogen storage diseases) or gluconeogenesis and the inability to oxidise fatty acids for energy production.
- Glycogen storage diseases (GSD) occur due to inherited deficiencies in specific enzymes of glycogen metabolism in both the liver and muscle. See Table 36.1.

1.4 Gluconeogenesis

- Gluconeogenesis is the pathway for the synthesis of glucose from noncarbohydrate sources such as lactate, glycerol and some amino acids like alanine (glucogenic amino acids) and propionyl-CoA. It occurs in the liver and kidney. Except for three regulatory steps, it is a reversal of glycolysis. It is an energy requiring process; the source of ATP is fatty acid oxidation.
- Cori's cycle: the conversion of lactate (generated in skeletal muscles during anaerobic glycolysis) into glucose; occurs in the liver and kidneys.
- Glucagon and epinephrine stimulate gluconeogenesis by activating the key enzymes:
    - Pyruvate carboxylase (pyruvate → oxaloacetate); inside the mitochondria
    - Phosphoenolpyruvate carboxykinase: (OAA → phosphoenolpyruvate); in the cytoplasm
    - Fructose-1,6-bisphosphatase (fructose-1,6-bisphosphate → fructose-6-phosphate)
    - Glucose-6-phosphatase (glucose 6-phosphate → glucose)

1.5 Hexose Monophosphate Pathway

- The hexose monophosphate pathway (HMP) is an alternative route for glucose metabolism, with no energy production.
- HMP produces nicotinamide adenine dinucleotide phosphate (NADPH) and ribose (a pentose sugar): NADPH is utilised for reductive biosynthesis: the synthesis of fatty acids, cholesterol and other steroid compounds. Ribose sugar (a pentose) is used for nucleotide and nucleic acid biosynthesis.
- The main enzyme is glucose-6-phosphate dehydrogenase (G6PD).
- Deficiency of G6PD causes haemolytic anaemia (due to the nongeneration of NADPH, which is required to maintain RBC membrane integrity). G6PD deficiency does not affect ribose production.
- The HMP pathway is especially active in tissues where reductive biosynthesis occurs such as the liver, adipose tissue, adrenal cortex, thyroid gland, RBCs, testes and lactating mammary glands.
- All cells synthesise ribose sugar.

1.6 Hexose Metabolism

1.6.1 Fructose

- High dietary fructose (sucrose and high fructose syrups) is rapidly absorbed from the intestine, taken up by liver cells and undergoes glycolysis (faster than glucose). This occurs because fructose bypasses the phosphofructokinase regulatory step in glycolysis, thus flooding the lipogenic pathways, causing increased fatty acid synthesis and their esterification to triacylglycerols in adipose tissues.
- Deficiency of fructokinase causes essential fructosuria, a rare and benign condition.
- Deficiency of hepatic aldolase B causes hereditary fructose intolerance (high levels of fructose-1-phosphate) and hypoglycaemia. It can be fatal if not treated.

1.6.2 Galactose

- Galactose can be synthesised in the body from glucose by the enzyme 4-epimerase.
- Galactose is required in the body as a constituent of glycolipids (cerebrosides), glycoproteins, proteoglycans and in lactating mammary glands.
- Dietary galactose is not essential for lactose synthesis during lactation.

Table 36.1 Glycogen storage diseases

Type	Defective enzyme	Organ affected	Glycogen in the affected organ	Clinical features
I Von Gierke	G-6-ptase or transport system	Liver and kidney	Increased amount; normal structure	Massive enlargement of the liver. Failure to thrive. Severe hypoglycaemia, ketosis, hyperuricemia, hyperlipaemia.
II Pompe	α-1,4-glucosidase (lysosomal)	All organs	Massive increase in amount; normal structure	Cardiorespiratory failure causes death; usually before age 2.
III Cori	Amylo-1,6-glucosidase (debranching enzyme)	Muscle and liver	Increased amount; short outer branches	Like type I, but milder course.
IV Andersen	Branching enzyme (α-1,4 → α-1,6)	Liver and spleen	Normal amount; very long outer branches	Progressive cirrhosis of the liver. Liver failure causes death, usually before age 2.
V McArdle	Phosphorylase	Muscle	Moderately increased amount; normal structure	Limited ability to perform strenuous exercise because of painful muscle cramps. Otherwise, patient is normal and well developed.
VI Hers	Phosphorylase	Liver	Increased amount	Like type I, but a milder course.
VII	Phosphofructokinase	Muscle	Increased amount; normal structure	Like type V.
VIII	Phosphorylase kinase	Liver	Increased amount; normal structure	Mild liver enlargement. Mild hypoglycaemia.

Types I to VII are inherited as autosomal recessives. Type VIII is sex linked.

Used with permission from Berg, J. M., Tymoczko, J.L., Stryer, L. (2012). *Biochemistry*, 7th ed., W. H. Freeman and Company

- Defects in galactokinase, galactose 1-phosphate uridyl transferase and/or 4-epimerase may lead to galactosaemia, which is characterised by failure to thrive, intellectual disability, liver failure and premature cataracts.

1.7 Polyol Pathway

- Persistent hyperglycaemia causes conversion of glucose to sorbitol in tissues such as the lens, peripheral nerves and renal glomeruli. NADPH and aldose reductase are required for this reaction. Sorbitol cannot diffuse out of cells, so it accumulates and causes osmotic swelling leading to cataract formation, neuropathy and nephropathy. Sorbitol can be further converted to fructose.

1.8 Diabetes Mellitus

- Diabetes mellitus (DM) is a group of metabolic disorders characterised by persistent hyperglycaemia, along with polyuria, polydipsia and polyphagia.
- It occurs due to complete or partial deficiency of insulin.
- If left untreated, it can lead to many complications:
    - acute complications: diabetic ketoacidosis (DKA), hyperosmolar hyperglycaemic coma
    - chronic complications: neuropathies, nephropathy, retinopathy, cardiovascular diseases
- Type I DM is the result of the absolute deficiency of insulin. It has an early onset, also known as juvenile diabetes. DKA is a common complication in untreated and uncontrolled states. Exogenous insulin supplementation is essential. Severe hypoglycaemia is common due to insulin overdose or missing a meal after insulin. Also known as insulin-dependent diabetes mellitus (IDDM).
- Type II DM is due to insulin resistance with hyperinsulinism. Glucose receptors on cell membranes do not respond to insulin for glucose uptake. Thus, cellular starvation occurs along with hyperglycemia. It is also known as noninsulin-dependent diabetes mellitus (NIDDM) and has an adult onset.
- Gestational DM occurs when pregnant women without a previous history of DM develop high blood glucose levels after 20 weeks of gestation.
- The categories of fasting plasma glucose (FPG) values are as follows:
    - FPG <100 mg/dL (5.6 mmol/L): normal fasting glucose; HbA1c <6.0%
    - FPG 100–125 mg/dL (5.6–6.9 mmol/L): IFG (impaired fasting glucose); HbA1c 6.0–6.4%
    - FPG <126 mg/dL (<7.0 mmol/L): impaired glucose tolerance; HbA1c 6.0–6.4
    - FPG ≥126 mg/dL (7.0 mmol/L): provisional diagnosis of diabetes; HbA1c >6.5
- The corresponding categories when the oral glucose tolerance test (OGTT) is used are as follows:
    - two-hour postload glucose <140 mg/dL (7.8 mmol/L): normal glucose tolerance
    - two-hour postload glucose 140–199 mg/dL (7.8–11.1 mmol/L): impaired glucose tolerance (IGT)
    - two-hour postload glucose ≥200 mg/dL (11.1 mmol/L): provisional diagnosis of diabetes

Used with permission from Geneva: WHO, 2006, 21.I SBN 978-92-4-159493-6

- Diagnosis of gestational DM (GDM) is made with a 100 g or 75 g glucose load. See Table 36.2.

1.9 Leptin Hormone

- Leptin is produced by adipose cells and helps to regulate energy balance by inhibiting hunger. Its deficiency can lead to obesity. Leptin acts on specific receptors in the hypothalamus to inhibit hunger (by counteracting the effects of neuropeptide Y and anandamide) and stimulate satiety (promoting synthesis of α-melanocyte stimulating hormone, which is a hunger suppressant).
- In fetal lungs, leptin is induced by parathormone-related peptide (PTHrP), acts on type II pneumocytes and causes surfactant expression.
- The placenta produces leptin, which inhibits uterine contractions.
- Leptin is also secreted into breast milk.

Table 36.2 Diagnosis of GDM with a 100 g or 75 g glucose load

	mg/dL	mmol/L
100 g glucose load		
Fasting	95	5.3
1 h	180	10.0
2 h	155	8.6
3 h	140	7.8
75 g glucose load		
Fasting	95	5.3
1 h	180	10.0
2 h	155	8.6

Two or more of the venous plasma concentrations must be met or exceeded for a positive diagnosis. The test should be done in the morning after an overnight fast of between 8 and 14 hours and after at least 3 days of unrestricted diet (≥150 g carbohydrate per day) and unlimited physical activity. The subject should remain seated and should not smoke throughout the test.

Used with permission from American Diabetes Association (2004). Diagnosis and classification of diabetes mellitus. Diabetes Care, 27 (suppl. 1),: s5–10

2 Protein Metabolism

- Dietary proteins are the primary source of nitrogen in the body. Amino acids, produced by the digestion of dietary proteins, are absorbed through intestinal epithelial cells and enter the circulation for assimilation.

2.1 Protein Digestion and Amino Acid Absorption

- Proteolytic enzymes or proteases break down dietary proteins into constituent amino acids. These enzymes are released in the stomach and intestine as zymogens (inactive, larger forms). In the intestinal lumen, zymogens are cleaved to produce the active forms.
- Chief cells secrete pepsinogen, and parietal cells secrete hydrochloric acid (HCl) into the stomach lumen. HCl (pH2–3) alters the conformation of pepsinogen such that it can autocleave itself, forming active pepsin.
- Dietary proteins are denatured by the acid in the stomach. Pepsin acts as an endopeptidase and cleaves peptide bonds between aromatic and acidic amino acids. Smaller peptides and free amino acids are the products of protein digestion that leave the stomach.
- The highly alkaline (due to bicarbonate ion) pancreatic secretions released into the small intestine neutralise the acidic gastric contents, and the various proteases (as inactive zymogens) cause further breakdown of proteins.
- Trypsinogen is cleaved to active enzyme trypsin by the action of a protease enteropeptidase or enterokinase, which is secreted from the brush-border cells of the small intestine.
- Trypsin in turn causes activation of other proteases:
  - chymotrypsinogen to chymotrypsin
  - proelastase to elastase
  - procarboxypeptidases to carboxypeptidases
- Trypsin plays a pivotal role in digestion as it breaks down dietary proteins and activates other pancreatic digestive proteases.
- Trypsin, chymotrypsin and elastase are serine proteases and act as endopeptidases. Trypsin is the most specific; it cleaves bonds at lysine or arginine. Chymotrypsin cleaves bonds at hydrophobic or acidic amino acids. Elastase degrades the protein elastin and bonds between small amino acids. The smaller peptides formed by the action of these enzymes are further attacked by the exopeptidases, which act on the ends of peptides and break one bond at a time; for example, carboxypeptidases (as procarboxypeptidases, activated by trypsin) remove amino acids from the carboxyl end of the peptide chain.
- Exopeptidases, aminopeptidases and intracellular peptidases bring about further breakdown of peptides into amino acids, which are absorbed into the circulation.

2.2 Absorption of Amino Acids

- Amino acids are absorbed from the intestinal lumen and brush border by secondary active sodium-ion-dependent transport, facilitated diffusion or through the γ- glutamyl cycle.
- Absorbed amino acids are taken up by cells, and utilised for protein synthesis or other nitrogen-containing compounds or oxidised for energy.

2.3 Protein Chemistry

- There are about 300 or more known amino acids in nature, but only 20 amino acids make proteins in our body. These are known as standard or

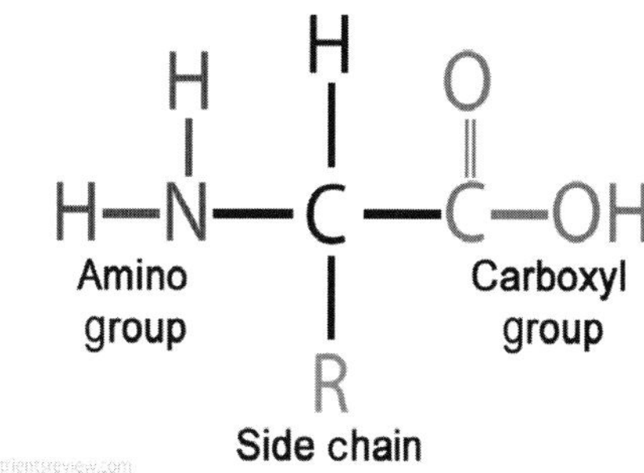

Figure 36.1 Amino acid structure. Source: Nutrientsreview.com

primary amino acids. Two more amino acids have been added to this list: selenocysteine and pyrrolysine, which are formed in the body during the translation process (co-translationally).

- All the mammalian amino acids are α-amino acids. They have an amino group (-NH_2), a carboxyl group (-COOH), a hydrogen atom (-H) and a side chain (-R), bound covalently to the central α-carbon atom. All the 20 amino acids differ in the side chains. See Figure 36.1.
- Glycine is the simplest amino acid, its R group being an H-atom.
- Valine, leucine and isoleucine are branched-chain amino acids. These, along with alanine, contain aliphatic side chains, so are also hydrophobic in nature.
- Phenylalanine, tyrosine and tryptophan have aromatic side chains.
- Methionine and cysteine contain a sulphur group (-SH); cystine is a dimer of cysteine having a disulphide bond (S-S).
- Threonine and serine contain a hydroxyl group (-OH).
- Glutamic acid and aspartic acid containing an extra – COOH group are the acidic amino acids, glutamine and asparagine being their amides respectively.
- Arginine and lysine have an extra amino group, hence are the basic amino acids.
- Histidine has an imidazole group and plays an important role in the buffering action of proteins.
- Proline contains an imino (-NH) group instead of an amino (-NH_2) group; thus is also known as an imino acid.
- Nutritionally, these have been divided into essential (not synthesised in the body, so have to be taken in the diet) and nonessential (synthesised in the body).

Table 36.3 Essential and nonessential amino acids

Essential or semiessential amino acids	Nonessential amino acids
Phenylalanine	Hydroxyalanine
Tryptophan	Serine
Valine	Glutamic acid
Leucine	Aspartic acid
Isoleucine	Proline
Lysine	Pyrolysine
Threonine	Tyrosine
Methionine	Glycine
Histidine	Cysteine
Arginine	Selenocysteine

- The eight essential amino acids are phenylalanine, tryptophan, valine, leucine, isoleucine, lysine, threonine and methionine. The two semi-essential amino acids are histidine and arginine. The remainder are nonessential. See Table 36.3.

2.4 Purification of Proteins

- A mixture of proteins can be separated or purified by various techniques such as chromatography and electrophoresis.
- High-pressure liquid chromatography is one of the most sensitive techniques for the separation of different proteins at a faster rate and at high resolution.
- Protein purity is assessed by polyacrylamide gel electrophoresis (PAGE), especially sodium dodecyl sulphate (SDS) PAGE. SDS is an anionic detergent, which imparts an overall negative charge to the polypeptide chains depending on their mass, such that proteins migrate on the polyacrylamide gel under the influence of electric current on the basis of their molecular weight.
- Isoelectric focusing is a technique that separates proteins depending on their isoelectric pH. Isoelectric pH is the pH at which the molecule or ion has zero net charge. Molecules or ions bearing zero net charge (i.e., having equal number opposite charges) are called zwitterions.

2.5 Synthesis of Proteins: Translation

- Translation is a process by which cells synthesise proteins. It occurs on ribosomes (attached to endoplasmic reticulum) and is guided by mRNA. It is an energy consuming process (in the form of guanosine-5-triphosphate (GTP)).

- The genetic message encoded in DNA is first transcribed into mRNA, and the nucleotide sequence of mRNA then determines the sequence of constituent amino acids in a protein.
- The portion of mRNA that specifies the amino acid sequence of a protein is read in codons. Codons are a set of three nucleotides, which specify specific amino acids. Initiation of the synthesis of a polypeptide chain starts with the codon AUG, which specifies the amino acid methionine. Codons on mRNA are read sequentially in the 5' to 3' direction, starting with 5'-AUG, which sets the reading frame, and ending with a 3'-termination (or stop) codons: UAG, UGA or UAA. The protein is produced from its N-terminus to its C-terminus.
- Specific tRNA carries amino acids to the ribosomal site of protein synthesis. Base-pairing between the anticodon of the tRNA and the codon on the mRNA ensures the insertion of the amino acid onto the growing polypeptide chain at the appropriate position as per the information on the DNA.
- The binding of initial methionyl-tRNA (methionine attached to its specific tRNA) to mRNA and the ribosome is called initiation and involves certain cytoplasmic proteins called initiation factors and GTP (the energy source).
- After initiation, sequential addition of specific amino acids according to the codon sequence on the mRNA, leads to the elongation of the polypeptide chain. Elongation involves three steps:
  1. Addition of an aminoacyl-tRNA to a site on the ribosome, where it binds and base-pairs with its next or the second codon on the mRNA.
  2. Formation of a peptide bond between the first and second amino acids.
  3. Translocation: movement of mRNA relative to the ribosome, so that another aminoacyl-tRNA can bind to the third mRNA codon and to the ribosome.
- Termination: the above three steps are repeated until a termination codon is reached on the mRNA. Release factors bind instead of a charged tRNA (aminoacyl-tRNA). This causes release of the completed polypeptide chain from the ribosome.
- As one ribosome moves along the mRNA, producing one polypeptide chain, a second ribosome may bind to the vacant 5'-end of mRNA. Many ribosomes can simultaneously translate a single mRNA, forming a complex called polysome.
- As the nascent polypeptide chain leaves the ribosome complex, it is folded into a three-dimensional conformation, which is the native or active form of the protein. This process requires action of some proteins known as chaperone proteins (e.g., hsp70, hsp60 or chaperonins).
- Posttranslational modification of some amino acid residues occurs in the newly formed proteins. This includes:
  - formation of a disulphide bond between two cysteine residues
  - glycosylation (addition of carbohydrate groups)
  - phosphorylation (addition of phosphate groups)
  - methylation (addition of methyl groups)
  - carboxylation (addition of carboxyl groups)
  - hydroxylation (addition of hydroxyl groups)
  - cleavage of peptide bonds, and so on

2.6 Inhibitors of Protein Synthesis in Prokaryotes

- Streptomycin: binds to the 30S prokaryotic ribosomal subunit and prevents initiation of protein synthesis. It also causes the misreading of mRNA and thereby disrupts the bacterial growth.
- Tetracyclin: binds to the 30S subunit and inhibits the binding of aminoacyl-tRNA to the A-site on the ribosome.
- Chloramphenicol: binds to the 50S subunit and inhibits peptidyltransferase.
- Erythromycin: binds to 50S and prevents translocation.

2.7 Protein Catabolism

- Human adults degrade 1–2% of body protein, mainly muscle protein, every day. Of the released amino acids, 75–80% are reutilised for new protein synthesis. The remainder are degraded and the nitrogen content is converted into urea.

2.8 Biosynthesis of Urea

Urea biosynthesis divided into four stages:

- transamination
- oxidative deamination
- ammonia transport
- urea cycle

2.8.1 Urea Cycle

The urea cycle consists of five enzymatically controlled steps, which are catalysed by carbamoyl phosphate synthetase, ornithine transcarbamylase, argininosuccinate synthetase, argininosuccinase and arginase.

1. Amino groups of all the released amino acids are used to form glutamate. This happens by the process of transamination.
   - In this, there is interconversion of a pair of amino acids and a pair of keto acids.
   - Enzymes required: transaminases or aminotransferases.
   - Coenzyme: pyridoxal phosphate; the active form of vitamin B_6.
   - Alanine transaminase (alanine-pyruvate transaminase) and glutamate transaminase (glutamate-α ketoglutarate transaminase) are the most common transaminases catalysing transfer of amino groups from all amino acids to form alanine and glutamate. Alanine in turn transfers its amino group to glutamate. This is important as L-glutamate is the only amino acid in mammalian tissues, which undergoes oxidative deamination at an appreciable rate.
   - Alanine aminotransferase is also known as glutamate pyruvate transaminase and aspartate aminotransferase as glutamate oxaloacetate transaminase. These are important diagnostic enzymes and play an important role in the diagnosis of liver and cardiac diseases.
2. Deamination: the removal of α-amino groups from amino acids as free ammonia of two types:
   - Oxidative deamination: glutamate is oxidatively deaminated to α-ketoglutarate and the amino group is liberated as free ammonia. Enzyme is glutamate dehydrogenase (GDH).
   - GDH is a zinc containing metallo-enzyme, present in mitochondria. It requires NAD^+ or $NADP^+$ as coenzyme. Oxidative deamination of glutamate by hepatic GDH is the major pathway for production of ammonia in mammals.
   - Oxidative deamination by L-amino acid oxidase is the minor pathway for ammonia production. It occurs in the mammalian liver and the kidneys.
3. The free ammonia consequently produced is then transported to the liver and kidneys in the form of glutamine.
   - Free ammonia ($NH^+{}_4$) is very toxic, especially to the central nervous system. Normal blood levels of free ammonia are 10–20μg/dL. An increase in its level leads to hyperammonaemia. It can lead to ammonia intoxication, causing slurring of speech, blurred vision and tremors. The brain is affected because of severe depletion of α-ketoglutarate, which impairs the function of the TCA cycle, leading to energy depletion in nervous tissues.
   - As such, free ammonia is 'trapped' as glutamine by the the enzyme glutamine synthase; the substrate is glutamate.
   - Glutamine transports ammonia to the liver and kidney, where another enzyme glutaminase acts on it and releases ammonia, which is then converted to urea.
4. Urea biosynthesis: urea is the major end product of nitrogen metabolism in humans. Animals that excrete amino nitrogen as urea are called ureotelic animals.
   - The urea cycle was discovered by Hans Kreb (who also discovered the TCA cycle) and Kurt Henseleit, so it is also known as the Krebs–Henseleit cycle.
   - It involves five steps/reactions: the first two in the mitochondria and the next three in the cytosol of the hepatic cells.
     a. Synthesis of carbamoyl phosphate: in the mitochondria of hepatocytes, ammonia ($NH^+{}_4$) and bicarbonate (CO_2) combine to form carbamoyl phosphate. The enzyme is carbamoyl phosphate synthetase I (CPSI). This is the rate-limiting step for urea synthesis. See Figure 36.2.

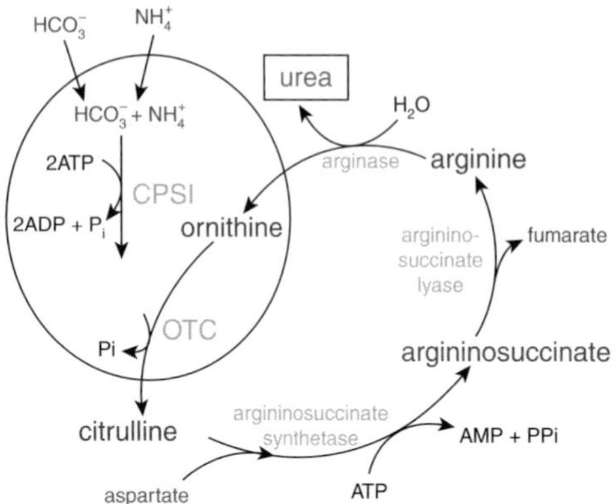

Figure 36.2 Urea cycle.

b. Synthesis of citrulline: carbamoyl phosphate combines with ornithine to form citrulline (enzyme: ornithine transcarbamoylase), which crosses the mitochondrial membrane and enters the cytoplasm.
c. Synthesis of arginosuccinate: citrulline in the cytosol then combines with aspartate to form arginosuccinate. Enzyme: arginosuccinate synthetase.
d. Arginosuccinate then cleaves into arginine and fumarate. Fumarate so formed enters the TCA cycle; thus, the urea cycle is linked to the TCA cycle through fumarate.
e. Finally, arginine cleaves to form urea and ornithine; ornithine being utilised again for urea synthesis.

5. Urea contains two amino groups: one from glutamine [glutamine → glutamate + free ammonia (NH_4^+)], and the second from aspartate.

2.8.2 Regulation of Urea Synthesis

- The first step catalysed by CPSI is the rate-limiting step.
- Normal levels of blood urea are 2.5–7.1 nmol/L (7–20 mg/dL).

2.9 Protein Metabolism During Pregnancy

During pregnancy, there is a positive nitrogen balance as it is a time of growth. There is increased uptake of amino acids for tissue growth, both maternal and fetal, with a decrease in urea synthesis. A low rate of leucine and other branched-chain amino acids (valine, leucine, isoleucine) transamination/oxidation has been observed during pregnancy, increasing their availability for fetal growth. Pregnancy is also associated with hypoaminoacidaemia, reflecting an enhanced placental uptake of amino acids. Placental uptake is an active process, using selective transporters and energy.

2.10 Special Products Formed from Amino Acids

1. Glycine: forms haem, creatine, purines, along with glutamate and cysteine forms glutathione, glycine conjugates. Glycine itself acts as an inhibitory neurotransmitter.
2. Methionine: forms S-adenosylmethionine (SAM), polyamines (spermine, spermidine). Along with glycine and arginine, methionine forms creatine.
3. Tryptophan: forms serotonin, melatonin, tryptamine and niacin (vitamin B_5).
4. Tyrosine: forms thyroid hormone (T3, T4), dihydroxyphenylalanine (DOPA), epinephrine, norepinephrine and melanin.
5. Glutamate: forms gamma-aminobutyric acid, which is an inhibitory neurotransmitter.

2.11 Disorders of Catabolism of the Amino Acid Carbon Skeleton

1. Phenylketonuria: the defective enzyme, phenylalanine hydroxylase, leads to hyperphenylalaninaemia as phenylalanine cannot be converted to tyrosine. In addition, alternative metabolites are produced: phenyl-pyruvate, phenyl-lactate, phenyl-acetate, and so on. These are excreted in urine, hence the name phenylketonuria. Intellectual disability occurs due to high phenylalanine levels, and skin tone is very fair due to low melanin levels. Treatment is with a phenylalanine-free diet until six years of age, when maximum brain growth occurs.
2. Alkaptonuria: defective enzyme homogentisate oxidase (in tyrosine catabolism). This leads to accumulation of homogentisate in tissues, causing pigmentation (ochronosis), and is excreted in the urine, which turns black on standing due to oxidation of homogentisate to alkapton. It is a benign condition.

3. Hartnup disease: an autosomal recessive condition, with defects in intestinal and renal transport of neutral amino acids including tryptophan. There is neutral aminoaciduria, causing a deficiency of tryptophan. This produces pellagra-like signs and symptoms due to decreased synthesis of niacin.
4. Maple syrup urine disease: an autosomal recessive condition with branched-chain ketonuria. The defective enzyme is α-keto acid decarboxylase, branched-chain amino acids and their keto acids elevated in blood and urine. Urine has the odour of burnt sugar or maple syrup.
5. Carcinoid syndrome: not related to amino acid catabolism. It is a paraneoplastic syndrome due to carcinoid tumours. There is increased endogenous secretion of serotonin and kallikrein. Tryptophan is diverted to serotonin synthesis, which is normally a minor pathway. Due to this, there is decreased synthesis of niacin, leading to pellagra-like symptoms along with the features of carcinoid syndrome.

3 Lipid Metabolism

3.1 Lipid Chemistry

- Lipids are a heterogenous group of compounds having common properties of the following:
  1. Relative insolubility in water
  2. Solubility in nonpolar solvents such as ether, chloroform and benzene
- Lipids include: fatty acids and triacylglycerols (TGs); glycerophospholipids and sphingolipids; eicosanoids; cholesterol, bile salts and steroid hormones; fat-soluble vitamins; and lipoproteins.
  - Fatty acids, stored as triacylglycerol in adipose tissue, are an efficient source of energy for the body. Fatty acids are saturated if they have no double bonds, monounsaturated with one double bond, and polyunsaturated with more than one double bond.
    - Essential fatty acids are polyunsaturated fatty acids (PUFAs), which cannot be synthesised in the body: linoleic acid, linolenic acid and arachidonic acid
    - Omega-3 fatty acids (e.g., linolenic acid) found in fish oils are cardioprotective by inhibiting platelet aggregation.
  - Glycerophospholipids and sphingophospholipids are important components of biomembranes, nervous tissue and lipoproteins.
    - Glycerophospholipids are synthesised from fatty acyl-CoA, which combines with glycerol 3-phosphate to form phosphatidic acid. Different groups are added to C-3 of g-3-p of phosphatidic acid to produce amphipathic compounds like phosphatidylcholine, phosphatidylinositol and cardiolipin (present in mitochondrial membrane and the only phospholipid that is antigenic in nature).
    - Plasmalogens (present in cardiac muscles) and platelet-activating factor are formed when a long-chain fatty alcohol links to glycerol 3-phosphate.
    - Phospholipids are broken down by phospholipases (found in pancreatic juice, cell membranes and lysosomes).
    - Sphingolipids are predominantly present in the brain and nervous tissues. They have sphingosine, an amino (serine) alcohol instead of glycerol, as the backbone to which acyl-CoA binds with an amide linkage: this is called a ceramide.
    - Sphingomyelin contains ceramide attached to phosphocholine or phosphoethanolamine as the polar head group. Sphingolipids are degraded by lysosomal enzymes.
    - Glycolipids or glycosphingolipids contain ceramide, to which sugar is attached. They are predominantly present in the brain and myelin sheath of nervous tissue. The sugar molecule can be glucose, galactose, sialic acid, and so on. They are further divided into cerebrosides and gangliosides:
      - cerebroside: ceramide plus a glucose or galactose molecule
      - gangliosides: ceramide plus sialic acid
  - PUFAs containing 20-carbons form eicosanoids, which regulate many cellular processes.
  - Cholesterol regulates the fluidity of biomembranes. It is a precursor for the synthesis of bile acids (required for digestion of dietary fats), a precursor for the synthesis of

steroid hormones and vitamin D and an important constituent of lipoproteins like low-density lipoprotein (LDL) and high density lipoprotein (HDL).
  - Fat-soluble vitamins A, D, E and K are involved in varied functions such as vision, cellular growth, calcium metabolism, antioxidant function and blood clotting.
  - Lipoproteins like chylomicron (CM), very low density lipoprotein (VLDL), LDL, and HDL are the transport forms of lipids.

3.2 Digestion and Transport of Dietary Lipids

- TGs are the main dietary lipids.
- Lipid digestion starts in the mouth: lingual lipase (from Ebner's glands in the tongue), then in the stomach: gastric lipase. Major digestion of lipids occurs in the small intestine, where pancreatic lipase acts on dietary lipids to form free fatty acids (FFAs) and 2-monoacyl glycerols (2-MAG). Pancreatic lipase requires action of bile salts and colipase for proper breakdown of lipids; bile salts cause emulsification of fats (the breaking down of fats into smaller droplets to allow complete action of the enzyme lipase). Colipase acts as an interface between water insoluble fats and water-soluble enzymes.
- The breakdown products (FFAs and 2-MAG) are taken up into the intestinal epithelial cells by simple diffusion, where triacylglycerols are reformed and transported into blood as CM, which transports TGs from intestine to liver. In circulation, CM is acted on by another lipase known as lipoprotein lipase (LPL). LPL is attached to the basement membrane of endothelial cells lining the capillaries, and digests TGs present in CM and other lipoproteins. The FFAs and glycerol released are taken up by the extrahepatic tissues for energy production.

3.3 *De Novo* Fatty Acid Synthesis (Lipogenesis)

- Site: the liver is the main site; other sites include the kidneys, brain, mammary glands and adipose tissue (not an important site in humans).
- Cellular location: cytoplasm.
- Enzymes required: acetyl-CoA carboxylase, fatty acid synthase (FAS) complex.

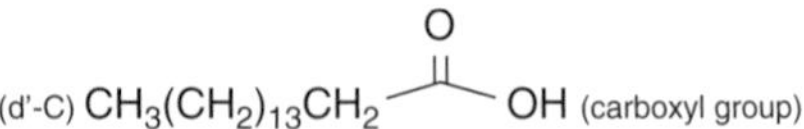

Figure 36.3 Structure of a saturated fatty acid with a carboxylic acid group and a long hydrocarbon chain consisting of carbon (C) and hydrogen (H) atoms.

- Coenzymes/cofactors: ATP, Mn^{2+}, biotin, HCO_3^+ and NADPH.
- Substrate: cytoplasmic acetyl-CoA.
- Product: free fatty acid (palmitate is the most common example with C-16) – see Figure 36.3.
- Fatty acid synthesis occurs in the fed state, when there is excess of carbohydrate. Excess dietary glucose undergoes glycolysis in the cytoplasm to form pyruvate, which is converted to acetyl-CoA in the mitochondria. Acetyl-CoA combines with oxaloacetate to form citrate. Citrate is transported to the cytoplasm by its specific transporter on the inner mitochondrial membrane. In the cytoplasm, citrate cleaves to form acetyl-CoA and oxaloacetate.
- In the cytoplasm, acetyl-CoA is used to synthesise the palmitic acid, 16-C saturated fatty acid. Acetyl-CoA carboxylase catalyses the rate-limiting step of conversion of acetyl-CoA to malonyl CoA. Malonyl CoA provides the acetyl-CoA moiety for fatty acid synthesis on FAS enzyme complex. See Figure 36.4.
- FAS is a multifunctional polypeptide chain; that is, a single polypeptide has multiple functional domains, which catalyse different reactions during the sequential addition of acetyl-CoA to the growing fatty acid chain.
- NADPH, produced by the HMP pathway and enzyme malate dehydrogenase, provide the reducing equivalents.

3.4 Overview of Fatty Acid Synthesis

- When the chain is 16-C long, it is released as palmitate.
- Further fates of palmitate include:
  - further elongation of the fatty chain (which occurs in peroxisomes)
  - desaturation (introduction of a double bond between C1 and 10 to form unsaturated fatty acid (FA))
  - esterification of fatty acids with glycerol to form TGs: major storage form of fuel (stored in adipose tissue)

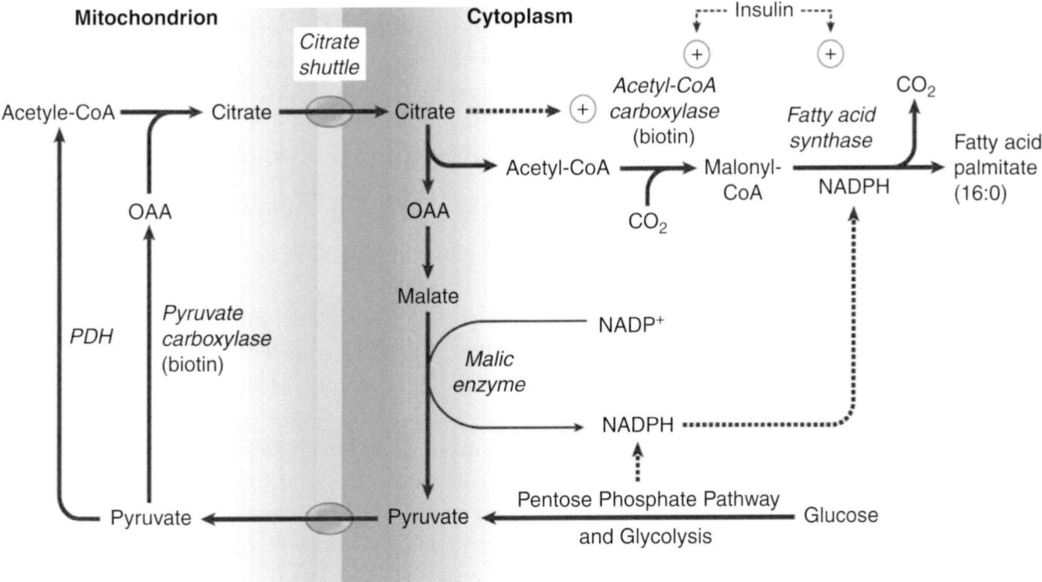

Figure 36.4 Pyruvate cycle.

 - esterification with cholesterol to form cholesteryl esters
- For these fates, the palmitate must be activated to palmitoyl CoA (by the enzyme acyl-CoA synthetase; requires ATP as energy source).

3.5 Regulation of Lipogenesis

- Rate-limiting reaction: acetyl-CoA carboxylase step.
- Short-term regulation:
  - Allosteric modification: citrate is the most important positive modulator and increases enzyme activity manifold by causing polymerisation of the enzyme.
  - FFA is the most important negative modulator and inhibits the enzyme by disrupting the polymerised form.
  - Covalent modification: the enzyme is active in dephosphorylated form, brought about by insulin (which has high concentrations in the fed state) by activating a specific phosphatase enzyme, which removes the phosphate group from the enzyme. In a starved state, glucagon is high and causes phosphorylation of the enzyme by activating a kinase enzyme and making carboxylase inactive.
- Long-term regulation: occurs by induction/repression of the carboxylase gene by insulin/glucagon during the fed/starvation state respectively.
- FAS enzyme undergoes induction and repression by insulin and glucagon, respectively.

3.6 Fatty Acid Oxidation (Breakdown)

- Fatty acid oxidation is the major source of energy for ATP synthesis in humans.
- Muscles use fatty acids for their energy needs during rest. The brain and RBCs do not use fatty acids as a source of energy. The β-oxidation pathway is not well developed in the brain and nervous tissues, and RBCs do not have mitochondria. Such tissues use glucose as their primary energy source; other tissues being the lens of the eye, the retina and the placenta.
- Fatty acid is oxidised in the mitochondria by a process known as β-oxidation.
- Fatty acid is first activated to fatty acyl-CoA, then enters mitochondrial matrix by a carnitine transport system present in mitochondrial membranes. The enzymes involved are carnitine-acyl (palmitoyl) transferase I (CPT I):
  - carnitine-acylcarnitine translocase (CAT)

- ◦ carnitine-acyl (palmitoyl) transferase II (CPT II)
- Deficiency of any or all of these enzymes can lead to decrease in β-oxidation, causing muscular weakness and hypoglycaemia.
- Once inside the mitochondria, fatty-acyl-CoA undergoes a series of four reactions repeatedly to cause breakdown of acyl chain in 2-C units sequentially from the carboxyl end of the fatty chain. This 2-C unit is acetyl-CoA. This process is known as β-oxidation, as the bond between α and β carbon atoms of acyl chain is broken. The four enzymes catalysing these steps are:
  1. acyl-CoA dehydrogenase, linked to FAD^+
  2. enoyl-CoA hydratase
  3. β-hydroxy acyl-CoA dehydrogenase, linked to NAD^+
  4. β-ketothiolase
- $NADH + H^+$ and $FADH_2$ produced in each cycle undergo oxidative phosphorylation for ATP generation: 2.5 ATP for each NADH and 1.5 ATP for each $FADH_2$.
- Acetyl-CoA cleaved off after every cycle goes to the TCA cycle for ATP generation: 10 ATP are generated from each molecule of acetyl-CoA.

3.7 Ketogenesis (Synthesis of Ketone Bodies)

- Organ: liver.
- Site: mitochondria of hepatocytes.
- Substrate: acetyl-CoA.
- Product: acetone, acetoacetate, β-hydroxybutyrate are the ketone bodies.
- Enzymes required: 3-hydroxy-3-methyl-glutaryl (HMG) CoA synthase, HMG CoA lyase, 3-hydroxybutyrate dehydrogenase.
- Ketone bodies serve as fuel for tissues such as muscles, especially cardiac muscle, slow-twitch muscle and renal cortex under normal conditions. During prolonged starvation, most of the tissues switch from glucose to ketone bodies as the primary source of energy, except RBCs, the lens, the retina and the fast-twitch muscle. The brain uses ketone bodies during prolonged starvation.
- Regulation of ketogenesis is maintained by (1) concentration of FFAs in the blood, (2) uptake by liver, (3) concentration of OAA in the TCA cycle. This is the deciding factor in mitochondria for acetyl-CoA to enter the TCA or ketogenesis pathway: adequate oxaloacetate (fed state) → acetyl-CoA enters the TCA; low OAA → it enters ketogenesis.

3.8 Utilisation of Ketone Bodies by Tissues During Starvation

- All tissues except the liver can utilise ketone bodies as a source of energy as they contain an enzyme called thiophorase (i.e., succinyl CoA-acetoacetate CoA transferase).
- Increased production of ketone bodies, causing an increase in blood ketone body levels, is ketonaemia. Normal blood values are 1 mmol/L. Excess is excreted in urine, ketonuria, which is seen in prolonged starvation, uncontrolled DM, heavy lactation and severe exercise.

3.9 Metabolism of Unsaturated Fatty Acids

- Monounsaturated fatty acids can be synthesised in the body as humans can introduce double bonds anywhere between C-1 (the carboxyl-C) and C-10, but not beyond it. The most common double bond is between C9 and C10. This process is facilitated by enzyme: desaturase; present in endoplasmic reticulum. The process also requires cytochrome b_5, NAD(P)H and oxygen O_2.
- PUFAs are essential in the diet as they cannot be synthesised in the body.
- Trans fatty acids are found in ruminant fat and are present in hydrogenated vegetable fat. In the body they behave as, and are metabolised as, saturated fatty acids. They also tend to raise blood levels of LDL and lower HDL levels, thus are atherogenic in nature. Trans fats tend to antagonise the metabolism of essential fatty acids (EFAs) and also exacerbate their deficiency.

3.10 Metabolism of Eicosanoids

- Arachidonic acid (from the plasma membrane) is the precursor for eicosanoids. They are prostaglandins (PGs), thromboxane (TX) (prostanoids), leukotriene (LT) and lipoxin (LX). They act as local hormones, having paracrine and autocrine effects.

- Prostanoids are synthesised by the cyclooxygenase (COX) pathway. The COX enzyme is inhibited by nonsteroidal anti-inflammatory drugs (NSAIDs), so inflammatory action of PGs can be inhibited by giving NSAIDs, which inhibits the enzyme cyclooxygenase irreversibly (suicidal inhibition).
- There are two isoenzymes of COX: COX-1 and COX-2. NSAIDS (e.g., aspirin) inhibit both isoenzymes. COX-1 has a gastro-protective action (decreases gastric acid secretion, but no effect on gastric mucus secretion), but since COX-1 is also inhibited, NSAID intake is associated with gastric irritation. Coxibs are drugs that selectively inhibit COX-2 and have gastro-protective action.
- Low-dose aspirin inhibits COX and prevents vasoconstriction and platelet aggregation (by inhibiting thromboxane, TX_2, synthesis) and promotes vasodilatation (uninterrupted role of PGI_2: prostacyclin).
- Omega-3 fatty acid, found in cod-liver oil, is very cardioprotective as it causes production of TX_3 and prostaglandin I_3 (PGI_3), whose overall effect is cardioprotective: leading to vasodilatation and decreased platelet aggregation. Additionally, levels of LDL, VLDL, triglycerides and cholesterol are also low in individuals who regularly consume omega-3 fatty acids in their diet.
- Prostaglandins (PGE and PGF) have roles as abortifacient, and for induction of labour in the term uterus.
- Leukotrienes and lipoxins are mediators of inflammatory reactions, synthesised by lipoxygenase enzyme system.

3.11 Phospholipids

- Lysolecithin is utilised for production of the lung surfactant, dipalmitoyl-phosphatidylcholine in lung alveoli. In babies born prematurely, concentration of lung surfactant is very low (L:S <2) and such babies are prone to develop infant respiratory distress syndrome (IRDS).
- Multiple sclerosis is a demyelinating disease, with loss of phospholipids and sphingolipids from white matter; thus, its lipid composition starts to resemble that of grey matter.
- Lipid storage diseases (sphingolipidoses) are a group of inherited diseases caused by a genetic defect in the catabolism of sphingolipids. There is accumulation of complex lipids in neurons, causing neurodegeneration and shortening of lifespan. The rate of synthesis of these lipids is normal. Treatment consists of enzyme replacement therapy, bone marrow transplant or gene therapy. Some of the important diseases are:

  1. Tay–Sachs disease: caused by deficiency of enzyme hexosaminidase A, leading to accumulation of gangliosides.
  2. Fabry disease: caused by deficiency of enzyme α-galactosidase, leading to the accumulation of a special ceramide. It is X-linked recessive in inheritance.
  3. Gaucher's disease: due to deficiency of the enzyme β-galactosidase, there is accumulation of glucosylceramide.
  4. Niemann–Pick disease: due to deficiency of the enzyme sphingomyelinase, there is accumulation of sphingomyelin.

- These diseases cause intellectual disability, hepatomegaly, skeletal deformities, and so on. Many are fatal in early life.

3.12 Cholesterol Metabolism

- Cholesterol is present in all cells and plasma either as free cholesterol or combined with a long-chain fatty acid as cholesteryl ester (the storage form). In plasma, both forms are transported as lipoproteins. It is an amphipathic molecule and an essential structural component of membranes. It gives rise to many important biomolecules in the body.
- The body gets cholesterol from the diet as well as it is synthesised in all nucleated cells in the body. The liver and intestine are the major sites of synthesis.

3.12.1 Cholesterol Synthesis

- Acetyl-CoA is the precursor molecule for cholesterol synthesis. See Figure 36.5.

3.12.2 Regulation of Cholesterol Biosynthesis

- HMG-CoA reductase is the rate-limiting and committed step in the cholesterol biosynthesis pathway.
- Statins are a group of drugs that inhibit cholesterol synthesis by competitively inhibiting HMG-CoA reductase.

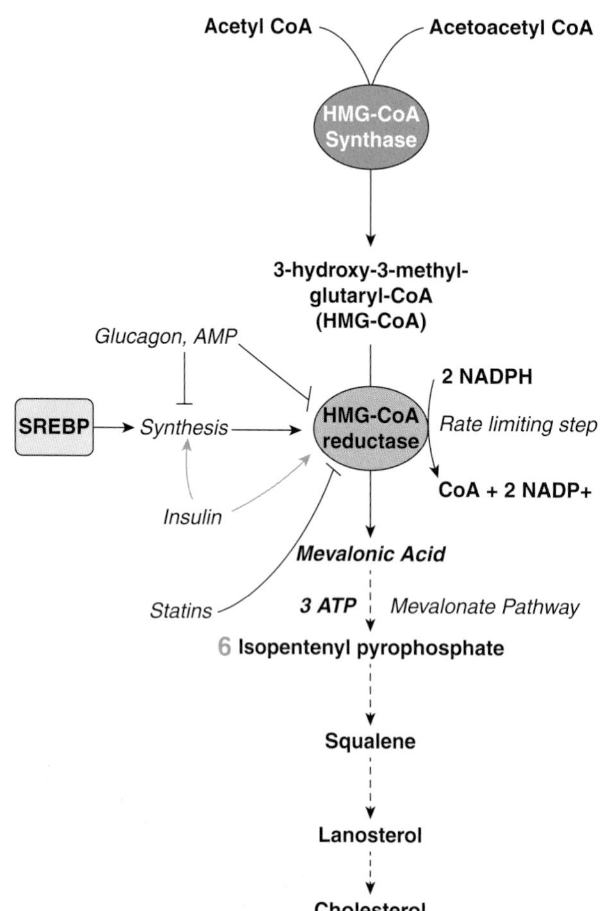

Figure 36.5 Biosynthesis of cholesterol.
SREBP – Sterol-regulatory-element-binding-protein

3.12.3 Cholesterol Balance at the Cellular Level

Intracellular cholesterol concentration is regulated by various factors:

1. An increase in cholesterol level is caused by: (a) an increase in cellular uptake of cholesterol-containing lipoproteins by specific lipoprotein receptors on the cell membrane; for example, LDL receptor or scavenger receptor, (b) uptake of free cholesterol from cholesterol-rich lipoproteins to the cell membrane, (c) cholesterol biosynthesis, (d) hydrolysis of cholesteryl esters by cholesteryl ester hydrolase.
2. A decrease in cholesterol level: (a) due to cholesterol efflux from the membrane to HDL via specific membrane receptors, (b) esterification of cholesterol by acyl-CoA: cholesterol acyl transferase, (c) utilisation of cholesterol for the synthesis of other steroid compounds such as steroid hormones, bile salts and vitamin D.

3.12.4 Transport of Cholesterol Between Tissues

- In blood, cholesterol is transported in lipoproteins, mainly as cholesteryl esters. LDL is the lipoprotein with maximum concentration of cholesterol.
- Dietary cholesterol equilibrates with plasma cholesterol in days, and with tissue cholesterol in weeks.
- Dietary cholesterol, as cholesteryl esters, is first hydrolysed to free cholesterol by the enzyme cholesteryl esterase, which is then absorbed by intestinal epithelium along with other lipids and fat-soluble vitamins. Dietary lipids and cholesterol are then incorporated, along with cholesterol synthesised in the intestinal epithelial cells, into chylomicrons. CM delivers most of the cholesterol to the liver in chylomicron remnants. Liver secretes most cholesterol in the form of VLDL, cholesterol is retained as VLDL transforms into intermediate density lipoprotein (IDL) and then into LDL. LDL is finally taken up by LDL receptors in liver and extrahepatic tissues.
- Excretion of cholesterol: cholesterol is excreted from the body as cholesterol in bile or as bile acids. The steroid nucleus cannot be degraded.

3.12.5 Synthesis of Bile Acids

- The primary bile acids are synthesised in the liver from cholesterol. They are cholic acid (major form) and chenodeoxycholic acid. They are conjugated with taurine and glycine to form taurocholic acid and glycocholic acid, and are stored in bile in the gall bladder.
- The rate-limiting enzyme is 7α-hydroxylase. It is a microsomal enzyme, requires oxygen, NADPH, cytochrome P450 and ascorbic acid (vitamin C).
- The bile acids or salts enter the intestine along with bile, where they are further metabolised by the intestinal bacteria and form secondary bile acids or salts, deoxycholic acid and lithocholic acid.
- Of the primary and secondary bile acids in the intestine, 98–99% are absorbed in the ileum and returned to the liver via portal circulation. This is called the enterohepatic circulation. The small fraction that escapes absorption is excreted in the

faeces. This is the only pathway for elimination of cholesterol from body.

3.12.6 Clinical Aspects Related to Cholesterol

- Normal serum cholesterol is less than 180 mg/dL. Values more than 200 mg/dL is a major risk factor in promoting atherosclerosis, which is characterised by deposition of cholesterol and cholesteryl esters present in lipoproteins into the artery wall. Prolonged elevated levels of blood VLDL, IDL, LDL (especially oxidised LDL) and CM remnants, due to diseases like DM, hypothyroidism, lipid nephrosis and hyperlipidaemia lead to atherosclerosis. Conversely, there is an inverse relationship between blood HDL (HDL_2) and the incidence of coronary heart disease. Thus, LDL:HDL cholesterol ratio is a good predictor to assess the risk of coronary artery disease (CAD).
- Diet and lifestyle changes have an important role to play in maintaining normal blood cholesterol.
- Although genetic factors are most important in determining an individual's blood cholesterol levels, dietary and environmental factors also play a part. Inclusion of polyunsaturated fatty acids (PUFAs) (corn oil and sunflower seed oil) and monounsaturated fatty acids (MUFAs) instead of saturated fatty acids (e.g., butter, palm oil, animal fat) is an important step towards a healthy lifestyle. Additionally, avoiding refined carbohydrates (sucrose, fructose, refined wheat flour, etc.) help in lowering triacylglycerols in blood.
- The cholesterol-lowering effect of PUFAs and MUFAs has been attributed to their role in upregulating LDL receptors on cell membranes, thereby increasing catabolism of LDL, which is the main atherogenic lipoprotein.
- Lifestyle factors such as excessive emotional stress, smoking, high blood pressure, male sex, postmenopausal women, abdominal obesity and heart disease increase the risk of atherosclerosis.
- When diet and lifestyle changes fail, then hypolipidaemic drugs help in reducing serum cholesterol and TG levels. Statins (atorvastatin, simvastatin, fluvastatin, etc.) are a group of drugs that act on HMG-CoA reductase enzyme and competitively inhibit the enzyme and also upregulate LDL receptor activity, thus reducing blood cholesterol.
- Ezetimibe reduces blood cholesterol by inhibiting its intestinal absorption.
- Dietary fibre has a major role to play in decreasing intestinal absorption of cholesterol, other fats, glucose, toxins, and so on by binding to it. Inclusion of dietary fibre in the diet is highly recommended as it has multiple beneficial effects: it is helpful in maintaining normal blood cholesterol, triglyceride and glucose levels, and it decreases the incidence of colon carcinoma by absorbing toxins and other oxidants implicated in carcinogenesis.

3.12.7 Hypercholesterolaemias

Familial hypercholesterolemia

- autosomal dominant inheritance
- defect in LDL receptor gene, leading to inhibition of cellular cholesterol uptake and increased LDL-cholesterol
- very high risk of developing CAD and myocardial infarction (MI)
- xanthomas (cholesterol deposits in skin), xanthelasma (deposits around eye), chest pain
- genetic mutation on chromosome 19
- blood total cholesterol levels are more than 250 mg/dL in children or >300 mg/dL in adults
- treatment includes drugs like statins, which inhibit cholesterol synthesis. Clofibrate decreases cholesterol absorption from intestine and, in severe cases, LDL-apheresis is used

3.12.8 Disorders of Plasma Lipoproteins

Defects in lipoprotein synthesis, transport or breakdown can lead to inherited primary dyslipoproteinaemias. There can be either hypo- or hyperlipoproteinaemia.

Secondary dyslipoproteinemias

Dyslipoprotenemias are associated with DM, hypothyroidism, nephrotic syndrome and atherosclerosis. See Figure 36.4.

Lipoprotein chemistry

- Dietary fats absorbed from the intestine, and lipids synthesised in the liver and adipose tissue have to be transported among the tissues and organs for utilisation and storage. Lipids are insoluble in water, so they need a hydrophilic medium for transportation. This is accomplished by associating the nonpolar

Table 36.4 Secondary hypercholesterolaemia

Endocrine:
• Hypothyroidism • Hypopituitarism • DM
Metabolic:
• Gaucher's disease • Glycogen storage disease • Tay–Sachs disease • Niemann–Pick disease
Renal:
• Nephrotic syndrome • Haemolytic uraemic syndrome
Liver:
• Hepatitis • Cholestasis (intrahepatic cholestasis, congenital biliary atresia)
Medication:
• Androgens • Diuretics • Glucocorticoids • Immunosuppressive agents (cyclosporine, tacrolimus) • Oral contraceptives • Retinoids
Miscellaneous:
• Anorexia nervosa • Systemic lupus erythematosus • Idiopathic hypercalcaemia • Klinefelter

TGs and cholesteryl esters with amphipathic lipids like phospholipids, cholesterol and proteins to make water-miscible lipoproteins. Thus, lipids are transported in plasma as lipoproteins.

- There are four major classes of lipids; namely, TGs (16%), phospholipids (30%), cholesterol (14%), cholesteryl esters (36%) and a very small fraction of unesterified long-chain fatty acids: FFAs (4%). FFAs are metabolically the most active fraction of plasma lipids.
- There are four major groups of lipoproteins, depending on the content of fat and protein. Fat is lighter than water, hence the density of a lipoprotein decreases as proportion of fat or lipid to protein ratio increases. Based on the density, they are classified into four classes:
  1. Chylomicron
  2. VLDL
  3. LDL
  4. HDL

Liver and lipid metabolism

The liver facilitates digestion and absorption of lipids by production of bile, which contains cholesterol and bile salts. Bile salts are synthesised in the liver. The liver actively synthesises and oxidises fatty acids. It also synthesises TGs and phospholipids (PLs). During prolonged starvation, the liver synthesises ketone bodies from fatty acids (ketogenesis); hence, it plays a pivotal role in the synthesis and metabolism of lipoproteins.

Fatty liver

- Extensive accumulation of lipids, especially TGs in the liver leads to fatty liver. Nonalcoholic fatty liver disease is the most common liver disorder in the world. Chronic fatty liver can lead to the development of inflammatory and fibrotic changes causing nonalcoholic steatohepatitis, which can progress to liver cirrhosis, hepatocarcinoma and liver failure.
- Categories of fatty liver:
  1. Chronic elevation of plasma FFAs:
     - high-fat diet
     - uncontrolled DM
     - starvation
  2. Metabolic block in production of plasma lipoproteins:
     - block in apolipoprotein synthesis
     - block in lipoprotein synthesis from apoprotein and lipids
     - lack of PLs found in lipoproteins
     - failure in secretion of lipoproteins

Causes of fatty liver

- Chemicals such as puromycin (an antibiotic), carbon tetrachloride (CCl_4), ethionine and chloroform.
- Metals such as lead, phosphorus, arsenic and orotic acid.
- Deficiency of antioxidant vitamins such as E, B complex, selenium and essential fatty acids
- Ethanol is an important cause of fatty liver.
- Alcoholic fatty liver is the first stage in alcoholic liver disease. This may lead to cirrhosis.
- Fat accumulation is due to impaired fatty acid oxidation and increased lipogenesis (due to increased energy production during alcohol

metabolism). The enzymes involved are alcohol dehydrogenase and aldehyde dehydrogenase.

- Substances that can prevent the onset of fatty liver are known as lipotropic factors.
- Many hormones promote lipolysis in adipose tissue by activating hormone-sensitive lipase (HSL) and increasing release of FFAs into the circulation. These are epinephrine, norepinephrine, ACTH, melanocyte-stimulating hormone, thyroid stimulating hormone, growth hormone and vasopressin. Glucocorticoids and thyroid hormones act as facilitatory factors.
- Adipose tissue secretes hormones such as adiponectin, and leptin. Adiponectin modulates glucose and lipid metabolism in muscle and the liver, and leptin tends to suppress appetite in the face of sufficient food intake. Lack of leptin secretion may lead to uncontrolled food intake, causing obesity.
- Brown adipose tissue is involved in metabolism when heat generation is essential. This tissue is active in hibernating animals (during arousal from hibernation), in animals exposed to cold (nonshivering thermogenesis), and in newborn human babies. It is responsible for diet-induced thermogenesis, where ATPs are not synthesised, but energy is dissipated as heat (to maintain body temperature in newborns).

Pregnancy and lipid metabolism

- There is an increased body fat accumulation during early pregnancy. It is associated with both increased dietary intake and lipogenesis.
- During late pregnancy, there is an increased lipolysis in fat depots; the FFAs and glycerol being used for fetal development.
- Maternal glucose, FFAs, ketone bodies and glycerol (in small quantities) easily cross the placenta and are used by the fetus as fuels for oxidative metabolism and as lipogenic substrates.
- Maternal cholesterol is a major source of cholesterol for the fetus during early gestation, but as the fetus grows, fetal tissues develop a high capacity to synthesise cholesterol during late pregnancy.
- There is maternal hypertriglyceridaemia, accumulating in VLDL, LDL and HDL. TGs do not cross the placental barrier, and there is presence of lipoprotein receptors, LPL, PLA_2 and intracellular lipase activity in the placenta. These allow release of long-chain PUFAs (particularly docosahexaenoic acid – DHA, 22:6 omega-3) and essential fatty acids from maternal lipoproteins to the fetus for its development.
- During the first two trimesters, lipid metabolism is mostly anabolic (an increase in lipogenesis and fat storage) promoted by maternal hyperphagia and an increased insulin sensitivity. In addition, there is an increase in levels of progesterone, cortisol, leptin and prolactin, which contributes to increased fat storage.
- In the third trimester, lipid metabolism is in a net catabolic phase, mainly due to insulin resistance, causing an increase in lipid breakdown. Additionally, increase in human placental lactogen stimulates lipolysis in adipose tissue.
- Dyslipidaemia during pregnancy may lead to preeclampsia or gestational DM in the mother, and poses a high risk of developing atherosclerosis later in life for the fetus.

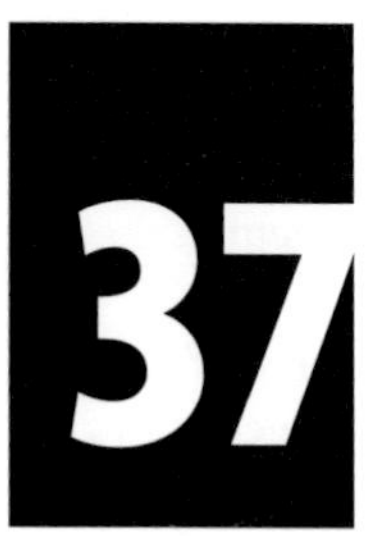

Enzymes and Signal Transduction

Neela Mukhopadhaya

1 Enzymes

- Enzymes are proteins that act as biological catalysts and accelerate chemical reactions in the body.
- Structure: the three-dimensional configuration of enzymes determines their activity and ability to act as catalysts. The three-dimensional structure is maintained by weak hydrogen bonds. Change of shape and loss of action is called denaturation (unfolding of the protein chains). This can happen when exposed to heat (50–60 degrees Fahrenheit). Organic solvents damage enzymes permanently. Change in pH can also denature enzymes. Enzymes contain proteins composed of amino acids, which are zwitterions and partially charged. A zwitterion is a molecule with functional groups, of which at least one has a positive and one has a negative electrical charge.
- Modes of action: enzymes act on substrates and change them into active substances, but remain unchanged themselves and do not get used up. They do not alter the equilibrium of reaction. The main mode of action is increasing the reaction rate by lowering the activation energy.

1.1 Function of an Enzyme

Enzymes serve a wide variety of functions. The main ones are as follows:

- Signal transduction and cell regulation, often via kinases and phosphatases.
- Movement of muscles: myosin hydrolyses ATP to generate muscle contraction.
- Transport of substances in the cell as part of the cytoskeleton. Other ATPases in the cell membrane are ion pumps involved in active transport.
- Viruses can also contain enzymes for infecting cells. Examples are HIV integrase and reverse transcriptase, or for viral release from cells, in influenza virus neuraminidase.
- Digestion: enzymes such as amylases and proteases break down large molecules (starch or proteins, respectively) into smaller molecules such as maltose and eventually glucose, which can then be absorbed. Different enzymes digest different food substances.

1.2 Enzyme Kinetics

- Enzyme kinetics involves the process of the enzyme binding to a substrate and converting this to the product. See Figure 37.1.
- Steps in enzyme action:
  1. Substrate binding: enzymes must bind their substrates before they can catalyse any chemical reaction. Enzymes are usually very specific and this then forms the enzyme substrate complex. Some enzymes are more specific than others. Examples of highly specific enzymes are DNA polymerase and RNA polymerase.
  2. Catalysis: the enzyme catalyses the reaction to lead to the release of the product and enzyme (remains unchanged).
- Enzyme saturation curve: the rate at which enzymes work depends on the solubility and concentration of the substrate. As the substrate concentration increases, the reaction rate increases too as more enzyme binds to the substrate. When the maximum reaction rate (V_{max}) is reached, all available enzyme is bound to all the substrate. The amount of substrate required to achieve a certain reaction rate is called Michaelis–Menten constant (K_m). Each enzyme has a characteristic (K_m) (see Figure 37.2).
- Enzyme catalysis: the enzyme binds to substrate to produce product.
- Enzyme inhibitors: there are five types of enzyme inhibition.

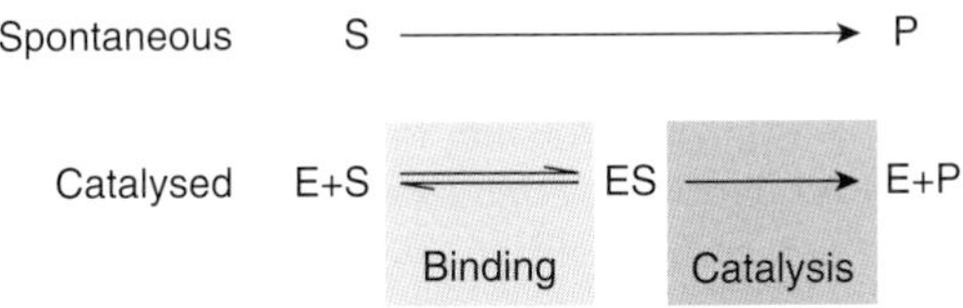

Figure 37.1 Enzyme substrate action.
E: enzyme; S: substrate; P: product

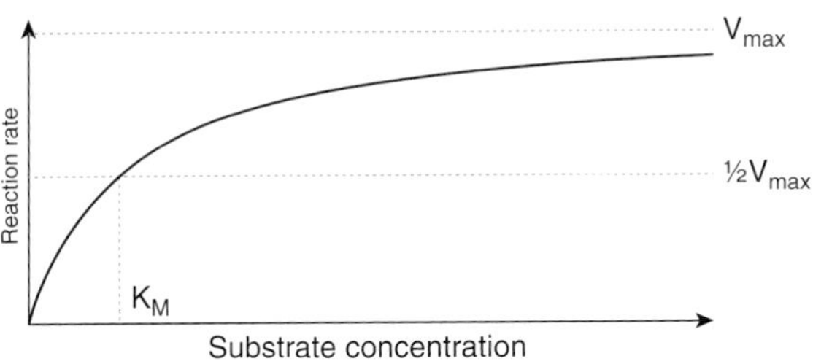

Figure 37.2 Enzyme kinetics.

1.3 Enzyme Inhibitors

1.3.1 Competitive Inhibitors

Competitive inhibitors strongly resemble the real substrate of the enzyme. They cannot bind to the enzyme at the same time. For example, the drug methotrexate is a competitive inhibitor of the enzyme dihydrofolate reductase, which catalyses the reduction of dihydrofolate to tetrahydrofolate. Other examples are statins used to treat hypercholesterolaemia and protease inhibitors used to treat retroviral infections such as HIV. This type of inhibition can be overcome with high substrate concentration.

1.3.2 Noncompetitive Inhibitors

A noncompetitive inhibitor binds to a different site to where the substrate binds. The substrate still binds with its usual affinity and hence K_m remains the same. However, the inhibitor reduces the catalytic efficiency of the enzyme so that V_{max} is reduced. While competitive inhibition can be overcome by increasing substrate concentration, noncompetitive inhibition cannot.

1.3.3 Uncompetitive Inhibitors

An uncompetitive inhibitor, contrary to the others, cannot bind to the free enzyme. It binds to the enzyme substrate complex only and is most effective at high substrate concentration. This kind of inhibition is rarely seen in humans.

1.3.4 Mixed Inhibitors

A mixed inhibitor binds to an allosteric site and the binding of the substrate and the inhibitor affect each other. The function of the enzyme is slowed down.

1.3.5 Irreversible Inhibitors

- An irreversible inhibitor permanently inactivates the enzyme, usually by forming a covalent bond to the protein of the enzyme. Some examples of drugs that work using this form of inhibition are penicillin and aspirin. Aspirin inhibits the cyclooxygenase (COX)-1 and COX-2 enzymes that produce the inflammation messenger prostaglandin. The poison cyanide is an irreversible enzyme inhibitor, which combines with the copper and iron in the active site of the enzyme cytochrome c oxidase and blocks cellular respiration.
- Inhibitors have an important role in humans where they act as part of a feedback mechanism. If an enzyme produces too much of one substance in the organism, that substance may act as an inhibitor for the enzyme at the beginning of the pathway that produces it, causing production of the substance to slow down or stop when there is sufficient amount. This is a form of negative feedback. An important example is the citric acid cycle.

1.4 Cofactors

- Some enzymes require additional nonprotein molecules to bind to in order to work fully. Cofactors are usually organic or inorganic compounds. Examples of inorganic cofactors are metal ions and iron-sulphur compounds. The cofactor acts by stabilising the active site. An example of an enzyme that contains a cofactor is carbonic anhydrase with a zinc cofactor bound as part of its active site.
- Organic cofactors can be either coenzymes, which are released from the enzyme's active site during the reaction (an example is flavin, and haem cofactors are often involved in redox reactions and biotin in enzymes such as pyruvate carboxylase).
- Coenzymes are small organic molecules, which can be loosely or tightly bound to an enzyme. Coenzymes transport chemical groups from one enzyme to another.
- Examples include:
    - NADH

- NADPH
- Adenosine triphosphate (ATP)

Some coenzymes are derived from vitamins. Examples are:

- flavin mononucleotide
- flavin adenine dinucleotide
- thiamine pyrophosphate
- tetrahydrofolate

- These coenzymes cannot be synthesised by the body *de novo*, and closely related compounds (vitamins) must be acquired from the diet. The chemical groups carried include:
  - the hydride ion (H^-), carried by NAD or $NADP^+$
  - the phosphate group, carried by adenosine triphosphate
  - the acetyl group, carried by coenzyme A
  - formyl, methenyl or methyl groups, carried by folic acid
  - the methyl group, carried by S-adenosylmethionine
- Contrary to enzymes, the structure of coenzymes is altered following an enzyme reaction; hence, they are considered a special class of substrates, or second substrates, which are common to many different enzymes. For example, about 1000 enzymes are known to use the coenzyme NADH.
- Coenzymes are usually continuously regenerated, and their concentrations maintained at a steady level inside the cell. For example, NADPH is regenerated through the pentose phosphate pathway and S-adenosylmethionine by methionine adenosyltransferase. This continuous regeneration means that small amounts of coenzymes can be used very intensively. For example, the human body turns over its own weight in ATP each day.

1.5 Role of Enzymes in Digestion

1.5.1 Protein

Stomach

- pepsinogen is secreted by the chief cells
- parietal (oxyntic) cells secrete hydrochloric acid
- the low pH causes hydrolysis of pepsinogen into pepsin
- pepsin is a specific enzyme, which acts on peptide bonds and hydrolyses them into amino acids, tryptophan, phenylalanine and tyrosine

Pancreas

- secretes three inactive precursors of protease enzymes: trypsinogen, carboxypeptidase and chymotrypsinogen
- secreted into the intestine via the pancreatic duct

Small intestine

- secretes enterokinase that converts trypsinogen to trypsin, which in turn activates carboxypeptidase and chymotrypsinogen
- chymotrypsinogen cleaves the bonds between amino acids and aromatic side chains
- trypsin cleaves next to lysine and arginine
- peptidases in small intestine cleaves the di- and tripeptides to single amino acids for absorption mainly in the duodenum and jejunum

Carbohydrate digestion

- salivary glands and the pancreas secrete amylases, which break starch into disaccharides (maltose and isomaltose)
- maltose, isomaltose, sucrose (composed of glucose and fructose) and lactose (composed of glucose and galactose) are broken down by respective enzymes (maltase, isomaltase, lactase and sucrase) secreted by mucosal villi into monosaccharides and transported in the blood
- transport of glucose and galactose is active and requires ATP; fructose is transferred passively

1.5.2 Fat Metabolism

- Mainly triglyceride (glycerol).
- Digestion starts in small intestine with the emulsification by bile salts.
- Bile is stored by the gall bladder after being produced in the liver and is released by the secretion of cholecystokinin.
- Cholecystokinin increases the surface area of the fat by creating droplets so that lipases (secreted by

pancreas) can act on the fat to form monoacylglycerols and fatty acids.

- Fat digestion is completed in the duodenum and jejunum.
- The epithelial cells in the intestine constitute the chylomicrons, which diffuse into the lacteals and into the lymphatic system.
- They finally enter the bloodstream when the thoracic duct flows into the left subclavian vein.
- Triglycerides and fatty acids can be released from tissue adipocytes when required and then they bind to albumin in the blood.

2 Signal transduction

Signal transduction is a process by which a chemical or physical signal is transmitted through the cell membrane, leading to a cellular response. There is phosphorylation of protein catalysed by protein kinase enzyme. At the molecular level, this means translation and transcription of genes and protein synthesis, which leads to cell modulation (cell growth, proliferation and metabolism).

2.1 External Reactions and Internal Reactions for Signal Transduction

- Signal transduction through membrane receptors takes place in four steps (see Figure 37.3):
  1. Primary messenger: an extracellular signalling molecule acts on the cell membrane of the target cell.
  2. Receptor protein: cells have cell surface receptor proteins, which bind to the primary messenger and cause phosphorylation of protein catalysed by protein kinase.
  3. Secondary messengers: these are signalling proteins, which help transmit the signal to the organelles of the cell leading to protein synthesis.
  4. Target proteins: the conformations or other properties of the target proteins are altered when a signalling reaction occurs, and this leads to the required action in the cell.
- There are three conformation states of acetylcholine receptor:
  1. Cell surface receptors: these are receptors that are embedded in the plasma membrane of the cell. There are different types of receptors in cells. They can be broadly divided into intracellular and extracellular.
  2. Extracellular receptors: these are integral transmembrane proteins and constitute the majority of receptors. They span the entire thickness of the cell membrane, one part is outside (this binds to the ligands or primary messengers) and the other inside (induces signalling pathways by causing enzyme activation, such as tyrosine kinase or phosphatase) or exposing binding sites for proteins, such as cyclic AMP (cAMP) or inositol phosphate 3 (IP_3).
  3. The cell membrane receptors can be further divided into two types: membrane and transmembrane receptors. They allow the signals from extracellular primary messengers to be conducted via the cell membrane to allow chemical change inside the cell. They are made of glycoproteins and lipoproteins. Membrane receptors are again divided by structure and function into three classes: the ion channel linked receptor, the enzyme-linked receptor and the G-protein-coupled receptor.
     - Ion channel linked receptors have ion channels for anions and cations, and are part of transmembrane proteins. They cause rapid signalling events usually found in electrically active cells such as neurons. They are also called ligand-gated ion channels. Opening and closing of ion channels is controlled by neurotransmitters.
     - Enzyme-linked receptors can be enzymes themselves, or can directly activate linked enzymes. Most of these are protein kinases.
     - G-protein-coupled receptors are very important integral membrane proteins, which possess seven transmembrane helices. These receptors activate a G-protein when the primary messenger binds to it, and the G-protein then triggers the intracellular signalling pathways.
- There are many receptors identified. Examples include:
  - adrenergic receptors
  - olfactory receptors
  - receptor tyrosine kinases

- epidermal growth factor receptors
- insulin receptors
- fibroblast growth factor receptors
- high-affinity neurotrophin receptors
- ephrin receptors
- integrins
- low-affinity nerve growth factor receptors
- N-methyl-D-aspartate (NMDA) receptors

- Tyrosine kinase receptor: this is a transmembrane protein with an extracellular domain, which binds ligands such as growth factors and insulin receptors. It causes phosphorylation (addition of a phosphate group) to tyrosine and this activates signal transduction, leading to release of intermediates (second messengers) and cell response. See Figure 37.4.
- Integrins: integrins are produced by many cells in the body. They help with attachment of cells (extracellular matrix) and in signal transduction from the extracellular matrix such as fibronectin and collagen. For example, fibronectin binds to integrin receptor and hyaluronan to CD44 receptor.
- Once the ligand or primary messenger binds to the integrin, change in cell conformation and signal transduction is activated. Integrins lack kinase activity; hence, integrin-mediated signal transduction is achieved through a variety of intracellular protein kinases and adaptor molecules such as integrin linked kinase. This then leads to apoptosis, proliferation and differentiation.
- Integrin signalling in circulating blood cells remains in an inactive state. When there is an inflammatory response, then the cell membrane integrins on leucocytes cause epithelial cell attachment. When activated in platelets, they produce thrombosis. Integrins on noncirculatory cells such as epithelial cells are in an active state and allow signal transduction for normal function of the cells.
- Ligand-gated ion channels: when a ligand binds to these receptors, these channels open, allowing transfer of ions, which relay signals such as that of a nerve synapse. Calcium ion is the commonest example of an ion that moves in and out of these channels. The other is sodium.
- Intracellular receptors: These are soluble proteins such as nuclear and cytoplasmic receptors. Lipophilic hormones (primary messengers) such as steroid hormones can pass through the plasma membrane by cell diffusion. They then bind to the nuclear receptor to cause alteration in gene expression.

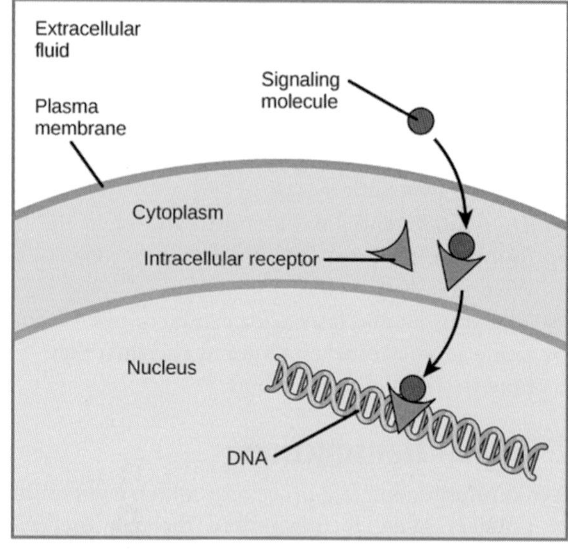

Figure 37.3 Action of signalling molecule on cell membrane receptors.

- The steroid receptors are a subtype of nuclear receptors that are free in the cytoplasm.
- The retinoic acid receptors are another subtype. They can be activated by retinol or prostaglandin. They are attached to the nuclear membrane.
- Messengers in signal transduction: there are two types of messengers – primary and secondary.

3 Primary Messengers or Ligands

The different types of chemical signalling are shown in Figure 37.5.

- Primary messengers, or ligands, are soluble molecules that bind to cell receptors. For example, the steroid hormones are derived from cholesterol and hence are lipid soluble. However, the majority of these substances will be transported in blood using a transport or binding molecules. A good example is sex hormone-binding globulin (SHBG) for estrogen and testosterone. Some examples of these substances include:
  - steroid hormones such as:
    - gonads: androgen, estrogen and progesterone

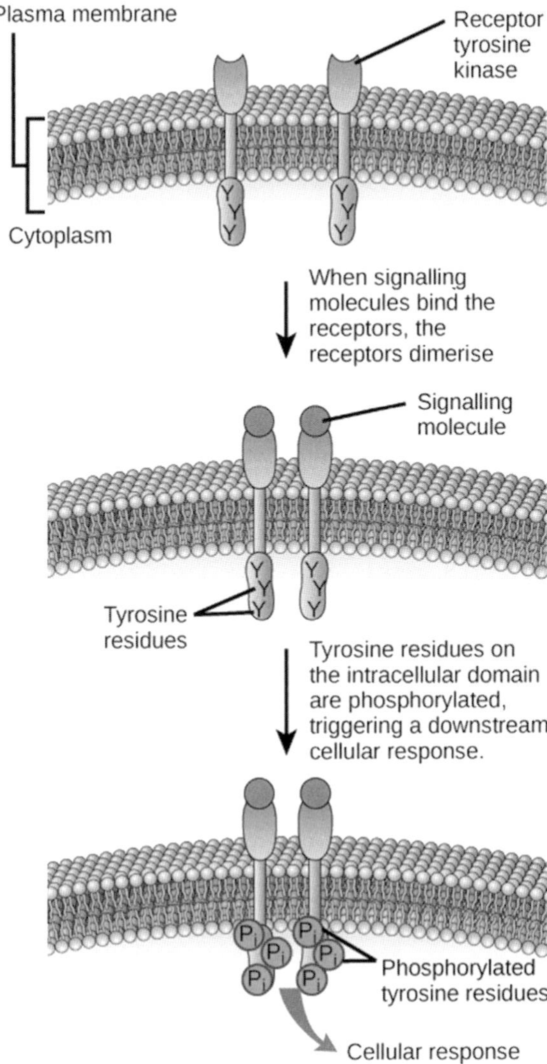

Figure 37.4 Signalling transduction.

  - adrenal cortex: aldosterone, cortisol and androgens
  - pregnancy: placental hormones like alkaline phosphatase (ALP)
- cytokines
- growth factors
- cell adhesion molecules
- nutrients
- neurotransmitters
- paracrine and autocrine agents
- fibronectin
- hyaluronan

- They reach the cell from extracellular fluid and bind to their specific receptors on the cell membrane.
- Secondary messengers: these are intermediary molecules such as nonlipid-soluble hormones. They cause change in cell activity and the benefit is the speed and amplification with which they act. The nonsteroid hormones are derived from proteins. No second messenger has been identified for insulin. The main examples are:
  - cAMP (main)
  - cyclic guanosine phosphate (cGMP)
  - inositol triphosphate
  - diacylglycerol
  - calcium

3.1 Cyclic AMP

- cAMP is the most important second messenger along with the calcium ion. It acts by activating the protein kinase A. It consists of four subunits: two catalytic and two regulatory.
- The cAMP-dependent pathway is necessary for all living organisms and life processes. This pathway is responsible for gene regulation and activation of enzymes. Many different essential cell responses are mediated by cAMP, such as:
  - increase in heart rate
  - cortisol secretion
  - breakdown of glycogen and fat
  - memory and brain function
  - relaxation in the heart muscles
  - water reabsorption in the kidney
- There are two main functions of cAMP: activation and deactivation of the cAMP pathways.

3.1.1 Activation

- Ligand binds to the receptor and exposes the G_s protein.
- Activated guanosine diphosphate (GPCR) causes the guanine nucleotide-binding (G_s) protein's affinity for guanosine diphosphate (GDP).
- Causes the alpha subunit to dissociate from the G_s complex, exposing the binding site for adenyl cyclase.
- Activated adenylyl cyclase converts ATP to cAMP.
- Molecules that activate cAMP pathway include:
  - cholera toxin: increases cAMP levels

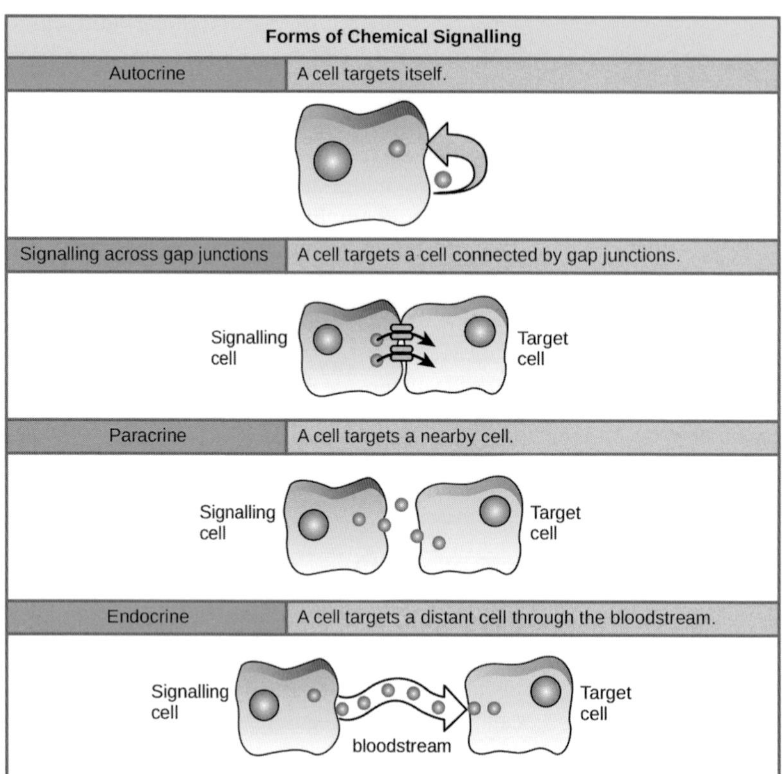

Figure 37.5 Chemical signalling. Used with permission from Lumen

- caffeine and theophylline inhibit cAMP phosphodiesterase, which degrades cAMP, thus enabling higher levels of cAMP than would otherwise be had
- clandestine (dibutyryl cAMP, dibutyryl (db) cAMP): also a phosphodiesterase inhibitor
- pertussis toxin: this increases cAMP levels by inhibiting Gi to its GDP (inactive) form; this leads to an increase in adenylyl cyclase activity, thereby increasing cAMP levels, which can lead to an increase in insulin and therefore hypoglycaemia

3.1.2 Deactivation

- The G_s alpha subunit slowly catalyses the hydrolysis of guanosine triphosphate (GTP) to GDP.
- This deactivates the G_s protein cAMP pathway shunts.
- The pathway may also be deactivated downstream by directly inhibiting inhibition of adenylyl cyclase or dephosphorylation of the proteins phosphorylated by phenylketonuria (PKU).
- Molecules that inhibit the cAMP pathway include:
  - cAMP phosphodiesterase converts cAMP into AMP by breaking the phosphodiester bond, in turn reducing the cAMP levels
  - G_1 protein, which is a G protein that inhibits adenylyl cyclase, reducing cAMP levels
- Calcium: calcium ions are released into the cytoplasm from the endoplasmic reticulum. It binds to signalling proteins and is then sequestrated by the smooth endoplasmic reticulum and the mitochondria:
  - intracellular 10^{-7} M; higher extracellular (10 $^{-3}$ M)
  - resting moles (Ca^{2+}) concentrations are kept low by the following:
    - — calcium-ATPases pump calcium out
    - — nerve and muscle cell has a pump, which couples sodium-ion (Na^{+}) influx to Ca^{2+} efflux
    - — mitochondria can pump Ca^{2+} inside
    - — calmodulin mediates Ca^{2+} regulated processes

   - calcium is used in many processes including muscle contraction, neurotransmitter release from nerve endings and cell migration

3.2 Nitric Oxide

- Nitric oxide (NO) is a free radical, which diffuses through the cell membrane and acts as a second messenger.
- It is produced from L-arginine by the enzyme NO synthase in the presence of cofactors and oxygen.
- It has a short half-life (5–10 s), converted to nitrates and nitrites.
- NO activates soluble guanylyl cyclase, which then activates cGMP.
- It is secreted by endothelial cells on blood vessels, diffuses into the muscle, reacts with iron on the enzyme guanylate cyclase → cGMP → muscle relaxation.
- It maintains blood pressure; vasodilatation in pregnancy is NO related.
- Reduced NO occurs in preeclampsia
- It regulates blood flow in the placenta; produced by the syncytiotrophoblast.
- cGMP acts by muscle relaxation in blood vessels and this lowers blood pressure. The action of NO is recognised in pregnancy, and lower levels are thought to be a factor in the pathogenesis of preeclampsia. The effect on blood vessels also explains the action of nitroglycerine in relaxing the blood vessels in the heart. Other functions of NO are apoptosis and penile erection.

3.3 Lipid Messengers

Some other lipid-based second messengers are diacylglycerol and ceramide. Diacylglycerol is activated by protein kinase C.

3.4 Redox Signalling

There are some more signal transducers similar to NO, which can activate some enzymes such as guanylate cyclase. Some examples are:

- carbon monoxide
- hydrogen peroxide
- hydrogen sulphide
- superoxide

3.5 Vascular Endothelial Growth Factor

- Vascular endothelial growth factor (VEGF) is a signal protein produced by cells that stimulates the formation of blood vessels.
- VEGF is a subfamily of growth factors; the platelet-derived growth factor family of cystine-knot growth factors. They are important signalling proteins involved in both vasculogenesis and angiogenesis.
- It is part of the system that restores the oxygen supply to tissues when blood circulation is inadequate such as in hypoxic conditions.
- Serum concentration of VEGF is high in bronchial asthma and diabetes mellitus.
- When VEGF is overexpressed, it can contribute to disease. Solid cancers cannot grow beyond a limited size without an adequate blood supply; cancers that can express VEGF are able to grow and metastasise. Overexpression of VEGF can cause vascular disease in the retina of the eye and other parts of the body. Drugs such as aflibercept, bevacizumab, ranibizumab and pegaptanib can inhibit VEGF and control or slow those diseases.

3.5.1 Types of VEGF Receptors

- VEGF family stimulate cellular responses by binding to tyrosine kinase receptors (the VEGFRs) on the cell surface, causing them to dimerise and become activated through transphosphorylation.
- VEGF-A is highly expressed in acute and subacute stages of central-nervous-system injury. VEGF-A has been implicated with poor prognosis in breast cancer. VEGF-A is also released in rheumatoid arthritis in response to tumour necrosis factor alpha (TNF-α), increasing endothelial angiogenesis permeability and swelling.
- In the kidney, increased expression of VEGF-A in glomeruli directly causes the glomerular hypertrophy that is associated with proteinuria.
- VEGF alterations can be predictive of early-onset preeclampsia.

4 Proteomics

- After genomics and transcriptomics, proteomics is the next step in the study of biological systems, especially proteins. It is more complicated than genomics because an organism's genome is more or less constant, whereas proteomes differ from cell to cell and from time to time. Distinct genes are expressed in different cell types, which means that even the basic set of proteins that are produced in a cell needs to be identified.

- In the past this phenomenon was assessed by RNA analysis, but it was found to lack correlation with protein content. Now it is known that mRNA is not always translated into protein and the amount of protein produced for a given amount of mRNA depends on the gene it is transcribed from and on the current physiological state of the cell. Proteomics confirms the presence of the protein and provides a direct measure of the quantity present.

4.1 Application of Proteomics

- The main application of proteomics is in identification of new drugs for the treatment of disease.
- Methods for studying proteins: the two main methods are by using antibodies (immunoassay) or not using antibodies (mass spectrometry).
- Protein detection with antibody can be of two types:
    - enzyme linked immunosorbent assay helps in the detection and quantification of proteins
    - western blot helps with the qualitative and quantitative assay of individual proteins and uses an initial step called SDG-PAGE (a variant of polyacrylamide gel electrophoresis, which uses sodium dodecyl sulphate).

4.2 Antibody Free Detection

- Mass spectrometry which uses high-resolution, two-dimensional electrophoresis and staining of differentially expressed proteins. This is the principle for the diagnosis of antibody free detection of recombinant proteins.

Section 7

Pathology

Nita Khurana and Mala Arora

Pathology of Clinical Sepsis

Varuna Mallya

Sepsis caused by infection is an amalgamation of biochemical, physiological and pathological abnormalities. In February 2016, the SEPSIS-3 group defined sepsis as organ dysfunction caused by dysregulated host response to infection. This is based on the quick sequential organ failure assessment score (quick SOFA score). It includes three criteria in which each is given a score of 1. See Table 38.1.

- A qSOFA score of greater than or equal to two is associated with an overall mortality of 10%.
- Septic shock is a subset of sepsis that is characterised by profound circulatory and cellular/metabolic abnormalities, which substantially increase mortality. These patients have persistent hypotension and require vasopressors to maintain mean arterial pressure (MAP) ≥65, lactate level of >2 mmol/L, despite volume resuscitation. These patients have a mortality of 40%. The term SIRS (systemic inflammatory response syndrome) is an old term, which includes two of the following:
  - respiratory rate >20/min
  - temperature >38 °C or <36 °C
  - white blood cell count >12 000 cells/mm^3 or <4000 cells/ mm^3, or more than 10% band forms
  - tachycardia >90 beats per minute (BPM)
- However, in pregnancy, these changes need to be differentiated from the normal physiological changes, which may produce mild tachycardia and leucocytosis.

1 Types of Sepsis

- during pregnancy, sepsis is termed as maternal sepsis, and can lead to chorioamnionitis
- postpartum/puerperal sepsis can occur within six weeks of delivery
- gynaecological infections of the genital tract can occur

Common predisposing factors:

- vaginal tampon usage: if the tampon is left in place too long, it may lead to toxic shock syndrome, which is caused by superantigens
- secondary to instrumentation like curettage, intrauterine contraceptive device (IUCD) insertion
- preexisting genital infections
- premature rupture of membranes
- retained products of conception
- postsurgical-like haematoma

Commonly implicated organisms include bacteria and viruses:

Bacterial

- Gram-positive bacteria such as group A streptococci; Staphylococcus; for example, *Staphylococcus aureus*: some Staphylococcus species may be methicillin resistant (methicillin-resistant *Staphylococcus aureus*: MRSA).
- Gram-negative bacteria such as *Escherichia coli*, klebsiella, proteus, *Haemophilus-Neisseria* and the enterococcus group.
- Some of these organisms may be beta-lactamase-producing organisms (also called extended spectrum beta-lactamase), which makes them resistant to commonly used beta-lactam antibiotics like penicillin, cephalosporins and carbapenem.
- Anaerobic organisms like *Chlamydia* are low virulence organisms, which are normally present in the vaginal microbiome. They are sensitive to metronidazole.

Viral

- Influenzae viruses, especially H1N1.

Table 38.1 Quick SOFA Score (qSOFA or Quick SOFA)

Assessment	qSOFA
Low blood pressure (SBP ≤100 mmHg)	1
High respiratory rate (≥22 breaths/min)	1
Altered mentation (GCS <15)	1

SBP: systolic blood pressure; GCS: Glasgow Coma Scale

1.1 Risk factors

- Risk factors include hyposplenism, cirrhosis, immune-compromised states like HIV, diabetes, alcoholism and extremes of age.
- Nonseptic sepsis may be seen in patients with severe acute pancreatitis or extensive burn injury.

2 Pathogenesis

2.1 Inflammatory mediators

- Receptors on neutrophils, monocytes and endothelial cells identify microbial products and are activated. This leads to release of tumour necrosis factor (TNF), various interleukins (IL-1, IL-12, IL-18), interferon gamma, reactive oxygen species, platelet-activating factor (PAF), high mobility group protein 1. These factors are all mediators of inflammation, which activate both the procoagulant and complement pathways.

2.2 Endothelial Cell Activation

- The proinflammatory cytokines and complement cascade cause endothelial cell activation. There is increased expression of tissue factor, coupled with reduced expression of anticoagulant factors such as tissue factor pathway inhibitor, thrombomodulin and protein C. Increased expression of plasminogen activator inhibitor 1 (PAI-1) prevents fibrinolysis. The effect of an increased level of procoagulants is magnified by the vascular stasis. This stasis also prevents removal of the coagulation factors. This eventually causes widespread microvascular thrombosis, leading to tissue hypoxia. In an attempt to maintain the ATP production in the absence of oxygen, the cells start anaerobic glycolysis, causing increased lactate levels, which decreases local pH.
- The haemorrhage, and increased vascular permeability, along with production of nitric oxide (NO) and vasoactive inflammatory mediators such as components of complement (C3a and C5a) and PAF results in oedema and vasodilatation and peripheral pooling of blood. This causes low intravascular volume with subsequent systemic hypoperfusion and hypotension, which we know is a criterion for sepsis according to SEPSIS-3.
- Metabolic abnormalities: there is gluconeogenesis attributable to stress and cytokine-induced release of glucagon, glucocorticoids and growth hormone. Insulin resistance occurs, along with reduced insulin release. Hyperglycaemia reduces neutrophil function, hence enhancing the detrimental effects. The effects are exaggerated in a diabetic patient.
- Immune suppression and systemic effects: anti-inflammatory mediators such as IL-10 and TNF receptor cause immunosuppression. TNF and IL-1 induce fever, leucocytosis, diminished myocardial contractibility and reduced cardiac output.
- Thus, microvascular thrombosis, increased vascular permeability, endothelial cell activation, hypotension and oedema lead to metabolic dysfunction, leading to multiple organ failure (multiple organ dysfunction syndrome).
- Lung: increased capillary permeability leads to oedema in both alveolar and interstitial compartments of the lung. Entrapped neutrophils lead to the release of cytokines, which cause acute lung injury and adult respiratory distress syndrome, characterised by inflammatory cell infiltrate, diffuse alveolar damage, hyperplasia of type 2 pneumocytes and hyaline membranes deposits along the alveolar ducts.
- GI tract: paralytic ileus occurs due to NO produced in septic shock, resulting in decreased uptake of nutrients and obstructive features: overgrowth of bacteria with aspiration into the lungs may lead to aspiration pneumonia. Impaired gut permeability may help the toxic products to spread into the systemic circulation.
- Liver dysfunction with elevated enzymes, decreased synthesis of proteins and coagulation factors, and decreased metabolism of toxins all contribute to the septic shock.
- Kidney: acute kidney injury can occur due to systemic hypotension, decreased intravascular

volume, direct toxic damage to kidney tubules and renal vasoconstriction. Glomeruli may show widespread fibrin thrombi if there is associated disseminated intravascular coagulation (DIC).

- Heart: interstitial oedema, myonecrosis and neutrophilic inflammation are evidence of myocarditis in cases of severe sepsis: these all contribute to decreased myocardial contractility and hypotension.
- Adrenals: extensive haemorrhagic necrosis (Waterhouse–Friderichsen syndrome) causes adrenal insufficiency and aggravates hypotension.
- Central nervous system: systemic hypotension with subsequent hypoperfusion to brain leads to encephalopathy. Meninges should be checked for inflammatory changes in case meningitis is the source of sepsis.
- Coagulopathy: subclinical coagulopathy with abnormal thrombin time and activated partial thromboplastin time are common in sepsis. In cases of septic shock, there may be DIC due to widespread endothelial cell activation and microthrombi formation with microangiopathic haemolytic anaemia, consumption of coagulation factors, thrombocytopenia and fibrin degradation products in the peripheral blood.
- Spleen: red pulp congestion with atrophy of white pulp and haemophagocytosis in the splenic macrophages.
- Bone marrow: may show myeloid hyperplasia and haemophagocytosis in the marrow macrophages.

In the puerperium, potential sites of sepsis should be specifically checked:

- Sites of surgical wound infection; for example, episiotomy/abdominal scar with evidence of necrotising fasciitis on the overlying skin.
- Postpartum endometritis with or without retained placental tissue.
- Vaginitis due to instrumentation.
- The breasts for evidence of mastitis
- Sites of local/regional anaesthesia.
- Urinary tract infection.
- Legs for evidence of deep vein thrombosis

Histopathology of Female Organs, Including Pituitary and Hypothalamus

Varuna Mallya

The interaction between the hypothalamus, pituitary and ovary (HPO axis) regulates the female reproductive system. The hypothalamus secretes the gonadotropin-releasing hormone (GnRH). This regulates the release of follicle stimulating hormone (FSH) and luteinising hormone (LH) from the gonadotroph cells in the anterior pituitary. These are released in pulses at an interval of one to four hours. They promote ovulation and stimulate the ovary to produce estrogen and progesterone.

Normal endometrium shows changes corresponding to the release of estrogen and progesterone from the ovary. The deep basal layer is nonresponsive, but is capable of regeneration following menstrual shedding. The superficial functionalis layer shows changes in both the glandular and stromal components. estrogens stimulate the endometrium to proliferate and the early phase, lasting from the fourth to seventh day, shows short narrow glands, compact stoma and few mitosis followed by a phase of increased mitosis, mild stromal oedema and columnar cell appearance in the mid-phase associated with progressive increase in the size of the ovarian follicle. The late proliferative phase from the tenth to fourteenth day shows abundant mitosis in endometrial glands and stroma and pseudostratification of the cells in the curving glands with simultaneous formation of the tertiary follicle in the ovary, which attains a large size up to 15–20 mm and progressively reaches the ovarian surface. Ovulation with release of ovum, atresia of the follicle and formation of corpus luteum in the ovary is associated with endometrial changes with subnuclear vacuoles in the glands on the sixteenth day and both sub- and supranuclear vacuoles by day 19. The mid secretory phase is characterised by tissue oedema and intraluminal secretions in the markedly tortuous glands with a saw-tooth appearance and, by day 23, the spiral arterioles can be easily seen with decidual stromal change around them the next day. Predecidualisation spreads to the rest of the endometrium, including the surface, in the next two days with the presence of polynuclear cells, haemorrhage and necrosis in the endometrium by day 27–28 (shedding of menstrual endometrium) in case the fertilised ovum is not received by the endometrium for implantation. In case there is implantation of the embryo, the endometrium exhibits gestational hyperplasia with simultaneous oedema, tortuous glands with large secretory columnar cells with vacuolated cytoplasm, intraluminal secretions and decidualisation. An exaggerated response is termed as the Arias-Stella reaction. In such cases, the ovary shows a large corpus luteum with bright yellow appearance and central cavitation: corpus luteum of pregnancy. The stratum basale, the surface-most layer and the endometrium in the lower uterine segment are not optimally responsive to the hormonal changes and so, in case the endometrial samples contain these fragments, they should not be considered for assignment of histological date. A correlation of chronological date and histological date is important to diagnose the luteal phase defect where there is more than two days' discrepancy between the chronological and histological date of the endometrium. The corpus luteum later involutes and forms corpus albicans, showing dense fibrosis.

- Exogenous hormone agents lead to hyperplastic features in case of only estrogen intake, while only progesterone therapy shows small tubular glands lined by cuboidal to flattened epithelium in an exaggerated decidualised stroma; also sometimes known as pill endometrium.
- Tamoxifen taken as hormonal therapy for breast carcinoma for its antiestrogenic action on hormone-receptor-positive tumour cells has a paradoxical pro-estrogenic effect on the endometrium and is associated with endometrial hyperplasia and, rarely, carcinoma on long-term use.
- Disorders of any of the organ in the HPO axis may result in a variety of diseases, which can present in different age groups.

1 Prepubertal and Pubertal Age Group

1.1 Delayed Puberty

Delayed puberty is the most common presentation and may be a cause of concern to the parents. Stimulation of the cyclic centre (medial preoptic area and medial eminence with arcuate nuclei) of the hypothalamus is crucial to switch on the reproductive function and lead to ovulation by secretion of GnRH and gonadotropins.

- Hypogonadotropic hypogonadism: occurs due to absent secretion of FSH and LH from pituitary, resulting in markedly decreased estrogen and progesterone levels. It could be isolated hypogonadotropic hypogonadism, also known as idiopathic or congenital hypogonadotropic hypogonadism, and may be due to defective development and migration of GnRH neurons (mutation of the KAL1 gene, as in Kallmann syndrome), defective GnRH secretion (mutation of the KISS1 gene) or resistance to GnRH action; all occurring at the level of the hypothalamus. In contrast, secondary hypogonadotropic hypogonadism arises due to pituitary adenoma, brain tumour, pituitary apoplexy, certain medications or trauma.
- Hypergonadotropic hypogonadism, also known as primary/gonadal hypogonadism, is due to the impaired response of the gonads to FSH and LH with normal blood levels of gonadotropins, indicating normal hypothalamus and pituitary function. It may be either congenital or acquired. The congenital causes include gonadal dysgenesis, as in Turner syndrome, and guanine nucleotide binding protein alpha stimulating (GNAS) gene mutation. Acquired causes are premature ovarian failure, ovarian torsion, infections, trauma, surgery and autoimmune oophoritis.

1.2 Precocious puberty

- Central gonadotropin dependent or true precocious puberty: arises from hypothalamic-pituitary-gonadal activation, causing progressive pubertal development, accelerated growth rate and advancing skeletal age. It can be idiopathic (90%) or caused by brain tumours, hydrocephalus, meningomyelocele, hypothalamic hamartoma (containing GnRH-secreting neurons), hypothyroidism (having both elevated TSH and gonadotropins). These patients have elevated serum FSH and LH levels.
- Peripheral/gonadotropin independent or pseudoprecocious puberty:
    - There is no activation of the hypothalamic-pituitary-gonadal axis. Causes include gonadal, extragonadal, adrenal or intra-gonadal sources of human chorionic gonadotropin (hCG) or exogenous hormone therapy. It could be one of the following:
        - isosexual or feminising:
            - McCune–Albright syndrome (this involves mutation in the GNAS gene, resulting in a G protein that causes constitutional activation of adenylate cyclase, leading to overproduction of hormones)
            - functional ovarian cysts
            - ovarian tumours: granulosa cell tumour, theca cell tumour, teratoma
            - exogenous estrogen administration or iatrogenic
        - heterosexual (masculinising)
            - congenital adrenal hyperplasia: 21-hydroxylase enzyme deficiency results in reduced synthesis of cortisol and aldosterone, leading to increased feedback secretion of adrenocorticotropic hormone (ACTH), causing adrenal hyperplasia and increased secretion of testosterone
            - adrenal tumours
            - ovarian tumours
            - exogenous androgen administration

2 Reproductive Age Group

- Polycystic ovarian syndrome: both the ovaries have a thick cortex with a dense fibrous capsule, multiple follicles; the theca interna layer is hyperplastic. Anovulatory cycles, obesity, hirsutism and insulin resistance are characteristic. Genetic factors, obesity and comorbidities result in increased pulsatile GnRH release by the hypothalamus. This causes high levels of LH and low levels of FSH by the pituitary, thus increasing the LH:FSH ratio. Low levels of FSH results in anovulatory cycles. High levels of LH causes theca lutein cells to produce androgens, which is eventually converted to estrogen. There is insulin resistance, which causes intraovarian androgen excess also contributing to arrest in follicle development. These patients are prone to develop endometrial hyperplasia and adenocarcinomas due to high levels of estrogen.

- Hypothalamic amenorrhea: decreased GnRH secretion affects the pulsatile release of FSH and LH, causing amenorrhea and anovulation. It is usually functional and is attributed to stress or malnutrition.
- Postpartum necrosis/Sheehan's syndrome: destruction of the anterior pituitary by infarction is mostly due to postpartum haemorrhage, leading to ischaemic shock.
- Postpartum thyroiditis: this develops due to an altered immune status. Postpartum, there is loss of placental immune suppression, hence activating intrathyroidal fetal immune cells. This results in a graft versus host reaction, activating the intrathyroidal autoreactive maternal T cells initiating the autoimmune process.

3 Postmenopausal Age Group

- Postmenopausal hyperandrogenism: the postmenopausal ovary is active, resulting in increased androgen and lower estrogen secretion. This is further enhanced by reduced sex hormone-binding globulin, increasing free androgen index. Insulin resistance and hyperinsulinemia enhances androgen secretion as insulin acts as a co-gonadotropin. This results in hyperandrogenism. The secondary causes of postmenopausal hyperandrogenism include androgen-secreting adrenal carcinomas and adenomas, granulosa cell tumours, Sertoli Leydig cell tumours and hilus cell tumours.

40 Placental Site Implantation

Varuna Mallya

The placenta is the organ that anchors the developing fetus to the uterine wall for providing nutrients and waste removal of the fetus. Normal placenta has a single chorionic plate and a fetal decidual portion. Under normal circumstances, it is implanted on the posterior wall in the upper part of the body of the uterus. On implantation of the blastocyst into the endometrium, the outer layer of the blastocyst forms the trophoblast. This trophoblastic layer differentiates into the outer syncytiotrophoblast layer and inner cytotrophoblastic layer. The cytotrophoblast is a cuboidal cell, which forms the syncytiotrophoblast, and the intermediate trophoblast. The syncytiotrophoblast is a multinucleated giant cell structure, which secretes human chorionic gonadotropin (hCG). The intermediate trophoblast anchors the placenta to the decidua and myometrium, replaces the spiral arteries of basal plate and helps establish the fetomaternal circulation.

1 Variants of Placental Morphology

- Single-lobed discoid: commonest.
- Bilobed discoid: there are two nearly equal sized lobes.
- Succenturiate lobe:
  - One or more accessory lobes connected to the main disc are called succenturiate lobes and predispose to haemorrhage and thromboemboli. It also predisposes to acute inflammation (chorioamnionitis) associated with premature rupture of membranes and ascending infection, leading to neonatal sepsis, stillbirth and perinatal mortality and morbidity.
- Circumvallate placenta: this has rolled placental edges with a smaller chorionic plate.
- Circummarginate: this is an uncommon variant. Chorionic membrane inserts inwards from the edge, but the edge is not thickened and there is no central depression.
- Placenta membranacea: this is a rare type and develops as a thin membranous structure occupying the entire periphery of the chorion.
- Placenta fenestrate: another rare variant where one or more areas of focal placental atrophy occurs with no villi and only chorionic membrane.

2 Morbidly Adherent Placenta

If placental villi are implanted without intervening decidua, this leads to firm adherence and is associated with severe postpartum haemorrhage. According to the extent of adherence, these may be termed as follows:

- Placenta accreta: partial absence of decidua with implantation on the superficial myometrial bundles. Detection by ultrasound in the first trimester has low sensitivity (41%), which increases in the second trimester (60%) and third trimester (83.5%). Typical ultrasound features are:
  - deficiency of retroplacental sonolucent zone
  - vascular lacunae
  - myometrial thinning
  - interruption of bladder line
- Placenta increta: when villi invade partial thickness of the myometrium. Placenta increta accounts for approximately 15–17% of all placenta abnormality cases.
- Placenta percreta: if the penetration is full thickness of the myometrium, this can be a reason for uterine rupture

Previous surgery, caesarean section, dilatation and curettage or uterine structural abnormalities are the predisposing causes. It may be associated with placenta praevia (implantation in the cervix or lower uterine segment).

3 Placental Location

- Placenta praevia: in this placental abnormality, the placenta overlies the internal cervical os of the uterus. In the third trimester and at term, abnormal bleeding can require caesarean delivery and can also lead to placental abruption. This condition occurs in approximately 1 in 200 to 250 pregnancies and risk factors include prior caesarean delivery, pregnancy termination, intrauterine surgery, smoking, multiple pregnancy, increasing parity and maternal age. Ultrasound screening during first and early second trimester includes placental localisation.
- Diagnosis is determined by abdominal and transvaginal ultrasound.
- Ultrasonic imaging techniques based on the location of the leading edge of the placenta in relation to the cervical os.
    - Grade I is a low-lying placenta
    - Grade II is a placenta that touches the edge of the cervical os
    - Grade III is a placenta that partially covers the cervix
    - Grade IV is a placenta that completely covers the cervix

4 Vasa Praevia

- Vasa praevia is a placental abnormality where the fetal vessels lie within the membranes overlying the internal cervical os. The diagnosis is by ultrasound and colour doppler in 98% of cases. Type II vasa praevia is defined as the condition where the fetal vessels are found crossing over the internal os connecting either a bilobed placenta or a succenturiate lobe with the main placental mass.
- Two main associations:
    - velamentous insertions (25–62%)
    - vessels crossing between lobes in succenturiate or bilobate placentas (33–75%)

5 Battledore Placenta

- Battledore placenta is a term describing a placenta where the umbilical cord is attached at the margin. Occurs 7–9% in singleton pregnancies and 24–33% in twin pregnancies and may affect placental function/fetal growth.

6 Molar Pregnancy

- Molar pregnancy is an abnormal placentation and generally caused by an abnormal fertilisation.

The World Health Organization (WHO) classifies the gestational trophoblastic diseases as follows:

- Molar lesions:
    - hydatidiform mole (complete/incomplete)
    - invasive mole
- Nonmolar lesions:
    - choriocarcinoma
    - diseases of implantation site intermediate trophoblast
        - exaggerated placental site
        - placental site trophoblastic tumour
    - diseases of chorionic type intermediate trophoblast
        - placental site nodule
        - epithelioid trophoblastic tumour

Hydatidiform mole

- Enlargement of chorionic villi occurs, accompanied by trophoblastic proliferation. Abnormal vasculogenesis is responsible for the swelling of villi.

Complete mole

- Develops from the fertilisation of an empty ovum by two haploid sperms (23,X) mostly showing a 46, XX karyotype. It is androgenic and diploid; that is, it is formed by dispermy. Grossly, placenta is grape-like due to the oedematous villi giving a snowstorm appearance on ultrasonogram. Microscopically, the villi show hydropic change (oedema), cisternal dilatation (accumulation of oedema fluid in the centre of the villi, leading to clear appearance and grape-like morphology), hypovascularity or avascularity and random and often circumferential prominent cyto- and syncytiotrophoblastic proliferation. No fetal parts or amnion is noted. Beta hCG levels are much higher than a normal pregnancy/partial mole.

Partial mole

- Triploid and diandric, formed by two sets of paternal chromosomes and a haploid maternal set. Mostly they are XXY, and could be XXX or XYY. Grossly, they show a mixture of oedematous and normal villi and may be accompanied by presence of fetal parts and amnion. The trophoblastic hyperplasia in partial mole is less as compared to complete mole. The villous stroma may show vessels containing nucleated red blood cells.

Invasive mole

- Characterised by large distended molar villi, and the trophoblastic cells are seen infiltrating the smooth muscles of the myometrium, grossly producing a haemorrhagic uterine lesion. May be the cause of persistent elevation of serum beta-hCG levels after evacuation. Presence of chorionic villi excludes the diagnosis of choriocarcinoma.

Choriocarcinoma

- Highly malignant tumour diagnosed after term pregnancy, miscarriage or hydatidiform mole. Grossly, the tumour is extensively haemorrhagic and necrotic, and lacks the chorionic villi. Microscopically, there is a biphasic appearance characterised by admixture of cytotrophoblastic and syncytiotrophoblast cells along with intermediate trophoblast. There is extensive necrosis, and no chorionic villi are noted. There is marked atypia with mitosis. Vascular invasion and distant metastases are common. The serum beta hCG levels are very high. On immunohistochemistry, the syncytiotrophoblast cells are strongly and diffusely beta hCG positive, the intermediate trophoblastic cells may show focal immunoreactivity for human placental lactogen (HPL).

Exaggerated placental site (EPP)/syncytial endometritis

- There is increase in implantation site trophoblastic cells infiltrating the endometrium and the myometrium. Can arise after miscarriage or normal pregnancy. As it resolves spontaneously, no treatment is required. Microscopically, intermediate site trophoblastic cells are seen invading the endometrium and myometrium. Many multinucleated forms are also seen. These trophoblastic cells are separated by hyaline, chorionic villi and decidual tissue. There is no necrosis or mitosis.

Placental site nodule

- Localised lesion, which may be detected incidentally in the reproductive age group. It is composed of sheets of intermediate trophoblast having a nodular and hyalinised appearance. It is surrounded by a rim of lymphocytes and decidualised cells. There is focal positivity of HPL or Mel-CAM (a cell adhesion molecule) supporting the intermediate trophoblast origin. A low proliferative Ki-67 index of <10% helps confirm the diagnosis.

Placental site trophoblastic tumour (PSTT)

- PSTT is a lesion arising from implantation-site trophoblastic cells, presenting with either amenorrhea or abnormal bleeding after a normal or molar pregnancy, or missed miscarriage. The beta hCG levels are low, but the HPL levels are increased. Grossly, the uterus is enlarged, with a tan-coloured mass having haemorrhage or necrosis in the uterine cavity and may invade the myometrium. Microscopically, single cell type of intermediate trophoblastic cells penetrate the myometrium. Cellular pleomorphism and atypia are noticeable, although villi are absent. There is deposition of fibrinoid material in the vessel walls, which these cells eventually invade.
- Both EPP and PSTT are positive for HPL and Mel-CAM, signifying the implantation site trophoblastic origin. However, the cell proliferation Ki-67 index is <1% in EPP, and >10% in PSTT.

Epithelioid trophoblastic tumour

- This is the neoplastic proliferation of intermediate trophoblast. It can be diagnosed after a miscarriage/termination or many years after a normal pregnancy. Seen in the uterus or cervix. There is elevation of beta hCG and HPL. The tumour is grossly nodular and brown with areas of haemorrhage and necrosis. Microscopically, nests and cords of intermediate trophoblast cells with large epithelial-like appearance and prominent anaplasia infiltrate the myometrium (squamous cell carcinoma is a microscopic differential diagnosis, hence its name). Necrosis and eosinophilic material are present in the centre of these nests and may show foci of calcification. Mitosis is usually present. The tumour cells are weakly positive for HPL and Mel-CAM, Ki-67 is >15%. Cyclin E is mostly positive.

Chorangiosis, chorangioma and chorangiomatosis

- Nontrophoblastic lesions characterised by placental hypervascularity.

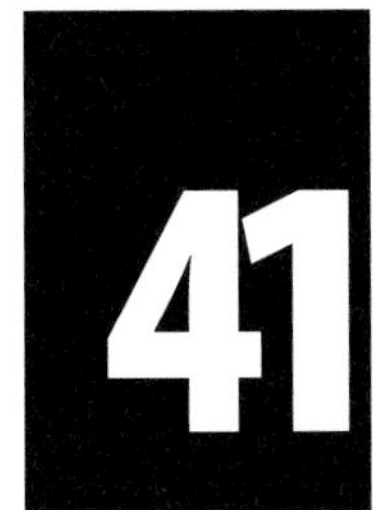

Teratogenesis

Varuna Mallya

The word 'teratogenesis' is derived from the Greek word 'tera', which means monster. Teratogenesis is the study of 'monster making'. Any factor, toxin, drug or chemical that can produce permanent abnormality in the structure and/or function, restriction of growth or death of the developing embryo or fetus is termed teratogen.

- Susceptibility of teratogenesis: the susceptibility of a fetus to a teratogenic agent is multifactorial and depends on the following:
  - The time of exposure to the teratogen. As the organogenesis takes place between the third and eighth week of gestation (the embryonic period), the susceptibility to cause abnormality is highest at this time. This is the time for differentiation, organisation and mobilisation. The first week of gestation is the resistant period and the period beyond the eighth week has a lowered susceptibility.
  - Genetic makeup of both the mother and fetus.
  - Dose of the toxin.
  - Duration of exposure.
  - Physical and chemical nature of the toxin.
  - Route of exposure and the ability of the toxin to cross the placenta.
  - The placenta is a great protective barrier and limits the entry of large-sized molecules and hydrophilic drugs. There is also presence of drug-metabolising enzymes in the placenta. However, it is not able to prevent the small molecules; those that bind the plasma proteins and lipophilic drugs and prevent them from entering the fetal circulation. Hence, over-the-counter prescriptions should be discouraged in pregnant women.
  - The screening of drugs and chemicals for the teratogenic potential involves the use of animal models and molecular studies to be able to produce safe drugs for use during pregnancy.
- The effect of teratogens may be:
  - immediate, resulting in death and spontaneous abortion
  - at the time of birth: functional defect or malformation
  - delayed, resulting in mutation and carcinogenesis
- The causes of teratogenesis include the following:
  - Genetic factors.
  - Known teratogenic drugs are thalidomide, androgens, progestins, tetracyclines, valproic acid, warfarin, retinoic acid, penicillamine, methotrexate, diethylstilbestrol, steroids, folic acid antagonists and alcohol.
  - Environmental toxins include radiation: lead, mercury and lithium poisoning.
  - Infections are teratogenic due to their ability to attach, penetrate and replicate in the cells; viral infections such as rubella, varicella, mumps, influenza and parvovirus may be the cause of abnormal fetal development. The gestational age at the time of infection is a major factor, which may be responsible for either early death and spontaneous abortion, or occurrence of a viable fetus with growth retardation, or functional or structural abnormalities.
  - Maternal conditions such as hyperthermia, where the body temperature is >38.9 °C exerts its teratogenic effect by being antimitotic. Obesity, diabetes, hypothyroidism, hyperthyroidism, hyperparathyroidism, iodine deficiency, phenylketonuria, myotonic dystrophy are other known associations.

1 Pathogenesis

A teratogen may exert its effect by one of the following mechanisms:

- Mutation: the nucleotide sequence of the DNA strand is altered in a mutation. If mutation occurs in the germ cells, it is heritable and termed a germinal mutation. If it involves the somatic cells, it is termed a somatic mutation.
- Chromosomal aberration: mostly results in spontaneous miscarriages as they are incompatible with life. These result from nondisjunction or loss or translocation of chromatids.
- Alteration of synthesis and function of nucleic acids is the mechanism seen mostly with exposure to the drugs, whereby they interfere with the expression of genetic information.
- Interference with the mitotic process: reduced DNA biosynthesis, disruption of formation of microtubules or formation and separation of chromatids could lead to interference with the mitotic activity.
- Decrease in the supply of precursors, substrates or coenzymes of the DNA synthesis such as folate deficiency.
- Enzyme inhibition: this interferes with metabolic pathways. Classically seen with dihydrofolate reductase enzyme, which is inhibited by drugs such as pyrimethamine and trimethoprim administration.
- Defective membrane transport: this changes the microenvironment and alters the transport of drugs and chemicals across cell membranes, hence predisposing the fetus to abnormal development.

2 Effects of Certain Common Teratogens

- Alcohol: causes fetal alcohol syndrome, whereby there is prenatal and postnatal growth retardation, facial anomalies and central nervous system dysfunction. The enzyme alcohol dehydrogenase converts alcohol to acetaldehyde, which is then converted by acetaldehyde dehydrogenase to acetone. In case of genetic polymorphisms in acetaldehyde dehydrogenase, which is associated with decreased activity of the enzyme, there is a decrease in the rate of conversion and high levels of acetaldehyde, which causes reduced DNA synthesis.
- Thalidomide: this is an immunomodulatory antiemetic drug classically known to cause phocomelia, in which there is shortened, or absent, long bones of limbs, anorectal stenosis and absence of external ears. Thalidomide intercalates into DNA at the guanine binding site, interfering with the production of integrin beta subunit 3, necessary for limb development. It also inhibits angiogenesis.
- Drugs that interfere with the metabolism of folic acid like hydantoin, carbamazepine, valproic acid and phenobarbital are associated with the occurrence of neural tube defects, cleft lip, cleft palate and cardiac defects in the fetus.
- Lead: poisoning leads to miscarriages and fetal growth restriction.
- Organic mercury: maternal exposure to mercury is associated with fetal neurological damage, blindness and deafness.
- Diabetes mellitus: maternal diabetes mellitus is associated with an increased risk of fetal cardiac, renal, gastrointestinal, neural and skeletal abnormalities.
- Phenylketonuria: mental disability, microcephaly and low birthweight are more often seen.
- Rubella: can cause congenital rubella syndrome in which there are neural, vascular, ocular and ear defects, along with fetal growth restriction.
- Syphilis: may result in spontaneous miscarriages or congenital infection, which may manifest in the fetus with hepatosplenomegaly, joint swelling, skin rashes, anaemia, jaundice, metaphyseal dystrophy, syphilitic rhinitis and periostitis.

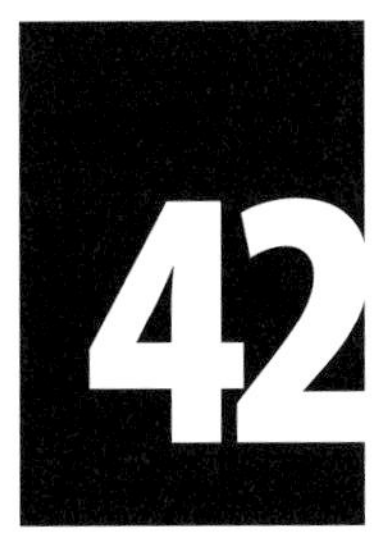

Pathological Conditions Related to the Uterus, Tubes and Ovaries

Varuna Mallya

1 Uterus

1.1 Endometritis

Acute endometritis is usually seen postpartum or post-termination due to retained placental tissue or instrumentation. It shows severe neutrophilic infiltrate with microabscess formation in the endometrial glands and stroma. Chronic endometritis occurs as part of pelvic inflammatory disease and is characterised by plasma cell presence in the endometrial tissue. Granulomatous inflammation can be seen in sarcoidosis (noncaseating granulomas), tuberculosis (caseating granulomas with acid-fast bacillus (AFB) positivity). Xanthogranulomatous endometritis is characterised by foamy histiocytes, giant cells and plasma cells, and is seen in elderly women with pyometra and cervical stenosis. In patients with an intrauterine contraceptive device, actinomyces may be the causative agent.

1.2 Endometriosis

The presence of functional endometrial tissue outside the uterus. The commonest site is the ovary followed by the uterine ligament, rectovaginal septum and pelvic peritoneum. Microscopically, it should contain two of the following: endometrial glands, stroma or evidence of haemorrhage in the form of haemosiderin laden macrophages. Malignant transformation is most commonly seen in the ovarian endometriosis. Retrograde menstruation, coelomic metaplasia of the lining epithelium and müllerian remnants are the probable theories for its origin.

1.3 Adenomyosis

This is the presence of endometrial glands and stroma (basal type) in the myometrium, at a distance of one low power field from the endomyometrial junction. It causes globular enlargement of the uterus. It is graded according to the depth of penetration (Molitor's criteria):

- grade 1: involving inner one-third of myometrium
- grade 2: involving middle one-third of myometrium
- grade 3: involving outer one-third of myometrium
- stromal adenomyosis (incomplete adenomyosis), characterised by presence of endometrial stroma and no glands

1.4 Endometrial Polyp

Polypoidal structure composed of irregularly spaced tubular or angulated endometrial glands with compact cellular stroma showing dispersed thick-walled vessels, and the surface shows endometrial lining on three sides. Common in the fundus, and in patients with unopposed estrogen levels or on tamoxifen therapy. Can show hyperplasia or harbour a focus of malignancy, the most common being serous carcinoma (especially in the stalk of the polyp). Could be functional, hyperplastic or neoplastic. Atypical polypoid adenomyoma is characterised by polypoidal growth with complex endometrial histology and atypia surrounded by smooth muscle and fibrotic stoma.

1.5 Endometrial Hyperplasia

Defined as increased proliferation of endometrial glands with increased gland to stroma ratio. It develops due to unopposed estrogen stimulation, polycystic ovarian syndrome, obesity, metabolic syndrome, hormone replacement therapy, estrogen or androgen-producing tumour. The World Health Organization revised classification divides endometrial hyperplasia into two groups based on the atypia:

- hyperplasia without atypia (showing a low level of somatic mutations)
- atypical hyperplasia/endometrioid intraepithelial neoplasia (harbours mutations seen in

endometrioid endometrial cancers such as in proto-oncogenes K-RAS, PTEN, and beta-catenin mutations, microsatellite instability and PAX-2 transcription factor inactivation)

1.6 Myometrium

1.6.1 Leiomyoma

Tumour of smooth muscle origin, seen arising in the myometrium. It is benign, well circumscribed and unencapsulated, in a submucosal, subserosal or intramural location. Microscopically composed of whorls and fascicles of smooth muscle cells with thin-walled vessels. Mitosis is less than 5 per 10 high power field (HPF). The smooth muscle origin is confirmed by immunohistochemistry as cells are positive for smooth muscle antibody (SMA), actin and caldesmon. Secondary changes include hyalinisation, myxoid change, mucoid degeneration, red degeneration (with pregnancy), calcification and infarction.

1.6.2 Malignant Leiomyosarcomas

Malignant leiomyosarcomas have two of the following features: mitosis >10/10 HPF, diffuse moderate-to-severe atypia and coagulative necrosis.

1.6.3 Smooth Muscle Tumour of Uncertain Malignant Potential

Those which cannot be categorised as definitely benign or malignant are classified as smooth muscle tumour of uncertain malignant potential (STUMP).

1.6.4 Disseminated Peritoneal Leiomyomatosis

Multiple tiny nodules of smooth muscle cells seen studding the peritoneum, measuring less than 2 cm. Symplasmic leiomyoma shows prominent atypia with bizarre cells, but lacks mitosis and necrosis. Cellular leiomyoma shows dense proliferation of smooth muscle bundles, but no atypia or necrosis.

1.6.5 Benign Metastasising Leiomyoma

Uterine leiomyoma associated with deposits of smooth muscle in lymph nodes, lungs and other organs. No evidence of atypia or mitosis.

1.6.6 Parasitic Leiomyoma

A uterine serosal leiomyoma, which gets detached from the uterus and is found only in the pelvis.

1.6.7 Intravascular Leiomyoma

Fragments of benign smooth muscle cells extending into vascular spaces.

2 Cervix

2.1 Nabothian Cyst

Seen in the cervix due to the obstruction of cervical crypts by squamous lining epithelium. The crypts are dilated, lined by flattened mucin-secreting epithelium and contain mucous. Obstruction results in acute and chronic inflammation of the cervix.

2.2 Papillary Endocervicitis

A form of chronic cervicitis with a predominant papillary architecture.

2.3 Squamous Papilloma

A polypoidal lesion composed of a fibrovascular core lined by stratified squamous epithelium showing hyperkeratosis, papillomatosis and acanthosis. Not associated with human papillomavirus.

2.4 Condyloma Acuminata

Associated with human papilloma virus (HPV) 6 and 11; it may involve the cervix.

3 Fallopian Tube

3.1 Acute Salpingitis

Infection of the fallopian tube; may progress to chronic salpingitis, and form a tubo-ovarian abscess. Caused by Neisseria, Chlamydia, Mycoplasma and *Mycobacterium tuberculosis*.

3.2 Salpingitis Isthmica Nodosa

Nodules smaller than 2 cm, seen in the tubal isthmus, composed of glands lined by tubal epithelium surrounded by hyperplastic smooth muscle cells. Chronic salpingitis, pelvic inflammatory disease, tubal ligation, tubal stricture, pelvic surgery, abnormal tubal motility predispose to ectopic pregnancy. The ampulla is the most common site. Rupture and shock are the associated complications. The rupture site shows chorionic villi and decidual change, while the endometrium shows Arias-Stella reaction.

3.3 Walthard Cell Nests

These are transitional or urothelial cell nests found on the serosal aspect of fallopian tube, mesosalpinx or mesovarium.

3.4 Paratubal Cysts

These are of müllerian origin, composed of a single layer of ciliated tubal epithelium.

3.5 Adenomatoid Tumour

This is the most common benign tumour occurring in the para-adnexal region, is of mesothelial origin, and is characterised by immunoreactivity to calretinin. Well circumscribed, usually <2 cm and is composed of gland-like spaces and cysts lined by cuboidal to flattened cells.

4 Ovary

4.1 Inflammatory

Oophoritis is either secondary to infection or of autoimmune origin.

4.2 Nonneoplastic Cysts

These are either functional or pathological.

4.2.1 Functional

- Follicular cysts may be >2 cm, and are lined by theca cells, which at times may be luteinised.
- Luteal cysts: these are lined by luteinised granulosa cells.

4.2.2 Pathological

- Chocolate cyst: endometriosis of the ovary; it is proposed to be caused either due to retrograde menstruation or metaplasia of lining cells. It is associated with elevated CA125 levels. The ovary is enlarged, thick-walled and contains brown fluid. Two out of the following three need to be identified histologically for confirmed diagnosis: endometrial glands, endometrial stroma and haemosiderin-laden macrophages (which is evidence of chronic haemorrhage).
- Atypia to be looked for as atypical endometriosis is a precursor for clear cell or endometrioid ovarian carcinoma.

4.3 Pathological Structures in Ovarian Tumours

- Schiller–Duval bodies → Yolk sac or germ-cell tumour
- Call–Exner bodies → Granulosa cell tumour
- Reinke's crystals → Leydig cell tumours
- Rokitansky nodule → Dermoid or mature teratoma
- Coffee bean nuclei → Mesonephroid tumours
- Psammoma bodies → Papillary serous adenoma
- Hobnail cells → Clear cell carcinoma

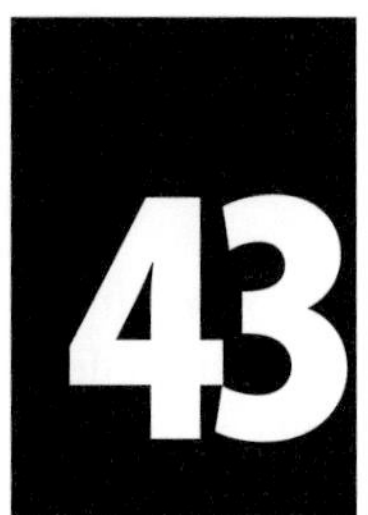

Gynaecological Cancers

Varuna Mallya

1 Tumours of the Uterine Corpus

Uterine corpus malignancies mostly arise from the endometrial glands, endometrial stroma and myometrium.

1.1 Endometrial Tumours

- Endometrial carcinoma (EC): presents as abnormal uterine bleeding, mostly in women above the age of 50 years old. Incidence (of endometrioid type of EC) is increasing due to obesity, increased life expectancy and treatment of breast cancer patients with tamoxifen. Most cases are sporadic. Women who develop inherited cancers usually house genetic mutations. It is extremely important that a proper family history is taken in these patients as genetics plays a pivotal role in their development. It is categorised into two types due to different risk factors: molecular pathogenesis and histologic features. See Table 43.1.
- The World Health Organization (WHO) classifies endometrial tumours into the following:
  - endometrioid adenocarcinoma
    - villoglandular
    - secretary
    - ciliated cell
  - serous
  - clear cell
  - mucinous
  - squamous
  - mixed type
  - undifferentiated
- Annual screening with transvaginal sonography (TVS) and endometrial biopsy is recommended by the British Gynaecological Cancer Society for high risk category women and their first-degree relatives. There is no recommendation to do endometrial biopsy in women with no genetic predisposition as a part of mass screening for early diagnosis of EC.
- The staging depends on the depth of myometrial invasion, involvement of either or both endocervical glandular or cervical stromal invasion and pelvic and extrapelvic extension.
- Gross morphologic types include papillary, polypoidal and ulcero-infiltrative.
- Tumour grade depends on the amount of combination of glandular and solid, morular or squamous component. Grade 1 is predominantly glandular with <5% solid areas. Grade 2 is with 6–50% solid areas, and tumours with >50% solid sheets of cells is grade 3 with an aggressive clinical course.
- The Cancer Genome Atlas Classification is a molecular classification:
  - copy number high: involving mutations of p53; includes serous carcinomas and high-grade endometrioid carcinomas
  - copy number low: involves mutations of phosphatase and tensin homolog (PTEN) protein and KRAS gene; includes low-grade endometrioid adenocarcinomas
  - microsatellite instability hypermutated (in these women, immunohistochemistry (IHC) based detection of mismatch repair genes or polymerase chain reaction (PCR)-based detection of microsatellite instability should be done)
- POLE: ultramutated type, seen in endometrioid type and associated with the best prognosis. Involve mutations in the exonuclease domain of DNA polymerase epsilon.
- Adenosarcoma: seen mostly in postmenopausal women, and may be associated with tamoxifen therapy. Composed of cytologically benign glands, surrounded by hypercellular stroma condensed around the gland with features of malignancy-like

Table 43.1 Characteristics of type 1 and type 2 endometrial carcinomas

Type 1 (80%)	Type 2 (20%)
• Grade I/ II, well-differentiated type • Seen in younger age groups • Includes endometrioid histological subtype • Low-grade tumours amenable to surgical resection, progesterone responsive and a better prognosis • estrogen dependent and increased risk in hyperestrogenic states like polycystic ovarian syndrome, obesity, late menopause, infertility and hormone replacement therapy • Associated with the following genetic mutations: loss of PTEN (a tumour suppressor gene located on 10q23; loss of this gene is an early event in tumour progression), RASi activation (activation of K-RAS, an oncogene associated with progression to EC) and microsatellite instability (seen in patients of Lynch syndrome or hereditary nonpolyposis colorectal cancer syndromes, an autosomal dominant defect characterised by defective DNA mismatch repair; also increases chances of colon and ovarian cancer)	• Grade III, poorly differentiated type • Seen in older age groups, usually includes clinically aggressive papillary serous and clear cell types • High-grade tumours: poor prognosis • estrogen independent • Multiparous, smokers and those treated with tamoxifen • Seen in atrophic endometrium • Associated with p53 (loss of p53, a tumour suppressor gene, is a late event in tumour progression and is mostly identified in clear cell histological subtype), HER2 neu (an oncogene that encodes tyrosine kinase and is involved in cell signalling; its overexpression is detected in serous cancers), E-cadherin mutations

anaplasia, hyperchromasia, mitosis and necrosis in the stromal spindle cell compartment only. An aggressive tumour with recurrences and haematologic spread, and metastasis is composed of sarcomatous component.

- Malignant mixed müllerian tumour: also known as carcinosarcoma, it is seen in postmenopausal women, most of them presenting at an advanced stage and older age. The lesion appears heterogenous with fleshy, haemorrhagic and necrotic areas: microscopically, both the glands (carcinomatous) and the stroma (sarcomatous) are malignant. The sarcomatous component may show homologous spindle cell cytologic appearance (leiomyosarcoma, fibrosarcoma, stromal sarcoma) or may show heterologous components like cartilage, bone, skeletal muscle or lipomatous (chondrosarcoma, rhabdomyosarcoma, osteosarcoma, liposarcoma) differentiation. The stromal component expresses epithelial membrane antigen and keratin on immunohistochemistry with mesenchymal markers of different differentiation, highlighting the homologous or heterologous components. A highly aggressive tumour with early dissemination and a poor prognosis.
- Endometrial stromal tumours:
  - May be benign (endometrial stromal nodule) or malignant (low grade, high grade). Composed of short spindled cells resembling compact endometrial stroma in the proliferative phase of the endometrium.
  - Endometrial stromal nodule (ESN) composed of localised proliferation of endometrial stromal cells; a circumscribed lesion with pushing margins, but not encapsulated, with no myometrial infiltration. Lacks lymphovascular invasion and necrosis. Mitosis less than 10/10 HPF.
- Endometrial stromal sarcoma:
  - Low grade: composed of oval cells in compact sheets with a prominent curvilinear vasculature. Shows tongue-like invasion into the myometrium, along with characteristic and prominent lymphovascular invasion (hence, also known as endolymphatic stromal myosis). It has extensive invasive capabilities despite low-grade histological features, but metastatic potential is low. The mitosis is less than 15/10 HPF. These can be differentiated from smooth muscle tumours as they express CD10 and lack smooth muscle actin on immunohistochemistry.
  - High-grade/undifferentiated endometrial stromal sarcoma: mitosis is more than 15/10 HPF, with marked atypia, pleomorphism, lymphovascular and extrauterine invasion and metastasis.
- The latest WHO 2014 classification takes into account translocations, particularly JAZF1-SUZ12 fusion, which is seen in ESN and low-grade endometrial stromal sarcoma. YWHAE-FAM22 translocation is noted in high-grade endometrial stromal sarcomas.
- Leiomyosarcoma occurs as *de-novo* rare sarcoma of the uterus, which presents as a rapidly growing fleshy mass, infiltrating and invading the uterine cavity in elderly women. This is characterised by at least two of three histologic features: high mitosis >10/10 HPF, coagulative tumour necrosis and marked atypia. The tumour has complex chromosomal aberrations and spreads though vascular dissemination, and the prognosis is poor. Tumours which do not fulfil the criteria of malignancy and which cannot be histologically characterised as benign are called STUMP: smooth muscle tumour of uncertain malignant potential.
- Other uterine sarcoma include rhabdomyosarcoma, with skeletal muscle differentiation (DESMIN, mYOD1 and myogenin reactive); perivascular epithelioid cell tumour (have myomelanocytic differentiation; SMA and HMB45 positive); sarcoma as component of mixed müllerian tumour (adenosarcoma, with benign epithelial component and carcinosarcoma, with malignant epithelial and mesenchymal component); and endometrial stromal sarcoma, low grade, high grade or undifferentiated.

2 Tumours of the Ovary

- Ovarian cancer is a heterogenous disease. Most hereditary ovarian tumours are associated with the breast cancer susceptibility gene BRCA1 and BRCA2 mutations. Sporadic high-grade serous carcinomas are associated with serous tubal intraepithelial carcinoma (STIC) and show similar molecular alterations in p53, p16. STICs progress to high grade serous carcinoma (HGSC), and show marked atypia, necrosis and a mitotic count of more than 12 per 10 HPF. HGSCs are positive on immunohistochemistry for p53, CK7, WT 1 and PAX 8; negative for CK20, CDX2 and CEA. It is proposed that extraovarian müllerian epithelium of the endometrium or fallopian tube is transformed and seeded on the ovary. Ovarian microenvironment promotes neoplastic transformation and propagation. Nulliparity, early menarche, late menopause and first childbirth after 35 years of age are other risk factors. It is important that details of family history and hormonal therapy are asked for. HGSC cases require BRCA testing as those that turn positive go into longer remissions and also require testing of their family members.

Based on the cell of origin, ovarian tumours are classified as follows:

2.1 Surface Epithelial

These are classified further as benign, borderline and malignant. The borderline or the atypical proliferative lesions show stratification, atypia and pleomorphism, but no invasion into the underlying ovarian stroma. The malignant tumours show invasion.

- Serous: lined by cuboidal cells with differentiation resembling fallopian tube lining.
- Mucinous: lined by mucin-secreting cells with differentiation resembling endocervical lining, classified as intestinal type (with goblet cells) or endocervical type. Mucinous carcinoma is associated with KRAS mutation.
- Seromucinous: show combination of both serous and mucinous differentiation.
- Endometrioid: microscopically, resembles endometrioid adenocarcinoma, often with squamous differentiation. May be associated with endometriosis/arise in the focus of adenomyosis or endometriosis, or with synchronous endometrial carcinoma, and is associated with beta-catenin/PTEN mutations.
- Clear cell: composed of cells with abundant clear to vacuolated cytoplasm and glandular arrangement such as in the secretory phase of the endometrium. Carry PIK3CA mutations. May be associated with endometriosis, hypercalcaemia or venous thromboembolism. Show WT1, p53 or Napsin A mutation.
- Transitional cell: Brenner: a type of ovarian tumour in which the epithelial component resembles the transitional epithelium.

All the above may be benign, borderline or malignant.

2.2 Germ-Cell Tumours

Seen in the younger age group. Elevated tumour markers; could be pure (single type or mixed).

- Dysgerminoma: large, solid, composed of nests of uniform cell population, separated by fibrous septa with extensive lymphocytic infiltrate. It occurs in young girls and adolescents. It is the ovarian counterpart of testicular seminoma, spreads to paraaortic lymph nodes and is radiosensitive. Placental type alkaline phosphatase (PLAP) and OCT3/4 are positive.
- Teratoma: the tumour shows differentiation towards all three germ layers. Could be solid/cystic and mature/immature/monodermal/teratoma with malignant transformation. Benign tumours with predominant ectodermal differentiation are called dermoid cysts. Those with immature tissues are graded from 1 to 3, depending on the amount of primitive neuroepithelium. The most common malignant transformation in a mature teratoma is squamous cell carcinoma. Monodermal teratoma with predominant thyroid tissue is called struma ovarii and the ones with carcinoid elements are called stromal carcinoids.
- Yolk sac tumour: has the characteristic Schiller–Duval body resembling mesodermal cores. Occurs in young girls, with elevated serum alpha fetoprotein (AFP) levels, which is secreted by the tumour cells.
- Choriocarcinoma: composed of cyto- and syncytiotrophoblast with extensive haemorrhage and necrosis. Rare in the ovary and has elevated beta hCG levels, which serve as a tumour marker.

2.3 Sex Cord Stromal Tumours

- May be functional (hormone secreting) or nonfunctional.
- estrogen-producing tumours are either granulosa cell tumours, adult type show Call–Exner bodies, theca cell tumours, androgen-producing tumours

such as Sertoli, Leydig cell tumours, hilar cell tumours.

- Fibroma: may be associated with ascites and pleural effusion: Meigs syndrome.
- Gynandroblastoma: composed of equal numbers of granulosa theca and Sertoli and Leydig cell tumours
- Gonadoblastoma: mixture of germ cell and sex cord stromal tumour: associated with gonadal dysgenesis and ataxia telangiectasia.
- Metastatic: most are bilateral, solid, multinodular. The endometrium, appendix, stomach, colon and breast are common primary sites. Modes of spread include haematogenous, transcoelomic, and direct and lymphatic routes.

3 Carcinoma of the Fallopian Tube

Primary fallopian tube malignancies are rare.

- arises from endosalpinx
- the uterus and ovary should be free from the tumour
- if the uterus and ovaries are involved in a primary fallopian tube malignant tumour, then the deposit should be similar to its fallopian tube counterpart
- presents in the sixth decade
- symptoms are vaginal bleeding and adnexal mass
- associated with BRCA1 and BRCA2 mutations
- histologically most common type is serous, followed by endometrioid and transitional

4 Carcinoma of the Cervix

Cervical cancers are classified as:

- epithelial (most common type; among these the most common subtype is squamous cell carcinoma and its variants followed by adenocarcinoma)
- mesenchymal
- mixed epithelial and mesenchymal
- melanocytic
- germ cell
- lymphoid/myeloid
- secondary

4.1 Squamous Cell Carcinoma (SCC)

A tumour characterised by squamous differentiation. The histology may be keratinising or nonkeratinising types and cell size can be large cell or small cell type.

- Most common type of cervical cancer, arises in sixth decade.
- More than 90% show association with human papillomavirus (HPV) (p53 and Rb genes play a role in tumorigenesis). HPV acts via E6 and E7 genes, which remain in episomes in condylomas while being integrated into the DNA in cases of high-risk strains, leading to preinvasive and invasive lesions. p16 immunoreactivity is considered as immunohistochemical surrogate marker for HPV if molecular testing is not available.
- HPV has multiple strains: these are high risk and low risk HPV strains.
- Low risk HPV 6 and 11 are associated with condyloma acuminatum, which are large exophytic papillary masses lined by hyperplastic epithelium with maintained maturation but show koilocytosis (raisin-like nuclear morphology, perinuclear clearing and peripheral condensation of the cytoplasm) indicative of HPV infection.
- High-risk HPV 16, 18, 31, 33 and other strains.
- HIV/human T cell lymphotropic virus 1 (HTLV-1) also implicated.
- Risk factors are multiple sexual partners, early age of first intercourse, multiparity, poor genital hygiene, other associated genital infections, cigarette smoking and non-circumcised male partner.
- Both squamous and adenocarcinoma may be preceded by preinvasive lesions making smear screening a good modality for early diagnosis.
- Histologically can be well, moderately or poorly differentiated.
- Immunohistochemically, tumour cells are positive for CK, CEA, p63 and progesterone. Histological variants include clear cell variant, glycogen rich, pseudoglandular, osteoclast giant cell rich, lymphoepithelial, basaloid and others.
- Prognostic factors other than clinical stage include lymphovascular invasion, neural infiltration, depth of invasion and parametrial involvement.

4.2 Adenocarcinoma

- Second most common cervical cancer, usually preceded by in situ lesions.
- Graded as well, moderately and poorly differentiated.
- A pattern-based classification system used: Silva system. This takes into account the pattern of stromal invasion (has prognostic significance):

  - Pattern A – Well demarcated glands, no destruction
  - Pattern B – Localized destruction of stroma
  - Pattern C – Diffuse destruction of stroma
- On immunohistochemistry, tumour cells positive for CK7, CEA and negative for ER, PR and p63.
- The cervical adenocarcinoma may be HPV related and has many histological variants: tubulopapillary, clear cell, mucinous, endometrioid, and so on. It needs to be differentiated from endometrioid carcinoma of endometrium extending to cervix using mucin stains and immunohistochemistry with vimentin, ER and PR and negative p16.
- Metastatic colorectal carcinoma should be excluded by careful physical examination and IHC reactivity with CK20 and CDX2.
- Mesonephric remnants and microglandular hyperplasia are benign mimics of adenocarcinoma cervix, which are potential diagnostic pitfalls.

5 Carcinoma of Vagina

5.1 Squamous Cell Carcinoma

Most common subtype; arises independent of cervix and vulva. Arises in sixth decade, with upper half of vagina being the commonest site. A strong association with HPV is noted. These tumours are positive for p16 on immunohistochemistry. It may be preceded by pre-invasive lesion (vaginal intraepithelial neoplasia; VAIN).

5.2 Adenocarcinoma

Could be associated with in utero exposure to diethylstilbestrol (DES) exposure type or could be non-DES type.

5.3 Clear Cell Adenocarcinoma

Has a bimodal age distribution with the peak in the third decade being DES type and the one in the fifth decade being non-DES type. It is a very aggressive tumour composed of clear cells and classic hobnail histology. These need to be differentiated from mesonephric adenocarcinoma, yolk sac tumour of vagina, extension of cervical adenocarcinoma, metastatic renal cell carcinoma and mucinous adenocarcinoma.

6 Carcinoma of Vulva

- vulval carcinomas are rare
- labia majora is the most common site
- mostly occurs after sixth decade
- most common type is squamous cell carcinoma
- vulval carcinomas have a strong association with HPV, similar to vaginal and cervical carcinoma, and considered to be a field effect of same carcinogen
- rare forms include adenocarcinoma, basal cell carcinoma, melanoma, Paget's disease of vulva

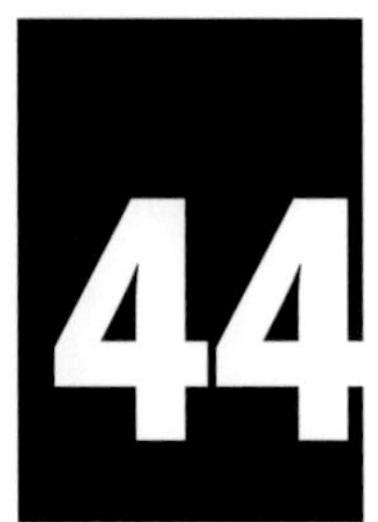

Pathophysiology of Pain

Varuna Mallya

- Pain is derived from the Latin word 'Poena', which means punishment from God.
- Pain could be acute or chronic.
  - Acute pain: defined as a normal time-limited response to a noxious experience. It is protective in nature, lasts less than three months and resolves on healing. It is the predicted physiological response to an adverse chemical, thermal or mechanical stimulus. It could be either visceral or somatic.
  - Chronic pain: persists beyond the normal tissue healing time, which is three months. It has no protective role to play and results in the degradation of health and body functions. Acute pain may become chronic. It occurs due to hyperactivity of the neurons owing to increased transmitters, increased responsiveness of the synaptic receptors and loss of inhibitory interneurons involved in pain modulation.
- Pain can be one of the following:
  - Nociceptive pain: related to damage of the somatic or visceral tissue. It arises due to trauma and inflammation of muscles, joint or skin, leading to localised nature of somatic pain. Hollow organs and smooth muscle are examples of visceral pain. Mediators of inflammation such as interleukins IL-1 and IL-6, and bradykinin are attributed to pain.
  - Neuropathic pain: arises from damage to the central or peripheral nerves, and is associated with features of numbness, tingling or hypersensitivity, like in diabetes mellitus, postamputation phantom limb pain and postherpetic neuralgia.
  - Sensory hypersensitivity: mostly arises from persistent neuronal dysregulation.

1 Pathophysiology

- The free nerve endings located in the skin, connective tissue, muscle and bone with cell bodies in the dorsal root ganglia are known as nociceptors. Inflammatory mediators such as serotonin, bradykinin, prostaglandins and cytokines released from the damaged tissues can stimulate the nociceptors.
- The first-order neurons are either A-delta type or polymodal-C type, which pick up the sharp and stinging or diffuse pain respectively.
- The first-order neurons synapse with the second-order neurons in the dorsal horn and release neuropeptides or amino acids. Glutamate and substance P play a role. These are either the nociceptive-specific or wide dynamic range type.
- The axons of both these types of neurons interact with the dorsal column medial lemniscus and the anterior lateral spinothalamic tract to synapse with the third-order neurons in the contralateral thalamus, transmitting signals to the somatosensory cortex, which is perceived as pain.
- A large area of the brain is activated during the pain experience; this is known as the pain matrix.
- The inhibition of pain transmission takes place via the descending inhibition.
- Descending inhibition: the periaqueductal grey in the midbrain and rostral ventromedial medulla are involved in descending inhibitory modulation. These contain high concentration of opioid receptors and endogenous opioids. They project to the dorsal horn, inhibiting pain transmission. Serotonin and noradrenaline are utilised in these pathways.

2 Pathophysiology of Labour Pain

- Labour pain is both visceral and somatic in nature. Although severe in nature, it is known to have a short memory.

- The first-stage pain is visceral and is due to dilatation of the cervix and distention of the lower uterine segment. It is dull, not localised, and is transmitted through small unmyelinated 'c' nerve fibres.
- The somatic component of the pain in the late first stage and second stage of labour is associated with distention of the perineal floor muscles and vagina, it is sharp and localised in character and is transmitted by fine type 'A' myelinated nerve fibres.
- Pain during menstruation or dysmenorrhoea may be primary (not attributable to any pelvic pathology), which has been attributed to increased myometrial contractility and decreased myometrial blood flow. Increase in prostaglandin F2-alpha stimulates muscle contractions and vasoconstriction, and it is thought that leukotrienes increase sensitivity of pain fibres.
- Secondary dysmenorrhoea can occur with adenomyosis, endometriosis, pelvic inflammatory disease or other pelvic pathology. Therefore, a complete workup is necessary in all cases of non-steroidal anti-inflammatory refractory dysmenorrhoea.
- Pelvic pain with high-grade fever and abnormal vaginal discharge indicates inflammatory pathology.
- Persistent nociceptive stimulation has been proposed to cause pain in endometriosis. Neuronal growth factors like neurotrophins and their receptors are overexpressed and subsequently an increased release of inflammatory cytokines and hyperinnervation leads to pain. There is nerve sprouting and increased vascularity (neuroangiogenesis) due to increased levels of interleukins and vascular endothelial growth factor secreted by the inflammatory cells, which are thought to be the cause of local and peritoneal inflammation, and associated pelvic pain.

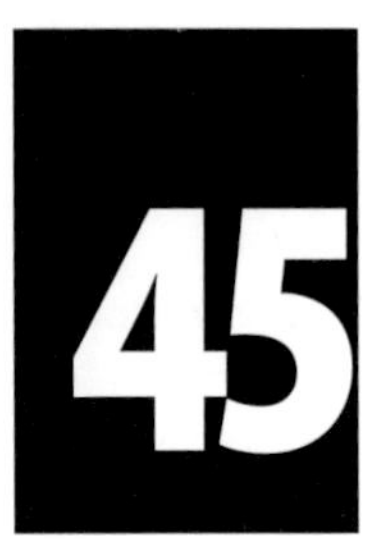

Pathology of the Bladder, Urethra and Vagina

Varuna Mallya

1 Bladder

1.1 Nonneoplastic

- Cystitis: acute bladder inflammation is usually caused by coliforms and is associated with infections of the urethra and vagina. Communication with the gut predisposes to anaerobic bacterial infection. Granulomatous inflammation is seen with *Mycobacterium tuberculosis* in association with renal tuberculosis and in patients with bladder carcinoma who have received Bacillus Calmette-Guerin (BCG) immunotherapy. *Schistosomia hematobium*-associated inflammation predisposes to squamous cell carcinoma (SCC) of the bladder. Interstitial cystitis, commonly seen in middle-aged women, is characterised by tiny pinpoint haemorrhages on the bladder wall. The associated painful bladder syndrome is poorly understood and variably attributed to autoimmunity, unidentified allergies, unidentified infectious agents, increased cytotoxicity to cationic metabolites, defective surface epithelial layer function, role of mast cells and genetic predisposition, among others. Emphysematous cystitis is associated with immune-compromised states, uncontrolled diabetes and neurogenic bladder, and shows gas-filled cysts. Classic haemorrhagic cystitis is a side effect of cyclophosphamide therapy.
- Malacoplakia: believed to be due to defective phagolysosomal function of the macrophages, leading to accumulation of histiocytes with intracellular round Michaelis–Gutmann bodies composed of iron and calcium with undigested bacterial glycolipids.

1.2 Neoplastic

- Bladder tumours are broadly classified (World Health Organization classification of urothelial tumours 2016) as urothelial tumours, squamous cell neoplasms, glandular neoplasms, urachal carcinomas, müllerian carcinomas, neuroendocrine tumours, melanocytic tumours, mesenchymal tumours, urothelial tract haematopoietic and lymphoid tumours, and miscellaneous tumours.
- The urothelial tumours are the most common and are further classified as noninvasive and invasive tumours. Noninvasive are further typed as papillary or flat based on morphology. The flat variant is high grade and is termed as carcinoma in situ. Papillary tumours include dysplasia, papillomas, papillary urothelial neoplasms of low malignant potential and low-grade and high-grade noninvasive papillary urothelial carcinoma. These types are based on the cytological and architectural features.
- Urothelial carcinoma is the most common type of bladder tumour, seen in the sixth to seventh decade, with a male preponderance. It can be multifocal and metachronous, and presents with haematuria. Cigarette smoking and exposure to arsenic and petroleum products are risk factors. Schistosomiasis, bladder diverticula, bladder calculus, indwelling longstanding catheters and bladder exstrophy predispose to SCC. Recurrent mutations of TP53, FGR3 and TERT genes are most common in bladder cancer, with FGR3 mutations seen in 80% of noninvasive low-grade papillary urothelial neoplasms. Histologic variants of invasive urothelial carcinoma include nested variant, microcystic, micropapillary, lymphoepithelioma-like and those with divergent differentiation. The most important prognostic feature is invasion into the muscularis muscle. Urothelial carcinomas are positive for CK7 and CK20.

2 Diseases of the Urethra

- Urethritis, commonly due to bacterial infection, presents with painful micturition. It could be a part of Reiter's syndrome (urethritis, conjunctivitis, arthritis).
- Urethral syndrome, characterised by sterile culture, dysuria and frequency, may be due to urethral stenosis, inflammation of paraurethral glands, hypersensitivity, traumatic coitus or reaction to gels, condoms or soaps.
- Urethral diverticula: commonly seen in women, secondary to infection, calculi or trauma. Lined by urothelium; may show squamous metaplasia/ carcinoma.
- Polypoid urethritis, leiomyoma and nephrogenic adenomas are other benign lesions seen in the urethra.
- Urethral carcinoma: primary tumours are more common in women. Classified as urothelial neoplasms, the most common is the urothelial type (seen in the proximal two-thirds). SCC is seen in the distal one-third. Adenocarcinoma may arise along the entire urethra. The most common risk factor is urethral irritation, secondary to stones, instrumentation or strictures. Urothelial carcinomas on immunohistochemistry (IHC) are positive for p53 and CK20.
- Clear cell carcinoma of urethra, commonly seen in women, arises in the diverticula.
- Melanoma: the urethra is the most common site of urinary tract melanoma. It presents as a pigmented polypoid mass in the distal urethra.

3 Diseases of the Vagina

3.1 Nonneoplastic Lesions

- Bacterial vaginosis is due to overgrowth of bacterial flora and shows presence of clue cells.
- Emphysematous vaginitis: shows multiple gas-filled cysts surrounded by multinucleated cells. It occurs in postpubertal women and is seen secondary to gardnerella or trichomonas infection.
- Vaginal adenosis: mostly seen after in utero exposure to diethylstilbestrol (DES), this drug stops the replacement of müllerian columnar epithelium by urogenital squamous epithelium. Grossly characterised by multiple cysts or reddish areas. Histologically, both DES and non-DES adenosis are characterised by the presence of müllerian epithelium in the vagina.
- Gartner cyst: a mesonephric cyst, located on the lateral or anterolateral wall, lined by cuboidal nonmucin-secreting epithelium.
- Mucous cyst: uniocular, lined by mucin secreting cells. It can be located anywhere in the vagina.

3.2 Neoplastic

- Stromal polyp: pedunculated; seen on the lateral walls of the lower one-third of the vagina. Microscopically, it is characterised by dense fibrovascular stroma, lined by squamous epithelium. Pleomorphic cells may be seen in the fibrovascular core, but do not exhibit mitosis.
- Vaginal rhabdomyoma sarcoma botryoides: commonly seen in middle-aged women. Nonencapsulated, composed of large spindle cells with enlarged nuclei, but no atypia. Cells with cross striations may be noted and are indicative of skeletal muscle differentiation.
- Angiomyofibroblastoma: more common in the vulva. It occurs as a submucosal, spongy, polypoidal, circumscribed, but unencapsulated, pink-to-yellow-coloured mass. It can attain a size up to 10 cm. It is most commonly seen after the fourth decade. It is characterised by hypo- and hypercellular areas, and prominent blood vessels. The stromal cells are ovoid to short spindled and swirl around the blood vessels, yet atypia and mitosis are not significant. The tumour cells are positive for estrogen and progesterone receptors.
- Aggressive angiomyxoma: commonly seen in the third and fourth decades. It measures up to 10 cm. It is characterised by spindle-shaped and stellate mesenchymal cells in a loose myxoid stroma and collagen bundles, thin-walled blood vessels and extravasated red cells. No necrosis or mitosis is seen, but it is prone to recurrences due to incomplete removal.
- Vaginal intraepithelial neoplasia (VAIN): seen in upper one-third of vagina. It is associated with human papillomavirus (HPV). It is common in postmenopausal women. It is graded as VAIN I, II or III based on whether the extent of dysplasia involves lower one-third, lower two-thirds or the entire thickness of the vaginal epithelium, respectively. It can progress to invasive SCC.

- SCC: the most common tumour of the vagina. It is commonly seen in postmenopausal women. It involves the upper one-third of the vagina, and is associated with HPV. It can present with associated cervical and vulval SCCs. It is grossly exophytic or ulcerative. Histologically, it may be keratinising or nonkeratinising.

  Other forms include the following:
- Verrucous carcinoma: well-differentiated SCC with pushing margins.
- Adenocarcinoma: can be the intestinal type, enteric type or mesonephric type.
- Clear cell adenocarcinoma: can be associated with in utero exposure to DES.
- Melanoma: usually pigmented. Composed of epithelioid and/or spindle cells, which are HMB-45 and S100 positive. Cells are highly pleomorphic and have prominent macronucleoli.
- Embryonal rhabdomyosarcoma: commonly seen in young girls under 5 years of age. It is characterised by a polypoidal, friable, grape-like mass occupying the vaginal cavity, arising from the anterior vaginal wall. Histologically, the malignant tumour shows skeletal muscle differentiation with spindle to oval cells concentrated just beneath the surface lining, (Nicholson's cambium layer) and extending into the deeper tissues. The cells show atypia and mitosis, and are positive for the markers of muscle differentiation: desmin, myogenin and MYOD1.

Section 8

Clinical Management and Data Interpretation

Neela Mukhopadhaya

This section addresses some of the clinical questions that are asked in the examination. You may be advised to refer to the Royal College of Obstetricians and Gynaecologists (RCOG) Green-top Guidelines to read the detailed clinical guidelines for some of the topics.

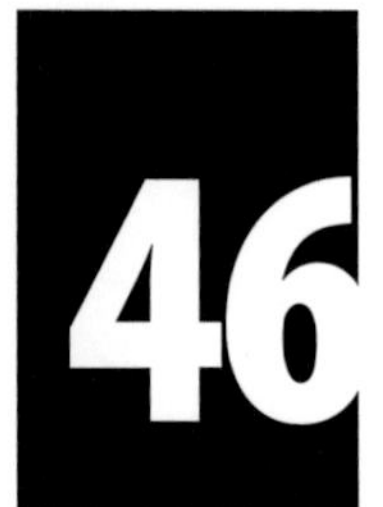

History and Physical Examination

Neela Mukhopadhaya

Introduce yourself to the patient/couple (name and designation) and explain what you are going to do. Follow a systematic approach and use a chronological order of events.

- personal information
- current problem
- history of current problem
- menstrual history
- past obstetric history
- past gynaecological history
- sexual history
- medical history
- surgical history
- family history
- social history
- drug and allergies history
- micturition and bowel

1 History

Always think:

- Is this patient pregnant or at risk of pregnancy?
- Every woman you see (10–60 years old) should be considered pregnant (or potentially so) until proved otherwise: then you will not miss one!

Personal information

- name, date of birth, age
- marital status
- occupation
- partner's details and occupation (relevant in infertility patients)

Current problem

- description of the problem
- severity, duration, periodicity (related to periods)
- aggravating and relieving factors
- use of any medication for the symptoms
- any treatment received in the past

Gravidity and parity

- gravidity: all previous pregnancies, regardless of gestation or outcome
- parity: number of pregnancies ≥24 weeks, regardless of outcome

2 Menstrual History

2.1 Date of First Day of Last Normal Period (LNMP)

- menarche/menopause as appropriate
- menstrual pattern

$$K = \frac{\text{Days of bleeding}}{\text{Length of cycle (day 1 of bleed to day 1 of the ne}}$$

- amount and character of bleeding; for example, flooding, clots
- any intermenstrual (IMB) or postcoital bleeding (PCB)
- any associated pain (dysmenorrhoea)
- use of contraception and details

3 Past Obstetric History

All pregnancies must be recorded, including miscarriages, ectopic pregnancies, termination of pregnancies (TOPs), molar pregnancies and successful pregnancies. Outcomes, gestation and mode of delivery, intrapartum or postpartum complications, children alive

Table 46.1 Summary of obstetric history

Pregnancy	Gestation	Outcome	Complications	Neonatal
1	6	Complete m/c	nil	
2	39	SVD	PPH 1000 ml	Male 4 kg A+W
3	40	Em LSCS	Fetal distress	Female 3.9 kg A+W
4	7	Ectopic preg	Right salpingectomy	
5	9	TOP	nil	

m/c: miscarriage; SVD: spontaneous vaginal delivery; PPH: postpartum haemorrhage; A+W: alive and well; Em LSCS: emergency lower segment caesarean section

and well, and birthweight should all be documented. See Table 46.1.

Remember all drugs in relation to (potential) pregnancy and lactation

- possible teratogenesis
- altered pharmacodynamics and pharmacokinetics
- toxicity in breast milk

4 Past Gynaecological History

- history of any other gynaecological problems, especially endometriosis, polycystic ovarian syndrome, infertility and any gynaecological surgery
- last cervical smear and result, including abnormalities

5 Sexual History

- dyspareunia: superficial or deep
- sexually transmitted infections
- any abnormal vaginal discharge
- Previous pelvic inflammatory disease

6 Micturition

- general enquiry: if urinary symptoms are disclosed or offered, explore:
  - frequency in both day and night
  - pain or burning sensation (dysuria)
  - urgency
  - incontinence stress (with any physical effort) or urge (occurs on urge)
  - haematuria

7 Bowels

- general enquiry: if bowel symptoms are disclosed or offered, explore:
  - regularity
  - use of laxatives
  - any pain or difficulty defecating
  - any rectal bleeding

8 Medical and Surgical History

- any medical conditions especially diabetes mellitus (DM), hypertension (HT), asthma and thromboembolism
- previous abdominal surgery is important

9 Drugs and Allergies

- details of all medication, doses and duration of use
- allergies to any medication
- use of folic acid in pregnancy

10 Family History

- especially DM, HT and thromboembolism where combined oral contraceptive pill (COCP) use considered
- familial cancers (e.g. breast, endometrial, ovarian and colonic) should be sought in gynaecology

11 Social History

- home conditions and relationships
- any history of domestic violence or safeguarding issues if relevant
- occupation and conditions of work
- smoking

- alcohol intake
- lifestyle issues; for example, drugs

12 Examination

12.1 General Examination

- height and weight
- body mass index $= \frac{\text{wt(kg)}}{\text{ht}^2(\text{m}^2)}$
- general look of the patient, signs of anaemia, breast examination in women over 35 years and systematic chest and cardiovascular examination

12.2 Abdominal Examination

Verbal consent should be obtained. The patient should be asked to empty her bladder. A chaperone should be offered routinely. The patient is asked to undress in privacy and cover herself with a sheet or light blanket. She should then lie on the couch.

12.3 Inspection

- skin quality
- abdominal distension
- surgical scars, umbilical (laparoscopy) or Pfannenstiel
- any visible masses

Gynaecological examination includes:

1. Abdominal examination:
   - inspection
   - palpation
   - percussion
   - auscultation
2. Pelvic examination:
   - inspection
   - speculum examination
   - bimanual examination
3. Rectal examination (where indicated)

12.4 Palpation

- superficial palpation for guarding, tenderness and rigidity
- deep palpation for any masses, especially with the left hand to detect those arising from the pelvis

12.5 Percussion

- dull if the mass is solid
- tympanic if bowel is distended
- shifting dullness and fluid thrill in case of ascites
- liver, spleen and kidneys should be palpated where indicated

12.6 Auscultation

- very rarely used in a routine gynaecological examination
- postoperatively used to auscultate for bowel sounds or intestinal activity

12.7 Pelvic Examination

Remember to obtain verbal consent and offer a full explanation of the examination you are about to perform. A chaperone should always be present and all equipment ready such as a warm speculum, lubricant, swabs, brush for smear and pipelle. Position the woman in either a dorsal, lithotomy or Sims' position. The Sims' position is a modification of the left lateral position and is ideal for the examination of a woman with a uterovaginal prolapse or a vesicovaginal fistula. The lithotomy position is generally used for vaginal surgery and involves abduction of both thighs and the feet suspended from lithotomy poles. The dorsal position is the most common position used in a gynaecological outpatient setting.

12.8 Inspection

Look for any swelling, inflammation or ulceration on the vulva and describe the mons pubis, hair distribution, labia majora, labia minora, the clitoris, urethral meatus and the vaginal introitus.

12.9 Speculum Examination

- This is an essential part of gynaecological examination. There are two types of speculums in use: Cusco's bivalve speculum and Sims' (duck-billed) speculum.
- Sims' speculum is used in the examination of uterovaginal prolapse. The Cusco's speculum is more frequently used in gynaecological examination. This consists of two limbs jointed at the handle. It is available in various sizes and also made in a disposable plastic form.

12.10 Digital Bimanual Examination

- The pelvic organs, uterus, cervix and the adnexa can be examined. The index and middle fingers of the right hand are introduced into the vagina using some lubricant. The fingers of the left hand should be placed on the abdomen and bimanual palpation done. The following should be assessed:
  1. Cervix
  2. Uterus
  3. Both adnexa
  4. Any tenderness
- Remember that a uterine mass usually moves if the cervix is moved, while an ovarian mass does not. A line of separation can be palpated between the ovarian mass and the uterus. This is absent when the mass arises from the body of the uterus, except in a pedunculated fibroid.
- Positive cervical excitation where there is pain in the adnexal area on moving the cervix, typically in an ectopic pregnancy.
- In an obese patient, it may be difficult to palpate the pelvic organs, and an ultrasound examination of the pelvis will be of value.
- Always check your gloves once the examination is over for any bleeding or discharge.
- Rectal examination is necessary in some cases only.
- A summary of history and findings should be an integral part of the examination, and this will help in the differential diagnosis of the problem with which the patient has presented to you.

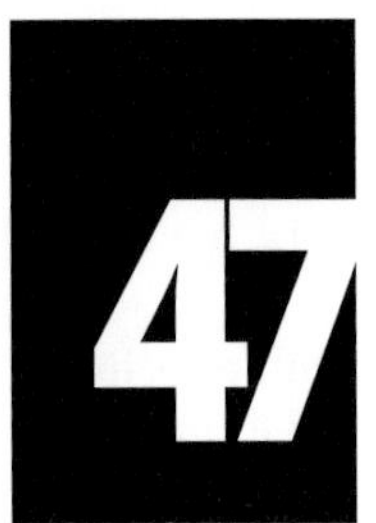

Fraser and Gillick Competence

Neela Mukhopadhaya

- In 1969, the Family Law Reform Act provided that 'a minor who has attained the age of 16 years could provide consent on their own behalf'. This, however, does not apply to minors under 16 years of age.
- In 1985, Mrs Gillick brought her concerns regarding guidance on contraceptive advice and treatment for girls under the age of 16 to the courts. There were two outcomes from the Gillick case. One was that it became lawful to provide contraceptive advice and treatment to girls under the age of 16, subject to certain guidelines (Fraser guidelines). The other was that, in certain circumstances, a child under the age of 16 could now give consent in their own right ('Gillick competence').
- Fraser guidelines refer to a specific set of guidelines that Lord Fraser proposed in the Gillick case. The guidelines state that contraceptive advice or treatment can be provided to a child under 16 without parental consent or knowledge provided that the healthcare professional is satisfied of the following:

1. That the girl will understand his or her advice
2. That he/she cannot persuade her to inform her parents or allow him/her to inform the parents that she is seeking contraceptive advice
3. That she is likely to begin or to continue having sexual intercourse with or without contraceptive treatment
4. That, unless she receives contraceptive advice or treatment, her physical or mental health, or both, are likely to suffer
5. That her best interests require him or her to give her contraceptive advice, treatment, or both, without parental consent

- Gillick competence, on the other hand, refers to the fact that some children under the age of 16 are able to give consent. The key to whether the child can give consent is their emotional and intellectual maturity, and their ability to understand the proposed treatment. Those children who are deemed by the healthcare professional to be Gillick competent are the ones who can provide consent for the proposed treatment.

Fluid Management in Pregnancy

Neela Mukhopadhaya

1 Haemorrhage

- Normal physiologic changes that occur during pregnancy allows women to tolerate the inevitable blood loss associated with delivery. In early haemorrhage, vascular tone, heart rate and myocardial contractility increases to improve oxygen delivery. Cardiac output is redistributed, selectively maintaining perfusion to the adrenal glands, brain and heart at the expense of other organs, including the uterus.
- Before delivery, this shunting may lead to fetal hypoxia and distress. With continued blood loss and delayed or inadequate resuscitation, secondary changes occur in the microcirculation. Initially, interstitial fluid enters the capillary beds and later capillary endothelial damage occurs. This results in increased permeability and leakage of fluid into the interstitial space. Prolonged hypoxia can cause tissue ischaemia and damage.

1.1 Use of Crystalloids

- The primary goal of treatment during haemorrhage is to restore and maintain oxygenation of tissues. This begins with aggressive replacement of intravascular volume. At the same time, supplemental oxygen should be added and strategies to control the cause of blood loss.
- Crystalloid solutions are most commonly used in initial fluid resuscitation. Hartmann's or lactated Ringer's and 0.9% sodium chloride (normal saline) are the two most common crystalloid solutions. They distribute primarily throughout the extracellular space, expanding both the intravascular and interstitial compartments. With the infusion of 1 L of lactated Ringer's solution, 200 ml will remain in the vasculature while 700 ml enters the interstitial spaces. Roughly 3 L of crystalloid are required for each litre of blood loss. Lactated Ringer's has the advantage of containing small quantities of additional electrolytes and lactate.
- The lactate is converted to bicarbonate by the liver. In theory, the bicarbonate may buffer some of the lactic acidosis produced from poor perfusion and offset acidosis resulting from dilution of existing buffers. Normal saline is a secondary choice because it can cause hyperchloraemic acidosis.

1.2 Use of Colloids

- Colloid solutions may be used as an alternative or an adjunct to crystalloids. Colloids are solutions containing large molecular weight substances. They cause intravascular volume expansion with little increase in the interstitial volume. There is a small risk of anaphylaxis (less than 0.04%).
- Albumin in a 5% solution is the colloid most commonly used for volume expansion. Adverse effects seen with albumin include a decrease in free calcium levels, which may be due in part to citrate binding. There is also a decrease in platelet aggregation as well as dilution of clotting factors, which may lead to prolongation of the prothrombin time and partial thromboplastin time.
- Usually, the risk of infections with HIV and Hepatitis B and C is small.
- Plasma protein fraction consists primarily of albumin with lesser amounts of alpha- and beta-globulins.
- Dextrans consist of high- and low molecular weight preparations: dextran 70 and dextran 40, respectively. These solutions have been associated with bleeding due to decreased platelet adhesion and dilution of clotting factors.
- Considerable controversy exists as to whether crystalloids or colloids are the optimal fluid for

initial resuscitation in hypovolaemic shock. Large volumes of crystalloids are required to achieve the effect that smaller quantities of colloids will require. Theoretically, this excess volume distributed within the interstitial space may impair oxygen transport to cells. Crystalloids have a shorter duration of action. The concern with decreasing capillary osmotic pressure (COP) combined with increasing hydrostatic pressure associated with volume replacement is that there will be a decrease in the gradient between COP and pulmonary capillary wedge pressure. This increases the risk of developing pulmonary oedema. When capillary permeability is increased, the high molecular weight substances may leak out into the extravascular tissue and increase the interstitial COP. This leads to worsened and prolonged pulmonary oedema.

- Renal function is also affected in patients being treated for hypovolaemic shock. Renal blood flow is increased with colloid solutions. However, this does not necessarily increase urine output or protect against acute tubular necrosis.

1.3 Fresh Frozen Plasma and Platelets Transfusion

- Fresh frozen plasma (FFP) is the plasma portion of a unit of whole blood frozen within eight hours of collection. It contains plasma protein and clotting factors, and is reserved for patients with clotting disorders. In the case of massive obstetric haemorrhage, where replacement of more than one blood volume has taken place over a few hours, FFP is transfused in the ratio of 1:1.
- Thrombocytopenia, defined as blood platelet count below 150 000/mm^3, is the second leading cause of blood disorders in pregnancy after anaemia. Gestational thrombocytopenia explains 70–80% of all cases of thrombocytopenia in pregnancy. Hypertensive disorders account for approximately 20% and immune thrombocytopenic purpura for about 3–4%.
- Vaginal delivery is safe when the platelet count is >30 000/mm^3. For operative vaginal or caesarean deliveries, the safe platelet count should be at least 50 000/mm^3.
- In the bleeding patient or a patient with thrombocytopenia in pregnancy, transfusion is indicated when the platelet count falls below 50 000/mm^3. Like FFP, platelets should not be given prophylactically with massive blood replacement. Prophylactic transfusions are appropriate preoperatively when the platelet count is less than 50 000/mm^3. In nonoperative situations where the count falls below 10 000/mm^3, prophylactic transfusions are indicated because of the increased risk of serious spontaneous bleeding involving the gastrointestinal tract or central nervous system. Platelet counts can be expected to rise by approximately 5000 to 10 000/mm^3 with each unit of platelet concentrate transfused.
- Spinal or epidural anaesthesia is contraindicated with platelet levels of <80 000/mm^3.
- Prophylactic pharmacological thromboprophylaxis is contraindicated in postoperative patients with platelet counts of <80 000/mm^3, but in high-risk cases, a risk-benefit discussion should take place.
- Immune thrombocytopenic purpura is not an indication for caesarean delivery.
- The immunoglobulin G (IgG) anti-glycoprotein platelet antibodies can cross the placenta and could induce neonatal thrombocytopenia (with an estimated risk of 5–10%).
- There is no correlation between maternal and fetal platelet levels, and maternal response to treatment does not protect the fetus from a possible neonatal thrombocytopenia.
- Neonatal platelet levels should be determined at birth and further daily monitored.
- When platelet count in the newborn is below 50 000/mm^3, the risk of intracranial haemorrhage is 0.5–1.5%.
- When the platelet count is between 30 000 to 50 000/mm^3, intravenous immunoglobulin G (IVIG) treatment should be started. With platelet count under 30 000/mm^3, platelet transfusion along with IVIG is recommended.

1.4 Fluid Replacement in Hyperemesis Gravidarum

- In cases of significant ketonuria, 1 L of 0.9% sodium chloride intravenously over two to four hours is used. Hartmann's can also be used.
- Thereafter, fluids should be reduced to 500 ml, 4–6 hourly, the regimen being guided by urea and electrolytes results, which should be performed

daily, particularly for monitoring potassium levels.

- Avoid glucose initially as it contains insufficient sodium and especially as Wernicke's encephalopathy may be precipitated unless thiamine is given first.

1.5 Fluid Management in Preeclampsia

- Preeclampsia can cause fluid and electrolyte imbalance, and can lead to accumulation of fluid in the extravascular spaces and interstitial spaces in the lungs and brain. This is a result of endothelial injury, leading to increased capillary permeability.
- A strict fluid input and output should be maintained in preeclampsia patients to prevent complications of pulmonary oedema and cerebral irritability, leading to eclamptic fits.
- Causes of pulmonary oedema in pregnant patients are due to increased preload in conditions like:
  - excessive fluid administration
  - resolving oedema in patients with preeclampsia in the postnatal period
  - cardiac causes such as diastolic dysfunction, cardiomyopathies and valvular heart disease
  - other cause such as essential hypertension, reduced oncotic pressure (preeclampsia/ nephrotic syndrome) and increased capillary permeability (sepsis)
- Untreated severe preeclampsia is associated with peripheral vasospasm and hypertension. The haemodynamic effect of bolus-dose intravenous fluids in untreated severe preeclampsia is a reduction in systemic vascular resistance, an increase in cardiac output and improved rates of peripheral oxygen delivery and consumption. This is accompanied by little, if any, change in blood pressure (the rise in cardiac output offsets the reduction in vascular resistance). See Table 48.1.

Table 48.1 Intravenous fluids in preeclampsia

Maintenance	Comments
Nil by mouth: 85 ml/h crystalloid	Reduce volume with co-administration of intravenous drugs; e.g., magnesium sulphate
Replacement	
Volume resuscitation: titrate to SBP >90 mmHg	Crystalloid or colloid
Anaemia and/or coagulopathy: appropriate blood products	Titrate primarily against volume deficit then laboratory indices. Consider invasive monitoring for patients in positive fluid balance.
Preloading	Fluid challenge prior to vasodilation (hydralazine) or regional anaesthesia: 300 ml crystalloid

Aim to maintain urine output ≥100 ml every four hours

Oliguria with positive fluid balance

- 300 ml colloid fluid challenge
- If no response: restrict fluids to match losses
- If continuing oliguria: low-dose dopamine
- Consider invasive haemodynamic monitoring

Oliguria with negative fluid balance

- 300 ml colloid fluid challenge
- Repeat every 30 minutes until in positive fluid balance or adequate urine output
- If persistent oliguria: restrict fluids
- If continuing oliguria: low-dose dopamine
- Consider invasive haemodynamic monitoring

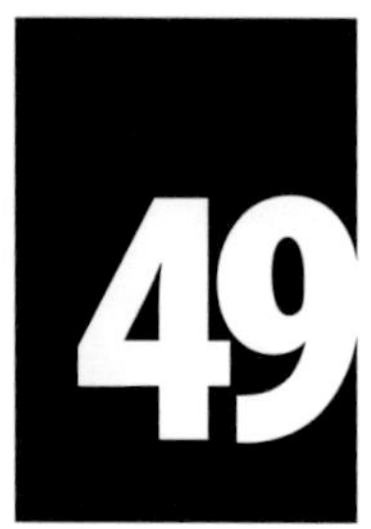

Coagulation

Neela Mukhopadhaya

There are several obstetric conditions that affect coagulation. Please refer also to the Physiology section.

1 Placental Abruption

See Table 49.1.

- Placental abruption occurs in one in 200 pregnancies.
- It causes 15% of intrapartum fetal deaths.
- The pathology is characterised by rupture of the maternal decidual artery, resulting in haemorrhage into the decidual–placental interface.
- It has also been shown that proinflammatory cytokines cause premature separation of the placenta.
- It is a poorly understood condition.
- Risk factors include smoking, preeclampsia, previous history of abruption, trauma in pregnancy, cocaine use and previous caesarean section.
- In preeclampsia, the maternal inflammatory response formed against trophoblasts results in a systemic endothelial dysfunction. Thus, vasodilator prostaglandins decrease and thrombocyte aggregation and uteroplacental ischaemia increases.

2 HELLP Syndrome

- This is a syndrome characterised by endothelial cell damage in the liver. It is thought to be caused by substances originating in the placenta, which cause an acute inflammation in the hepatic endothelial cells.
- Typically, there are raised liver enzymes and low platelets.

3 Septic Abortion

- This causes disseminated intravascular coagulation (DIC) by triggering the release of inflammatory substances, which cause disruption of the coagulation cascade. Studies showed that endothelial dysfunction plays a key role in the pathophysiology of septic abortion.
- It is common for patients with severe sepsis to develop a coagulopathy and thrombocytopenia. If the patient is not actively bleeding and no invasive procedures are planned it may be possible to tolerate the abnormal laboratory clotting results. If the platelet count falls to 5 $x10^9$/L, platelets should be given regardless of bleeding. If there is significant risk of bleeding or if surgery or invasive procedures are planned, platelets will be required to maintain the count above 50 $x10^9$/L. Red blood cells should be given when the haemoglobin is less than 7.0 g/dL with the aim of achieving a target haemoglobin of 7–9 g/dL. If the woman has any significant cardiac or respiratory comorbidities, it may be necessary to have a higher transfusion trigger to maintain tissue oxygenation while avoiding an excessive increase in the cardiac workload.

Table 49.1 Disseminated intravascular coagulopathy

Obstetric causes	Nonobstetric causes
Amniotic fluid embolism	Sepsis
Abruptio placentae	Trauma
Placenta praevia	Leukaemia
Postpartum bleeding	Acute fatty liver
HELLP syndrome	Toxic and immunological causes
Preeclampsia/eclampsia	Narcotic drugs
Septic abortion/intrauterine sepsis	ABO incompatibility
Acute fatty liver of pregnancy	Transplant rejection

HELLP: haemolysis (H), elevated liver enzymes (EL), low platelet count (LP)

4 Amniotic Fluid Embolism

- Amniotic fluid embolism is a rare condition, which can be observed during delivery and postpartum up to 48 hours. It has been reported that 70% of cases occur prepartum. The clinical features are hypotension, cardiac arrhythmias, cyanosis, dyspnoea, altered mental status and bleeding. Maternal mortality is as high as 70%.

Surgical Complications

Neela Mukhopadhaya

1 Bladder and Ureteric Injury

1.1 Course of the Ureters

- The abdominal ureter becomes the pelvic ureter as it crosses over (see Figure 50.1):
  - the pelvic brim
  - the bifurcation of the common iliac arteries
- It passes lateral to the cervix and under the uterine vessels.
- The intravesical ureter travels obliquely inside the wall of the bladder.

1.2 Ureteric Injuries

- A common site of ureteric injury is at the pelvic brim where the ureter is close to the infundibulopelvic ligament and lateral to the uterine artery where the uterine artery/cardinal ligament/uterosacral ligament is divided during hysterectomy.
- The ureter is damaged less commonly in the ovarian fossa.

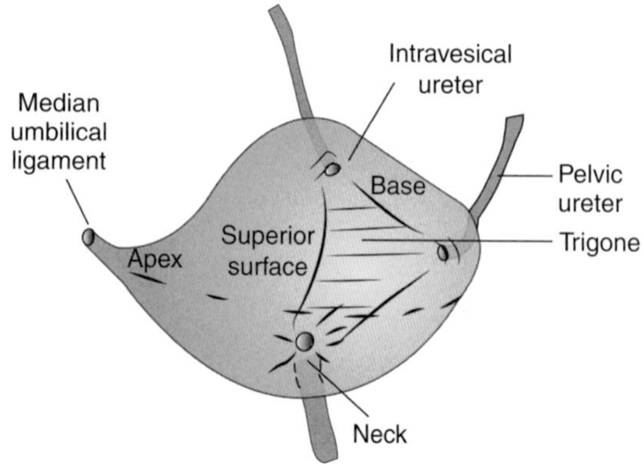

Figure 50.1 Course of the ureter in the pelvis.

1.3 Bladder Injuries

- The most common visceral injury during laparoscopic surgery is bladder injury (0.02–8.3%).
- This occurs most commonly during vaginal surgery or abdominal surgery while dissecting the bladder off the cervix.
- The most common cause of injury is inadvertent electrosurgical injury.
- The injury clinically manifests around 48 hours after surgery.
- Thermal injury to the bladder usually presents in 10–14 days with a uroperitoneum or vesicovaginal fistula.
- A biochemical marker of rising creatinine after a bladder or ureteric injury is raised creatinine, which is absorbed by the peritoneum.
- Bladder injury in the cave of Retzius is managed conservatively.
- Fistula formation after bladder injury occurs in about 5% of cases (usually <1–2%, but up to 20% with deep infiltrating endometriosis (DIE)).

2 Haemorrhage

- Major obstetric haemorrhage (MOH) is a challenge for anaesthetists and obstetricians. Worldwide haemorrhage remains a major cause of maternal death: it is estimated that between one-quarter and one-half of preventable maternal deaths are secondary to haemorrhage.
- Antepartum haemorrhage (APH) complicates 3% of pregnancies. Placental abruption refers to abnormal separation of the placental lining from the uterus. Bleeding may occur per vagina or be concealed in a retroplacental clot. Significant bleeding can compromise fetal oxygenation and cause fetal distress or stillbirths.

- one-third of APHs are due to placental abruption
- one-third of APHs are due to placenta praevia
- one-third of APHs are due to other causes such as uterine rupture

- Causes of postpartum haemorrhage (PPH) are commonly ascribed to the 'four Ts' (see below): uterine atony is responsible for 70% of cases. PPH is more commonly associated with placenta praevia, multiple pregnancy, polyhydramnios, previous PPH, Asian ethnicity, anaemia, obesity, prolonged labour, induction and augmentation of labour and primipara over 40 years:
  - tone (uterine atony)
  - trauma
  - tissue (retained placenta)
  - thrombin (coagulopathies)
- PPH secondary to trauma may follow delivery by caesarean section (more common with emergency than elective), mediolateral episiotomy, operative vaginal delivery and delivery of a neonate >4 kg.
- Preexisting coagulopathy may be congenital or the result of anticoagulant use. Disseminated intravascular coagulation occurs early after massive abruption and amniotic fluid embolism and may develop after intrauterine death, when products are retained for more than two weeks. Coagulopathy may also occur after haemorrhage due to haemodilution and loss of clotting factors.

2.1 Initial Management of Severe Bleeding in Pregnancy

1. High-flow oxygen.
2. Place the woman in the left lateral position if antepartum, or head down if postpartum.
3. Intravenous access: two large-bore cannula (≥16 g). Start infusion of crystalloid (warmed) until blood is available.
4. Send blood for group-specific/crossmatched blood (six units), and fresh frozen plasma (FFP) (4–6 units), full blood count, clotting, and urea and electrolytes.
5. Put out 'MOH call' to alert anaesthetist, obstetrician, senior midwife, blood bank and porters.
6. If blood loss is ongoing:
   a. Aim to replace losses with blood and products as soon as possible and to warm all fluids
   b. Give O Rh negative blood if group-specific/crossmatched blood is not available in the presence of worsening cardiovascular instability
7. If blood loss has stopped:
   a. Give fluid replacement with crystalloid and blood products until clinical signs of normovolaemia are seen
   b. Monitor haemoglobin with point-of-care tests (HemoCue or blood gas)
8. Consider transfer to a critical-care area for monitoring.
9. Further steps will depend on the cause of haemorrhage, and treatment should be tailored to individual patients.
10. In the obstetric patient, the aim should be to keep fibrinogen >2 g/L.
11. Fibrinogen is present in FFP and cryoprecipitate and as a small volume in fibrinogen or prothrombin complex concentrate (PCC). The much smaller volume of cryo, fibrinogen and PCC compared with FFP avoids haemodilution or overload, and concentrates do not require defrosting.
12. The National Institute for Health and Care Excellence cautiously recommends cell salvage in obstetrics, and the Royal College of Obstetricians and Gynaecologists (RCOG) recommends its use when ≥1500 ml blood loss is expected. Separate suction should be used for the removal of amniotic fluid before the cell savage and a leucodepletion filter is required. Significant hypotension during re-transfusion of salvaged blood possibly related to infusion of cell fragments may be expected.
13. Activated factor VIIa has been used in the management of MOH complicated by coagulopathy. It requires adequate concentrations of fibrin (>1 g/L) and platelets (>20 x10^9/L). Evidence for its use is limited, and concerns remain regarding increased risk of thrombosis and lack of effect in the face of major haemorrhage. Factor VIIa may be acceptable to Jehovah's Witnesses.

2.2 Pharmacotherapy in Major Obstetric Haemorrhage

- Syntocinon: synthetic oxytocin
- Ergometrine: an ergot alkaloid
- Syntometrine: a combination of oxytocin and ergometrine
- Carboprost: a prostaglandin $F2_{\alpha}$
- Tranexamic acid: competitive inhibitor of plasminogen activation
- Misoprostol: a synthetic prostaglandin E1 analogue

2.2.1 Ergometrine

- recommended as a second-line uterotonic
- acts on uterine muscle
- it may cause diarrhoea, nausea and vomiting
- contraindicated in preeclampsia or other hypertensive conditions
- duration of action is 3 hours after intramuscular dose
- ergometrine can be given as 500 μg intramuscularly or 250–500 μg slow intravenously

2.2.2 Carboprost

- given by deep intramuscular injection
- not licensed for intrauterine injection
- 250 μg may be given intramuscularly at 15-minute intervals up to a maximum of 2 mg or eight doses
- it may precipitate bronchospasm and is contraindicated in asthmatics

2.2.3 Misoprostol

- is active via rectal, sublingual and oral routes
- the dose is 400 μg to 1 mg
- it is inexpensive and does not need refrigeration, and is therefore useful as a resource outside of the hospital setting

2.3 Surgical and Other Interventions

- intrauterine balloon tamponade (Bakri balloon)
- uterine compression sutures (B-Lynch sutures)
- interventional radiology (IR) (intra-arterial balloon occlusion and arterial embolisation)
- pelvic vessel ligation (internal iliac, uterine, hypogastric or ovarian arteries)

3 Laparoscopic Injuries

RCOG recommends using the following terminology:

- very common: 1/1 to 1/10 (a person in a family)
- common: 1/10 to 1/100 (a person in a street)
- uncommon: 1/100 to 1/1000 (a person in a village)
- rare: 1/1000 to 1/10 000 (a person in a small town)
- very rare: less than 1/10 000

3.1 Frequent Risks

- wound bruising
- shoulder-tip pain
- wound gaping
- wound infection

3.2 Serious Risks

- the overall risk of serious complications from diagnostic laparoscopy are approximately two women in every 1 000 (uncommon)
- damage to the bowel, bladder, uterus or major blood vessels which would require immediate repair by laparoscopy or laparotomy is uncommon
- failure to gain entry to abdominal cavity and to complete intended procedure
- hernia at the site of entry (<1:100)
- death: 3–8 women in every 100 000 undergoing laparoscopy die as a result of complications (very rare)

3.3 Risks During Surgical Management of an Ectopic Pregnancy

Frequent risks include:

- inability to identify an obvious cause for the presenting complaint (negative laparoscopy)
- bruising
- shoulder-tip pain
- wound gaping
- wound infection
- persistent trophoblastic tissue when salpingotomy performed (4–8 in 100)
- hernia at site of entry
- any extra procedures which may become necessary during the procedure
- laparotomy
- salpingectomy

- repair of damage to bowel, bladder, uterus or blood vessels
- blood transfusion
- oophorectomy

3.4 How to Prevent Bowel Injury During Laparoscopy

- the primary incision for laparoscopy should be vertical from the base of the umbilicus
- a disposable needle is recommended
- the operating table should be horizontal (not in the Trendelenburg tilt) at the start of the procedure
- the abdomen should be palpated to check for any masses and for the position of the aorta before insertion of the Veress needle
- two audible clicks are usually heard as these layers are penetrated
- excessive lateral movement of the needle should be avoided as this may convert a small needlepoint injury in the wall of the bowel or vessel into a more complex tear
- once the laparoscope has been introduced through the primary cannula, it should be rotated through 360 degrees to check visually for any adherent bowel
- when the Hasson open laparoscopic entry is employed, confirmation that the peritoneum has been opened should be made by visualising bowel or omentum
- secondary ports must be inserted under direct vision perpendicular to the skin, while maintaining the pneumoperitoneum at 20–25 mmHg
- during insertion of secondary ports, the inferior epigastric vessels should be visualised laparoscopically to ensure the entry point is away from the vessels
- the Hasson technique or insertion at Palmer's point is recommended for the primary entry in women who are very thin
- women at highest risk of vascular injury are the young, thin, nulliparous women with well-developed abdominal musculature
- patients with severe anorexia are at particular risk. The aorta is less than 2.5 cm below the skin in very thin women

4 Surgical Risks During Hysteroscopy

- the risk of uterine perforation is 1%, rising to 2.5% in postmenopausal women
- serious risks are uncommon
- the overall risk of serious complications from diagnostic hysteroscopy is approximately two women in every 1000 (uncommon)
- damage to the uterus is uncommon
- damage to the bowel, bladder or major blood vessels is rare
- failure to gain entry to the uterine cavity and to complete intended procedure (uncommon)
- infertility is rare
- out of every 100 000 women undergoing hysteroscopy, 3–8 die as a result of complications (very rare)
- frequent risks include infection and bleeding

5 Uterine Perforation

- with evacuation of retained products of conception (ERPC), uterine perforation is reported at about 0.002–1.7%
- with hysteroscopy, uterine perforation is reported in up to 1.6%
- the commonest cause of perforation is surgical termination of pregnancy (STOP)
- when perforation is caused by a 5 mm hysteroscope, dilator, coil insertion, polyp forceps or curette, further monitoring and/or procedures may be needed to prevent complications; the main actions are:
    - alert team
    - +/− catheterise
    - antibiotics
    - senior help
    - observe
    - if bleeding is observed, then laparoscopy is indicated
- if perforation is caused by a 10 mm hysteroscope, avulsion attempted or resection loop/laser, a laparotomy should be performed
    - laparoscopy suggests a small perforation: observe
    - laparoscopy suggests a large perforation: observe or suture/repair

6 Postoperative Complications

Deep vein thrombosis (DVT)

- Patients undergoing abdominal surgery who are at risk due to the procedure or due to personal risk factors should receive thromboprophylaxis with mechanical methods unless contraindicated and either subcutaneous low molecular weight heparin, unfractionated heparin or fondaparinux.
- All women should be assessed for risk factors for venous thromboembolism (VTE) when booking for antenatal care and at each subsequent maternity contact.
- All patients presenting with VTE should have a full clinical history and examination undertaken to diagnose thrombosis and assess for thromboprophylaxis.
- Testing for inherited forms of thrombophilia (antithrombin, protein C, protein S deficiency, factor V Leiden and prothrombin G20210A) does not influence the initial management of VTE and should not be performed routinely.

Superficial thrombophlebitis

- Patients with clinical signs of superficial thrombophlebitis affecting the proximal long saphenous vein should have an ultrasound scan to exclude concurrent deep vein thrombosis.
- Patients with superficial thrombophlebitis should have anti-embolism stockings and can be considered for treatment with prophylactic doses of low molecular weight heparin for up to 30 days or fondaparinux for 45 days.
- If low molecular weight heparin is contraindicated, 8–12 days of oral nonsteroidal anti-inflammatory drugs should be offered.

Risk factors

- age: incidence of first VTE rises exponentially with age
- obesity: 2–3-fold VTE risk if obese (body mass index >30 kg/m^2)
- varicose veins: 1.5 to 2.5-fold risk after major surgery
- family history of VTE: a history of at least one first-degree relative having had VTE
- cancer: compared with the general population, overall 5–7-fold risk of first VTE and increased risk of recurrent VTE
- severe acute infection
- chronic HIV infection, inflammatory bowel disease, nephrotic syndrome, myeloproliferative disease, paraproteinaemia, Behcet's disease, paroxysmal nocturnal haemoglobinuria, sickle cell trait and sickle cell disease, combined oral contraceptives (COCs), hormone replacement therapy and antiestrogens
- COCs: compared with nonusers, COC users have 3–6-fold increased risk
- compared with users of COCs containing second-generation progestogens (levonorgestrel), users of COCs containing third-generation progestogens (desogestrel, norgestimate) have a further 1.7-fold increase in VTE risk
- progestogen-only oral contraceptives are not associated with increased VTE risk, but high-dose progestogens used to treat gynaecological problems may be associated with a 6-fold increased VTE risk
- oral estrogen hormone replacement therapy (HRT) users have 2.5-fold increased VTE risk, but not transdermal estrogen HRT users
- heritable thrombophilia further increases VTE risk in COC and oral estrogen HRT users
- raloxifene and tamoxifen are associated with a 2–3-fold increased VTE risk
- there is approximately a 10-fold increased risk during pregnancy compared with nonpregnant women and a 25-fold increased risk compared with nonpregnant/nonpuerperal women; pregnant and puerperal women with thrombophilia have increased risk of VTE compared to pregnant and puerperal women without an identified thrombophilia
- offer VTE prophylaxis to patients undergoing gynaecological surgery
- start mechanical VTE prophylaxis at admission: choose any one of:
    - anti-embolism stockings
    - intermittent pneumatic compression devices
    - unfractionated heparin (UFH) (for patients with severe renal impairment or established renal failure)

Pulmonary embolism

- up to 15% of patients with DVT will have a pulmonary embolism (PE)

- approximately 51% of deep venous thrombi will embolise to the pulmonary vasculature, resulting in a PE
- Computed tomography (CT) pulmonary angiography is the preferred method of diagnostic imaging in patients with a clinical risk score indicative of PE because it provides a high-resolution image and is as accurate as, and less invasive than, pulmonary angiography; which was the previous 'gold standard' test

7 VTE in Pregnancy

- Any woman with symptoms and/or signs suggestive of VTE should have objective testing performed expeditiously and treatment with low molecular weight heparin (LMWH) given prophylactically.
- Compression duplex ultrasound should be undertaken where there is clinical suspicion of DVT.
- If ultrasound is negative and there is a low level of clinical suspicion, anticoagulant treatment can be discontinued.
- If ultrasound is negative and a high level of clinical suspicion exists, anticoagulant treatment should be discontinued but the ultrasound should be repeated on days three and seven.
- Women presenting with symptoms and signs of an acute PE should have an electrocardiogram (ECG) and a chest X-ray performed.
- In women with suspected PE without symptoms and signs of DVT, a ventilation/perfusion (V/Q) lung scan or a computed tomography pulmonary angiogram (CTPA) should be performed.
- When the chest X-ray is abnormal and there is a clinical suspicion of PE, CTPA should be performed in preference to a V/Q scan.
- Anticoagulant treatment should be continued until PE is definitively excluded. Women with suspected PE should be advised that, compared with CTPA, V/Q scanning may carry a slightly increased risk of childhood cancer, but is associated with a lower risk of maternal breast cancer.
- D-dimer testing should not be performed in the investigation of acute VTE in pregnancy.
- Before anticoagulant therapy is commenced, blood should be taken for a full blood count, coagulation screen, urea and electrolytes and liver function tests.
- The woman on LMWH for maintenance therapy should be advised that, once she is in established labour or thinks that she is in labour, she should not inject any further heparin.
- Where delivery is planned, either by elective caesarean section or induction of labour, LMWH maintenance therapy should be discontinued 24 hours prior to planned delivery.
- Regional anaesthetic or analgesic techniques should not be undertaken until at least 24 hours after the last dose of therapeutic LMWH.
- LMWH should not be given for four hours after the use of spinal anaesthesia or after the epidural catheter has been removed, and the epidural catheter should not be removed within 12 hours of the most recent injection.

8 Fluid Balance Postsurgery

- Fluid loss happens in numerous different ways such as bleeding, drainage of ascites, urination, insensible water loss and 'third space losses'.
- Dehydration and bleeding should be considered when urine output is low postoperatively.
- Bowel lumen, peritoneal and pleural cavities are examples of the third space.
- Overhydration with saline and surgical trauma cause endothelial dysfunction and interstitial oedema due to fluid shift to extracellular volume.
- Infusion of large volumes of fluids to patients who do not have enough preload reserves may result in unbalanced fluid shift to interstitial tissue, with no effect on tissue perfusion.
- Central venous pressure (CVP) is widely believed to indicate general intravascular volume status of the patient.

9 Intravenous Access

- the best site for intravenous access is usually in the hand
- dorsal arch veins: the princeps pollicis artery lies in the first interspace on the dorsum and is the branch of the dorsal carpal branch of the radial artery

- the cephalic vein lies in the anatomical snuffbox
- cubital fossae: risk of damaging the median nerve and brachial artery in the same area:
- median antecubital vein
- cephalic vein
- basilic vein
- intraosseous access: generally in neonates; the main sites are
- distal femur
- sternum
- proximal tibia
- humeral head

10 Respiratory Distress With Morphine (Pain Relief)

See Chapter 38.

- opioid-induced respiratory depression (OIRD): can cause cardiorespiratory arrest with subsequent hypoxia and hypercapnia
- OIRD is directly related to the activation of opioid receptors expressed on respiratory neurons in the central nervous system
- naloxone, which is an opioid receptor antagonist, is used to treat OIRD
- naloxone has a short half-life (its elimination half-life is 15 to 20 minutes)

Common Disorders of Pregnancy

Neela Mukhopadhaya

Most common disorders of pregnancy are covered in the rest of the book (see, for example, Section 3, Physiology, and Section 5, Endocrinology):

- preeclampsia
- hyperemesis gravidarum
- diabetes in pregnancy
- hypothyroidism
- hyperthyroidism
- cardiac conditions
- respiratory disorders
- haematological disorders

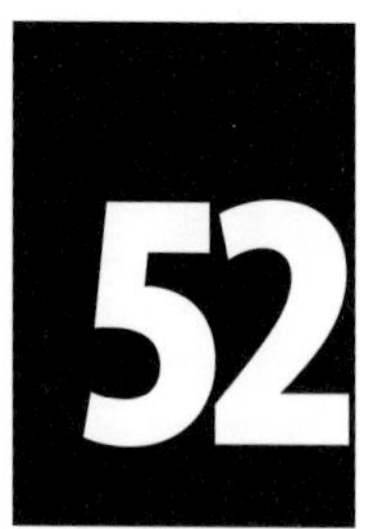

Management of Labour

Neela Mukhopadhaya

1 Fluid Management

- oral fluids are encouraged in labour
- close input and output should be maintained
- IV fluids should be given when the fetal heart monitoring on the cardiotocography (CTG) is suspicious
- usually Hartmann's (Ringer's lactate solution) should be given
- preload before regional analgesia
- IV access should be secured in high-risk women such as induction of labour, anaemia, risk of postpartum haemorrhage (PPH)
- catheter: to manage output and bladder care if not passing urine
- careful hydration in preeclampsia (85 ml/hour); risk of pulmonary oedema

2 Pain Management

See Chapter 63.

- Women need emotional support in labour and a birthing partner is recommended.
- Upright position: rocking, swaying or leaning forwards helps with the axis of the pelvis and in vaginal delivery.
- Transcutaneous electrical nerve stimulation (TENS): generally, TENS is applied at high frequency (>50 Hz) with an intensity below motor contraction (sensory intensity) or low frequency (<10 Hz) with an intensity that produces motor contraction. The noninvasive nerve stimulation reduces both acute and chronic pain. It is generally applied at the level of T10–S2 where the nerve pathways to the uterus, vagina and perineum enter the spinal cord. The mechanism of action is poorly understood, but it is thought that the electrical impulses block the pain impulses. A secondary benefit may be related to the release of endorphins.

2.1 Entonox

- Nitrous oxide (N_2O) is itself active (does not require any changes in the body to become active), and so has an onset of action in roughly the lung–brain circulation time with a half-life of 3.5 minutes.
- It is a combination of nitrous oxide and oxygen in a fixed 1:1 ratio.
- This gives it a peak action 30 seconds after the start of administration.
- Entonox should thus be used accordingly; that is, inhalation should start 30 seconds before a contraction becomes painful in labour.
- It is removed from the body unchanged via the lungs, and does not accumulate under normal conditions, explaining the rapid offset of around 60 seconds.
- It is a weak anaesthetic in high concentrations and an anxiolytic and analgesic at low concentrations. It suppresses the reticuloendothelial system activity and increases endogenous endorphins, corticotropin and dopamine.
- N_2O should not be used in patients with bowel obstruction, pneumothorax, middle ear or sinus disease.
- Prolonged exposure of >5 hours per week in healthcare workers can lead to vitamin B_{12} deficiency, preterm labour and subfertility.

2.2 Epidural/Combined Epidural

- Epidural is an injection into the epidural space (the area between the dura mater (a membrane) and the vertebral wall, containing fat and small blood vessels. The space is located just outside the dural sac, which surrounds the nerve roots and is filled with cerebrospinal fluid). See Table 52.1.
- In adults, the spinal cord terminates around the level of the disc between L1 and L2, below which

Table 52.1 Boundaries of the epidural space

Superiorly	Fusion of the spinal and periosteal layers of dura mater at the foramen magnum
Inferiorly	Sacrococcygeal membrane
Anteriorly	Posterior longitudinal ligament, vertebral bodies and discs
Laterally	Pedicles and intervertebral foramina
Posteriorly	Ligamentum flavum, capsule of facet joints and laminae

lies a bundle of nerves known as the cauda equina ('horse's tail'). Hence, lumbar epidural injections carry a low risk of injuring the spinal cord.

- A study (Shen, 2017) published in the journal *Obstetrics & Gynaecology* showed that the use of epidural analgesia in the second stage of labour made no difference to duration of labour.
- The results show epidural also had no effect on normal vaginal delivery rate, incidence of episiotomy, the position of the fetus at birth or any other measures of fetal wellbeing. The study compared the effects of catheter-infused, low-concentration epidural anaesthetic to a catheter-infused saline placebo in this double-blinded, randomised trial of 400 women.
- Drugs used in epidural or spinal anaesthetic are local anaesthetics like bupivacaine, opioids like fentanyl, and often used with epinephrine and morphine.
- Regional anaesthetic usually lasts for 4–8 hours.
- Side effects: severe headache can be caused by leakage of spinal fluid (<1%) and will require a blood patch if symptoms persist: nausea, shivering, backache and difficulty in micturition.

2.3 Opioids

- Drugs used are pethidine, diamorphine (given by midwife) and remifentanil (given by anaesthetist).
- They can cause CTG changes with 'sleep pattern' in fetuses, reduced variability and accelerations.
- The neonate can take up to six days to eliminate pethidine.
- It can cause symptoms such a poor feeding, respiratory depression, hypothermia and altered crying.

2.4 Other Modalities of Pain Relief

- Water birth: water birth is known to help with pain relief and is recommended for low-risk labours.
- Complementary therapies: acupuncture, aromatherapy, reflexology, yoga, self-hypnosis and massage are different pain-relief modalities used.

3 Monitoring in Labour

3.1 Intermittent Auscultation

- Intermittent auscultation of the fetal heart rate is offered to women at low risk of complications in established first stage of labour.
- Either a Pinard stethoscope or Doppler ultrasound should be used.
- Intermittent auscultation should be performed immediately after a contraction for at least 1 minute, at least every 15 minutes, and recorded as a single rate.
- Maternal pulse should be recorded hourly.

Advise continuous cardiotocography if any of the following risk factors are present at initial assessment or arise during labour:

- maternal pulse over 120 BPM on 2 occasions 30 minutes apart
- temperature of 38 °C or above on a single reading, or 37.5 °C or above on 2 consecutive occasions 1 hour apart
- suspected chorioamnionitis or sepsis
- pain reported by the woman that differs from the pain normally associated with contractions
- the presence of significant meconium
- fresh vaginal bleeding that develops in labour
- severe hypertension: a single reading of either systolic blood pressure of 160 mmHg or more or diastolic blood pressure of 110 mmHg or more, measured between contractions
- hypertension: either systolic blood pressure of 140 mmHg or more or diastolic blood pressure of 90 mmHg or more on 2 consecutive readings taken 30 minutes apart, measured between contractions

- a reading of 2+ of protein on urinalysis and a single reading of either raised systolic blood pressure (140 mmHg or more) or raised diastolic blood pressure (90 mmHg or more)
- confirmed delay in the first or second stage of labour
- contractions that last longer than 60 seconds (hypertonus), or more than 5 contractions in 10 minutes (tachysystole)
- oxytocin use
- do not offer continuous cardiotocography to women who have nonsignificant meconium if there are no other risk factors
- telemetry is offered to women who need continuous monitoring or those using water birth

Normal labour: you are expected to know the basic sciences around the following topics. Most of these have been covered in other chapters in this book:

- vaginal delivery
- caesarean section
- PPH
- preterm premature rupture of membranes (PPROM)
- preterm labour
- group B Streptococcus (GBS) prophylaxis
- antibiotics
- sepsis

4 Fetal Blood Sampling

- do not take a fetal blood sample during or immediately after a prolonged deceleration
- take fetal blood samples with the woman in the left lateral position
- use either pH or lactate when interpreting fetal blood sample results
- use the classifications shown in the box for fetal blood sample results

pH:

- normal: 7.25 or above
- borderline: 7.21 to 7.24
- abnormal: 7.20 or below

or

lactate:

- normal: 4.1 mmol/L or below
- borderline: 4.2 to 4.8 mmol/L
- abnormal: 4.9 mmol/L or above

Interpret fetal blood sample results, taking into account:

- any previous pH or lactate measurement
- the clinical features of the woman and baby, such as rate of progress in labour

5 Paediatric Resuscitation/Basic Life Support

- basic life support comprises the following elements: initial assessment, airway maintenance, breathing and circulation (ABC) which includes cardiopulmonary resuscitation (CPR)
- CPR should be administered to a person who is not breathing normally and who shows no signs of life by combining chest compressions with 'effective rescue breaths'
- in an adult: chest compression of 5–6 cm
- in a child (1 year to onset of puberty) compress at least one-third of the chest's depth (5 cm), using one hand
- in an infant (0–1 years of age), compress at least one-third of the chest's depth (4 cm), using two fingers
- the rate of compression should be 100–120 compressions per minute.
- after completing 30 chest compressions, two effective breaths should be administered

Bibliography

Shen, X., Li, Y., Wang, N., et al. (2017). Epidural analgesia during the second stage of labor: a randomized controlled trial. *Obstet Gynecol*, **130**(5), 1097–1103.

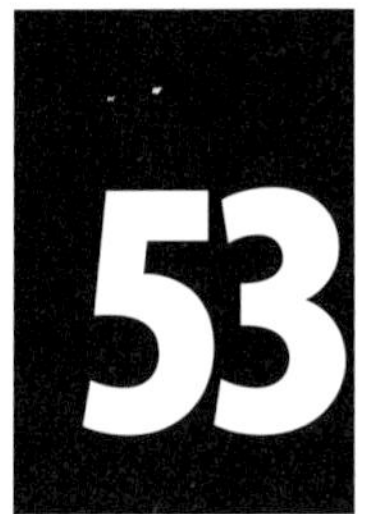

Operative Delivery and Perineal Tears

Neela Mukhopadhaya

You are required to have a basic knowledge of vacuum and forceps delivery, instruments and the technique.

1 Forceps

- forceps are used when labour needs to be expedited for maternal or fetal reasons

Advantages of forceps
- avoidance of caesarean and its complications
- reduction of decision to delivery time

1.1 Indications

Maternal factors
- maternal exhaustion
- prolonged second stage
- maternal illnesses such as heart disease, hypertension, glaucoma and aneurysm, or other factors that make pushing difficult or dangerous
- haemorrhage
- analgesic drug-related inhibition of maternal effort (especially with epidural/spinal anaesthesia)

fetal factors
- suspicious or pathological cardiotocograph (CTG)
- after-coming head in breech delivery

Complications to mother
- bruising to the perineum
- perineal tears
- increased risk of perineal lacerations, pelvic organ prolapse and incontinence
- increased postnatal recovery time and pain
- increased difficulty evacuating during the recovery time

Complications to baby
- cuts and bruises
- occasionally (usually temporary) facial nerve injury can occur
- rarely, clavicle fracture
- intracranial haemorrhage
- improper twisting of the neck can cause damage to cranial nerve VI, resulting in strabismus
- severe and rare complications (occurring less frequently than 1 in 200) include nerve damage, skull fractures and cervical cord injury

2 Ventouse

- ventouse is used in the second stage of labour if it has not progressed adequately
- it may be an alternative to a forceps delivery and caesarean section
- it is contraindicated in breech position or for premature births

2.1 Indications

- maternal exhaustion
- prolonged second stage of labour
- fetal distress in the second stage of labour, generally indicated by changes in the fetal heart rate (usually measured on a CTG)
- maternal illness where prolonged 'bearing down' or pushing efforts would be risky (e.g., cardiac conditions, blood pressure, aneurysm, glaucoma)

2.2 Advantages and Outcomes

- an episiotomy may not be required
- the force applied to the baby can be less than that of a forceps delivery, and leaves no marks on the face

- the risk of maternal trauma is slightly lower than forceps and caesarean section
- the baby will be left with a temporary lump on its head, known as a chignon
- there is a possibility of cephalohaematoma formation, or subgaleal haemorrhage
- there is a higher risk of failure to deliver the baby than forceps, and an increased likelihood of needing a caesarean section

Perineal tears

- first-degree tear: laceration is limited to the fourchette and superficial perineal skin or vaginal mucosa
- second-degree tear: laceration extends beyond the fourchette, perineal skin and vaginal mucosa to the perineal muscles and fascia, but not the anal sphincter
- third-degree tear: the fourchette, perineal skin, vaginal mucosa, muscles and anal sphincter are torn; third-degree tears may be further subdivided into three subcategories:
  - 3a: partial tear of the external anal sphincter involving less than 50% thickness
  - 3b: greater than 50% tear of the external anal sphincter
  - 3c: internal sphincter is torn
- fourth-degree tear: fourchette, perineal skin, vaginal mucosa, muscles, anal sphincter and rectal mucosa are torn

Urogynaecology, Fertility and Early Pregnancy Complications

Neela Mukhopadhaya

1 Urodynamics

- Urodynamic tests are used to diagnose patients who have urinary incontinence or other urinary symptoms.
- These tests are given to both men and women. A urodynamic test is used to measure nerve and muscle function, pressure around and in the bladder, flow rates and other factors.
- The tests are to see if the bladder has involuntary contractions that cause urine leakage.
- The tests comprise:
  - uroflow test or uroflowmetry
  - postvoid residual volume
  - cystometry (cystometrogram or filling cystometry)
  - electromyography
  - voiding pressure study
  - videourodynamics
  - basic fertility investigations; bloods for ovulation and ovarian function (covered in Section 3, Physiology, and Section 5, Endocrinology)

2 Tubal Patency Tests

- Hysterosalpingogram: a radiocontrast dye is injected through the cervix, and X-rays taken to check for filling and spillage from both fallopian tubes. It is important to do these tests in the early follicular phase of the cycle and ensure that patients continue with a reliable contraception. Pregnancy test should be done before these tests.
- Hysterosalpingo contrast sonography: is done under ultrasound guidance when an echo contrast dye (Echovist) is injected through the cervix and shows spillage from the tubal ends.
- Laparoscopy and dye test: this is the 'gold-standard test' and spillage of methylene blue is seen under direct laparoscopic views. It also provides an opportunity to treat any additional pathologies like endometriosis and adhesions.

Ultrasound scan, semen analysis and clomiphene ovulation induction are covered in other chapters.

3 Early Pregnancy Complications

3.1 Miscarriages

- spontaneous loss of pregnancy at or before 24 weeks

3.1.1 Threatened Miscarriage

- per vaginal bleeding and pain
- uterus is expected size
- cervical os closed
- ultrasound: intrauterine pregnancy
- twenty-five percent of pregnancies will go on to miscarry

3.1.2 Inevitable Miscarriage

- per vaginal bleeding and pain
- cervical os open
- ultrasound: intrauterine pregnancy

3.1.3 Incomplete Miscarriage

- per vaginal bleeding and pain
- cervical os open
- ultrasound: retained products of conception

3.1.4 Complete Miscarriage

- pain and bleeding has resolved
- uterus is no longer enlarged
- cervical os closed
- ultrasound: no retained products of conception

3.1.5 Missed Miscarriage

- may or may not have pain and bleeding
- uterus is smaller than expected
- cervical os is closed
- ultrasound: fetal pole is present, but no fetal heartbeat; or gestational sac is present, but no fetal pole

3.2 Causes of Miscarriage

- maternal age
- chromosomal abnormalities
- previous miscarriages
- medical/endocrine disorders
- polycystic ovarian syndrome (PCOS)
- progesterone deficiency
- hypothyroidism
- uterine structural abnormalities
- infection, usually bacterial vaginosis (BV)
- drugs/chemical

3.3 Recurrent Miscarriage

Three or more consecutive first-trimester pregnancy losses or the loss of one or more pregnancies in the second trimester:

- affects 1 in 100 women
- in the majority of cases there will be no specific cause

3.3.1 Risk Factors

- epidemiological: age-related risk is highest in those aged over 45 (93%) and for couples where the female is over 35 years old and the male is over 40 years old
- antiphospholipid syndrome: most important treatable cause
- genetic factors: parental chromosomal rearrangements (balanced structural chromosomal abnormalities; e.g., Robertsonian translocation): embryonic chromosomal abnormalities account for 30–57% and increase with advancing maternal age
- anatomical factors: septate uterus, arcuate uterus, submucosal fibroids and cervical weakness
- endocrine factors: diabetes mellitus and thyroid dysfunction, PCOS
- infective agents: any severe infection causing bacteraemia and viraemia can cause sporadic miscarriage: BV in the first trimester is RF for the second trimester miscarriage and preterm delivery
- genetic thrombophilias: Factor V Leiden, activated protein C/S deficiency, antithrombin III and prothrombin gene mutation

3.4 Investigations and Management

- Karyotyping of fetal products.
- Pelvic ultrasound scan to assess uterus and ovaries.
- Thrombophilia screen.
- Infection screen.
- Antiphospholipid antibodies taken 12 weeks apart if positive.
- Genetic abnormalities: prenatal diagnosis or IVF with preimplantation testing.
- Hysteroscopy for septate uterus and submucosal fibroids.
- Maintaining normal body mass index in PCOS.
- For antiphospholipid syndrome: 75 mg aspirin daily (from positive pregnancy test) and 4500 IU/mL subcutaneous heparin once fetal heart activity is seen on ultrasound.
- Cerclage for cervical weakness; transvaginal ultrasound scan (TVUSS) surveillance.
- Antibiotics for BV.
- Offer reassurance and additional support in pregnancy: there is no evidence for routine use of steroids in pregnancy, which can cause complications such as development of gestational diabetes. Patients will be understandably anxious, so will need extra support throughout pregnancy. You can offer serial growth scans and regular clinic reviews.
- There has been some evidence that steroids can reduce levels of natural killer cells. There is no national guidance about management of abnormal levels.
- No investigation is required after two miscarriages. No need for thrombophilia in the presence of risk factors such as OCP. A family history of diabetes does not increase the risk of miscarriage.
- Uncontrolled glycaemic control in someone known to have diabetes can increase the risk of miscarriage, congenital abnormalities, risk of preeclampsia and growth problems.

3.5 Management of Miscarriages

- expectant
- medical
- surgical
- management depends on whether the miscarriage is complete or incomplete

3.5.1 Medical

- speeds up the process of missed or delayed miscarriage, or helps to empty the uterus after incomplete miscarriage
- two stages: mifepristone (200 mg by mouth); 48 hours later: misoprostol (4 x 200 μg = 800 μg per vaginum)
- give painkillers
- ultrasound scan and assess every two weeks until miscarriage is complete

If miscarriage is not complete by four weeks, consider alternative options such as surgery.

3.5.2 Surgical

- evacuation of retained products of conception
- cervix dilated and products of conception removed by suction under general anaesthetic
- risks: infection (2 in 100), uterine perforation (1 in 100), adhesions (<1 in 100)

3.5.3 Anti-D

Nonsensitised rhesus (Rh) negative women should receive anti-D immunoglobulin in the following situations:

- all ectopic pregnancies
- all miscarriages over 12 weeks of gestation (including threatened)
- all miscarriages where the uterus is evacuated (whether medically or surgically)

3.6 Ectopic Pregnancy

3.6.1 Causes

- iatrogenic
  - intrauterine contraceptive device
  - IVF
  - pelvic surgery (including past caesarean)
  - sterilisation
  - diethylstilbestrol exposure in utero
  - emergency contraception use (current pregnancy)
- infections
  - pelvic inflammatory disease (PID)
  - sexually transmitted diseases (STIs) (chlamydia, gonorrhoea)
- smoking
- multiple sexual partners
- advanced maternal age
- lower socioeconomic status

3.6.2 Diagnosis

- no intrauterine pregnancy (IUP) on scan with positive pregnancy test: could be early IUP
- if ectopic pregnancy: could rupture
- if human chorionic gonadotropin (hCG) >1000 IU/L with empty uterus on transvaginal (TV) scan or hCG >6500 IU/L with empty uterus on transabdominal (TA) scan, consider laparoscopy
- otherwise, repeat hCG in 48 hours and plan management
- serial serum hCG assay is particularly useful in the diagnosis of asymptomatic ectopic pregnancy
- at levels above 1500 IU/L, an ectopic pregnancy will usually be visualised with TV scan
- a doubling of hCG titre is often expected: this can vary depending on gestation

3.6.3 Management

- expectant
- medical: methotrexate
- surgical: laparoscopic salpingectomy or laparoscopic salpingostomy (selected cases)

3.6.3.1 Expectant Management

- the success rates are 57–100%
- should be considered in patients with hCG <1000 IU/L
- a decreasing beta hCG is a predictor of successful outcome

3.6.3.2 Medical

See Table 54.1.

- systemic single dose methotrexate can be used if:

Table 54.1 Medical management of ectopic pregnancy

Indications	Contraindications
• Previous good health	• Rupture
• Low hCG	• Abdominal bleeding
• Comorbidities preventing GA	• Infection
• Pelvic adhesions	• Anaemia
• Embryo implanted at neck of the uterus	• Kidney problems
	• Liver problems
	• HIV
	• Peptic ulcers
	• Ulcerative colitis

  - patient has no significant pain
  - ectopic pregnancy is unruptured
  - no intrauterine pregnancy on scan
  - there is no cardiac activity
  - hCG levels are below 3000 IU/L
- hCG levels are then monitored to confirm no trophoblast tissue remains:
  - <15 IU/L confirms ectopic resolution
- if levels remain high, a second dose or surgery may be required in 3–27% of patients
- if serum hCG levels fail to fall:
  - 10% chance repeat surgery for persisting ectopic is required
- patients should be counselled regarding future pregnancies:
  - on becoming pregnant again, an early scan is required to ensure it is not ectopic
  - there is a 10% chance of further ectopic pregnancy
  - give information on the signs of an ectopic pregnancy to increase awareness

3.6.3.3 Surgical Management

In the haemodynamically unstable patient
- surgical management by the most expedient method; laparotomy is an acceptable approach

Salpingectomy
- laparoscopy is preferable to laparotomy:
  - faster recovery
  - reduced rate of repeat ectopic pregnancy
  - similar rate of subsequent intrauterine pregnancy

Salpingotomy or salpingectomy
- salpingotomy preferred option if contralateral tube is damaged
- no evidence that it is superior if contralateral tube is healthy and future fertility is desired
- higher recurrent ectopic pregnancy rates (18% versus 8%)

Salpingectomy
- definitive: use if haemodynamically unstable
- may reduce future intrauterine pregnancy rates (limited data)

3.6.4 Methotrexate: Mode of Action and Use

- prevents division of rapidly dividing cells
- stops early pregnancy developing into a fetus
- works by inhibiting enzymes involved in folate metabolism; this prevents DNA and protein synthesis
- single intramuscular dose; based on height and weight
- additional dose if hCG has not fallen after follow-up
- overall 90% success rate
- abdominal pain usually occurs for first two days (but pain should be reported to health professional in case of rupture)
- bleeding can occur up to six weeks after
- tiredness
- sore mouth and throat
- hair loss
- gastrointestinal problems: nausea, diarrhoea, indigestion
- changes in blood count (bone marrow suppression)
- pneumonitis
- liver and kidney dysfunction

3.6.5 Follow-up

- hCG monitored every 2–3 days, usually days 4 and 7
- hCG rise on day 4, but a 15% decrease by day 7

- advise patient on avoiding:
    - breastfeeding for at least 4 weeks
    - pregnancy for at least 2 period cycles

3.7 Pregnancy of Unknown Location

- pregnancy of unknown location: no signs of either intra- or extrauterine pregnancy or retained products of conception in a woman with a positive pregnancy test
- pregnancy of 'uncertain viability': intrauterine sac (<25 mm mean diameter) with no obvious yolk sac or fetus or fetal pole <7 mm crown–rump length with no obvious fetal heart activity
- to confirm or refute viability, a repeat scan at a minimal interval of one week is necessary

4 Pelvic Inflammatory Disease

4.1 Symptoms and Signs

- pelvic or lower abdominal pain
    - usually bilateral
- deep dyspareunia
- abnormal vaginal or cervical discharge
    - may be transient/slight
- right upper quadrant (RUQ) pain due to perihepatitis (Fitz-Hugh–Curtis syndrome):
    - occurs in 10–20% of women with PID
    - development of adhesions between the liver and the peritoneum, causing RUQ pain
- lower abdominal tenderness:
    - usually bilateral
- adnexal tenderness:
    - with or without a palpable mass
- cervical excitation/uterine tenderness
- abnormal cervical/vaginal mucopurulent discharge
- temperature >38 °C:
    - although may be normal

4.2 Differential Diagnosis

- ectopic pregnancy
- threatened miscarriage
- ruptured corpus luteal cyst
- complications of an ovarian cyst
- acute appendicitis
- endometriosis
- gastrointestinal disorders; for example, irritable bowel syndrome
- urinary tract infection
- mittelschmerz pain

4.3 Investigations

- pregnancy test
- endocervical swabs for *Chlamydia trachomatis* and *Neisseria gonorrhoeae*:
    - a positive result supports a diagnosis of PID
- need to treat sexual partners:
    - a negative result does not exclude PID
- high vaginal swab:
    - endocervical or vaginal pus cells: if absent, a diagnosis of PID is unlikely
- erythrocyte sedimentation rate, C-reactive protein and white cell count:
    - nonspecific, but if elevated, support a diagnosis of PID
- laparoscopy: gold standard, but is invasive

4.4 Treatment

- start empirical antibiotics as soon as possible after a clinical diagnosis of PID is made:
    - do not wait for swab results
- usually treat as outpatient
- ensure STI screening of partners/contact tracing
- avoid intercourse during treatment
- ibuprofen or paracetamol for pain relief
- commonly used antibiotics:
    - ofloxacin
    - metronidazole
    - ceftriaxone
    - doxycycline
    - >2x antibiotics to cover all potential causative organisms
- taken for 14 days
- if high risk of gonococcal infection, avoid ofloxacin:
    - quinolone resistance

Benign Conditions of the Genital Tract

Neela Mukhopadhaya

1 Vulval Neoplasms

1.1 Ectopic Tissues

- endometriotic lesions may be found on the vulva, especially on an episiotomy wound
- ectopic breast tissue can be seen on the vulva presenting during pregnancy as a firm mobile lump

1.2 Cysts of the Vulva

- Bartholin's cyst arises from blocked Bartholin's duct, usually in the subcutaneous tissue in the lower third of the labia majora. This may present as an acute abscess after infection. The treatment is incision and marsupialisation with adequate drainage of the pus, which should be checked for culture and sensitivity. Antibiotic treatment should be commenced. Always check for gonococci in the urethra and cervix as some of these abscesses are due to gonococcal infection.
- Boils and carbuncles may be seen in women with glycosuria and diabetes.
- Sebaceous cysts are common cysts of the vulva and if symptomatic should be treated by incision and drainage. They generally tend to recur.
- Cysts of the canal of Nuck appear in the anterior part of the vulva (from the peritoneum being carried into the vulva by the round ligament).
- Mucinous cysts may arise from the minor vestibular glands.
- Mesonephric cysts are generally seen on the labia majora.

1.3 Nonepithelial Tumours

- Lipomas, fibromas and melanomas are benign tumours of the vulva and the diagnosis is by histopathological examination of the mass.

1.4 Epithelial Tumours

- Skin tags or squamous papillomata are common benign masses of the vulva.
- Secondary syphilis presents as a maculopapular rash, but condyloma lata may be seen as sessile papules on the vulva and perianal skin. A generalised lymphadenopathy is commonly associated at this stage.
- Condylomata acuminata caused by human papillomavirus 6/11 commonly presents as a sessile polypoidal mass on the vulva. First-line patient-applied treatment includes imiquimod, podophyllotoxin and sinecatechins. The treatment involves application of 80% trichloroacetic acid. Laser or electro diathermy under local anaesthesia is reserved for larger lesions.
- Keratoacanthoma presents with a smooth papule and a plug of keratin in the centre, but the diagnosis is again on histological grounds.

2 Urethra

2.1 Urethral Caruncle

- This is seen more commonly in postmenopausal women or children as a bright red, tender swelling at the posterior margin of the urethral meatus. Patients may present with dysuria, bleeding and dyspareunia. The treatment is excision using diathermy.
- A differential diagnosis is prolapse of the urethra.
- It presents as a red lesion involving the entire circumference of the urethral meatal margin. It may be acute or chronic. Again, diathermy of the prolapsed mucosa is curative.

3 Vagina

- Benign neoplasms in the vagina are fairly uncommon.

- Condylomata acuminata of the vagina is a viral condition caused by human papillomavirus and tends to be multifocal. It is generally benign, but rare subtypes may cause cervical or vaginal cancers. It is sexually transmitted, and the virus can be transmitted from the mother to a baby during vaginal birth. Lesions have a 'wart-like' appearance. It turns acetowhite with application of acetic acid and should be biopsied before treatment. Rarely verrucous carcinoma may be present. Treatment is medical or surgical, with laser vaporisation or cryotherapy. Podophyllin and 5-fluorouracil may be used too.
- Endometriotic deposits presenting as small brown-black deposits are common. They may be embedded in an episiotomy wound.
- Simple mesonephric cysts (Gartner's cysts) or paramesonephric cysts usually appear in fornices of the vagina. If symptomatic they should be marsupialised rather than excised.
- Adenosis: multiple mucinous vaginal cysts is a rare condition. Adenosis vaginae can be found in the female offspring of a mother exposed to diethylstilbestrol.
- Inclusion cysts can arise where the vaginal epithelium is embedded under the surface during a perineal surgery. Treatment is only warranted when patients are symptomatic.

4 Uterus

4.1 Uterine Fibroids

- These are the most common benign tumours arising from the myometrium of the uterus. Also called leiomyomata, these tumours are composed primarily of smooth muscles, but may contain fibrous tissue as well. Uterine fibroids can present in 20–40% of women in the reproductive age group with a higher prevalence in women over the age of 40 years. It has a higher incidence in American and African women and those with a family history of fibroids. Women present with symptoms of dysmenorrhoea and menorrhagia. Infertility may be associated and in <10% of cases, solely caused by the fibroids. In addition, pressure symptoms and pain are often reported by women.

4.1.1 Types of Uterine Fibroids

- Submucous: they project into the uterine cavity and present as >50% projection into the endometrial cavity. These can be type 0, 1 or 2.
- Intramural: these are located within the myometrium.
- Subserous: they occur when >50% of the fibroid mass extends outside the uterine contours.
- Cervical: relatively uncommon, these tumours arise from the cervix and can cause surgical difficulty due to the proximity to the bladder and the ureters.
- The Federation of International Gynaecology and Obstetrics (FIGO) classification system, which is commonly used for classifying the myomas, retains the original submucosal relationship of types 0–2, but extends staging to an additional six categories. Type 3 fibroids abut the endometrium but are completely intramural. Type 4 describes a completely intramural fibroid; types 5 and 6 are defined by the relationship to the serosal layer; type 7 describes fibroids that are pedunculated on the subserosal surface; and type 8 refers to fibroids found in ectopic locations such as the cervix. FIGO staging subclassifies fibroids that traverse multiple layers of the myometrium; for instance, a fibroid with less than half of its volume in the uterine cavity and extending to the subserosal layer could be labelled type 2–5.

4.1.2 Diagnosis

- Transvaginal or abdominal ultrasound can differentiate the types and dimensions of the fibroids. Magnetic resonance imaging may be needed when the scan is inconclusive.

4.1.3 Treatment

Conservative

- Routine six-monthly ultrasound under close surveillance and review of patient symptomatology is an option for women wishing to avoid treatment.

Surgical Myomectomy

- In women who especially wish to preserve their fertility, and when the fibroids are distinctly isolated on ultrasound, myomectomy may be an option. Fibroids generally tend to recur in these women.

Hysterectomy

- Women who have either completed their family or those over 45 years of age benefit from hysterectomy.

Hysteroscopic resection

- This can be undertaken if they are submucosal.

Uterine artery embolisation

- This is a technique in gynaecology and involves an interventional radiologist. Uterine artery is catheterised generally using the unilateral approach. Polyvinyl alcohol powder or gelatin sponge is used as the embolic material. The main advantage is that it is a minimally invasive procedure with avoidance of a general anaesthetic.

4.2 Endometrial Polyps

- These are more common in women over 40 years of age, but may occur at any age. They are focal overgrowth of the endometrium and are malignant in <1% patients. Treatment is usually resection during hysteroscopy and the polyp should be subjected to histological assessment.

5 Cervix

5.1 Cervical Polyps

- These are common and caused by overgrowth of the endocervical mucosa. Sometimes they arise in the endometrium, but get pedunculated and protrude from the cervix. These are very rarely malignant (1:6000). However, they should be removed and a hysteroscopy performed to rule out further polyps.

5.2 Nabothian Cysts

- These are mucous-retention cysts, caused by blockage of endocervical mucous glands. They may be associated with chronic cervicitis. Treatment is not required unless they are infected, when point cryotherapy or cautery should be done.

6 Fallopian Tubes

- Hydrosalpinx, pyosalpinx and tubo-ovarian masses following pelvic inflammatory disease or endometriotic adhesions may present as a benign mass in the pelvis. The diagnosis is essentially by ultrasound and laparoscopy. Most tumours of the fallopian tubes are malignant, although very rare.

7 Ovarian Neoplasms

- Ovarian enlargement is often silent and symptomless. This is because of the space in the pelvis that can accommodate the enlarged ovary until pressure symptoms appear. Pain is not a common presenting symptom of ovarian disease and nor is vaginal bleeding.
- Common symptoms:
  - abdominal distension
  - pressure symptoms from pressure on the bladder, rectum and lymphatic system
  - pain associated with torsion, haemorrhage, infection or rupture, leading to peritoneal irritation
  - secretion of hormones, leading to vaginal bleeding features of androgenisation like hoarseness of voice, facial hair and menstrual irregularities

7.1 Benign Ovarian Masses

- Follicular cysts: these are the most common cysts on the ovaries.
- Corpus luteum cysts: these are lined with luteal cells derived from the granulose layer. Most resolve spontaneously, but some may persist and cause amenorrhea or pain.
- Haemorrhagic cysts: these could result from bleeding into a corpus luteum or a graafian follicle. Pain may be a presenting feature, but often they remain asymptomatic.
- Theca luteal cysts: these are associated with raised human chorionic gonadotropin (hCG) levels such as with:
  - hydatidiform mole
  - choriocarcinoma
  - gonadotropin therapy

7.2 Ovarian Tumours

- These are classified as:
  - epithelial tumours
  - sex cord/stromal tumours
  - germ-cell tumours
  - embryonic tumours

- miscellaneous
- metastatic

8 Nongynaecological Causes

- other benign masses due to nongynaecological conditions in the pelvis should always be considered as a differential diagnosis
- bladder tumours
- intestinal tumours
- diverticular disease
- inflammatory bowel disease

56

Cancer Screening in Gynaecology

Neela Mukhopadhaya

Definition: Screening is a test designed to identify and eliminate those asymptomatic individuals who are not affected by a disease.

The intention of screening is an early identification of a disease, prompt referral for diagnostic tests and appropriate intervention and management. A screening test does not necessarily diagnose a condition or disease, but can reduce the incidence, mortality and morbidity from the disease.

World Health Organization (WHO): Principles of screening (1968) still apply:

- the condition should be an important public health problem
- an effective intervention should be available
- facilities for diagnosis and treatment should be available
- there should be a clear, recognisable early stage of the condition
- there should be a suitable screening test available
- the test should be acceptable to the population
- the natural history of the condition should be adequately understood
- the benefits of the test should outweigh the risks from the test
- there should be an agreed policy on who to treat
- the total cost of finding a case should be economically balanced in relation to the medical expenditure on the whole
- case finding should be a continuous process, not just a 'once-for-all' project

An effective screening test should:

- have a high sensitivity and specificity
- be acceptable to patients
- be cost effective
- be reproducible

- Sensitivity is defined as the proportion of subjects tested, who are positive for the screening test and have the condition.
- Specificity is defined as the proportion of subjects who test negative for the condition and do not have it.
- A valid screening test should therefore have an acceptable sensitivity (detects most people with the target disorder) and have high specificity (excludes most people without the disorder). Specificity is especially important in a screening programme.
- Positive predictive value is the proportion of subjects with a positive test result, who have the disorder.
- Negative predictive value is the proportion of subjects with a negative test result, who do not have the disorder.
- Odds ratio is the number of subjects with a positive screening test result for each person with the confirmed disorder.
- Likelihood ratio is the value that the result has in predicting the presence of the disorder. It is important in determining the clinical utility of a test.

1 Screening for Cervical Premalignancy

1.1 Background

The foundation for cervical screening is based on Papanicolaou's publication in 1941 when he showed that exfoliated cervical cells could be collected, spread, fixed and stained on slides for examination under the microscope. During the 1960s, a population screening programme in British Columbia showed reduction in the incidence and death rates from cervical cancer. The 1970s saw a large increase in the numbers of abnormal cervical cytology and the discovery of a correlation with human papillomavirus (HPV) infection. The National Health Service Cervical Screening Programme (NHSCSP) was streamlined in the 1980s and this has since shown a 50% reduction in the death rates from cervical cancer. Regular cervical screening reduces (but does not eliminate) the risk of death from cervical carcinoma by 75%.

1.2 Target Age Group

In the UK, the incidence of cervical cancer is extremely low in women less than 25 years of age; less than 40 cases are recorded each year. The new screening programme aims to screen all women between 24.5 and 49 years at 3-yearly intervals and 5-yearly until the age of 64 years; after which it is not necessary to screen any further. Three-yearly screening identifies more than 95% of abnormalities tested by annual screening and so is more cost effective.

1.3 Procedure

The cervix is visualised by a speculum examination. The brush is inserted into the cervix and rotated through 360 degrees at the external cervical os. This is then inserted into a preservative liquid. At the laboratory the liquid is treated to remove other elements such as mucus before a layer of cells is placed on a slide.

- Since October 2003, NICE recommends the liquid-based cytology for the cytological preparation of cervical cells. The UK screening programmes changed their cervical screening method from the Pap test to liquid-based cytology in 2008. This was found to give a cleaner preparation, was easier to read, inadequate cytology could be cut by 80% and it would be cost effective.
- In 2019, HPV primary screening has replaced the cytology-based guidelines.
- In the UK, 9–13-year-old girls are offered two doses of HPV vaccine to prevent HPV infection.

1.4 Terminology of cervical premalignancy

- The original Bethesda terminology is not used in the UK. This classification groups lesions into high grade and low grade.
- Grading of smears is based on examination of cells from the squamocolumnar junction (SCJ). These are the cells that are undergoing metaplasia from columnar to squamous and are most likely to undergo metaplastic changes. The changes that the cytologists are looking for are:
  - nuclear/cytoplasmic ratio (amount of cytoplasm should be twice that of the nucleus)
  - shape of the nucleus (poikilocytosis: abnormal shape)
  - density of the nucleus (koilocytosis: abnormal density)
  - inflammation, infection and mitosis

Original classification (based on smears)

- mild dysplasia
- moderate dysplasia
- severe dysplasia
- carcinoma in situ

1.4.1 Terminolgoies Used

- inadequate: no cells seen from the SCJ for assessment
- inflammatory: excessive numbers of leucocytes, candida or trichomonas may be seen
- borderline: indeterminate changes seen in the nucleus
- mild dyskaryosis: cells have irregular, enlarged nuclei, dense chromatin or irregular nuclear membrane pattern
- moderate dyskaryosis: the nucleus is enlarged to <50% of the cell size
- severe dyskaryosis: the nucleus is enlarged to >50% of the cell size
- possible invasive carcinoma: mitotic figures seen

Richart's classification (1967) based on histological diagnosis

- HPV changes
- CIN I
- CIN II
- CIN III

CIN: cervical intraepithelial neoplasia

- Cervical intraepithelial neoplasia (CIN) I: the outer one-third of the epidermis contains cells with a reduced cytoplasmic:nuclear ratio and increased nuclear density.
- CIN II: the outer two-thirds contain abnormal cells.

- CIN III: the entire depth of the epidermis contains abnormal cells, but the basement membrane is intact.
- Microinvasion: the entire depth of the epidermis contains abnormal cells and there are breaches in the basement membrane with abnormal cells invading to a depth of <3 mm.
- Screening is based on the natural course of cervical cancer where premalignancy precedes overt malignancy and CIN is a progressive condition. However, in reality, CIN may also revert to normal. Routine screening carries a 50–70% sensitivity to detect CIN III. Failure to adequately sample the lesion and failure by cytoscreeners to detect cytological abnormalities can lead to increase in false-negative results.
- Squamous intraepithelial lesion (SIL) is the abnormal growth of squamous cells on the surface of the cervix.
- Low-grade SIL: the changes are thought to be just starting. The changes can be in the size, shape or number of cells that are on the surface of the cervix. In these low-grade lesions, the cells have only a few abnormal characteristics, but are still somewhat similar to the normal cells. Other common names for this low-grade SIL are mild dysplasia or cervical intraepithelial neoplasia type I (CIN 1).
- High-grade SIL: the cells look very abnormal under the microscope. However, these cells are still only on the surface of the cervix. They are not invading the deepest parts of the cervix yet. These lesions are also called moderate or severe dysplasia, CIN II or III or carcinoma in situ (CIS).

1.5 Human Papillomavirus Triage and Test of Cure

See Table 56.1.

This section is not clinically relevant due to change in guidelines, and it is only for noting.

- Under the high risk-human papillomavirus (HR-HPV) triage protocol, women whose cervical samples are reported as showing borderline changes (of squamous or endocervical type) or low-grade dyskaryosis are given a reflex HR-HPV test. Those who are HPV positive are referred to colposcopy; those who are HR-HPV negative are returned to routine recall.
- Women whose cervical sample is reported as high-grade dyskaryosis or worse are referred straight to colposcopy without an HR-HPV test.
- Under the HR-HPV 'test of cure' protocol, after treatment for all grades of CIN, women are invited for screening six months after treatment for a repeat cervical sample in the community.
- A woman whose sample is reported as negative, borderline change (of squamous or endocervical type) or low-grade dyskaryosis is given an HR-HPV test. If the HPV test is negative, the woman is recalled for a screening test in three years (irrespective of age) and can be returned to routine recall if the subsequent test result is cytologically negative. Those who are HR-HPV positive are referred back to colposcopy.
- Women whose cytology is reported as high-grade dyskaryosis or worse are referred straight to colposcopy without an HR-HPV test.

Table 56.1 Cancer wait and referral standards applicable to the NHSCSP

• Patient's smear that was taken in the general practitioner surgery was reported inadequate	• Repeat in three months
• Patient with borderline squamous nuclear changes with HPV unreliable	• Repeat in six months with HPV test
• Patient with low-grade changes with HPV unreliable	• Refer to colposcopy to be seen in six weeks
• High-grade dyskaryosis: moderate or severe	• No need for HPV test; direct referral to colposcopy in two weeks
• Patient with borderline squamous/borderline endocervical changes	• Needs HPV test done at the same time
• With low-grade changes with HPV test positive and after referral colposcopic assessment of cervix is normal	• Discharged to routine recall
• Failed test of cure	• Negative smear with high-risk HPV test positive
• After a low-grade change	• Two negative smears before being discharged to routine recall
• After cervical glandular intraepithelial neoplasia (CGIN) treatment: test of cure	• Two negative smears with HPV test not detected 12 months apart before being discharged to routine recall
• After CGIN treatment, as part of test of cure, if smear is negative and high risk HPV positive	• Needs colposcopy assessment and if normal repeat assessment in 12 months

1.6 Colposcopy

The cervix is visualised using a bivalve speculum. Any discharge should be cleaned using cotton wool. Five percent acetic acid is applied on the cervix liberally and gently. This turns abnormal epithelium white: so-called acetowhite lesions. Examination of the cervix and vaginal wall is done using a microscope under low power magnification. Treatment of suspicious lesions is based on a see-and-treat policy. Selective punch biopsies and large loop excision of transformation zone are the most commonly used excisional treatment options.

1.7 Role of HPV Testing

- Nearly 20% of women aged 25–30 years may test HPV positive. Papillomaviruses are a group of double-stranded DNA viruses that infect epithelial cells. HPV-6 and 11 cause benign genital warts and respiratory papillomatosis, while persistent infection with highly oncogenic strains such as HPV-16 and 18 together account for nearly 70% of cervical cancers across the world. Other high-risk types are HPV-31, 33 and 45. The importance of HPV testing lies in the high sensitivity to detect high-grade CIN in women positive for the virus. Women who test negative have a low risk of having high-grade CIN.
- Cell cycle molecular markers that could be assessed using immunochemistry are another challenge in the future.

1.8 HPV Vaccines

- Vaccination is a means of primary prevention and is particularly useful in developing countries where the screening programme cannot be effectively practised. Also, a small proportion of women who have been screened for cervical cancer are still likely to have the disease. Gardasil (Merck) is a quadrivalent vaccine offering protection against four virus strains: HPV-6, 11, 16 and 18. A pilot trial showed 89% reduction in infection in the vaccinated group of women. Although further trials are being done, Gardasil has received a European licence and is available in the UK. Cervarix, a bivalent vaccine against HPV-16 and 18 is also under trial presently. Both vaccines are safe and have minimal adverse effects such as localised tissue reaction. It will take at least 20 years before one can see a reduction in actual incidence of cervical cancer following the use of vaccines.

2 Vulval Intraepithelial Neoplasias

- Medical therapy reported to be effective in at least some cases of vulval intraepithelial neoplasia (VIN)/ SIL, and is useful for treating a field area prone to multifocal disease. Options include the following:
  - Imiquimod cream, applied three times weekly for 12 to 20 weeks. This results in red, inflamed and eroded tissue often accompanied by considerable discomfort.
  - 5-fluorouracil cream, applied twice daily for several weeks. This causes quite severe inflammation (several weeks) and will not be tolerated by all women. It is less effective than imiquimod cream.
  - Photodynamic therapy requires specialised equipment and can also be very painful.
  - Cidofovir has been described to be useful in some patients.

3 Ovarian Cancer Screening

Ovarian carcinoma usually presents with advanced disease in nearly 75% of cases. This therefore necessitates the need for a reliable screening test. Cancers of the ovary are less well studied compared to other gynaecological malignancies and only a few aetiological factors have been identified. The main factors that predispose one to epithelial cancers of the ovary are parity, use of estrogen hormone replacement therapy (HRT) and family history. There is lack of robust evidence regarding other factors like age at menarche, menopause and first childbirth.

Parity: decreasing risk with increasing parity
Oral contraceptive use: reduction in risk with use (risk ratio 0.40 if used for >36 months)
Years of ovulation: increases with number of years of ovulation.
Little effect of age of menarche and menopause (most cycles are anovulatory)

3.1 Genetic Factors

- If a first-degree relative develops ovarian cancer at an age less than 50, the risk increases by 6–10-fold.
- If two or more close relatives were affected, the lifetime risk rises to 40%.

- Possibly 1% of families in the UK may belong to a very high-risk group and this familial risk is associated with a mutation of the BRCA1 gene on chromosome 17, but other loci may also be involved. However, the absolute risk remains small.
- Several mutations are required to cause cancer. The genetic changes occur in somatic cells. Some individuals develop oncogenic mutations in the germ cells that can be passed to a progeny.
- BRCA1 and BRCA2 have been identified in almost all families with both breast and ovarian cancer and in 40% of families with breast cancer alone.
- Genetic advice to women with one of the above genes should be given by clinical geneticists.
- The efficacy of screening for ovarian cancer is not proven.

3.1.1 Investigations and Management

- Ultrasound examination of the pelvis can reveal cysts on the ovaries. While most of these in a young woman will be physiological, features suggestive of malignancy are large size of cyst, internal septa and solid areas in the cyst and increased blood flow on Doppler examination. Operator expertise is extremely important in the screening process.
- CA125 is a glycoprotein shed by 85% of epithelial tumours. Normal levels are 30 to 65 IU/L, but false positives are commonly seen in other malignancies (liver, pancreas), endometriosis, pelvic inflammatory disease and early pregnancy. Sensitivity is improved using serial measurements and the trends. Up to 50% of stage 1 tumours will present with a CA125 level of <30 IU/L.
- Both ultrasound examination and CA125 estimation can give rise to a false-positive result in nearly 2–3% of postmenopausal women. The use of the two tests together reduces the chance of false positives.
- Women with a family history of ovarian cancers in one first-degree relative should be reassured. Although their risk of ovarian cancer is increased the absolute risk remains small (lifetime risk of 2–5% versus 1% in the general population).
- Oophorectomy should not be used as a primary procedure, but may be considered in women who have a strong family history and have completed their family. The risk of other peritoneal cancers cannot be ruled out in these women.
- The results from a large UK Collaborative Trial of Ovarian Cancer Screening funded by the Medical Research Council (MRC), Cancer Research UK and NHS research and development are awaited. At the present time any screening offered to women for ovarian cancer should be as part of a clinical trial.

3.2 Risk of Malignancy Index

Risk of malignancy index (RMI) combines three pre-surgical features: serum CA125 (CA125), menopausal status (M) and ultrasound score (U). The RMI is a product of the ultrasound scan score, the menopausal status and the serum CA125 level (IU/mL).

RMI = U x M x CA125

- The ultrasound result is scored 1 point for each of the following characteristics: multilocular cysts, solid areas, metastases, ascites and bilateral lesions. U = 0 (for an ultrasound score of 0), U = 1 (for an ultrasound score of 1), U = 3 (for an ultrasound score of 2–5).
- The menopausal status is scored as 1 = premenopausal and 3 = postmenopausal.
- The classification of 'postmenopausal' is a woman who has had no period for more than one year or a woman over 50 who has had a hysterectomy.
- Serum CA125 is measured in IU/mL and can vary between zero and hundreds or even thousands of units.

4 Endometrial Cancer Screening

There are no screening strategies available for endometrial cancer screening. Ultrasound assessment of endometrial thickness and sampling of the endometrium have been described, but there is no evidence to use these as screening methods in clinical practice.

Malignancy and Premalignancy of the Genital Tract During Pregnancy

Neela Mukhopadhaya

1 Introduction

The incidence of cancer in pregnancy is about 1:6000 live births. This is much lower (about 50%) than that in nonpregnant women because fewer women would fall pregnant if they were aware of the diagnosis. The diagnosis can often be delayed in pregnant women as symptoms such as vomiting, abdominal pain, backache and feeling unwell can be attributed to the pregnancy itself. In addition, often treatment may have to be delayed to achieve fetal maturity and this is mostly guided by the woman's wishes. Despite these facts, there does not appear to be any difference in the stage-for-stage survival and mortality figures and the prognosis. The recent CEMACH report introduced a new section on maternal deaths due to cancers, summarising the lessons learnt as most deaths were either indirect or late; many not being reported as patients lost touch with the midwifery team. Overall, 28 cases were reported to the enquiry in the last triennium. Some cancers, particularly those that are hormone dependent, can grow rapidly in pregnancy, but factors related to tumour growth in relation to the dynamic changes in the endocrine and physiological changes in pregnancy is still poorly understood.

2 Cervical Carcinoma in Pregnancy

There is no UK data on the occurrence of cervical cancer in pregnancy. Many authors have reported an incidence of 1:2000 pregnancies. It is the most common cancer of the genital tract to present in pregnancy. There is a decline in the incidence of invasive carcinoma of the cervix in the western world and this may be attributed to the cancer screening programme.

2.1 Presentation

It is believed that pregnancy does not accelerate the progression of cervical intraepithelial neoplasia (CIN) to invasive disease. Prognosis of cervical cancer is dependent on the duration between diagnosis and treatment. Treatment can be delayed to achieve fetal maturity and this is not known to worsen prognosis. Nearly 7% of women are diagnosed with having carcinoma of the cervix at the time of their pregnancy confirmation. Most (up to 65%) of women at presentation are asymptomatic. The diagnosis may follow the assessment of an abnormal smear or colposcopy. Patients presenting with a history of vaginal bleeding or postcoital bleeding in pregnancy should have further investigations to rule out threatened miscarriage and antepartum haemorrhage: this sometimes leads to the diagnosis of cervical cancer. Any contact bleeding or uncertainty in diagnosis should prompt a colposcopy and directed biopsy. Staging of the disease is often difficult when the uterus is enlarged. Intravenous urography should be withheld to avoid exposure of the fetus to radiation, but magnetic resonance imaging (MRI) is acceptable.

2.2 Management

Treatment has to be individualised according to the histological stage, grade and gestational age.

Early invasive disease

Local excision using cone biopsy is the treatment of choice but does not necessarily remove the whole lesion. If no residual tumour or CIN is seen at the margins of the cone, then this treatment may be adequate with no need for pelvic lymph node sampling. There is a risk of haemorrhage, infection, miscarriage, preterm labour and premature rupture of membranes. Of pregnancies, 80% are term deliveries and fetal survival is over 90%.

Stage 1a and 1b

In the first and second trimesters, radical hysterectomy and lymphadenectomy can be performed with the fetus in utero. In late midtrimester (usually above 24 weeks of gestation based on the individual hospital neonatal survival rates) corticosteroids can be administered and caesarean performed followed by radical hysterectomy and lymphadenectomy. A classical section has the advantage of reduced risk of encroaching into the tumour and its vascularity. Although there is little evidence to suggest any benefit, if the patient presents in labour, an emergency section may be performed to reduce dissemination of the disease. If the disease is diagnosed at gestation less than 24 weeks, treatment should not be delayed. If radiotherapy is used, miscarriage usually follows, but a termination of pregnancy may be required to facilitate brachytherapy (intravaginal system).

Advanced disease

Treatment should not be delayed. If the pregnancy is beyond 24 weeks of gestation, the baby should be delivered by classical caesarean section and radiotherapy instituted.

2.3 Prognosis

Cervical cancer is preventable by early detection and treatment of CIN2/3. Conservative management with large loop excision of the transformation zone and conisation is the accepted treatment for high-grade CIN. Five-year survival rate for CIN is 84–90%; if the tumour diameter is <3 cm, 95% of these patients should remain disease free. Prognosis ranges from 15% 5-year survival rate in stage IV to 62% for stage II. There is no evidence to suggest that, when early-stage disease is diagnosed during pregnancy, the prognosis is worse compared with nonpregnant individuals. However, 5-year survival in pregnant women with advanced disease is lower compared with their nonpregnant counterparts. It is thought that this difference could be due to radiation dosimetry during or soon after pregnancy.

2.4 Preinvasive Disease

The national cervical screening programme in the UK ensures that the majority of women have routine cervical screening and proper timely referral for colposcopy and follow-up after an abnormal cytology. This allows most women to plan their pregnancies if they have had an abnormal cytology. It may be slightly more difficult to interpret a cytology result in a pregnant woman and quite often a routine test is deferred until about six weeks postpartum. However, where indicated clinically, referral for colposcopy should be made. It is more difficult to interpret changes in the colour of the cervix following application of acetic acid due to the increased vascularity and accentuation of the neoplastic acetowhite areas. Biopsy of the cervix can lead to brisk bleeding, but this generally stops with pressure. Risk of miscarriage or preterm labour is low. If CIN is diagnosed by histology, repeat colposcopy is undertaken at 36 weeks, and then 6–12 weeks postpartum. There is no evidence to suggest that there is increased progression of preinvasive disease to invasive disease in pregnancy. Therefore, the approach is generally conservative.

3 Ovarian Tumours

The incidence of ovarian or an adnexal cyst in pregnancy is about 1:80–1:2500. The majority of these are functional cysts, benign cystadenomas and dermoids. Only 3–6% of the tumours that require surgery are malignant; nearly a third are dysgerminomas, teratomas or endodermal sinus tumours (germ-cell tumour).

3.1 Presentation

Most tumours are asymptomatic and are discovered during fetal viability scans. Only a quarter are greater than 10 cm. Some will present as abdominal pain due to torsion or leakage (torsion complicates 10–15% of tumours). Torsion usually occurs in the early second trimester.

3.2 Management

If a cyst is identified in the first trimester, it should be rescanned around 14 weeks. Most corpus luteal cysts involute by this time. If the cyst has not increased to more than 5 cm, a conservative approach is acceptable. However, where the cyst was 5–10 cm in diameter, a close watch on the size by repeated scans should be kept and any symptoms or change in size and morphology should prompt a surgery.

Where there are signs of malignancy in the tumour, surgery can be limited to unilateral oophorectomy, but a complete staging should be performed. If staging at laparotomy is suggestive of spread beyond the ovary, or if histology determines the need for chemotherapy then a multidisciplinary approach is taken. There is limited evidence in this area especially about the administration of bleomycin, etoposide and cisplatin for germ-cell tumours and whether these agents can be given during pregnancy. Chemotherapeutics are known to be teratogenic in the first trimester and where indicated, detailed counselling regarding termination of the pregnancy should be undertaken. Each case has to be individualised based on the gestation, tumour histology and patient choice. Where there is evidence of extracapsular invasion, a total hysterectomy, bilateral salpingo-oophorectomy and pelvic node sampling should be considered.

4 Vulval Carcinoma

Eighty percent occur in those over 65 years. Vulval intraepithelial neoplasia is seen in younger women.

4.1 Presentation

Most patients with preinvasive disease are asymptomatic. Nearly 70% present with pruritis vulvae; 57% may present with a mass or an ulcer. Bleeding occurs in a quarter of the patients. Two-thirds are located in the anterior labia majora and the rest on the clitoris, posterior fourchette and the perineum. Diagnosis is usually after colposcopic assessment, excision biopsy with groin node sampling and histological findings.

4.2 Management

Preinvasive disease

Treatment can be delayed until delivery and usually a wide local excision is sufficient.

Invasive disease

Treatment is same as in a nonpregnant woman. Wide local excision for stage Ia tumours (excision includes a 10 mm margin of normal tissue both laterally and deep to the tumour). For lateralised lesions (stage Ib/II) wide local excision with ipsilateral groin node dissection is carried out. Contralateral lymph node sampling is essential if the ipsilateral nodes are positive. This can be carried out with minimal effect on the pregnancy in the first and second trimester. However, if the pregnancy is 36 weeks or more, the treatment can be delayed until delivery. There is no evidence on the mode of delivery in such a situation. Where the wound on the vulva has healed there is no contraindication to a vaginal delivery. Adjuvant radiotherapy is indicated where more than two groin nodes are positive (microscopic involvement) or one is involved (macroscopic).

4.3 Prognosis

Generally, 5-year survival is said to be 80% if the groin nodes are negative, but falls to 40% where groin nodes are positive. Predictive factors for nodal disease are: clinically suspicious groin nodes, grade of tumour (well differentiated versus poorly differentiated), age of patient (old versus young) and presence of lymphatic or vascular space involvement.

Bibliography

Kerr, M. (1972). Cited by Donald I. *Practical Obstetric Problems*, 4th ed., Lloyd-Luke, 224.

Abdominal Incisions, Sutures, Diathermy and Latex Allergies

Neela Mukhopadhaya

1 Abdominal Incisions

Please refer to the section on abdominal incisions in Chapter 1.

1.1 Types of Abdominal Incisions

- Kustner incision: also referred to as a 'modified Pfannenstiel incision', involves a slightly curved skin incision beginning below the level of the anterior superior iliac spine and extending just below the pubic hairline. This involves a risk of injury to the superficial branches of the inferior epigastric artery or vein.
- Cherney incision: this involves transecting through the rectus muscles at their insertion on the pubic symphysis.
- Maylard incision: this is a muscle-cutting incision, in which all layers of the lower abdominal wall are incised transversely approximately 5 cm above the symphysis, depending on the patient habitus and indication for surgery. The fascia is also transected and not separated.
- Joel-Cohen incision: this is a straight transverse incision through the skin, 3 cm below the level of the anterior superior iliac spines. Blunt dissection is used to separate the rectus muscles vertically and then open the peritoneum.
- If transverse incision is extended laterally beyond the edge of the rectus muscles and into the substance of the external and internal oblique muscles, injury to the iliohypogastric and ilioinguinal nerves can occur. This results in a neuroma. See Figure 58.1. See Figure 58.2 for details of different suture materials.

2 Latex Allergy

- this is a type 1 hypersensitivity reaction
- symptoms suggesting possible latex allergy include:
  - itching, swelling or redness of the skin immediately or soon after contact with rubber
  - swelling, itching of eyes/lips/mucous membranes on contact with rubber
  - sneezing/itching of nose/wheezing on contact with rubber or near to airborne rubber; for example, powdered rubber gloves

Latex may be found in many different products within the hospital:

- gloves
- airways maintenance products
- intravenous tubing
- catheters
- dressings/bandages
- rubber bungs on multidose vials

If a patient is identified as having a latex allergy, then:

- label patient's notes with an allergy sticker
- provide an allergy wrist band (red) and input an alert on the patient administration system
- alert medical staff who may arrange appropriate investigations
- alert other staff who may be in contact with the patient
- ensure relevant information on request forms
- ensure that natural rubber latex (NRL)-free products are used.

Theatre, reception, recovery, intensive care unit, day surgery and endoscopy:

- first on the list wherever possible
- ensure that all staff are aware if a patient is latex allergic
- warning notices should be placed at the entrance to theatre
- ensure NRL-free gloves are available for staff
- remove or cover all NRL products

Table 58.1 Advantages and disadvantages of transverse and midline incisions

Incision	Advantage	Disadvantage
Transverse	• Better cosmetic results • Less painful • Less discomfort and pain with postoperative respirations • Greater tissue strength	• More time consuming • More bleeding • Less access to upper abdominal cavity • Division of multiple layers of fascia and muscle and nerves, may result in potential spaces with haematoma, neuroma or seroma
Midline	• Excellent exposure • Easily extendable • Less bleeding • Minimum nerve damage • Rapid entry into abdomen	• Wound dehiscence • Hernia • Poorer cosmetic results • Higher infection rate

Table 58.2 Sutures

Name	Type	Material	Tissue strength	Time taken to dissolve (days)
Dexon	Braided or monofilament	Polyglycolic acid	Good	90–120
Vicryl	Monofilament	Polyglactin	Good	60–90
Vicryl rapide	Monofilament	Polyglactin 910	Low	7–14
Polydioxone suture (PDS)	Monofilament	Polydioxanone	High	180–210
Monocryl	Monofilament	Poliglecaprone	Low	90–120
Maxon	Monofilament	Polytrimethylene	Good	180–210
Silk	Braided	Silk	Low	Nonabsorbable
Nylon	Monofilament	Nylon	High to low	Nonabsorbable
Prolene	Monofilament	Polypropylene	Good–Poor	Nonabsorbable
Mersilene	Braided	Polyester	High–Good	Nonabsorbable

3 Principles of Electrosurgery

For further information on this subject, see Chapter 72.

3.1 Bipolar

- active and return electrode functions at the site of surgery
- tissue grasped between the forceps is included in the electrical current
- no patient return electrode is needed

3.2 Monopolar

- active electrode is in the surgical site
- return electrode is in the pad attached to patient
- current passes through the patient's body

3.3 Electrosurgical Tissue Effects

- cutting: cut with intense heat at the surgical site
- fulguration: sparking with coagulation waveform
- desiccation: by touching the tissue with cutting current, less heat is generated and no cutting occurs; the tissue dries up
- cut effect: low voltage waveform, 100% duty cycle
- coagulation effect: high voltage waveform, 6% duty cycle

Factors affecting diathermy effects:

- size: the smaller the electrode, the higher the current
- time: longer the time spent, the more heat is generated

- manipulation: can cause vaporisation or coagulation
- type of tissue: tissues vary in resistance
- eschar: eschar is a poor conductor, hence high resistance to heat; keep electrodes clean

3.4 Pad Position

- well vascularised muscle
- avoid areas of vascular insufficiency
- avoid bony prominences
- avoid irregular body contours
- consider incision site
- patient position
- consider other equipment

3.5 Radiofrequency Ablation

- alternating current passes through tissue and creates a friction on a molecular level
- causes increased intracellular temperature
- localised interstitial heating
- temperatures more than 60 °C causes denaturing of proteins and coagulation

3.6 Safety Consideration With Diathermy

- direct coupling: active electrode touches a metal and current flows
- insulation failure: insulation barrier is breached and current flows
- capacitative coupling: electrical current is transferred from active electrode through intact insulation to adjacent conductive tissue or trocar

59 Data Interpretation

Neela Mukhopadhaya

Questions under this section will be presented with some data such as blood results, electrocardiogram trace, blood gases, fetal blood results, cardiotocograph (CTG), laparoscopic images, hysteroscopic images, hCG levels and culture results. These questions will be contextualised within obstetrics and gynaecology clinical conditions. You are advised to familiarise yourself with the other conditions covered in the rest of the book.

1 Clinical Conditions

- menstrual disorders
- pelvic pain
- polycystic ovarian syndrome
- contraception
- oral contraceptive pills
- long-acting reversible contraceptives (LARC)
- sterilisation
- vasectomy
- endometriosis
- urinary incontinence
- infertility
- miscarriages

2 Emergency Admissions

These are all dealt with in various parts of the book:

- postoperative wound infections
- miscarriages
- ectopic pregnancy
- hyperemesis gravidarum
- molar pregnancy
- pelvic inflammatory disease

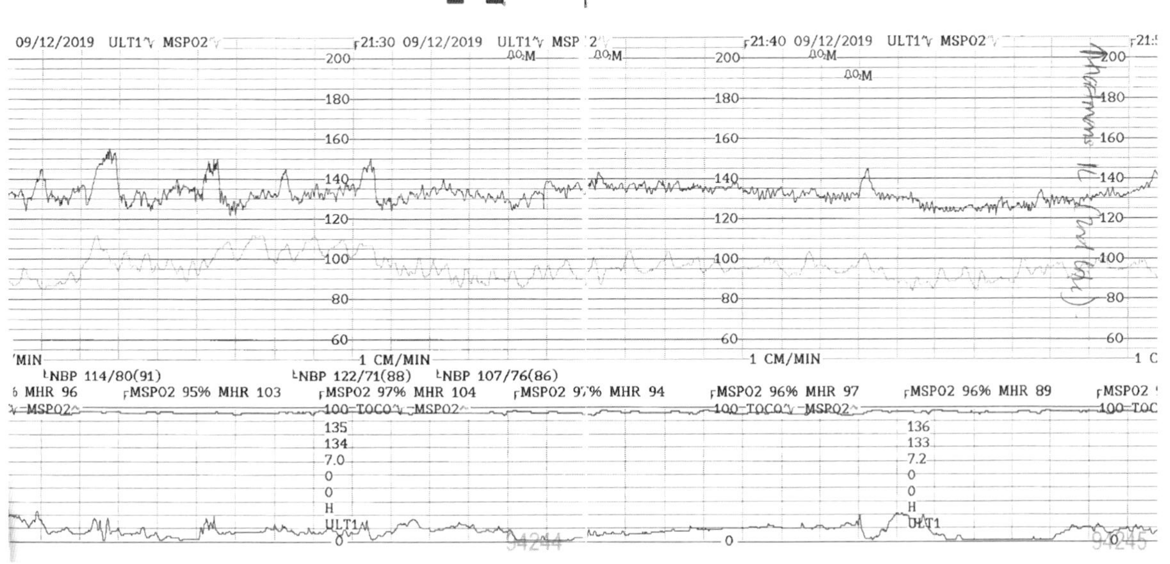

Figure 59.1 CTG interpretation.

- urinary tract infections: nitrofurantoin, trimethoprim, methicillin-resistant *Staphylococcus aureus*, penicillinase resistant
- perforated intrauterine contraceptive device
- retained products
- ovarian torsion
- ovarian hyperstimulation syndrome (OHSS)
- ovarian cyst accidents

This section refers to interpretation of clinical knowledge and will be presented as information. The topics have been covered in the rest of the book but readers are advised to take note of the various data interpretation that they do in day-to-day clinical practice and consider further reading on areas that they feel are lacking in knowledge.

Suggested Reading

CTG: you will be asked to identify the baseline rate, variability, accelerations, decelerations, and contractions and give an opinion on whether normal, suspicious or pathological (see Figure 59.1).

Blood gases interpretation

Blood tests interpretation

Ultrasound scan and X-ray interpretation

Swab results/microbiology reports/culture reports

Laparoscopic findings

Hysteroscopic findings

Statistical interpretation from Forrest plot, ROC, data provided

Histological examination/slides

Family tree interpretation in genetics

Images of anatomical structures/identifying structures

ECG interpretation

Section 9 Pharmacology

Mala Arora

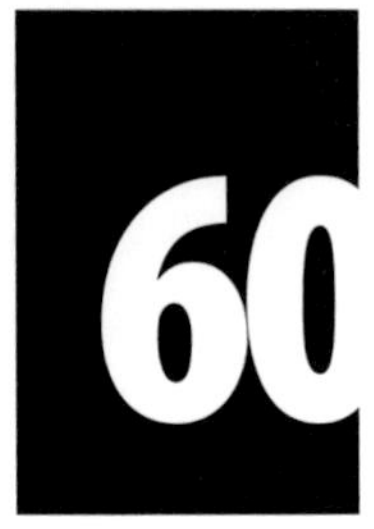

Pharmacokinetics and Pharmacodynamics

Sahil Kumar and Vandana Tayal

Most pharmacokinetic changes can also translate into an alteration in the action of drugs (pharmacodynamics); hence, these two are linked.

1 Physiological Changes in Pregnancy Affecting Pharmacokinetics

- Taken together, gastrointestinal changes in pregnancy have an overall minimal effect on the bioavailability and therapeutic effect of most oral drugs, especially with repeated dosing (Feghali et al., 2015). See Table 60.1.
- The activities of CYP3A4 (50–100%), CYP2A6 (54%), CYP2D6 (50%) and CYP2C9 (20%) are all increased during pregnancy, induced by progesterone (Loebstein et al., 1997; Feghali et al., 2015). See Tables 60.2, 60.3 and 60.4.

Table 60.1 Absorption

Physiological change of pregnancy	Pharmacokinetic consequence	Remarks/examples
Nausea and vomiting in early pregnancy	Decreased amount of drug available for absorption following oral administration	Oral medications should be administered when nausea is minimal; usually during the evening
Gastric acid production is decreased, whereas mucus secretion is increased	• Increased ionisation of weak acids and their reduced absorption • Weak bases diffuse more readily since they are primarily unionised	• Acidic drugs: penicillin, sulphonamides, ampicillin, ibuprofen • Basic drugs: atropine, imipramine, chlorpheniramine, quinine, metoprolol, lignocaine
Increase in plasma progesterone level reduces intestinal motility and reduces gastric and intestinal emptying time by 30–50%	Delay in absorption and increase in bioavailability of most drugs	–
Pulmonary absorption increases as cardiac output and tidal volumes are increased; there is hyperventilation and increased pulmonary blood flow	Alveolar uptake is favoured; dose requirements for volatile drugs likely to be reduced	Demonstrated for halothane, isoflurane and methoxyflurane (Loebstein et al., 1997)

2 Role of Pharmacokinetics in Lactation

- Neonates are sensitive to drug-induced haemolysis by drugs like chloroquine, quinine, nitrofurantoin, quinidine, dapsone and sulpha drugs (due to G6PD enzyme deficiency): these should be avoided in lactation (Sharma and Sharma, 2017).
  See Table 60.5.

3 Pharmacodynamics

- The effects of drugs on the reproductive tissues (breast, uterus, etc.) of the pregnant woman are sometimes altered by the endocrine environment appropriate for the stage of pregnancy.
- Under the influence of estrogen, the sensitivity of the myometrium to the effects of oxytocin changes markedly during pregnancy (mediated by changes

Table 60.2 Physiological changes in pregnancy and pharmacokinetic consequences

Physiological change of pregnancy	Pharmacokinetic consequence	Remarks/examples
40–50% expansion in plasma volume. Increase in total body water is 8 L, distributed 60% to the placenta, fetus and amniotic fluid, and 40% to maternal tissues	Increased volume of distribution for hydrophilic drugs, leading to lower plasma concentrations	Most drugs are hydrophilic, e.g., ranitidine, penicillin, cefazolin, chlorpheniramine
Albumin decreases; moreover, steroid and placental hormones occupy protein binding sites	Unbound fraction of acidic drugs increases (acidic drugs bind to albumin)	• Acidic drugs: penicillin, sulphonamides, ampicillin, ibuprofen • A more thorough approach is to monitor free drug concentrations and adjust drug dosing accordingly
α1-acid glycoprotein also decreases	Unbound fraction of basic drugs increases (basic drugs bind to α1_ acid glycoprotein)	Basic drugs: atropine, imipramine, lignocaine, chlorpheniramine, quinine, metoprolol
Increase in uterine perfusion and the addition of the fetoplacental compartment occurs	• Placental membranes are lipoidal and allow free passage of lipophilic drugs, while restricting hydrophilic drugs • However, restricted amounts of hydrophilic drugs, when present in high concentration or for long periods in maternal circulation, gain access to the fetus	Lipophilic drugs: imipramine, fluoxetine, progesterone, cholecalciferol, morphine (given just before delivery can reach the fetus)
Some influx transporters also operate at the placenta. The transport role is mediated by the syncytiotrophoblast	Most xenobiotics cross the placental barrier by simple diffusion; thus, it is an incomplete barrier	• P-glycoprotein (P-gp) and breast cancer resistance protein (BCRP) are the most important placental drug transporters • Substrates for P-gp: glyburide, digoxin, loperamide, ritonavir and St John's wort • Substrates for BCRP: glyburide, statins, porphyrins, methotrexate

Table 60.3 Metabolism

Enzyme	Pregnancy-induced change	Potential substrates in obstetrics
CYP3A4	Increased	Glyburide, nifedipine and indinavir
CYP2D6	Increased	Metoprolol, dextromethorphan, paroxetine, duloxetine, fluoxetine and citalopram
CYP2C9	Increased	Glyburide, NSAIDs, phenytoin and fluoxetine
CYP2C19	Decreased	Glyburide, citalopram, diazepam, omeprazole, pantoprazole and propranolol
CYP1A2	Decreased	Theophylline, clozapine, olanzapine, ondansetron
UGT1A4	Increased	Lamotrigine
UGT1A1	Increased	Paracetamol

UGT: uridine 5′-diphospho-glucuronosyltransferase; NSAIDs: nonsteroidal anti-inflammatory drugs

in the density and affinity of oxytocin receptors). Oxytocin receptors in the myometrium increase 100-fold by 32 weeks and 300-fold by term. Failed induction and postdated pregnancies are associated with a decreased concentration of oxytocin receptors. Oxytocin thus does not act as a

Table 60.4 Excretion

Physiological change of pregnancy	Pharmacokinetic consequence	Remarks/examples
GFR is 50% higher by the first trimester and continues to increase until the last week of pregnancy	If a drug is solely excreted by glomerular filtration, its renal clearance is expected to parallel changes in GFR during pregnancy	Cefazolin and clindamycin exhibit increased renal elimination during pregnancy (Feghali et al., 2015)
	Differences in secretion or reabsorption can result in differing effects on renally cleared drugs	Clearance of lithium is doubled, digoxin is 20–30% higher, atenolol is 12% higher across pregnancy (Feghali et al., 2015)

GFR: glomerular filtration rate

Table 60.5 Pharmacokinetics in lactation

Physiology	Pharmacokinetic consequence	Remarks/examples
Human milk is more acidic than plasma	Acidic drugs are ionised at plasma pH (as plasma is relatively basic) and diffuse very little across mammary epithelium; hence, chances of their elimination into breast milk are less	• Sodium/potassium salts of phenytoin, phenobarbitone and salicylate • Certain acidic drugs (although less secreted) are better avoided during lactation: sulphonamides (kernicterus, haemolysis), penicillin (allergy), ampicillin (diarrhoea)
	Basic drugs are unionised at plasma pH, diffuse across mammary epithelium and are accumulated in breast milk as they get ionised in the acidic pH of milk (called 'ion trapping'), eventually being excreted	Morphine hydrochloride, chloroquine sulphate and atropine sulphate
	Certain nonelectrolytes can pass through filtration; cause toxicity	Ethanol
	Small molecular weight electrolytes (<100 Da) can pass through filtration; cause toxicity	Lithium

labour stimulant before term, possibly due to lack of adequate oxytocin receptors.

- Drug effects on other maternal tissues (heart, lungs, kidneys, central nervous system, etc.) are not changed significantly by pregnancy.

Bibliography

Blackburn, S. T. (2012). *Maternal, Fetal, & Neonatal Physiology: A Clinical Perspective*, 4th ed., Elsevier.

Davison, J. M., Dunlop, W. (1980). Renal hemodynamics and tubular function normal human pregnancy. *Kidney Int*, **18**(2), 152–61.

Feghali, M., Venkataramanan, R., Caritis, S. (2015). Pharmacokinetics of drugs in pregnancy. *Semin Perinatol*, **39**(7), 512–19.

Katzung, B. G., ed. (2017). *Basic & Clinical Pharmacology*, 14th ed. McGraw-Hill.

Loebstein, R., Lalkin, A., Koren, G. (1997). Pharmacokinetic changes during pregnancy and their clinical relevance. *Clin Pharmacokinet*, **33**(5), 328–43.

Murphy, M.M., Scott, J. M., McPartlin, J. M., Fernandez-Ballart, J. D. (2002). The pregnancy-related decrease in fasting plasma homocysteine is not explained by folic acid supplementation, hemodilution, or a decrease in albumin in a longitudinal study. *Am J Clin Nutr*, **76**(3), 614–19.

Qasqas, S. A., McPherson, C., Frishman, W. H., Elkayam, U. (2004). Cardiovascular pharmacotherapeutic considerations during pregnancy and lactation. *Cardiol Rev*, **12**(4), 201–21.

Sharma, H. L., Sharma, K. K. (2017). *Principles of Pharmacology*, 3rd ed., Paras Medical Publisher.

Tripathi, K. D. (2013). *Essentials of Medical Pharmacology*, 7th ed., Jaypee.

Vasicka, A., Lin, T. J., Bright, R. H. (1957). Peptic ulcer and pregnancy, review of hormonal relationships and a report of one case of massive gastrointestinal hemorrhage. *Obstet Gynecol Surv*, **12**(1), 1–13.

Waldum, H. L., Straume, B. K., Lundgren, R. (1980). Serum group I pepsinogens during pregnancy. *Scand J Gastroenterol*, **15**(1), 61–3.

61 Antibiotic Prophylaxis

Vandana Tayal

Appropriately administered antibiotic prophylaxis reduces the incidence of surgical wound infection. Prophylaxis is uniformly recommended for all clean-contaminated, contaminated and dirty procedures. It is considered optional for most clean procedures, although it may be indicated for certain patients and clean procedures that fulfil specific risk criteria. Timing of antibiotic administration is critical to efficacy. The first dose should always be given before the procedure, preferably within 15–60 minutes before incision. Re-administration at one to two half-lives of the antibiotic is recommended for the duration of the procedure. In general, postoperative administration is not recommended. The duration of administration is extended only in special circumstances, such as gross contamination secondary to a ruptured viscus or severe trauma. Antibiotic selection is influenced by the organism most commonly causing wound infection in the specific procedure and by the relative costs of available agents.

1 Selection and Administration of Antibiotics

An appropriate prophylactic antibiotic should:

1. Be effective against microorganisms anticipated to cause infection
2. Achieve adequate local tissue levels
3. Cause minimal side effects
4. Be relatively inexpensive
5. Not be likely to select virulent organisms

- In general, a first-generation cephalosporin fulfils these criteria and is regarded as sufficient prophylaxis for the majority of procedures.
- Cefotaxime, ceftazidime and ceftriaxone are 'third generation' cephalosporins with greater activity than the 'second generation' cephalosporins against certain gram-negative bacteria. However, they are less active than cefuroxime against gram-positive bacteria, most notably *Staphylococcus aureus*. For procedures of the alimentary tract, genitourinary tract and hepatobiliary system, coverage should be additionally influenced by site-specific flora, such as gram-negative and anaerobic microorganisms. In such cases, a third generation cephalosporin and metronidazole is preferred.
- For coverage of gram-positive as well as gram-negative bacteria, third-generation cephalosporins are preferable. For patients with documented allergy to cephalosporins, vancomycin is a reasonable alternative for coverage of *Staphylococcus*, and metronidazole or clindamycin and an aminoglycoside may be used for coverage of anaerobic and gram-negative organisms, respectively. A quinolone, such as ciprofloxacin, may also be effective for coverage of gram-negative organisms, although data for the context of prophylaxis are not available. Aztreonam can be combined with clindamycin, but not with metronidazole in the same setting.
- For covering anaerobic organisms, metronidazole, and clindamycin are preferred.
- For *Chlamydia trachomatis*, doxycycline and azithromycin are preferred.
- For treating secondary fungal infections, systemic coverage with fluconazole or a related drug should be added.

Antibiotic prophylaxis is recommended for the following:

- All women undergoing caesarean section. The antibiotic (commonly cefuroxime) is administered immediately before knife to skin to avoid exposing the newborn to antibiotics. If the patient has a penicillin allergy, clindamycin or erythromycin can be used. Broad-spectrum antibiotics effective against endometritis and urinary tract and wound infections, which occur in about 8% of women who have had a caesarean section, should be used. Co-amoxiclav should not be given before delivery of the baby due to the risks associated with necrotising enterocolitis in the baby.

- All women undergoing an abdominal or vaginal hysterectomy.
- All women undergoing laparoscopic hysterectomy or laparoscopically assisted vaginal hysterectomy.
- If an open abdominal procedure is lengthy (e.g., >3 hours), or if the estimated blood loss is > 1500 mL, an additional dose of the prophylactic antibiotic may be given 3 to 4 hours after the initial dose.
- All women undergoing surgery for pelvic organ prolapse and/or stress urinary incontinence should receive a single dose of first-generation cephalosporin.
- All women undergoing an induced (therapeutic) surgical abortion should receive prophylactic antibiotics to reduce the risk of postabortal infection:
  - 200 mg doxycycline within two hours before the procedure, or
  - 500 mg azithromycin within two hours before the procedure
- There is no need for antibiotic prophylaxis in women undergoing HSG and known to be chalmydia negative. Women with dilated tubes found at the time of hysterosalpingography are at higher risk, and prophylactic antibiotics, for example, doxycycline or quinolones with metronidazole, should be given.
- For the reduction of infectious morbidity associated with repair of third- and fourth-degree perineal injury (cefuroxime and metronidazole, depending on local protocol).
- Manual removal of the placenta.

Antibiotic prophylaxis is not recommended for the following:

- Laparoscopic procedures that involve no direct access from the abdominal cavity to the uterine cavity or vagina.
- Hysteroscopic surgery.
- Following surgery for a missed or incomplete abortion.
- Insertion of an intrauterine device. However, healthcare professionals could consider screening for sexually transmitted infections in high-risk populations.
- There is insufficient evidence to support the use of antibiotic prophylaxis for an endometrial biopsy.
- Urodynamic studies in women at low risk, unless the incidence of urinary tract infection is >10%.
- Administration of antibiotics solely to prevent endocarditis is not recommended for patients who undergo a genitourinary procedure.
- For operative vaginal delivery.
- Postpartum dilatation and curettage, unless clinically indicated.

1.1 Special Circumstances

- For genital sepsis, it is important to cover gram-negative bacilli as well as anaerobes while awaiting culture and sensitivity reports.
- Resistant or recurrent urinary sepsis is usually treated after advice from the local microbiologist. Piperacillin/tazobactam is a combination medication containing the antibiotic, piperacillin, and the β-lactamase inhibitor, tazobactam. The combination has activity against many gram-positive and gram-negative bacteria including *Pseudomonas aeruginosa*. Another drug that may be used is secreted in urine such as fosfomycin (this is currently not licensed in the UK). Fosfomycin is a novel class of antibacterial drug with a chemical structure unrelated to other known antibiotics. It is a bactericidal drug, which disrupts cell wall synthesis by inhibiting phosphoenolpyruvate synthetase and thus interferes with the production of peptidoglycan.
- Breast abscess requires coverage against gram-positive cocci.
- For recurrent vaginitis, long-term probiotics like *Lactobacillus rhamnosus* are recommended.

Bibliography

Van Eyk, N., van Schalkwyk, J. Infectious Diseases Committee. (2012). Antibiotic prophylaxis in gynaecologic procedures. *J Obstet Gynaecol Can*, **34**(4), 382–91.

Woods, R. K., Patchen Dellinger, E. (1998). Current guidelines for antibiotic prophylaxis of surgical wounds. *Am Fam Physician*, **57**(11), 2731–40.

Drugs Used in Obstetrics and Postpartum Haemorrhage

Vandana Tayal

1 Oxytocin

A polypeptide hormone secreted from the posterior pituitary gland.

Indications

1. Induction of labour
2. Augmentation of labour
3. Reduction of postpartum bleeding: drug of choice for active management of third stage of labour
4. Reduce bleeding during miscarriage and termination of pregnancy
5. Action of oxytocin on the uterine musculature and breast

- in small doses there is increase in frequency and force of uterine contractions, similar to physiological uterine contractions
- increase in contraction is restricted to the fundus and the body of uterus: facilitates relaxation of the cervix due to fetal descent
- in the breast it causes engorgement and milk ejection
- nonpregnant uterus is resistant to its action

2 Carbetocin

A newer analogue of oxytocin.

Indications

1. Postpartum haemorrhage
2. Uterine atony

- Advantages are rapid onset and longer duration of action. The half-life is much longer (45 min) as compared to oxytocin (5 min).

2.1 Adverse effects

- Nausea, vomiting, diarrhoea, headache, hypertension and bronchospasm.

2.2 Contraindications

- Should not be used in patients with cardiovascular, pulmonary, hepatic and renal diseases.

3 Ergot Derivatives: Ergometrine and Methylergometrine

- Acts directly on myometrium and causes tonic uterine contractions of both upper and lower segment without any relaxation in between. Action is through the partial agonistic action on $5\text{-HT}_2/\alpha$-adrenergic receptors.
- Onset of action of ergometrine is quicker (45–60 s) than methylergometrine (90 s).
- Duration is similar (3 h).

Indications

1. Postpartum haemorrhage: for prevention and treatment
2. Caesarean section and instrumental delivery: in cases of uterine atony
3. The use of ergotamine in modern obstetrics is a second-line one, mainly due to the side effects

- Note: not to be used for induction of labour/abortion

3.1 Adverse drug reactions

- nausea, vomiting, headache, hypertension, blurring of vision, dizziness, seizures, retinal detachment and gangrene of toes after prolonged use.

3.2 Contraindications

- eclampsia, rhesus negative mothers, heart disease, during pregnancy and before the third stage of labour

Table 62.1 Pharmacology of oxytocin

Mechanism of action	Onset and duration of action	Side effects	Contraindications
• Mobilisation of bound intracellular calcium from sarcoplasmic reticulum to activate the contractile protein. • Oxytocin also increases local prostaglandin production	**Onset:** Immediate (IV), 3–5 min (IM) **Duration**: 1 h (IV), 2–3 h (IM)	• Safe when used judiciously • In high doses: 1. Fetal distress 2. Placental abruption 3. Rupture of the uterus 4. Water intoxication (due to its antidiuretic effect): hyponatraemia, heart failure, seizures, death 5. Hypotension (with bolus injection)	1. Unfavourable fetal positions (transverse lie, which are undeliverable without conversion prior to delivery) 2. Obstetrical emergencies 3. Fetal distress where delivery is not imminent 4. Adequate uterine activity fails to achieve satisfactory progress 5. Uterus is already hyperactive or hypertonic 6. Active herpes genitalis 7. Total placenta praevia, vasa praevia 8. Prolapse of the cord 9. Cephalopelvic disproportion

IV: intravenous; IM: intramuscular; h: hour

Oxytocin is preferred over ergometrine because:

1. Short biological half life: action can be easily terminated
2. Normal relaxation of uterus allowed: good fetal oxygenation
3. Lower segment not affected: descent free
4. More physiological action

4 Prostaglandins

Enhance uterine contractility and cause vasoconstriction.

- PGF2α (carboprost): given intramuscularly
- PGE1 (misoprostol): given by intravaginal, oral or rectal routes
- PGE2 (dinoprostone): mainly used in induction of labour (long-acting propess)

Indications

1. Induction of abortion
2. Induction/augmentation of labour
3. Control of postpartum haemorrhage

Clinical effects

- myometrial contraction
- softening and dilatation of the cervix
- inhibition of secretion of progesterone by the corpus luteum
- response of the uterus to prostaglandins is maximum in the middle trimester (thirteenth to twentieth weeks)
- prior administration of mifepristone (antiprogestin drug) sensitises the uterus to the action of prostaglandins

Adverse effects

- nausea, vomiting, diarrhoea, fever, flushing and bronchospasm
- cardiovascular side effects: tachycardia, increased mean arterial pressure and pulmonary artery pressure

Contraindications

- bronchial asthma, uterine scar, cardiac, renal or hepatic diseases

5 Drugs Used in Obstetrics

See Tables 62.2, 62.3 and 62.4.

Table 62.2 Drugs considered safe for use in obstetric patients

Drug class/condition	Safer alternative
Antiemetics (morning sickness, other types of vomiting, GORD)	Promethazine, dicyclomine, prochlorperazine, metoclopramide
Drugs for peptic ulcer disease/GORD	Ranitidine, famotidine, omeprazole, pantoprazole
Laxatives (constipation)	Dietary fibre, lactulose
Antidiarrhoeals	Oral rehydration salt
Analgesic	Paracetamol, codeine phosphate, opioid analgesics like Tramadol (reserved for severe pain)
Common-cold remedies	Xylometazoline, oxymetazoline, budesonide: all nasal drops
Antiallergics	Chlorpheniramine, promethazine
Antibacterials	Penicillin G, ampicillin, amoxicillin-clavulanate, flucloxacillin, piperacillin, cephalosporins, erythromycin
Antitubercular	Isoniazid, rifampicin, ethambutol
Antiprotozoal	Diloxanide furoate, paromomycin
Antimalarial	Chloroquine, artisunate, mefloquine, proguanil, quinine (safe only in first trimester), pyrimethamine plus sulphadoxine (only single dose)
Antihelminthic	Piperazine, praziquantel, niclosamide
Antifungal	Clotrimazole, nystatin, tolnaftate: all topical
Antiretroviral	Zidovudine, lamivudine, nevirapine, nelfinavir, saquinavir
Antihypertensives	Methyldopa, hydralazine, labetalol, atenolol, metoprolol, nifedipine
Haematinics	Oral iron salts, iron dextran, folic acid, cyanocobalamin
Antidiabetics	Insulin, metformin, glyburide
Corticosteroids	Inhaled/topical corticosteroids, oral prednisolone (low dose)
Thyroid hormone	Levothyroxine
Antithyroid drugs	Propylthiouracil
Antipsychotics	Haloperidol, trifluoperazine
Antidepressants	Amitriptyline, imipramine, SSRIs (fluoxitine, sertraline, citalopram)
Anticoagulants	Heparin (unfractionated/ LMWH)
Anti-asthmatics	Salbutamol/salmeterol, ipratropium bromide, beclomethasone, budesonide, sodium cromoglycate: all inhaled

GORD: gastro-oesophageal reflux disease; LMWH: low molecular weight heparin; SSRI: selective serotonin receptor inhibitor

Table 62.3 Antibiotics, their modes of action and important side effects

	Antibiotic	Mode of action	Static/cidal	Adverse effects
1	Penicillins (ampicillin, ticarcillin and clavulanic acid)	Inhibits cell wall synthesis	Bactericidal	Hypersensitivity reactions
2	• Cephalosporins • Cephamycins	Inhibits cell wall synthesis	Bactericidal	Hypersensitivity, diarrhoea, mild liver function test abnormalities and neutropenia
3	Monobactams (aztreonam)	Inhibits cell wall synthesis	Bactericidal	Rashes and transaminase elevations
4	Carbapenems (imipenem)	Inhibits cell wall synthesis	Bactericidal	Hypersensitivity reactions, nausea and phlebitis
5	Vancomycin	Inhibits cell wall synthesis	Bactericidal	Rapid infusion may cause flushing of the upper body (called 'red neck' or 'red-man syndrome')
6	• Amphotericin B • Colistin • Nystatin • Polymyxin B	Damages fungal cell membranes	Fungicidal	Acute reactions including fever, shaking chills, hypotension, nephrotoxicity
7	Aminoglycosides (streptomycin, gentamicin, tobramycin, kanamycin, amikacin, and netilmicin)	Inhibits protein synthesis through 30S subunit of ribosomes	Bactericidal	Nephrotoxicity, ototoxicity and neuromuscular blockade
8	Macrolides (erythromycin, azithromycin, clindamycin)	Inhibits protein synthesis through 50S subunit of ribosomes	Bacteriostatic	Gastrointestinal upset, pain at injection sites, hypersensitivity reactions, headache, dizziness, mild liver function abnormalities
9	Sulphonamides (sulfisoxazole, combination of trimethoprim/ sulfamethoxazole)	Interferes with bacterial synthesis of folate	bacteriostatic	Neonatal hyperbilirubinaemia with kernicterus, hemolytic anaemia in G6PD deficiency, skin rashes
10	Fluoroquinolones (norfloxacin, ciprofloxacin, ofloxacin)	Damages DNA	Bactericidal	Pain, burning, tingling, numbness, weakness; symptoms affecting tendons, muscles and joints, including swelling, pain and tendon rupture
11	Metronidazole	Inhibits nucleic acid synthesis by disrupting the DNA of microbial cells	Bactericidal	Gastrointestinal upset, metallic taste, headache, vertigo, disulfiram-like reaction to alcohol

Table 62.4 Mode of action and drug interactions of different antihypertensives and antiepileptics

		Mode of action	Drug interaction
A	**Antiepileptics**		
1	Lamotrigine	Selectively binds sodium channels, stabilising presynaptic neuronal membranes and inhibiting glutamate release	• Antidepressants and antipsychotics (chlorpromazine, clomipramine, sertraline); increases the serum concentration • Oral contraceptives induce metabolism and reduce serum concentrations
2	Levetiracetam	Modulation of synaptic neurotransmitter release through binding to the synaptic vesicle protein SV2A in the brain	-
3	Gabapentin	Inhibition of the alpha 2-delta subunit of voltage-gated calcium channels	Antacids decrease absorption
4	Clonazepam	Facilitates GABAergic transmission in the brain, inhibition of neuronal firing	Antihistamines, central-nervous-system depressants, alcohol, lamotrigine; increase dizziness, drowsiness, confusion and difficulty concentrating
B	**Antihypertensives**		
1	Methyldopa	**Alpha**-2 adrenergic receptor agonist, stimulates the brain to decrease the activity of the sympathetic nervous system	• Absorption of methyldopa is decreased by iron products (such as ferrous sulphate, ferrous gluconate) • Symptoms of lithium toxicity when given with lithium • Hypertensive crisis with mono amine oxidase (MAO) inhibitors • Increase in drowsiness with sedatives, antihistamines, muscle relaxants
2	Clonidine	**Alpha**-2 adrenergic receptor agonist; stimulates the brain to decrease the activity of the sympathetic nervous system	• Increase in drowsiness with sedatives, antihistamines, antidepressants and muscle relaxants • The hypotensive effect of clonidine may be reduced with tricyclic antidepressants • Slow heartbeat, headaches, dizziness (sinus bradycardia) with beta blockers such as acebutolol, atenolol and calcium channel blockers, including amlodipine and diltiazem
3	Hydralazine	Peripheral vasodilating effect through a direct relaxation of vascular smooth muscle	• Hypotension with MAO inhibitors • Aspirin/NSAIDs decrease the hypotensive effects
4	Nifedipine	Calcium channel blockers; cause peripheral arterial vasodilation	• CYP3A inducers such as rifampin reduce the bioavailability and efficacy of nifedipine • Potentiation of the antihypertensive action and neuromuscular blockade of magnesium sulphate • Aspirin/NSAIDs decrease the hypotensive effects
5	Labetalol, atenolol, metoprolol	• Beta blockers: block peripheral sympathetic nervous system activity, decreased peripheral vascular resistance • Labetalol in addition has alpha blocking activity	• Aspirin/NSAIDs decrease the hypotensive effects • Increase the risk of hypoglycaemia with sulfonylureas • Ampicillin and rifampicin decrease the hypotensive effects • MAO inhibitors can cause rebound hypertension on withdrawal of beta blockers

SV2A: Synaptic vesicle glycoprotein 2A; GABA: γ-aminobutyric acid; MAO inhibitor: monoamine oxidase inhibitors

Pain Relief in Labour and Puerperium

Bhupinder Kalra and Vandana Tayal

In at-risk pregnancies, due to fetal, obstetric or maternal factors, analgesia is mandatory and always required. For women who request pain relief for labour and/or delivery, there are many effective analgesic techniques available. The primary goal is to provide an adequate maternal analgesia with minimal motor block (e.g., achieved with the administration of local anaesthetics at low concentrations with or without opioids).

1 Systemic Analgesia

Analgesia during labour can be administered through a systemic or regional route.

1. Systemic analgesia is effective, but there is a risk of affecting uteroplacental blood flow and the fetus. It includes the following:
   a. Gaseous drugs like 50% nitrous oxide (N_2O) in oxygen and sevoflurane. Currently, sevoflurane is not part of clinical practice, whereas N_2O is being widely used for labour analgesia. These drugs have rapid onset of action and rapid elimination with minimal metabolism in the body. Adverse effects like vertigo, nausea and drowsiness may occur with its use.
   b. Opioids like morphine and pethidine were widely used, but with the availability of fentanyl and remifentanil, their use in obstetric analgesia is less popular, although they are still used. The problem with morphine and pethidine are difficulty in dose titration and altered cardiorespiratory physiology in the neonate.

1. Fentanyl is a highly lipid-soluble synthetic opioid more potent than morphine and pethidine. It has a short duration of action and rapid onset.
2. Patient-controlled intravenous analgesia (PCA) may be used if regional analgesia is contraindicated. Remifentanil PCA is used for labour. Since there is a risk of respiratory depression and sedation, it is recommended that pulse oximetry and the continuous presence of trained personnel should be available.
3. Diamorphine, a more potent drug than pethidine, is increasingly used for labour analgesia in the UK. It is administered intramuscularly in the dose of 5–7.5 mg. See Table 63.1.

2 Regional Analgesia

- Neuraxial blockade (epidural or intrathecal) provides the most effective form of pain relief in labour. Low-dose epidurals combining the local anaesthetic (bupivacaine, 2–2.5 mg) with an opioid (commonly fentanyl 15–25 μg) and using a combined spinal epidural (CSE) technique is presently being practised.
- Advantages of CSE are fast onset of action (1–5 min), minimal observable leg weakness, markedly reduced failure rate and low incidence of postpuncture headache and hypotension. CSE provides the advantages of a spinal (speed of onset) with the ability to prolong labour analgesia with an epidural catheter.
- Adverse effects of regional analgesia include increased use of urinary catheterisation, maternal fever (noninfective) and pruritus due to neuraxial opioids.

The main contraindications for epidural analgesia are:

- coagulations disorders
- local or systemic sepsis
- hypovolaemia
- lack of trained staff
- severe back deformity

3 Patient controlled anaesthesia

If regional analgesia is unavailable or contraindicated, then PCA is a useful method of pain control if the equipment and staffing are available. Many opioids

Table 63.1 Drugs used in labour analgesia

Drug	Dose/route of administration	Onset of action	Duration of action	Adverse effects	Remarks
Morphine	5-20 mg: IM, IV every 4 h	20–60 min	4–5 h	Neonatal respiratory depressive effects	Use lower dose in patients with asthma
Pethidine	100–150 mg (IM), 25–50 mg (IV) every 4 h	1–15 min	2–3 h	• Maternal sedation, vomiting and nausea, constipation and neonatal respiratory depression • Affects newborn neuroadaptive score and breastfeeding behaviour	• Accumulation of active metabolite leading to CNS toxicity • Pethidine is contraindicated in patients with renal dysfunction
Fentanyl	0.025–0.05 mg IV	3–5 min	30–60 min	Maternal sedation, nausea, vomiting, decreased gastrointestinal motility	Low placental transfer; low fetal plasma levels and lacks active metabolite like pethidine
Remifentanil	PCA with varying doses	0.5–1 min	20 min	Potent maternal respiratory depressant	Dose at beginning of uterine contraction
Butorphanol	IV: 1–2 mg every 3–4 h IM: 1–2 mg every 3–4 h	IV: 2–3 min IM: 10–20 min	4–6 h	Nausea, confusion, sedation, incidence of constipation is less	Maternal ceiling effect on respiratory depression and analgesia
Naloxone	0.1 mg/kg, IV	2 min	20–60 min		For reversal of respiratory depression induced by opioids

IM: intramuscular; IV: intravenous; CNS: central nervous system have been used in PCA devices: drugs currently used include fentanyl and, more recently, remifentanil, which is an ultra-short-acting opioid, is rapidly hydrolysed by blood and tissue esterases and does not accumulate even after prolonged infusions.

4 Nonpharmacological Methods

Transcutaneous electrical nerve stimulation, continuous support in labour, touch and massage, water bath, intradermal sterile water injections, acupuncture and hypnosis may all be beneficial for the management of pain during labour. See Chapter 52.

5 Pain relief in puerperium

- Paracetamol and codeine
- Nonsteroidal anti-inflammatory drugs (NSAIDS) are avoided, especially when there has been significant bleeding, or in women with asthma.
- Morphine

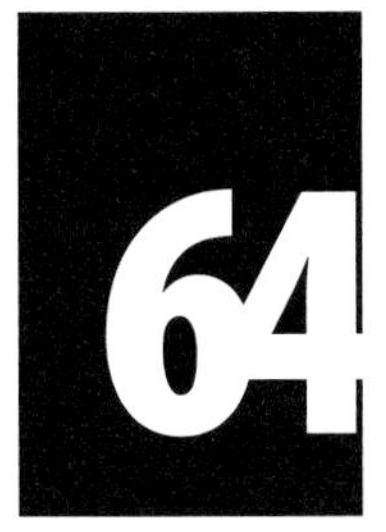

64 Contraception and Drugs Used in Gynaecology

Siddharth Dutta and Vandana Tayal

1 Contraception

There are various options available for contraception (see Table 64.1).

1. **Oral contraceptives:**
   a. **Monophasic**: no phasic increase or decrease in estrogen/progesterone content over 21 days
   Started on day 5 of menstrual period; taken for 21 days; then 7 days' pill-free period
   b. **Biphasic**: fixed dose estrogen plus two-phase doses of progesterone (day 1–10 lower dose and day 11–21 higher dose)
   c. **Triphasic**: mimics the hormonal changes during the menstrual cycle as physiologically as possible: slightly higher dose of estrogen near midcycle plus increased dose of progesterone in three successive phases – see Table 64.1
   d. **Quadriphasic**: more physiological since they simulate the woman's natural cycle – see Table 64.2
   - estrogen–estradiol valerate (E2V) along with newer progestin (dienogest: DNG) is used
   - Step-down doses of estrogen and step-up doses of progestin preparation are used
   - 26/2 regimen, which provides reliable contraception together with a good bleeding profile
   - See Table 64.2.

   e. **Extended cycle oral contraceptive pill (OCP)**: newer extended-cycle regimens involve taking active pills continuously for one year and can stop all menstrual bleeding. This can be for 84 days or continuous (365 days) used for menstrual suppression, endometriosis and dysmenorrhoea
   f. **Daily progestin tablet**: examples are norethindrone 0.35 mg, norgestrel 0.075 mg daily and desogestrel 0.075 mg daily

   Started on fifth day of menstruation normally
   Desogestrel pill has a 12 h window
   Strict compliance is needed (<3 h window)

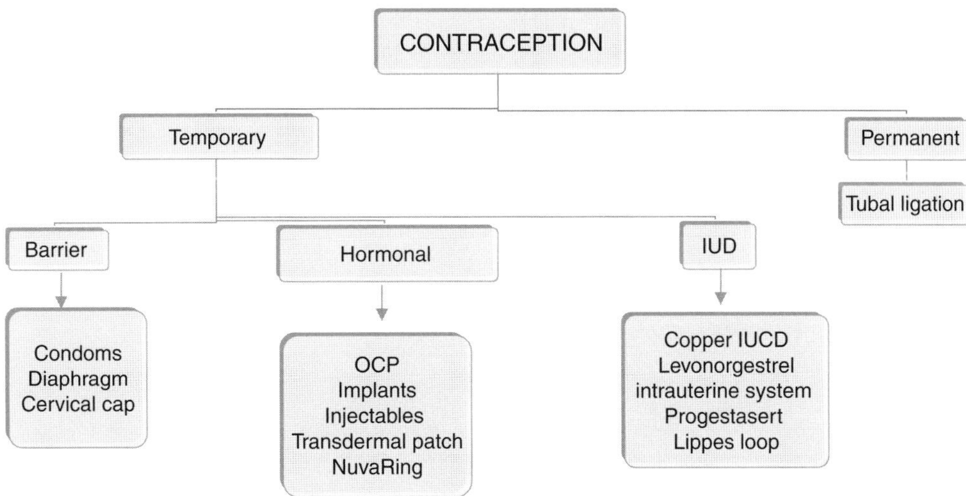

Figure 64.1 Contraceptive options.

Can be used in postpartum period and soon after miscarriage and termination

Can be used during lactation

2. **Contraceptive transdermal patch**: estrogen plus progesterone: to apply one patch per week
3. **Implantable progestin**: Implanon/Norplant: subcutaneous implantation
4. **Intrauterine device (IUD)**: Nonhormonal (copper IUCD) and hormonal (progesterone)
5. **Injectable progestin**: depot medroxyprogesterone acetate (DMPA), norethindrone enanthate (NET-EN)
6. **Vaginal ring (NuvaRing)**: used for 21 days in a cycle, removed and a new one inserted on day 5 of menstruation.
7. Emergency contraception for unprotected sexual intercourse (UPSI):
   a. Levonorgestrel: 0.75 mg, two doses 12 hours apart, or 1.5 mg single dose taken as soon as possible, but before 72 hours of unprotected intercourse
   b. Levonorgestrel: 0.5 mg plus ethinylestradiol, 0.1 mg, two doses at 12-hour intervals within 72 hours of exposure
   c. Ulipristal: 30 mg single dose as soon as possible, but within 120 hours of intercourse
   d. Mifepristone: 600 mg single dose taken within 72 hours of intercourse
   e. Copper IUCD: within 5 days of UPSI
8. Contraceptives in development:
   a. Nestorone gel: applied daily
   b. Nestorone (NES): metered dose transdermal system
   c. Cyclofem: monthly injectables
   d. C31G Glyminox 1% gel: vaginal microbicide (carrageenan, beta-cyclodextrin) contraceptive along with spermicidal agent (nonoxynol-9)

- Mild adverse effects: no need to withdraw (see Table 64.3)
- Moderate adverse effects: may warrant discontinuation
- Severe adverse effect: needs stoppage immediately

2 Drugs that Modulate estrogen Function

Selective estrogen receptor modulators (SERMs)

- Tissue-selective actions: beneficial effects on bone, brain and liver; and prevents detrimental effects on uterus and breast

Table 64.1 Dosing of estrogen and progesterone in triphasic contraceptive pills

Type	estrogen	Progesterone
Triphasic	EE: 30 µg (D1–6)	Levonorgestrel 50 µg
	EE: 40 µg (D7–11)	Levonorgestrel 75 µg
	EE: 30 µg (D12–21)	Levonorgestrel 125 µg

EE: ethinyl estradiol; D: day

Table 64.2 Dosage of estrogen and progesterone in quadriphasic contraceptive pills

Type	Days	E2V	DNG
Quadriphasic	1–2	3 mg	
	3–7	2 mg	2 mg
	8–24	2 mg	3 mg
	25–26	1 mg	
	27–28	Placebo	

Table 64.3 Adverse effects of hormonal contraceptives

	Mild	Moderate	Severe
estrogen	• Nausea, vomiting, breast tenderness, mild oedema, migraine	• Vertigo, leg and uterine cramps, diabetes mellitus	• Thromboembolism, cholestatic jaundice, cholelithiasis, hepatic adenoma
Progesterone	• Increased appetite, weight gain, acne, hirsutism, decrease in libido, increased body temperature	• Breakthrough bleeding, monilial vaginitis, amenorrhea	• Myocardial infarction, cerebrovascular thrombosis • Depression

- ◦ Clomifene: facilitates ovulation and treats infertility
- ◦ Tamoxifen, droloxifene, toremifene: treatment of breast carcinoma; increase the risk of endometrial carcinoma and thromboembolism
- ◦ Raloxifene and bazedoxifene: used for postmenopausal osteoporosis; increased risk of thromboembolism
- ◦ Ormeloxifene: approved for dysfunctional uterine bleeding

Selective estrogen receptor (ER) downregulator

- Fulvestrant: pure estrogen antagonist. Inhibits ER dimerisation and prevents ER interaction with DNA. Used for metastatic ER-positive breast cancer in postmenopausal women.

Selective tissue estrogen activity regulators (STEARs)

- Tibolone-estrogenic, progestogenic and weak androgenic property
- Tissue selective mode of action (no endometrial stimulation is noted)
- Alternative to HRT: used in decreasing vasomotor symptoms and postmenopausal osteoporosis

Aromatase Inhibitors

- Blocks the conversion of testosterone to estradiol
  - ◦ Type 1: steroidal/irreversible inhibitors: formestane, exemestane
  - ◦ Type 2: nonsteroidal/reversible: anastrozole, letrozole, fadrozole, vorozole
- Used in ER+ breast cancer; resistant to tamoxifen and precocious puberty

3 Drugs that Modulate Progesterone Function

Progesterone receptor blockers

- Mifepristone: also has antiandrogenic and anti-glucocorticoid activity used for medical termination of pregnancy, emergency contraception, fibroids and endometriosis, and treatment of Cushing's syndrome for patients with ectopic adrenocorticotropic hormone secretion
- Onapristone: pure progesterone receptor antagonist is used for the treatment of endometrial, breast and ovarian cancer. It is also undergoing trials for treatment of prostate cancer.
- Gestrinone: also has androgenic and antiestrogenic activity
  - ◦ Approved to treat endometriosis
  - ◦ Also used for treating fibroids and abnormal uterine bleeding

Selective progesterone receptor modulators (SPRMs)

- A mixed profile of action.
- Leads to stimulation or inhibition in tissue-specific manner; agonist in some tissues, while antagonist in others.
- Asoprisnil: first SPRM that was developed for treatment of uterine fibroids, but due to risk of endometrial changes, development was stopped.
- Ulipristal: approved for treating uterine fibroids, endometriosis and emergency contraceptive; risk of hepatotoxicity has been observed. At the time of writing, there are restrictions on the use of ullipristal acetate for fibroids. It has been temporarily withdrawn from the market in the UK due to liver damage.

Table 64.4 Urogynaecology drugs

	Urogynaecological drugs	Mode of action	Adverse effects	Interactions
1	Mirabegron	Selective agonist for beta-3 adrenergic receptors; relaxes the detrusor smooth muscle to allow for a larger bladder capacity	Increased blood pressure, tachycardia, headache, dizziness, urinary retention	• Mild prolongation of Q-T interval with sotalol, erythromycin, clarithromycin, haloperidol • Increased levels of drugs metabolised by CYP2D6 such as thioridazine, flecainide, propafenone, desipramine, metoprolol
2	Oxybutynin	Tertiary amine anticholinergic drug, which exerts antimuscarinic, as well as direct antispasmodic action on smooth muscle	Dry mouth, constipation, tiredness, headache, urinary tract infections, blurred vision and difficulty in micturating	• Increased frequency and/or severity of anticholinergic side effects such as dry mouth, constipation, confusion, blurred vision, urinary retention and an increased heart rate, with drugs having anticholinergic effects (diphenhydramine, dimenhydrinate, scopolamine, benztropine, disopyramide, thioridazine, amitriptyline)
3	Tolterodine	Competitive muscarinic receptor antagonist	Dry mouth, constipation, tiredness, headache, urinary tract infections, blurred vision, difficulty urinating, allergic reaction, hallucinations	• Increased frequency and/or severity of anticholinergic side effects with drugs having anticholinergic effects • Prolongation of Q-T interval with sotalol, erythromycin, amiodarone, dofetilide

Table 64.4 (cont.)

4	Darifenacin	Selective antagonist of the M3 receptor (the major subtype that modulates urinary bladder muscle contraction)	Dry mouth, constipation, tiredness, headache, urinary tract infections and difficulty urinating	• Increased levels when co-administered with potent CYP3A4 inhibitors (e.g., ketoconazole, itraconazole, ritonavir, nelfinavir, clarithromycin and nefazadone) • Increased frequency and/or severity of anticholinergic side effects with drugs having anticholinergic effects
5	Propiverine	Anticholinergic drug, which exerts antimuscarinic as well as direct antispasmodic action on smooth muscle by modulating calcium influx	Dry mouth, headache, accommodation disorder, constipation, abdominal pain, dyspepsia, fatigue, restlessness, dizziness, vertigo	• The risk or severity of hypotension can be increased when propiverine is combined with amiodarone • Amisulpride may increase the central nervous system (CNS) depressant activities of propiverine

4 Drugs Used in Urogynaecology

See Table 64.4.

5 Newer Drugs such as DHEA used in Vulvovaginal Atrophy

Treatment for vulvar-vaginal irritation and pelvic support issues has been traditionally limited to lubricating creams and over-the-counter options, herbal therapies, estrogen therapies and other prescriptions, Kegel/pelvic-strengthening exercise and surgery.

Dehydroepiandrosterone (DHEA) is an androgen-like testosterone. Androgens are important to the integrity of skin, muscle and bone (in both males and women) and have a role in maintaining libido.

DHEA can be introduced vaginally or through topical application around the vulva. It is an inactive precursor, which leads to the production of active sex hormones like androgens or estrogens in specific cells and tissues.

Topical DHEA has been found to have favourable effects on skin health and appearance due to the production of collagen. If DHEA is delivered directly to the vagina (6.5 mg), the tissues transform DHEA to the estrogen, estradiol. This natural production of estradiol occurs without a significant release of estrogens systemically in the blood.

In November 2016, the US Food and Drug Administration (FDA) approved the first product containing the active ingredient prasterone, also known as DHEA.

The research surrounding vaginally applied DHEA has shown it to:

- Reduce vaginal dryness and irritation
- Strengthen vaginal musculature
- Increase bone mineral density
- Decrease pain during intercourse
- Increase arousal and libido, as well as sexual satisfaction

Prasterone seems to be very safe. The endometrium is not affected by DHEA because the enzymes required to transform DHEA into estrogens are absent in the endometrium. Although no systemic increase of estrogen level has been reported, a history of breast cancer remains a contraindication.

6 Bioidentical Hormones

Bioidentical hormones are artificial hormones derived from plant estrogens (chemically synthesised), which have exactly the same chemical and molecular structure as hormones that are produced in the human body (US Endocrine Society definition). estrogen, progesterone and testosterone are among those most commonly replicated and used in treatment.

17β-estradiol is by far the most studied bioidentical estrogen. It is approved by the FDA for the management of many menopausal symptoms, vulvar or vaginal atrophy, hypestrogenism, prostate cancer, prevention of osteoporosis and palliation in metastatic breast cancer.

Two branded forms of bioidentical progesterone are approved by the FDA. The first, crinone, was approved in 1997 and is used for luteal phase support during in vitro fertilisation. The second, prometrium, was approved in 1998 for relief of postmenopausal symptoms and for the prevention of endometrial hyperplasia.

The use of testosterone in women has been controversial. Although a variety of testosterone products are approved by the FDA, they are approved for use in women only for the palliative treatment of metastatic breast cancer and, with two branded formulations combined with estrogen, for the treatment of menopausal vasomotor symptoms.

Though bioidentical hormone therapy offers a favourable adverse-effect profile over conventional hormone replacement therapy, and is equally effective in managing menopausal symptoms, long-term studies are needed to assess the safe duration of use of all bioidentical hormone therapy.

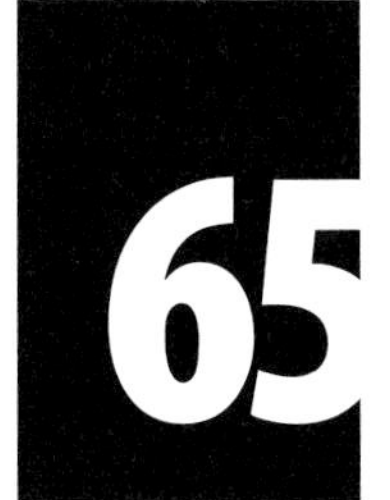

Teratogenic Drugs

Sahil Kumar and Vandana Tayal

Teratogenicity: the capacity of a drug to cause fetal abnormalities when administered to a pregnant mother.

To be considered teratogenic, a candidate substance should:

1. Result in a characteristic set of malformations, indicating selectivity for certain target organs
2. Exert its effects at a particular stage of fetal development; for example, during the limited time period of organogenesis of the target organs
3. Show a dose-dependent incidence

- The thalidomide disaster (1958–61) focused attention onto the teratogenic potential of drugs.

Drugs can affect the fetus in three stages:

1. **Fertilisation and implantation**: conception to 17 days: failure of pregnancy, often goes unnoticed
2. **Organogenesis**: 18 to 55 days of gestation: most vulnerable period; deformities produced
3. **Growth and development**: 56 days onwards: developmental and functional abnormalities; for example, ACE inhibitors can cause hypoplasia of lungs and kidneys; androgens and progestins cause masculinisation of female fetus; anti-thyroid drugs and lithium can cause fetal goitre

- The type of malformation depends on the drug as well as the stage at which exposure to the teratogen occurred. fetal exposure depends on the blood level and duration for which the drug remains in maternal circulation.
- The teratogenic potential is to be considered against the background of congenital abnormalities occurring spontaneously, which is ~2% of all pregnancies. Some drugs have been clearly associated with causing fetal abnormalities in human beings. See Table 65.1.
- The US Food and Drug Administration (FDA) has attempted to quantify teratogenic risk into five categories, from A (safe) to X (definite human teratogenic risk). This system has been criticised as inaccurate and impractical, and not adequately updated. See Table 65.2.
- Presently the US FDA is changing its system from the A, B, C grading system to narrative statements, which will summarise evidence-based knowledge about each drug in terms of fetal risk and safety.
- Frequency of spontaneous, as well as drug-induced, malformations, especially neural tube defects, may be reduced by folate therapy during pregnancy.

The mechanisms by which different drugs produce teratogenic effects are poorly understood and are probably multifactorial:

1. There may be a direct effect on maternal tissues with secondary effects on fetal tissues.
2. Drugs may interfere with the passage of oxygen or nutrients through the placenta and therefore have effects on the most rapidly metabolising tissues of the fetus.
3. There may be direct actions on the processes of differentiation in developing tissues. For example, vitamin A (retinol) has been shown to have important differentiation-directing actions in normal tissues. Several vitamin A analogues (isotretinoin, etretinate) are powerful teratogens, suggesting that they alter the normal processes of differentiation.
4. Deficiency of a critical substance. For example, folic acid supplementation during pregnancy appears to reduce the incidence of neural tube defects (e.g., spina bifida).

Table 65.1 Teratogenic drugs

Drug	Trimester	Effect
ACE inhibitors	All	Renal damage
Androgens	Second, third	Masculinisation of female fetus
Antidepressants, tricyclic	Third	Neonatal withdrawal symptoms have been reported in a few cases with clomipramine, desipramine and imipramine
Barbiturates	All	Chronic use can lead to neonatal dependence
Carbamazepine	First	Neural tube defects
Cocaine	All	Increased risk of spontaneous abortion, abruptio placentae and premature labour; neonatal cerebral infarction, abnormal development and decreased school performance
Diazepam	All	Chronic use may lead to neonatal dependence
Diethylstilbestrol	All	Vaginal adenosis, clear cell vaginal adenocarcinoma
Ethanol	All	Risk of fetal alcohol syndrome and alcohol-related neurodevelopmental defects
Isotretinoin	All	Extremely high risk of CNS, face, ear, other malformations
Lithium	First	Ebstein's anomaly
Methadone	All	Chronic use leads to neonatal dependence
Methotrexate	First	Multiple congenital malformations
Methylthiouracil	All	Hypothyroidism
Metronidazole	First	May be mutagenic (from animal studies; there is no evidence for teratogenic effects in humans)
Misoprostol	First	Möbius sequence
Mycophenolate mofetil	First	Major malformations of the face, limbs and other organs
Phencyclidine	All	Abnormal neurologic examination, poor suck reflex, poor suck reflex and feeding
Phenytoin	All	fetal hydantoin syndrome
Propylthiouracil	All	Congenital goitre
Smoking	All	IUGR, prematurity, sudden infant death syndrome, perinatal complications
Streptomycin	All	Eighth nerve toxicity
Tamoxifen	All	Increased risk of spontaneous abortion or fetal damage
Tetracycline	All	Discoloration and defects of teeth, altered bone growth
Thalidomide	First	Phocomelia (seal limbs: shortened or absent long bones of the limbs) and many internal malformations
Valproic acid	All	Neural tube defects, cardiac and limb malformations
Warfarin	First Second Third	Hypoplastic nasal bridge, chondrodysplasia CNS malformations Risk of bleeding; discontinue use one month before delivery

CNS: central nervous system; IUGR: intrauterine growth restriction

Bibliography

Katzung, B. G., ed. (2017). *Basic & Clinical Pharmacology*, 14th ed., McGraw-Hill.

Tripathi, K. D. (2013). *Essentials of Medical Pharmacology*, 7th ed., Jaypee.

Table 65.2 Teratogenic risk categories of drugs by the FDA

FDA category	Description	Example
A	Well-controlled studies in humans show no risk to the fetus	Folate, $MgSO_4$, levothyroxine, niacin
B	No well-controlled studies in humans; animal studies show no risk to the fetus	Penicillin V, amoxicillin, metronidazole, cefotaxime, erythromycin, paracetamol, lignocaine, ondansetron
C	No well-controlled studies in humans; animal studies have demonstrated an A/E to the fetus; caution advised	Morphine, codeine, atropine, corticosteroids, adrenaline, thiopentone, bupivacaine, albuterol, sertraline, fluoroquinolones
D	Positive evidence of risk; in some cases benefits may outweigh risks	Full-dose aspirin, paroxetine, phenytoin, carbamazepine, valproate, lorazepam
X	Absolutely contraindicated in pregnancy	Methotrexate, estrogens, ACEi, thalidomide, isotretinoin

A/E: adverse effect; Inj.: injectable; MgSO4: magnesium sulphate; ACEi: ACE inhibitor

Section 10

Microbiology

Neela Mukhopadhaya

Infections in Pregnancy and Fetal Impact of Maternal Infection

Tanuja Mokashi

1 Bacterial Infections

See Figure 66.1 for the classification of different microorganisms.

1.1 Bacteria

- prokaryotic (no membrane bound organelles)
- have cell membrane and cell wall
- classified in three groups depending on staining properties – see Table 66.1

Gram-positive bacteria: stain blue due to peptidoglycan – see Figure 66.2

- gram-negative bacteria: stain pink (thin cell wall, consists of outer layer of lipo polysacharide (LPS), and periplasmic layer contains β-lactamase)

1.2 Encapsulated Bacteria or Polyosides

- The polysaccharide capsule that surrounds bacterial species such as *Haemophilus influenzae*, *Streptococcus pneumoniae*, *Neisseria meningitidis* and *Salmonella typhi* is a potent virulence factor by protecting the bacteria from phagocytosis.
- The host responds with antibody production and specific antibodies plus complement binding to the capsule facilitate opsonisation of the microorganism, which is phagocytised and eliminated.
- In conditions such as sickle cell disease that are hyposplenic, there is an increased risk of infections with encapsulated bacteria. See Table 66.2.

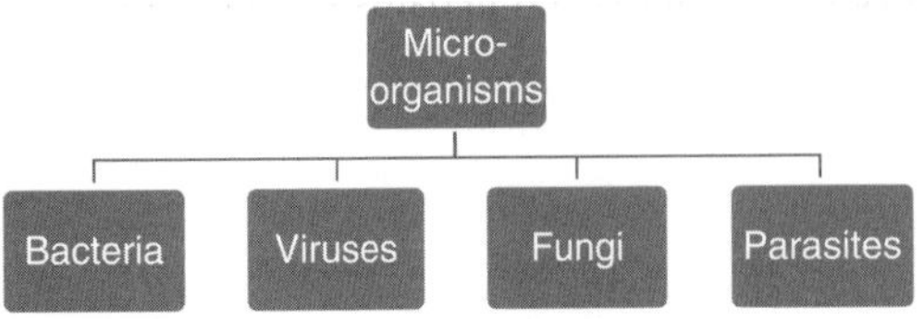

Figure 66.1 Classification of microorganisms.

1.3 Bacterial Toxins

1. Endotoxins:
   - feature of gram-negative bacteria
   - released on cell death/lysis
2. Exotoxins:
   - secreted by organisms
   - feature of gram positive and negative organisms
   - form toxoids

1.4 *Streptococcus*

- Facultative anaerobes
- Form chains
- Divided in three groups:
  1. β-haemolytic: cause complete haemolysis of red cells in agar. Group A, C, G (associated with toxic shock syndrome, necrotising fasciitis, vaginitis), Gr B (can cause chorioamnionitis, neonatal sepsis, endometritis), Gr F (can cause abscesses).
  2. α-haemolytic: cause partial haemolysis of red cells causing green/brown discoloration. Examples are *S. viridans* and *Enterococcus, pneumococcus.*
  3. γ-haemolytic: nonhaemolytic. An example is *Enterococcus faecalis* (Group D).

1.5 Group B *Streptococcus* (GBS)

- *S. agalactia*
- found in 20–35% of pregnant women
- maternal to fetal transmission rate: 80%
- invasive neonatal disease 1:2000 births
- early-onset GBS causes neonatal mortality in 6%

Table 66.1 Groups of bacteria

Gram stainable	Acid fast	Nonstainable/unusual
• Gram positive; e.g., *Staphylococci, Streptococci* • Gram negative; e.g., *Escherichia coli, Klebsiella* • Gram variable; e.g., *Gardnerella vaginalis*	• Cell wall has high lipid content, difficult to stain; e.g., *Mycobacterium*	• Have no peptidoglycans; e.g., *Chlamydia*

Table 66.2 Encapsulated bacteria

Cocci	Bacilli	Spirochaetes	Vibrio
• *Neisseria gonorrhoeae* • *Neisseria meningitidis* • *Moraxella catarrhalis*	• *Haemophilus influenzae* • *Klebsiella pneumoniae* • *Legionella*	• *Leptospira* • *Borrelia* • *Treponema*	• *Cholera*

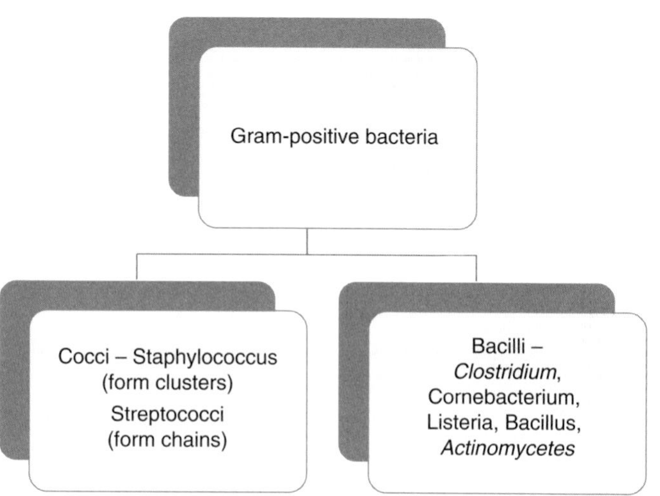

Figure 66.2 Gram-positive bacteria.

- indications for GBS prophylaxis in labour:
  - previous baby affected with GBS
  - GBS urinary tract infection (UTI) in current pregnancy
  - positive vaginal swab for GBS in current pregnancy
  - preterm labour <37 weeks of gestation irrespective of carrier state
- no routine testing for all women for GBS recommended
- treatment:
  - benzyl penicillin 3 g IV loading dose followed by 1.5 g every 4 hours until delivery
  - clindamycin 900 mg IV every eight hours if penicillin allergic

1.6 *Streptococcus pneumoniae*

- forms pairs
- it is optochin sensitive
- it is bile soluble
- causes: meningitis, pneumonia and primary bacterial peritonitis

1.7 *Listeria monocytogenes*

- causes: meningitis and hepatosplenomegaly (listeriosis)
- transmission of infection:
  - contaminated food
  - from mother to fetus: transplacental transfer and ascending infection

- fetal mortality rate: about 50%
- treatment:
  - amoxycillin
  - gentamicin if penicillin sensitive

1.8 *Staphylococcus aureus*

- gram-positive, facultative anaerobe
- *S. aureus* (30% of population can be nasal carriers with no symptoms) potential pathogen: produces coagulase; causes serum to clot
- *S. epidermidis* (skin): less virulent, does not produce coagulase (coagulase negative staphylococci)
- grape-like bunches
- causes:
  - toxic shock syndrome in tampon users; systemic infection by staphylococcal toxin
  - scalded skin syndrome
  - cellulitis, boils and surgical-site wound infection
  - bacteraemia, endocarditis and osteomyelitis
- treatment: most resistant to penicillin due to beta-lactamase production; can be treated with flucloxacillin: not degraded by beta-lactamase
- methicillin-resistant *S. aureus*: cause of severe infection in postoperative patients; have a mutant penicillin-binding protein in cell wall; can be treated with vancomycin

2 Sexually Transmitted Infections

2.1 *Actinomycetes israelii*

- anaerobic bacillus, nonacid fast
- can cause ascending infection in women with intrauterine contraceptive device devices
- causes granulomatous lesions; pus contains sulphur granules
- treatment: penicillin; may need long-term treatment

2.2 *Neisseria*

- Diplococci, aerobic, gram negative.
- Oxidase positive.
- *N. meningitidis:* causes meningitis; spread by respiratory droplets and saliva. Serogroups based on capsular polysaccharide: A, B and C most common. MenC vaccine widely used in the UK. Penicillin sensitive: drug of choice.
- *N. gonorrhoeae:*
  - causes gonorrhoea
  - infects mucus membranes (endocervix, urethra, rectum, pharynx, conjunctiva), causes pelvic inflammatory disease (PID)
  - ophthalmia neonatorum in babies if mother has active genital infection
  - treatment: ceftriaxone 250 mg intramuscular stat followed by cefixime 200 mg PO for 2 weeks

2.3 Syphilis

- Caused by the spirochaete, *Treponema pallidum*

2.3.1 Stages of Disease

See Figure 66.3.

- primary: chancre appears 10–90 days after exposure; persists for 4–6 weeks
- secondary: occurs 1–6 months after primary infection
  - — mucus patches around mouth or genitals
  - — nonitchy rash on body
  - — condyloma lata
- tertiary: occurs 1–10 years after initial infection
  - — gummas
  - — neurosyphilis tabes dorsalis; generalised paralysis of insane (GPI) or paralytic dementia is a severe neuropsychiatric disorder, classified as an organic mental disorder and caused by the chronic meningoencephalitis, which leads to cerebral atrophy in late-stage syphilis; Argyll Robertson pupil

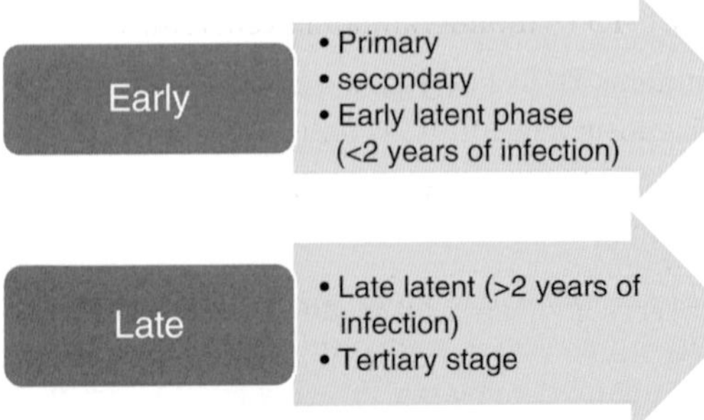

Figure 66.3 Classification of Syphilis disease.

2.3.2 Diagnosis

- cannot be cultured
- difficult to distinguish from yaws and pinta on serology
- nonspecific tests: the venereal disease research laboratory (VDRL) test, rapid plasma regain and Wassermann reaction
- specific tests: fluorescent treponemal antibody-absorption test and treponema pallidum agglutination test
- false positive in nonspecific tests occurs in viral infections, tuberculosis, malaria, pregnancy and lymphoma

2.3.3 Treatment

- penicillin G 2.4 million units intramuscular
- doxycycline if penicillin sensitive

2.4 *Mycoplasma*

- unusual as have no cell wall; thus, penicillin and cephalosporins ineffective in mycoplasma infections
- colonies: fried-egg appearance
- present in about 20% sexually active women
- causes atypical pneumonia, PID, postpartum pyrexia and chorioamnionitis
- treatment:
  - doxycycline
  - clindamycin

2.5 *Chlamydia*

- obligate intracellular, gram negative
- three subgroups:
  - A–C (follicular conjunctivitis)
  - D–K (genital: vaginitis, cervicitis, PID, urethritis in males)
  - L1–L3 (lymphogranuloma venereum)
- contains DNA and RNA
- diagnosis: cell culture is difficult; cannot be grown on solid media; diagnosed by enzyme immunoassay detection of antigen or amplification of nucleic acid (can use urine instead of cervical or urethral swabs)
- treatment: azithromycin, doxycycline, erythromycin and ofloxacin
- test of cure (repeat testing 3–4 weeks after completing therapy) is recommended in breastfeeding and pregnant women

2.6 Bacterial Vaginosis

- polymicrobial condition of the vagina characterised by variable degrees of depletion of protective lactobacilli and marked increase in other organisms: anaerobes like *G. vaginalis* and *Mobiluncus*
- can be associated with midtrimester miscarriage, preterm birth, premature rupture of membranes and postpartum endometritis
- symptoms: fishy-smelling vaginal discharge; more so after intercourse
- Amsel criteria for diagnosis: vaginal discharge, presence of clue cells, vaginal pH >4.5 and fishy odour with 10% potassium hydroxide (KOH) on wet mount (whiff test)
- treatment: metronidazole 400 mg three times daily (TDS) for 7–10 days

2.7 *Trichomonas Vaginalis*

- flagellate genital protozoan, pear-shaped, 10 x 7 μm
- sexual spread
- symptoms: green/yellow frothy vaginal discharge, intense itching/irritation and fishy odour
- male patients generally asymptomatic
- on examination: strawberry cervix
- can cause preterm delivery
- diagnosis: clinical, wet prep, polymerase chain reaction (PCR), culture
- treatment with metronidazole 400 mg TDS for 7–14 days

3 Viruses

General facts:

- no organelles and no cytoplasm
- host-dependent for:
  - energy
  - protein synthesis
- have a nucleic acid (RNA or DNA) surrounded by protein coat (capsid: composed of capsomeres)
- viral genome plus capsid: naked viruses (more resistant)

- viral genome plus capsid plus lipid/protein membrane: enveloped viruses (more susceptible)
- viral infections can cause latent infection, remain dormant in host cells and are reactivated when host defence is lowered; for example, herpes simplex virus (HSV) (cold sores), varicella zoster (shingles)
- some viruses cause chronic infection without cell death with continued viral replication over months/years; for example, hepatitis B and C
- viruses associated with malignancies: transform host cells by inducing uncontrolled cell growth; for example, Epstein–Barr virus (Burkitt's lymphoma), parvovirus (cervical cancer), hepatitis B (hepatocellular carcinoma)
- fetal transmission rate generally increases with gestation
- form inclusion bodies in host cells:
    - Negri bodies in rabies
    - Cowdry type A in varicella zoster and herpes simplex
    - Cowdry type B in polio and adenovirus
    - Torres in yellow fever
    - Owl's eye appearance in cytomegalovirus (CMV)
    - Warthin–Finkeldey in measles
    - Guarnieri and Paschen in smallpox
- classification:
    - depends on genetic material – see Table 66.3

4 Fetal Infections

4.1 *Cytomegalovirus*

- forty to eighty percent of women are seropositive
- acute illness with fever, malaise, headache and mild hepatitis

Table 66.3 Types of viruses

RNA	DNA
• Rubella	• CMV
• Human immunodeficiency virus (HIV)	• Varicella virus
• Hepatitis A, C, D, E, G	• Parvovirus
• Ebola	• Herpes
• Coronavirus	• Hepatitis B
	• Human papillomavirus

- Fetomaternal transmission rate is 40%: increases with gestational age
- Causes symptoms in 10% of affected infants
- Causes congenital defects:
    - microcephaly
    - hearing loss
    - cerebral palsy
    - hepatosplenomegaly
    - thrombocytopenia
    - intracranial calcification
    - intrauterine growth restriction (IUGR)
- diagnosis of infection in mother:
    - maternal immunoglobulin G avidity: high avidity signifies old infection

4.2 Herpes Simplex Virus

- HSV 1: usually affects mouth and face, spread by oral/salivary contact. Primary infection in childhood, latent infection re-emerges as cold sores. Causes 30% of genital infections in the UK.
- HSV 2: affects the genital area and spread by sexual contact. Seventy percent of genital infections in the UK present as recurrent painful genital lesions.
- Fetal transmission:
    - high if primary infection occurred in the last trimester with rate of >40%
    - if secondary infection during labour, transmission rate is 1–3%
- Incubation period: 21 days.
- Affects skin, eyes, mouth and central nervous system (CNS).
- High fetal mortality.
- Treatment with acyclovir from 36 weeks onwards recommended to suppress the recurrence of lesions if patient has had primary infection in early pregnancy.
- Very rarely, caesarean section is indicated in presence of primary active lesions at onset of labour with intact membranes.

4.3 Varicella Zoster

- causes chicken pox as primary infection; latent infection re-emerges as shingles
- infection in pregnancy can be severe with pneumonitis and encephalitis

- fetal transmission: congenital varicella syndrome
  - first 20 weeks of gestation
  - incidence 1% (0.4% up to 12 weeks and 2% >12 weeks)
- fetal varicella syndrome is characterised by:
  - CNS abnormality: microcephaly and cortical atrophy
  - limb hypoplasia
  - eye defects: microphthalmia, cataracts and chorioamnionitis
- risk of neonatal varicella if maternal infection occurs within 10 days of birth
- maternal complications: pneumonia, encephalitis and hepatitis
- treatment:
  - if maternal infection occurs: acyclovir
  - maternal exposure to varicella infection: varicella zoster immunoglobulin (VZIG) administration (not effective in patients with chicken pox)

4.4 Rubella

- German measles, togavirus group
- single-stranded RNA genome enclosed in a capsid
- spreads via droplets
- incubation period 2–3 weeks, coryzal prodrome followed by lymphadenopathy and maculopapular rash
- can be prevented by measles, mumps, rubella (MMR) vaccine
- congenital rubella syndrome:
  - eyes: cataracts and glaucoma
  - heart: patent ductus arteriosus (PDA), ventricular septal defect (VSD) and pulmonary stenosis
  - sensorineural hearing loss
  - haematological manifestations: thrombocytopenic purpura, haemolytic anaemia and lymphadenopathy
- fetomaternal transmission rate: decreased risk of transmission after 16 weeks:
  - first trimester: 90%
  - second trimester: 30%
- fetal defect rates:
  - first trimester: 90%
  - second trimester: 20%
  - >16 weeks: risk of deafness only
  - >20 weeks: no increased risk

4.5 Parvovirus B19

- the only single-stranded DNA virus
- infection spreads by respiratory droplets
- fifth disease/slapped cheek syndrome/erythema infectiosum in children
- adults can present with pain and swelling in the joints
- virus infects red cell precursors; may cause aplastic crisis is some patients
- maternal infection causes miscarriages (6–10% risk of fetal loss), hydrops fetalis due to fetal anaemia (small risk); most infections in pregnancy have no ill effects on the baby
- does not cause congenital defects
- fetal transmission mostly in first trimester; rate of transmission about 30%
- fetal hydrops can be treated with intrauterine blood transfusion

4.6 Zika Virus

- transmitted by bite of *Aedes* (*A. egypti* and *A. albopictus*) mosquito, sexually transmitted and from mother to the fetus
- symptoms: mild viral-illness-type symptoms: fever, headache, malaise, joint pain and conjunctivitis
- investigations: blood test for symptomatic pregnant women in Zika risk area or recent travel to Zika risk area. A test called a reverse transcriptase polymerase chain reaction (RT-PCR) will check for the virus in the blood and urine if it has been two weeks or fewer since being exposed to Zika. If it has been 2–12 weeks after a possible exposure, then immunoglobulin M is tested for.
- Zika risk areas: Africa, Asia, South America, Mexico, Central America, the Caribbean
- congenital Zika syndrome:
  - severe microcephaly
  - brain damage with decreased brain tissue
  - retinal damage
  - skeletal deformities
  - seizures, blindness and deafness

4.7 *Toxoplasma Gondii*

- zoonotic infection, mainly by cats (undergo sexual reproduction in the gastrointestinal tract of cats: definitive host)
- oocytes excreted by cats in faeces: ingested by other animals: trophozoites exit and migrate in the body forming tissue cysts
- human infection by handling cat faeces or ingesting undercooked meat containing cysts
- acute infection subclinical; may present as glandular-fever-like illness
- can affect muscles, neural tissue; cysts persist in tissues and reactivate in immunocompromised states such as HIV and mostly present as toxoplasma encephalitis
- transmission from mother to baby: transplacental in primary infection or reactivated infection
- maximum risk between 26 weeks of gestation to term (earlier infection is more severe)
- lowest risk 10 to 24 weeks
- congenital infection:
  - stillbirth
  - cerebral calcification, microcephaly, hydrocephalous
  - chorioretinitis
  - cerebral palsy
  - epilepsy
  - hepatosplenomegaly
  - thrombocytopenia
- treatment: spiramycin or sulfadiazine
- toxoplasma immunoglobulin M can persist for three years after eradication of infection

5 Other Infections

5.1 Measles

- belongs to *Paramyxoviridae*; RNA virus
- incubation period: 10–14 days
- prodromal coryzal symptoms: patient starts shedding virus from this stage
- Koplik's spots develop from late coryzal stage (on oral mucosa)
- erythematous maculopapular rash spreads from face to trunk and extremities
- major complications: pneumonia (more common) and encephalitis (rare)

5.2 Mumps

- *Paramyxoviridae* family
- spread by respiratory droplets, mainly affects unvaccinated children
- can be prevented by MMR vaccine
- incubation period of 2–4 weeks
- unilateral parotitis, rarely meningitis and encephalitis
- adult males can develop epididymo-orchitis (testicular atrophy usually unilateral: rarely can cause male subfertility)

5.3 HIV

- retrovirus family, has reverse transcriptase enzyme
- two copies of single-stranded RNA enclosed by a capsid
- capsid composed of viral protein P24, surrounded by a matrix composed of viral protein P17
- viral envelope surrounds the matrix; composed of phospholipids and glycoproteins (GP120 and GP41)
- glycoprotein enables virus to attach and fuse with target cells
- primarily infects T cells (CD4 molecule) via glycoprotein envelope GP41, macrophages and dendritic cells
- viral RNA enters host cell and is transcribed into DNA by reverse transcriptase; viral DNA is incorporated in host DNA and serves as template for viral replication
- infection is followed by seroconversion illness a few weeks later: fever and rash followed by long latency period; gradual decrease in CD4 cell count with failure of immune system manifested by secondary infections (low virulence opportunistic pathogens)
- transmission by:
  - sexual contact: female to male: 0.04%

    male to female: 0.08%

    anal intercourse: 1.7%
  - blood and blood products: blood transfusions and IV drug abusers
  - perinatal transmission
- prevalence in antenatal women in the UK: 0.17%
- one-third of infections are due to HIV-1 and two-thirds due to HIV-2

- fetal transmission rate: 15% without treatment and <1% with treatment
- increased rate of vertical transmission:
  - high maternal viral load
  - low maternal CD4 count
  - prolonged rupture of membranes
  - presence of chorioamnionitis
  - breastfeeding
- Autoimmune deficiency syndrome (AIDS) occurs when CD4 count is $<200/mm^3$
- increases risk of miscarriages, preterm delivery and IUGR
- complications of AIDS include *Pneumocystis carinii pneumonia*, Kaposi's sarcoma, non-Hodgkin's lymphoma
- HIV can be controlled, but not eradicated, by antiretroviral drugs in combination (nucleoside, nucleotide and nonnucleotide reverse transcriptase inhibitors and protease inhibitors)
- prevention of parent to child transmission (PPTCT) by suppression of maternal viraemia using combination antiretroviral medications (highly active antiretroviral therapy (HAART)), avoiding prolonged rupture of membranes, elective caesarean section if appropriate and avoiding breastfeeding

5.4 Malaria

- mosquito-borne infection, caused by bite of female Anopheles mosquito
- exists in tropical and subtropical countries
- infects red blood cells
- causative organism: *Plasmodium falciparum* (severe infection), *P. vivax* and *P. ovale* (form hypnozoites and cause relapsing fever), *P. malariae* (milder but may persist for many years) – see Figure 66.4
- clinical features in mother: fever, arthralgia, splenomegaly, hepatomegaly, haemoglobinuria and renal failure, cerebral malaria and convulsions
- high maternal mortality
- fetal effects: placental parasitaemia, miscarriage, IUGR, preterm labour and stillbirth
- diagnosis: thick and thin blood films
- treatment: chloroquine, quinine
- chemoprophylaxis (when travelling to endemic area): doxycycline, mefloquine, Malarone, quinine

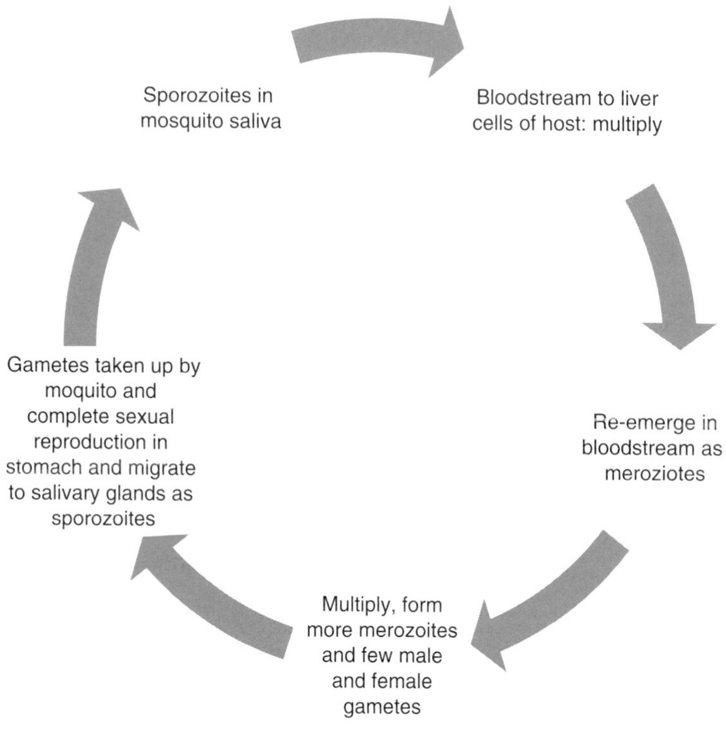

Figure 66.4 Life cycle of *Plasmodium*.

Sporozoites in mosquito saliva

Bloodstream to liver cells of host: multiply

Re-emerge in bloodstream as meroziotes

Multiply, form more merozoites and few male and female gametes

Gametes taken up by moquito and complete sexual reproduction in stomach and migrate to salivary glands as sporozoites

- vector control: insecticides (dichlorodiphenyltrichloroethane (DDT), permethrin), mosquito nets and skin repellents (50% DEET)

5.5 *Candida albicans*

- small oval measuring 2-4 μm
- gram-positive yeast with single bud; sometimes seen as pseudo hyphae on staining
- found in humans as commensal in mucosal surfaces of oropharynx and vagina
- infection common in immunocompromised status like HIV, diabetes and pregnancy
- cause vulvovaginitis, oropharyngeal infections, pneumonia and rarely meningitis

5.6 Coronavirus

- RNA virus
- spherical to pleomorphic enveloped particles
- cause upper respiratory tract infections; rarely pneumonitis
- spread via airborne droplets to the nasal mucosa

5.7 Ebola Virus

- Ebola and Lassa viruses cause haemorrhagic fevers, and have been reported mainly in Africa
- RNA virus: the recent epidemic suggested a higher rate of miscarriages, preterm delivery and maternal and neonatal mortality in pregnant women affected by the Ebola virus

Human Papillomavirus and Other Viral Infections

Tanuja Mokashi

1 Human papillomaviruses

- single-stranded DNA viruses affecting the skin and mucus membrane cells
- more than 70 subtypes, including:
  - plantar and common warts: human papillomavirus (HPV) 1, 2
  - recurrent respiratory papillomatosis: HPV 6, 11
  - conjunctival papillomas/carcinomas: HPV 6, 11, 16
  - genital warts: HPV 6, 11, 30, 42
  - cervical intraepithelial neoplasia: low-risk HPV 6, 11; high-risk HPV 16, 18
  - cervical carcinoma: HPV 16, 18
- transmission by skin-to-skin and sexual contact; common in people with multiple sexual partners
- affects mostly women aged 18–30 years
- affects cells during greatest metaplastic activity; for example, puberty and pregnancy
- increased rate of cervical intraepithelial neoplasia and cancers after 35 years of age; implies slow progression from infection to cancerous changes in cells
- immunocompromised women with, for example, HIV and renal transplant, more likely to progress to development of cancer as primary immune response to HPV is cell mediated
- common presentations:
  - anogenital warts: in both males and women; usually asymptomatic, do not lead to cancer and generally disappear within 3–4 months spontaneously; treatment is ablation/excision or podophyllin
  - asymptomatic: no cytological changes, but positive for HPV 6 and 11
  - active infection with high-risk HPV 16 and 18, causing intraepithelial neoplasia in cervical, vaginal, urethral, penile or vulval cells; can develop cervical cancer
- vaccine:
  - Gardasil protects against HPV 6, 11, 16 and 18
  - offered to girls aged 12–18 years in the UK on NHS
  - first dose at 12 years, followed by second dose 6–12 months later
  - if first dose after 15 years of age, 3 doses needed instead of 2
  - no routine vaccine for boys as are protected by herd immunity in girls
  - for homosexual males, vaccine available on NHS from 15 to 45 years of age; 3 doses given 1–3 months apart

2 Hepatitis

- A to G subtypes

2.1 Hepatitis A

- related to enteroviruses
- rare maternofetal transmission
- incubation period: one month
- jaundice develops; no chronic infection state
- once infected, gives lifelong immunity
- diagnosis by detection of immunoglobulin M (IgM)
- effective vaccines available: can be used during outbreaks

2.2 Hepatitis B

- only enveloped DNA virus in hepatitis family

- spread via blood and sexual contact
- hepatitis B vaccine to those at high risk of infection such as healthcare workers and sexual contacts of patient with infection
- incubation period: six weeks to six months
- detection of antigens in blood: HBsAg, followed by HBcoreAg, followed by HBeAg
- detection of antibodies in blood: the sequence is IgM core, followed by eIgE followed by surface antibodies
- immunity confirmed by anti-surface IgM
- prevalence in UK pregnant women: 0.5%
- mother-to-child transmission occurs via vertical transmission during pregnancy, labour and lactation; transplacental transmission accounts for 5% of transmissions
- mother-to-child transmission rates: depend mainly on viral load and antigen profile:
    - mother HBsAg positive: 20%
    - mother HBeAg positive: 90%
    - transmission during first trimester: 10%
    - transmission during last trimester: 90%
- treatment in pregnancy: lamivudine, interferon γ
- prophylaxis for neonate born to HBeAg positive mother: hepatitis B vaccine and immunoglobulins

2.3 Hepatitis C

- enveloped RNA virus
- present in blood and other fluids
- common in intravenous drug abusers; spread via unsterile injection equipment
- most infections asymptomatic; high incidence of chronicity
- no vaccine
- ribavirin plus interferons can halt progression of chronic hepatitis
- prevalence in UK: 0.3–0.7%
- increases risk of obstetric cholestasis
- vertical transmission: 3–5%

2.4 Hepatitis E

- RNA virus
- risk of maternal mortality: 5%
- risk of fulminant hepatic failure in pregnancy: 25–30%

Puerperal Infections and Surgical-Site Infections

Tanuja Mokashi

1 Puerperal Infections

- Most common causative organisms: group A *Streptococcus*, *Escherichia coli*, *Staphylococcus aureus*, *S. pneumoniae*, methicillin-resistant *S. aureus* (MRSA), *Clostridium*.
- Definition: any bacterial infection in a woman after childbirth or miscarriage/termination of pregnancy. Most common site is genital tract; less common is urinary tract infection, pneumonia, and so on.
- Bacteraemia: presence of viable bacteria in the blood.
- Sepsis: systemic response to infection characterised by two or more of the following plus infection:
  - temperature: >38 °C or <36 °C
  - heart rate: >90 BPM
  - respiratory rate: >20 BPM or pCO_2: <32 mmHg
  - white blood cell count: >12 x 10^9/L or <4 x 10^9/L or with >10% immature forms
- Severe sepsis: sepsis plus hypoperfusion/organ dysfunction/hypotension/lactic acidosis, oliguria or alteration in mental state
- Septic shock: sepsis-induced hypotension (systolic blood pressure (SBP) <90 mmHg or reduction in SBP >40 mmHg from baseline) despite adequate fluid resuscitation, along with presence of perfusion abnormalities.
- Investigations: to be done within first hour of suspected sepsis:
  - full blood count, liver and renal function tests, coagulation screen
  - blood cultures, urine culture, wound swab if appropriate, high or low vaginal swab
  - arterial blood gas including serum lactate (>4 mmol/L indicates hypoperfusion of tissues)
  - sputum, throat swab, stool for ova/parasite, lumbar puncture depending on suspected source of infection
- Treatment: to be initiated within the first hour of suspected sepsis:
  - intravenous fluids
  - broad-spectrum antibiotics: reassess in 48–72 hours; microbiologist opinion if no improvement
  - oxygen if hypoxia
- To remove any suspected source of infection: wound debridement, drainage of pelvic collection/abscess, removal of drains, and so on.

2 Surgical-site Infections

- Infections occurring at incision site for invasive procedures.
- Usually localised to incision site; may spread to deeper tissues.
  - Superficial: localised to surgical site and subcutaneous tissue; signs of redness and swelling.
  - Deep incisional: in fascia and muscle; can form pus/abscess, fever, tenderness; gaping in the wound exposing deeper tissues.
  - Organ or space infection: any part of an organ that is opened during the surgery; for example, bowel or uterus. Can form abscess or pus; detection by radiology or during reoperation.
- Most acquired by inoculation of patient's own flora at the time of surgery.
- Exogenous factors: from contaminated surgical instruments, ventilation in theatres and poor scrub practices.

Section 11

Immunology

Jodie Lam

Principles of Reproductive Immunology

Jodie Lam

The human body relies on its sophisticated and complex immune system to protect it against disease and harm. It can distinguish between self and foreign antigens, and, if appropriate, generates an immune response. The immune system has two different components that can either operate independently or act in synergy to produce an effective response (see Table 69.1):

Innate system

- naturally occurring immune system, which exists from birth
- forms the 'first-line' response that is mobilised rapidly after a potential threat is recognised
- nonspecific antigen recognition

Table 69.1 Types of immunity

Innate immunity	Adaptive immunity
Rapid activation within seconds/minutes (first-line response)	Activates in days
Able to interact with foreign antigens directly	Requires help from other immune cells to detect pathogens; i.e., antigen processed and then presented to them
Nonspecific, but recognises general groups/patterns of molecules	Highly specific with the ability to distinguish between similar pathogens
Able to fully differentiate between self and foreign antigens	Occasionally can target self-antigens and cause autoimmune disease
Forms the same response when exposed to the same antigen	Able to retain memory and form a more rapid and aggressive response with repeat exposure
Monocytes, macrophages, neutrophils, mast cells, NK cells, complement system	B cells, T cells, antigen-presenting cells

- composed of leucocytes (natural killer (NK) cells, monocytes/macrophages, neutrophils, basophils, eosinophils) and mast cells
- cytokines and the complement system are groups of signalling molecules, which allow communication between the various cells of the immune system; they are involved in cell activation, recruitment and destruction of infected cells

Adaptive system

- more refined and sophisticated immune response
- able to distinguish between different antigens; that is, demonstrates specificity
- able to exhibit memory, and responds more quickly and more aggressively if exposed to the same microbe later
- composed of B cells and T lymphocytes
- activated B cells produce antibodies to target specific antigens and mark them for destruction
- T cells with CD8 surface markers are cytotoxic; they recognise and destroy infected cells
- T cells with CD4 surface markers help to regulate the immune system by secreting cytokines: Th1 secretes interleukin 2 (IL-2), interferon gamma (IFN) and tumor necrosis factor (TNF) alpha, and help inflammatory responses; Th2 secretes IL-4, IL-5, IL-10 and IL-13, and helps antibody-mediated responses
- specialised T cells called regulatory T cells are immunosuppressive in nature and prevent recognition of self-antigens

An antigen is any substance capable of triggering an immune response:

- exogenous antigen: substance not found naturally within the body
- endogenous antigen: may either be a self-antigen (autologous) or from a different species (heterologous), but sharing strong similarities

Major histocompatibility complex (MHC) is a group of genes that encode for cell-surface glycoproteins important for cell recognition and differentiation from foreign cells.

- Class I MHC is expressed by all nucleated body cells
- Class I MHC presents endogenous antigens, which originate from within the cell to cytotoxic T cells; that is, allow infected/damaged cells to be identified and destroyed
- Class II MHC is primarily expressed by antigen presenting cells and B lymphocytes
- Class II MHC presents exogenous antigens, which originate extracellularly to T helper cells, and thereby activate antibody production

The absence of MHC class I in the placenta should make it a target for maternal NK cells. However, a different MHC molecule is present and deactivates the NK cells, escaping elimination.

70 Immunology of Pregnancy

Jodie Lam

Pregnancy is an immunological mystery and it is not fully understood why/how the body permits fetal cells to invade, persist and grow without any long-term adverse effect to the mother.

- Immunological changes commence from the time of fertilisation to protect the newly formed blastocyst. This is necessary to permit normal and successful implantation and prevent rejection in the form of miscarriage.
- Invading fetal trophoblast cells ultimately differentiate into the highly specialised syncytiotrophoblasts (placenta). They secrete factors such as TNF alpha, which disrupts normal cell–cell adhesion, collagenases and endopeptidases to aid invasion of maternal tissue.
- During this process, trophoblasts produce and release factors into the maternal circulation and cause widespread activation, especially of the innate immune system.
- High progesterone levels are immunosuppressive, and are produced initially by the corpus luteum, and subsequently the placenta. Low levels are thought to be a contributing factor to early pregnancy failure.
- There is a general shift of balance between proinflammatory and anti-inflammatory components of the immune system; for example, greater number of anti-inflammatory T helper type 2 (Th2) cells and upregulation of anti-inflammatory cytokines IL-4 and IL-10.
- Natural killer (NK) cells are necessary for regulating normal trophoblast invasion and spiral artery remodelling, the absence of which leads to suboptimal implantation and placentation, ultimately increasing the risk of developing complications such as preeclampsia or fetal growth restriction.
- There is immunomodulation of the maternal immune system; for example, factors released that cause widespread activation of the innate system and expression of human leucocyte antigen (HLA)-G to inhibit NK cells.
- There is release of immunosuppressive agents; for example, prostaglandin E2 (PGE2), interleukin-1 (IL-1)-alpha, IL-6, interferon (IFN)-alpha, human chorionic gonadotropin (hCG) and platelet activating factor (PAF).
- There is greater tolerance shown towards foreign material demonstrated by the increased numbers of regulatory T cells.

1 Placenta

The main interface between mother and fetus occurs at the placenta. It is an important site of complex interactions and processes:

- the primary site for transport of essential nutrients necessary for fetal development and growth (glucose, amino acids, fatty acids)
- production of peptide hormones; for example, hCG, human placental lactogen, growth factors and steroid hormones such as progesterone and estrogen
- synthesis of glycogen and cholesterol for metabolism
- it contains high levels of lymphocytes, cytokines and NK cells from the innate system
- acts as a physical barrier between the two circulations and protects against bloodborne pathogens from the maternal circulation entering and infecting the fetus
- selective transfer of maternal immunoglobulins to the fetus, providing passive immunity against infection

1.1 Passive Immunity

- The placenta acts as a physical barrier isolating/ protecting the developing fetus from the mother

Table 70.1 Immunoglobulins

Type	Structure	Heavy chain	Location	Function
IgA	Dimer	α	Mucosal cells like gastrointestinal tract, respiratory tract and urogenital tract, and found in secretions like tears, saliva, breast milk	Prevents colonisation by pathogens
IgD	Monomer	δ	Antigen receptors on B cells not exposed to antigens	Activates mast cells and basophils to produce antimicrobial factors
IgE	Monomer	ε	Synthesised by plasma cells and located in lymph nodes	Binds to allergens and triggers histamine from mast cells and basophils
IgG	Monomer	γ	Exists in four forms	Provides immunity against infections and crosses the placenta to give passive immunity to fetus
IgM	Pentamer	μ	Expressed on B cells and exists as pentamers	Has high avidity and fights infections in early stages before IgG is sufficient

and any pathogens in her circulation. However, infection can still occur.

- Transplacental passage of antibodies depends on maternal concentration, antibody type and gestational age.
- Immunoglobulin G (IgG) is the only isotype (preferentially IgG-1) of maternal immunoglobulins that can cross the placenta via specific Fc receptors and provide passive immunity to the fetus. See Table 70.1.
- fetal IgG concentration is much lower than maternal concentration in the first half of pregnancy, but increases from 50% of maternal levels around 28 weeks of gestation to exceed maternal levels at full term.
- Maternal antibodies only remain in the fetus temporarily (4–6 months) and start declining after the first few weeks.
- After birth, breastfeeding can also provide passive immunity to the newborn through the presence of immunoglobulin A (IgA) in colostrum and breast milk.

2 Infection in Pregnancy

- Maternal infection and severe sepsis are risk factors for miscarriage or preterm labour.
- Pregnant women are relatively immunosuppressed compared to nonpregnant women, and are severely affected by other infections; for example, cytomegalovirus, herpes simplex virus and malaria.
- The majority of infections are limited to the mother and resolve without any consequences, but some can cause more serious complications to the vulnerable fetus; for example, parvovirus causes fetal hydrops.
- Although the maternal immune response changes during pregnancy, most pregnant women experience healthy pregnancies.
- The changes in maternal immune responses are also reflected by changes in autoimmune diseases; for example, rheumatoid arthritis often goes into remission during pregnancy.
- When considering maternal vaccination for neonatal immunity, the ideal timing is in the early third trimester; for example, whooping cough vaccine.
- Vaccination against preventable diseases is recommended prior to pregnancy. However, it is warranted when the risk of exposure is high, the infection poses risks to the mother and/or fetus and the vaccine is unlikely to be harmful.
- There is no evidence of harm to pregnant women or fetuses from administration of inactivated vaccines; for example, influenza.
- In some situations, after exposure to an infectious agent that has potentially serious complications, immunoglobulins can be administered to provide both the mother and fetus with passive immunity

with the aim of limiting severity; for example, postvaricella exposure

There has been increasing interest in the role of NK cells in early pregnancy failure and infertility. At the time of writing, there is limited evidence for the routine testing. There are two types of NK cells: uterine NK (uNK) cells and peripheral blood NK cells. They express a variety of surface receptors, including CD16 and CD56.

3 Natural Killer Cells

There has been some evidence showing elevated number of uNK cells within endometrium in women with poor pregnancy outcomes; that is, pregnancy failure or recurrent miscarriage. It is unclear whether the presence of uNK cells affects the remodelling of spiral arteries, and so increasing the risk of developing pre-eclampsia in the pregnancy.

- The detection and measurement of uNK cells require an endometrial biopsy and immunostaining of the tissue.
- Levels of peripheral blood NK cells can be easily measured by venepuncture.
- The levels of peripheral blood and uNK cell levels are not directly correlated.
- They may have different physiological/pathological roles in pregnancy, but further research is required.

3.1 Treatment

- In the presence of elevated NK cells, there is no recognised national guidance about management to improve pregnancy outcomes.
- Most information at the time of writing comes from small studies, which have not demonstrated a statistical difference from treatment. Further research in this field is required.
- The use of intravenous immunoglobulin for treating high NK cells to improve pregnancy outcomes is not evidence based, and not recommended.
- Small studies have shown steroids can reduce numbers of NK cells, but it is unclear whether this directly improves live birth rate.
- NK cells play an important role in normal pregnancy, and they regulate trophoblast invasion.
  - uNK cells are the predominant leucocytes within the decidua
  - they are recruited in response to high progesterone and IL-15 levels
  - levels rise during the luteal phase of the menstrual cycle, but regress if implantation does not occur
  - they secrete granulocyte macrophage colony stimulating factor and angiogenic factors
  - levels are highest in the first trimester and fall with advancing gestation

Section 12

Biophysics

Neela Mukhopadhaya

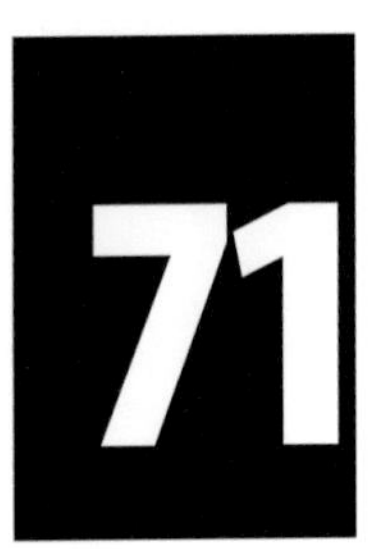

Imaging Modalities in Obstetrics and Gynaecology

Rachana Shukla

1 Principles of Imaging

Diagnostic imaging employs various forms of energy sources: X-ray radiation, gamma radiation, radiofrequency and sound. It exploits the properties of several elements and compounds to help visualisation of anatomical structures.

Of these, X-rays and gamma radiation are capable of cell damage by stochastic (deterministic or dose dependent) effects. These risks must be balanced against the potential benefit to the patient. Consideration must also be given to the use of other imaging modalities that do not involve ionising radiation.

The exposure to radiation in the UK is regulated using the Ionising Radiation (Medical Exposure) Regulations (IR(ME)R): these set out the responsibilities of duty holders (the employer, referrer, IR(ME)R practitioner and operator) for radiation protection.

The main aims of the IR(ME)R principles are (see Table 71.1):

- minimising unintended, excessive or incorrect medical exposures
- ensuring the benefits outweigh the risks of each exposure (justification)
- keeping doses in diagnostics 'as low as reasonably practicable' for their intended use (optimisation)

Breaches of IR(ME)R can result in civil or criminal proceedings.

IR(ME)R requires that the referrer provides sufficient clinical data so that the exposure can be justified and adequate demographic data so the referred patient can be correctly identified. This should include full name, date of birth and address.

A diagnostic imaging referral should also include:

- clinical diagnosis
- clinical findings on examination
- any available histology and relevant previous imaging investigations

The safety of nonionising medical diagnostic imaging is regulated by the Medicines and Healthcare products Regulatory Agency (MHRA).

2 Imaging Modalities

2.1 X-rays

Principle: X-rays represent a form of electromagnetic radiation. They are produced by the X-ray tube. High voltage is used to accelerate the electrons produced by the cathode. The electrons interact with the anode producing X-rays.

Table 71.1 IR(ME)R regulations

	IR(ME)R regulation	Consider
a.	The specific objectives of the exposure	What is to be gained by carrying out the exposure? How may the outcome affect the management of the patient?
b.	The characteristics of the individual involved	Such as previous imaging, medical history, age or pregnancy status of the patient and body habitus
c.	The potential or therapeutic benefits to the individual from the exposure	What is the expected benefit of the medical exposure? Will the patient's treatment be altered?
d.	The detriment the exposure may cause	What is the possible detriment from the associated radiation dose?
e.	The efficacy, benefits and risk of alternative techniques having the same objective, but involving no or less exposure to ionising radiation	What other imaging modalities are available that could answer the diagnostic question, but involve no or less radiation?

2.1.1 Advantages

- easily accessible
- fast image production and interpretation
- does not require patient preparation
- low dose (0.1 mSV for a chest X-ray compared to 7 mSV for a computed tomography (CT) scan of the chest)

2.1.2 Disadvantages

- exposure to ionising radiation: the cumulative dose would be relevant in patients having repeated exposures for a chronic condition
- limited spatial resolution: remember, this is a two-dimensional representation of a three-dimensional object

2.1.3 Common Clinical Indications in Obstetrics and Gynaecology

- chest X-ray is the first-line investigation in unexplained cough or chest pain: remember the pregnant patient with suspected pulmonary embolism: a baseline X-ray is indicated prior to specialist imaging
- abdominal X-rays: first-line investigation in suspected bowel obstruction or toxic megacolon; erect chest X-ray in suspected perforation
- an abdominal X-ray will also be indicated to evaluate for a missing intrauterine contraceptive device (IUCD) in the presence of a negative ultrasound scan to exclude uterine perforation by the IUCD

2.2 Ultrasound

Principle: the ultrasound beam originates from mechanical oscillations of numerous crystals in a transducer, which is excited by electrical pulses (piezoelectric effect). The transducer converts one type of energy into another (electrical to mechanical/sound).

The ultrasound waves (pulses of sound) are sent from the transducer, propagate through different tissues and then return to the transducer as reflected echoes. The returned echoes are converted back into electrical impulses by the transducer crystals and are further processed to form the ultrasound image presented on the screen.

2.2.1 Advantages

- Ultrasound uses nonionising sound waves and has not been associated with carcinogenesis. This is particularly important for the evaluation of fetal and gonadal tissue.
- Ultrasound is more readily available than more advanced cross-sectional modalities such as CT or magnetic resonance imaging (MRI) in most UK hospitals.
- Ultrasound examination is less expensive to conduct than CT or MRI.
- There are few (if any) contraindications to use of ultrasound, compared with MRI or contrast-enhanced CT.
- The real-time nature of ultrasound imaging is useful for the evaluation of physiology as well as anatomy (e.g., fetal heart rate).
- Doppler evaluation of organs and vessels adds a dimension of physiologic data.
- Ultrasound images may not be as adversely affected by metallic objects, as opposed to CT or MRI (e.g., hip replacement prosthesis).
- An ultrasound exam can easily be extended to cover another organ system or evaluate the contralateral extremity.

2.2.2 Disadvantages

- Training is required to accurately and efficiently conduct an ultrasound exam and there is nonuniformity in the quality of examinations ('operator dependence').
- Ultrasound is not capable of evaluating tissue types with high acoustical impedance (e.g., bone, air).
- The high frequencies of ultrasound result in a potential risk of thermal heating or mechanical injury to tissue at a micro level. This is of concern in fetal imaging in the first trimester.
- Ultrasound has its own set of unique artifacts (Radiopaedia), which can potentially degrade image quality or lead to misinterpretation.
- Some ultrasound exams may be limited by abnormally large body habitus.
- Deeper collections can be difficult to detect due to tissue impedance, especially in a patient with large body habitus.

2.2.3 Common Clinical Indications in Obstetrics and Gynaecology

Pelvic ultrasound is the first-line investigation for most common clinical presentations in obstetrics and gynaecology; for example, pelvic pain, menorrhagia, dysmenorrhoea, postmenopausal bleeding, fetal evaluation and retained products of conception.

2.3 Computed Tomography Scanning

CT scanning, also known computerised axial tomography (CAT) scanning in older literature, is a diagnostic imaging procedure that uses X-rays to build cross-sectional images ('slices') of the body. Cross-sections are reconstructed from measurements of attenuation coefficients of X-ray beams in the volume of the object studied.

CT is based on the fundamental principle that the density of the tissue passed by the X-ray beam can be measured from the calculation of the attenuation coefficient. Using this principle, CT allows the reconstruction of the density of the body, by two-dimensional section perpendicular to the axis of the acquisition system.

The emitter of X-rays rotates around the patient and the detector, placed in diametrically opposite side, picks up the image of a body section (beam and detector move in synchrony).

Unlike X-ray radiography, the detectors of the CT scanner do not produce an image. They measure the transmission of a thin beam (1–10 mm) of X-rays through a full scan of the body. The image of that section is taken from different angles, and this allows retrieval of the information on the depth (in the third dimension).

The density of various structures is measured using a standardised scale and is described in Hounsfield Units (HU) (Sir Godfrey Hounsfield invented the CT scan in 1967).

Hounsfield chose a scale that affects the four basic densities, with the following values:

- air = −1000 HU
- fat = −60 HU to −120 HU
- water = 0 HU
- compact bone = +1000 HU

Dual-energy CT utilises two separate energy sets to examine the differing attenuation properties of matter, having a significant advantage over traditional single-energy CT. Independent attenuation values at two energy sets can create virtual noncontrast images from contrast-enhanced imaging, as well as delineate the composition of renal calculi and arterial plaque.

2.3.1 Advantages

- rapid acquisition of images – less prone to breathing artifact
- can acquire images of a large portion of the body in a relatively short time
- three-dimensional extrapolation of images (multiplanar reconstructions) provides a wealth of clear and specific information
- not as dependent on body habitus of the patient: deeper structures can be imaged

2.3.2 Disadvantages

- The principle disadvantage of CT scanning is the radiation dose of CT; for example, a contrast-enhanced CT of the abdomen and pelvis is associated with a radiation dose of 20 mSV; equivalent to seven years of background radiation. This becomes especially relevant for the patient with postoperative complications who can end up having multiple scans. This is also relevant in the evaluation of the pregnant patient with fetal radiation to be considered. Exposure to 10 mSv ionising radiation, such as from a CT chest or a CT abdomen, increases one's lifetime attributable risk of cancer by 0.1 %, and this risk is cumulative with serial CT scans performed over one's lifetime. The fetus is more sensitive to carcinogenesis than children and adults, and has a longer life expectancy in which cancers may manifest. The main radiation-induced cancer in childhood is leukaemia, but in utero exposure also increases the risk for solid organ cancers.
- There is limited tissue differentiation for solid pelvic organs; for example, the depth of myometrial invasion in endometrial carcinoma cannot be quantified on CT scan.
- There is limited functional/physiological assessment; for example, differentiation between a fibrous lesion and tumour deposit.

2.3.3 Common Clinical Indications in Obstetrics and Gynaecology

- staging of carcinoma with chest and upper abdominal evaluation
- evaluation of the postoperative patient for surgical complications
- evaluation of the patient with sepsis of unknown origin
- evaluation of deep collections/bowel evaluation
- CT pulmonary angiogram (CTPA) in suspected pulmonary embolism: a ventilation/perfusion (V/Q)

scintigraphy is the preferred first-line investigation in the young/pregnant patient with suspected pulmonary embolism; CTPA being reserved in the indeterminate cases

2.4 Magnetic Resonance Imaging

Principle: MRI is an imaging modality that uses non-ionising radiation to create useful diagnostic images.

In simple terms, an MRI scanner consists of a large, powerful magnet in which the patient lies. A radio-wave antenna is used to send signals to the body and then receive signals back. These returning signals are converted into images by a computer attached to the scanner.

To obtain an MR image of an object, the object is placed in a uniform magnetic field, B_0, of between 0.5 and 3 Tesla. As a result, the object's hydrogen nuclei align with the magnetic field and create a net magnetic moment, M, parallel to B_0.

Next, a radiofrequency (RF) pulse, B_{rf}, is applied perpendicular to B_0. This pulse causes M to tilt away from B_0, as in Figure 71.1

Once the RF signal is removed, the nuclei realign themselves such that their net magnetic moment, M, is again parallel with B_0. This return to equilibrium is referred to as relaxation. During relaxation, the nuclei lose energy by emitting their own RF signal (see Figure 71.1(B)). This signal is referred to as the free-induction decay (FID) response signal. The FID response signal is measured by a conductive field coil placed around the object being imaged. This measurement is processed or reconstructed to obtain 3D greyscale MR images.

2.4.1 Advantages

- ability to image without the use of ionising X-rays, in contradistinction to CT scanning
- images may be acquired in multiple planes (axial, sagittal, coronal or oblique) without repositioning the patient
- MR images demonstrate superior soft-tissue contrast as compared to CT scans and plain radiographs, making it the ideal examination of the brain, spine, joints and other soft tissue body parts
- some angiographic images can be obtained without the use of contrast material, unlike CT or conventional angiography
- advanced techniques such as diffusion, spectroscopy and perfusion allow for precise tissue characterisation, rather than merely 'macroscopic' imaging
- functional MRI allows visualisation of both active parts of the brain during certain activities and understanding of the underlying networks

2.4.2 Disadvantages

- MRI scans are more expensive than CT scans.
- MRI scans take significantly longer to acquire than CT, and patient comfort can be an issue, possibly exacerbated by:
    - MR image acquisition is noisy compared to CT
    - MRI scanner acquisition tunnels tend to be more enclosed than CT, with associated claustrophobia
- MR images are subject to unique artifacts, which must be recognised and mitigated against.
- MRI scanning is not safe for patients with some metal implants and foreign bodies. Careful attention to safety measures is necessary to avoid serious injury to patients and staff, and this requires special MRI-compatible equipment and stringent adherence to safety protocols.
- In the UK, the MHRA does not recommend MRI in the first trimester of pregnancy.

2.4.3 Common Clinical Indications in Obstetrics and Gynaecology

- local (regional) staging of pelvic cancers: carcinoma endometrium, cervix, vulva and vagina

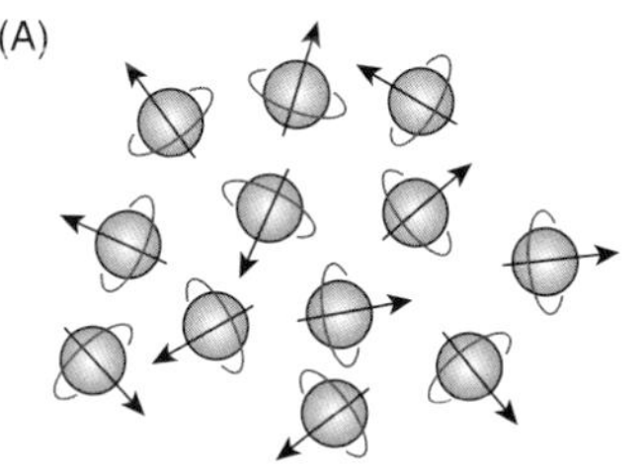

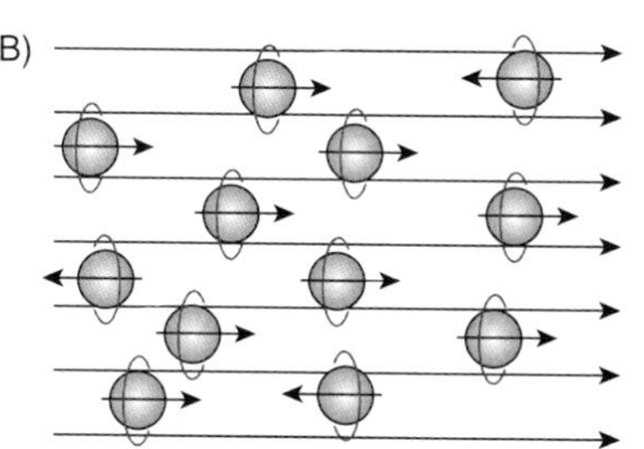

Figure 71.1 Principles of MRI.
Used with permission from www.schoolphysics.co.uk/age16-19/Atomic%20physics/Atomic%20structure%20and%20ions/text/MRI/index.html?PHPSESSID=4efb7b210aababb8e14bd5e7c386b2a1

- staging endometriosis
- characterisation of indeterminate adnexal lesions
- planning for fibroid embolisation
- second-line investigation for suspected fetal anomalies on ultrasound
- characterisation of müllerian duct anomalies

2.5 Nuclear Scintigraphy

Principle: a radionuclide is administered to the patient; the type of radionuclide administered depends on the organ being imaged. Gamma radiation emitted from a radionuclide administered to the patient (most commonly, Tc-99m) travels in all directions. A fraction of the radiation travels towards the gamma camera. The gamma camera contains a large rectangular crystal of sodium iodide doped with thallium: NaI(Tl). The crystal can stop incoming gamma rays and convert part of the deposited energy into scintillations. When the gamma photon strikes the crystal, a light photon is produced; this light photon is then converted into an electrical signal by the photomultiplier. The amount of light reaching the photomultiplier is proportional to the electrical signal produced.

Analogue-to-digital converters then convert the signal and determine the X, Y and Z planes of the signal produced. The X, Y and Z signals are then processed and displayed on a computer.

Gamma cameras may be found in isolation (scintigraphy) or in combination with a CT scanner (single photon emission computed tomography).

Positron emission tomography (PET) is a modern noninvasive imaging technique for quantification of radioactivity in vivo. A radiolabelled biological compound such as 2-deoxy-2-(^{18} F) fluoro-D-glucose (FDG) is injected intravenously.

Uptake of this compound followed by further breakdown occurs in the cells. Tumour cells have a high metabolic rate, and hence this compound is also metabolised by tumour cells.

FDG is metabolised to FDG-6-phosphate, which cannot be further metabolised by tumour cells, and hence it accumulates and concentrates in tumour cells. This accumulation is detected and quantified.

With single photon emission computed tomography (SPECT) and PET imaging, data can be reconstructed and displayed as a three-dimensional image. This is in contrast to scintigraphy, which yields planar data which can only be used to create a two-dimensional image.

Although the physiologic information afforded by PET and SPECT imaging is invaluable, the quality of obtained data is poor/noisy and limits imaging spatial resolution. For this reason, scans are often combined with CT imaging, allowing correlation between functional and anatomical imaging ('hybrid imaging').

2.5.1 Advantages

- Physiological information; for example, tumour activity. Therefore, differentiation between radiation necrosis and recurrence is possible.
- Obscure tumour deposits can be identified, useful for staging cancers and detecting response to treatment.
- Lower radiation dose in V/Q scintigraphy compared to CTPAs makes it the preferred modality for first-line assessment of pulmonary embolism in the pregnant patient. See Table 71.2 and Table 71.3.

2.5.2 Disadvantages

- limited spatial resolution: this is improved by combining with a CT scan as in SPECT and PETCT
- false-positive FDG uptake can be seen in granulomatous disease, abscess, postoperative changes, foreign body reaction and inflammation

2.5.3 Common Clinical Indications in Obstetrics and Gynaecology

- staging gynaecological cancer recurrence
- evaluation of pulmonary embolism in the young/pregnant patient

Table 71.2 Radiation exposure to mother

Maternal dose	Lung	Breast
CTPA	39.5 mGy	10-60 mGy
V/Q	5.7–13.5 mGy	0.98–1.07 mGy

Table 71.3 Radiation exposure to fetus

	CTPA	V/Q
Fetal dose	3.3 mGy to 130 mGy (increases from first to third trimester)	0.32 mGy to 0.74 mGy (constant for all trimesters)

3 Conclusion

It is important for the clinician to be aware of the principles of imaging and the advantages and disadvantages of various imaging modalities. Use local and national guidelines to request the most appropriate investigation for your patient. The Royal College of Radiologists has a useful online guide called iRefer, which is a helpful tool to ensure that you ask for IRMER appropriate investigations

Bibliography

Bier, V. (1990). *Health Effects from Exposure to Low Levels of Ionizing Radiation.* National Academy Press.

Brenner, D. J., Hall, E.J. (2007). Computed tomography–an increasing source of radiation exposure. *N Engl J Med*, **357** (22), 2277–84.

Coursey, C.A., Nelson, R.C., Boll, D.T., et al. (2010). Dual-energy multidetector CT: how does it work, what can it tell us, and when can we use it in abdominopelvic imaging? *Radiographics*, **30**(4), 1037–55.

Cook, J.V., Kyriou, J. (2005). Radiation from CT and perfusion scanning in pregnancy. *BMJ*, **331**(7512), 350.

Doll, R., Wakeford, R. (1997). Risk of childhood cancer from fetal irradiation. *Br J Radiol*, **70**, 130–9.

ter Haar, G. R., Abramowicz, J. S., Akiyama, I., et al. (2013). Do we need to restrict the use of doppler ultrasound in first trimester pregnancy. *Ultrasound in Med. & Biol*, **39**(3) 374–80.

McKeighen, R. A. (1980). Review of gamma camera technology for medical imaging. *Int Urogynecol J*, **27**(3), 119.

Medicines and Healthcare Products Regulatory Agency (2015). *Safety guidelines for magnetic resonance imaging equipment in clinical use.* MHRA.

Radiopaedia. *Ultrasound artifacts* (online). https://radiopaedia.org/articles/ultrasound-artifacts-3

Royal College of Radiologists. (2015). (online). *A guide to understanding the implications of IRMER in diagnostic and interventional radiology.* https://www.rcr.ac.uk/sites/default/files/bfcr152_irmer.pdf

Scheuler, B. A. (1998). Clinical applications of basic X-ray physics principles. *Radiographics*, **18**(3), 731–44.

Wagner, L., Applegate, K. (2008). *ACR practice guideline for imaging pregnant or potentially pregnant adolescents and women with ionizing radiation.* 1–15.

Wagner, L. K. (1997). *Exposure of the pregnant patient to diagnostic radiations: a guide to medical management.* Medical Physics Publishing.

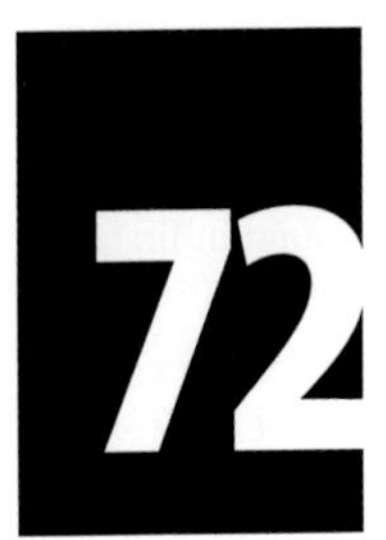

Laser and Electrosurgery

Rachana Shukla

1 Electrosurgery

1.1 Definition

The use of electric current (flow of electrons) to cut, coagulate, desiccate and fulgurate tissue.

1.2 Electrosurgery Unit

A machine that converts low-frequency alternating current to high-frequency alternating current to produce the desired surgical effect. See Tables 72.1, 72.2 and 72.3.

1.3 Components of an Electrosurgery Unit

A closed circuit contains the following components:

1. generator
2. active electrode
3. return electrode

1.4 Waveforms and Tissue Effects

1.4.1 Cutting

- uses low voltage but constant waveform duty cycle (duty cycle 100% on)

Table 72.1 Current and frequency

	Low frequency	High frequency
Value	50 cycles per second	>200 000 cycles per second
Use	Standard household appliances	Electrosurgery
Reason	Slow change of current direction → ionic exchange across cell membrane → neuromuscular stimulation in human body	Rapid change of current direction → No ionic exchange across cell membrane → No neuromuscular stimulation in human body

→: leads to

Table 72.2 Monopolar versus bipolar electrosurgery

	Monopolar	Bipolar
Circuit pathway	Generator → active electrode → tissue → patient → patient return electrode → generator	Generator → active electrode → tissue (conducting medium) → return electrode → generator
Uses	Cutting and coagulation	Coagulation only
Types of active electrodes	Blade, ball, needle tip, open/closed loop The smaller the electrode tip, the greater the concentration of current at the tip	Forceps: one blade is the active electrode and the other blade is the return electrode
Disadvantage	Less safe than bipolar	Can only coagulate

→: leads to

Table 72.3 Grounded versus isolated electrosurgery systems

	Grounded system	Isolated system
Age	Older system	Modern system
Circuit	Circuit completes via an earth/ground system separate from the generator	Circuit completes through the generator rather than the earth/ground
Risks	If conductive objects touch patient → current may not travel via patient return electrode → may cause alternate site burns	Current travels via patient return electrode only → No alternate site burns

→: leads to

- the electrode should be held near, but not in contact with, the tissue
- current arcs between the electrode and the tissue, and produces rapid rise in temperature, which leads to vaporisation of cells (cells explode into clouds of steam)
- current dissipates rapidly so less surrounding tissue trauma
- minimal collateral coagulation: clean cut with no haemostasis

1.4.2 Coagulation (Pinpoint)

- uses high voltage but intermittent waveform duty cycle (duty cycle 6% on, 94% off)
- tissue cools down between heat bursts, so it does not vaporise but instead coagulates
- the higher the voltage plus the longer the modulation interval, the greater the haemostatic effect
- avoid long duration of electrode activation as this can lead to electrode sticking to coagulum and tearing off the coagulum from the vessel
- reasonably good collateral coagulation: carbonisation of adjacent tissue

1.4.3 Blended Cutting

- interrupted duty cycle: examples: 50% on/50% off, 25% on/75% off
- produces both cutting (low voltage) and coagulation (high voltage) effects

1.4.4 Fulguration (Forced Coagulation)

- high current is used to coagulate or carbonise a larger bleeding area by creating a sparking or spray effect
- wider electrodes applied without touching the tissue
- leads to deeper coagulation than normal
- use in special circumstances only

1.4.5 Desiccation

- tip of electrode must touch tissue
- leads to dehydration of intracellular fluid when the cell is heated to 70–100 °C
- can use either monopolar or bipolar diathermy
- can use either cutting (more common) or coagulation mode

1.5 Safety of Electrosurgery

1.5.1 Built-in Safety Mechanisms

- generator monitors low frequency current leakage
- generator alerts when there is an incomplete application of return electrode
- dual return electrodes: if there is difference in resistance between the two, the generator shuts off
- power output display for surgeon to be aware of the power used (30 watts, 35 watts)

Monopolar system has three potential hazards:

1. Direct coupling
2. Insulation failure
3. Capacitive coupling

Direct coupling

- Occurs when surgeon activates the generator when the active electrode is near another conductive instrument.
- Example:
  - the active electrode is activated when it touches the camera. The camera acts as a conductive instrument and injures the nearby bowel.

Insulation failure

- Occurs when the coating which insulates the active electrode is broken.
- Example:
  - There is a break in the insulation covering the bipolar electrode. When the electrode is activated, the voltage is pushed through the break and injures the nearby bowel.

Capacitive coupling

- Occurs when a capacitator is inadvertently created by two conductors separated by a nonconductor.
- The capacitator creates an electrostatic field between the two conductors so when current is running through one conductor, it travels to the second conductor.
- Highest risk when using a metal plastic hybrid trochar system.
- Example:
  - An active electrode (conductor) with insulated protector (nonconductor) is placed through

a metal trochar (conductor). Current can travel to the metal trochar, which can injure tissue in proximity of the trochar.

1.5.2 Safety Practices for Electrosurgery

- check individual instruments before surgery
- use the lowest voltage setting for the clinical effect
- activate electrode only when needed
- do not activate electrode when it is in proximity with a metal or conductive object
- use either all metal or all plastic cannula/trochar system: avoid hybrid cannula
- bipolar electrodes are safer than monopolar electrodes

2 Laser

Stands for Light Amplification by the Stimulated Emission of Radiation.

2.1 Properties of Laser

- emits photons, which are used to vaporise, cut and coagulate tissue
- has natural sterilisation effect against bacteria, viruses and fungi
- seals nerve endings: reduces postoperative pain
- types of lasers: gas (carbon dioxide or argon ions), solid state
- endoscopic lasers are class 4 lasers: can cause fire, burns and retinal injury
- interact with tissues in four ways: photothermally, photochemically, photomechanically and photoablatively

2.2 Carbon Dioxide (CO_2) Gas Laser

- wavelength 10 600 nm
- highly absorbed by soft tissues that contain water
- offers precise cutting, limited depth of penetration and limited lateral thermal damage
- invisible to human eye: require additional aiming laser
- operation system is expensive

2.3 Solid State Lasers

- made by covering crystalline solid host with ions
- examples:
  - Nd:YAG laser: neodymium-doped yttrium aluminium garnet laser
  - KTP laser: passing Nd:YAG beam through a crystal of potassium titanyl phosphate

2.4 Nd:YAG Laser

- wavelength 1064 nm
- can be transmitted down a fibreoptic cable
- can cut, coagulate and vaporise
- if transmitted down a bare quart fibre can penetrate tissue deeply: useful for hysteroscopy
- ensure beam focuses at the tip to limit lateral tissue damage

2.5 KTP Laser

- wavelength 532 nm
- produces a visible beam
- beam characteristics lies between CO_2 laser and Nd:YAG laser
- penetrates tissue depth 1–2 mm
- can cut, coagulate and vaporise

2.5.1 Monopolar and Bipolar

Remember some instruments use monopolar and some bipolar:

1. Blade: bipolar
2. Needle tip: monopolar
3. Forceps: monopolar
4. Ball: bipolar
5. Loop: bipolar

Section 13

Epidemiology and Statistics

Jane Ding

73 Statistical Methods Used in Clinical Research

Jane Ding

1 Basic Statistics

Table 73.1 Scale

Scales	Description	Example
Nominal	Categorical variable	• Blonde, brunette, black, red • Male, female
Ordinal	Ordering of variables	• Low, medium, high • Unsatisfied, neutral, satisfied
Interval	• The interval between two neighbouring points is the same as the interval between another two neighbouring points • Can be below zero	• £1000, £1500, £2000 • -5 °C, 0 °C, 5 °C, 10 °C
Ratio	Interval scale with an absolute zero	• 20 kg, 40 kg, 60 kg • 1.5 cm, 2 cm, 2.5 cm

Table 73.2 Measurement

Concepts of measurement	Description
Accuracy	Measurement that matches the true value
Precision	Measurement that has small random errors
Reliability	Measurement that has minimal variations when repeated
Validity	Measurement that gives true information about what is being tested

Table 73.3 To describe the central tendency of a large data set

Measure	Description	Example
Range	Spread of data	7, 2, 8, 10, 5, 3, 6 Range = 2–10
Mode	Value occurring most frequently	9, 2, 5, 4, 10, 6, 7, 9 Mode = 9
Median	Middle value of ranked data	6, 3, 5, 1, 4, 8 Median = 4.5
Mean	Average	4, 7, 3, 9, 7 Mean = 6

2 Types of Data Distributions

1. Normal distribution
2. Binomial distribution
3. Poisson distribution

2.1 Normal (Gaussian) Distribution

1. Single peak (unimodal)
2. Symmetrical: equal number of observations to the left and right of midpoint

- Symmetry does not always mean normality
- Examples:
  - Sparse distribution around the mean (i.e., curve is heavy tailed)
  - Concentrated distribution around the mean (i.e., curve is peaked)

3. Same mode, median, mean
4. Described by mean and standard deviation
5. Two tests that assesses normality:

   a. Shapiro–Wilk
   b. Kolmogorov–Smirnov

2.2 Measures of Spread in a Normal Distribution

2.2.1 Variance (s^2)

- The average amount by which a measurement differs from the mean
- The greater the variance the greater the range of the data
- variance =

$$\frac{\Sigma(x - \bar{x})^2}{n - 1}$$

($\bar{x}$ = mean, n = number of observations)

2.2.2 Standard Deviation (s or SD)

- Describes the scatter or spread in a Sample
- Easier to use than variance

$\sqrt{variance}$

- Different from POPULATION standard deviation (σ)
- In a normal distribution with $n \geq 30$ → can assume SAMPLE mean ($\bar{x}$) and standard deviation (s) is similar to POPULATION mean (μ) and standard deviation (σ)
- Normal score or standard normal deviate (z) = the number of standard deviations from the mean μ (i.e., 1 = 1 σ, 2 = 2 σ)

2.2.3 Coefficient of Variation (COV)

- Useful for determining reliability of repeated measurements
- Coefficient of variation $= \frac{s}{\bar{x}} \times 100$

Table 73.4 Normal distribution

Standard deviation	Area covered under the curve	Area lies outside the range	Area from μ (each side)
± 1σ	68%	32%	16%
± 2σ	95%	5%	2.5%
± 3σ	99.8%	0.2%	0.1%

2.2.4 Standard Error of the Mean (SEM)

- Useful for determining how close a sample mean is to the population mean
- The smaller the SEM, the closer the sample mean to the population mean
- Standard error of the mean $= \frac{s}{\sqrt{n}}$

- The mean ($\bar{x}$) age at booking is 35 years old (yo)
- The standard deviation (s) is 12yo
- If n = 100, SEM $= \frac{12}{\sqrt{100}} = 1.2$yo

2.2.5 Confidence Interval (CI) for the Difference Between Two Means

- The probability (90% or 95%) that the true population mean lies between a specific range of values
- Used with normal distribution with $n \geq 30$
- The 95% CI gives similar information to a p-value <0.05
- Confidence interval $= \bar{x} \pm (2 \times \text{SEM})$
- Example:

The mean ($\bar{x}$) age at booking is 35yo

The sample size is 100

SEM is 1.2yo

95% CI = 35 ± (2 × 1.2) = 33–37yo

Interpretation: 95% probability that the true population mean lies between 33 and 37yo odds ratio (OR); 5% probability that the true population mean lies outside the age range.

2.3 Non-normal Distribution

2.3.1 Skewed Data

- Skewed data are not normally distributed
- In skewed data the distribution of sample means still can approach a normal distribution: this means SEM can still be used
- Skewed data may sometimes be transformed into normal distribution by the following methods:

1. Logarithm (log x)
2. Square root ($\sqrt{x}$)
3. Squaring (x^2)
4. Reciprocal ($\frac{1}{x}$)

2.3.2 Binomial Distribution

- Used for counts of data on a dichotomous scale (i.e., pregnant/not pregnant, yes/no)
- When $n > 30$ binomial distribution approaches normal distribution
- Standard deviation of $a = a \times (1 - a)$
- Standard error $= \sqrt{\frac{a \times (1-a)}{n}}$
- Therefore $\bar{x} = 10\%$ and $a = 0.1$
- Example:

There are 100 pregnant women

Ten admitted smoking

Therefore $\bar{x} = 10\%$ and $a = 0.1$

SEM $= \sqrt{\frac{0.1 \times (1-0.1)}{100}} = 0.03$

95% CI = 0.1 ± (2 × 0.03) = 0.04–0.16 or 4–16%

Interpretation: 95% probability that the true population mean lies between 4 and 16%.

2.3.3 Poisson Distribution

- Useful for counting the number of events occurring over a period of time (e.g., daily number of admissions from Accident and Emergency to the gynaecology ward)
- Always whole numbers
- Useful for rare events as it allows for calculation of probability of event per unit of time (e.g., gynaecology admission number on a single day)
- When the mean is close to zero (i.e., lots of zero admissions), distribution is skewed
- As the mean increases, the distribution approximates to normal
- Variance = mean

3 Comparative Statistics

3.1 Null Hypothesis (H0)

- Definition: there is no significant difference between the two variables in the hypothesis
  - Example: there is no difference in heart rate between Group 1 and Group 2
- p-value (aka alpha value) is used to support or reject the null hypothesis
- The smaller the p-value, the higher the probability of a true difference between the two groups
- Null hypothesis is rejected if $p < 0.05$

3.2 Sample Size ($_n$)

- Needs to be big enough to detect real difference in variables as being statistically significant
- Takes into account alpha (α) and beta (β) errors
- Power (beta value) is directly related to sample size
- Minimal sample size is determined in advance to give a power of 80–90%

3.3 Types of Errors

- Type 1 (alpha) error:
  - When H0 is wrongly rejected
  - In practice, when a difference in mean is found when there is none
  - Due to p-value set at 0.05: so error occurs in 1 in 20 times
- Type 2 (beta) error:
  - When the H0 is wrongly accepted
  - Due to small sample size

3.4 Types of Tests

- Nonparametric analyses: no assumption of normal distribution of the data is required
- Table 73.5 shows the tests for data with normal distribution (parametric) and the equivalent for distribution-free (nonparametric)

Table 73.5 Types of tests

Parametric tests	Nonparametric tests	Measures
Student's t-test (paired)	Wilcoxon test	Mean
Student's t-test (unpaired)	Mann–Whitney U test	Mean
Fisher's test	Chi-square (χ^2) test	Categorical variables
Pearson's *r* test	Spearman's rho (ρ) test	Correlation
Analysis of variance (one or more way)	Kruskal–Wallis analysis of variance (one way)	Variance

3.5 Chi-square (χ^2) Test

- Compares two categorical variables in a continency table to determine if they are related
- Simplest type is using a 2 x 2 contingency table, but can be applied to larger contingency tables
- Cannot be used:
  - When expected number of observations <5
  - When total number of observations <20
  - With proportions
- Example for using the χ^2 test:

  A doctor has reviewed 1000 patients with high blood pressure: 800 were men; 200 were women. Is high blood pressure gender related?

3.6 t-Tests

- Compares means of samples
- Paired: measurements made on the same subjects at two different time points:
  - Example: comparing blood pressure of 100 patients, measured at 12 weeks of gestation and at 30 weeks of gestation.
- Unpaired: measurements made on different groups of subjects:
  - Example: comparing a new drug (50 patients) against placebo (50 patients) to determine if it lowers blood pressure.
- CI for difference between means:
  - If CI includes 0 → then no significant difference between means

3.7 Pearson's and Spearman's Correlation Tests

- Determines whether two continuous variables are associated
- Correlation coefficient:
  - Pearson's r or Spearman's ρ
  - Tests degree of association between variables
  - Essentially measures the scatter around a linear trend
- Perfect positive correlation between variables → Pearson's $r = 1.0$
- Perfect negative correlation between variables → Pearson's $r = -1.0$
- Correlation ≠ causal
- Example:

  Is blood pressure correlated with age in 100 patients?

  $r = 0.6$, $r^2 = 0.36$, $p<0.001$

  Interpretation: 36% of blood pressure variation can be accounted for by difference in age.

4 Statistical Interpretation

Incidence: rate of new cases of disease per population

Prevalence: frequency of existing disease at a given time

In a stable condition:
prevalence = incidence × duration of disease

Crude proportion: value that is not standardised by confounders; that is, death rate

Standardised proportion: value that is standardised or adjusted by confounders

4.1 Odds Ratio (OR)

- Odds that the outcome (i.e., getting the disease) will occur, comparing the exposed group to the control group
- If OR is reported with a confidence interval including 1, then the OR is not significant
- Can be calculated from prospective or retrospective study – see Table 73.6
- Odds ratio

$$= \frac{\text{odds of having the disease in the exposed group}}{\text{odds of not having the disease in the exposed group}}$$

- Example:

Table 73.6 Interpretation of odds ratio

OR	Interpretation	Example
1	The odds of the outcome occurring is the same for the exposed compared to the control	
>1	The odds of the outcome occurring is higher for the exposed compared to the control	OR 2.2 – 2.2 times more likely to have the disease compared to the control
<1	The odds of the outcome occurring is lower for the exposed compared to the control	OR 0.7 – 30% less likely to have the disease compared to the control

Table 73.7 Interpretation of odds ratio

		Smoker		
		Yes	**No**	**Total**
Preeclampsia	***Yes***	20	170	190
	No	80	900	980
	Total	100	1070	1270

Are smokers at higher risk of developing preeclampsia compared to nonsmokers?

Exposure: smoking

Control: not smoking

Odds of a patient having preeclampsia being a smoker = $\frac{20}{170}$ = 0.117

Odds of a patient not having preeclampsia being a smoker = $\frac{80}{900}$ = 0.08

$$\text{OR} = \frac{0.117}{0.08} = 1.46$$

Interpretation: smokers have 46% higher chance of developing preeclampsia compared to nonsmokers (assuming that CI does not include 1) – see Table 73.7

4.2 Relative Risk

- Probability of getting the disease in an exposure group divided by the probability of getting the disease in an unexposed (control) group
- Calculated from prospective study only.
- Relative risk $= \dfrac{\frac{TP}{TP+FP}}{\frac{FN}{FN+TN}}$

4.3 Risk matrix

A chart used to assess the chance of a risk arising and consequence of it.

4.4 Likelihood Ratio (LR)

See Tables 73.8 and 73.9.

- The effectiveness of a test to confirm or exclude the diagnosis
- Likelihood ratio $= \dfrac{\text{sensitivity}}{\text{specificity}}$

4.5 Positive Likelihood Ratio (LR+)

- If the test is positive, how much does that increase the odds of having the disease?

Table 73.8 Interpretation of likelihood ratios

LR	Interpretation
>10	Test result has **large** effect on **increasing** the probability of having the disease
5–10	Test result has **moderate** effect on **increasing** the probability of having the disease
<5	Test result has **small** effect on **increasing** the probability of having the disease

- Positive likelihood ratio $= \dfrac{\text{sensitivity}}{1 - \text{specificity}}$
- Interpretation: see Table 73.8

Table 73.9 Interpretation of likelihood ratios

LR	Interpretation
<0.1	Test result has **large** effect on **decreasing** the probability of having the disease
0.5–0.1	Test result has **moderate** effect on **decreasing** the probability of having the disease
>0.5	Test result has **small** effect on **decreasing** the probability of having the disease

4.6 Negative Likelihood Ratio (LR-)

- If the test is negative, how much does that decrease the odds of having the disease?
- Negative likelihood ratio $= \dfrac{1 - \text{sensitivity}}{\text{specificity}}$
- Interpretation: see Table 73.9

Table 73.10 Levels of Evidence

1a	Systematic review or meta-analysis of randomised controlled trials
1b	At least one randomised controlled trial
2a	At least one well-designed controlled study, without randomisation
2b	At least one other type of well-designed, quasiexperimental study
3	Well-designed descriptive studies
4	Expert committee reports or opinions OR Clinical experience of respected authorities

Table 73.11 Grade of evidence

Grade	Description	Level of evidence equivalent
Grade A	At least one randomised controlled trial	1a, 1b
Grade B	Well-controlled study but no randomised controlled trial	2a, 2b, 3
Grade C	Expert reports or opinions Clinical experience of respected authorities	4

4.7 Number Needed to Treat (NNT)

- The average number of patients who need to receive the treatment for one of them to get the positive outcome in a specified time frame
- The lower the NNT, the more effective the treatment/intervention
- Example: NNT = 5

  Interpretation: five patients need to receive the cancer drug for one person to be cleared from the cancer.

4.8 Number Needed to Harm (NNH)

- The average number of patients who need to receive the treatment for one of them to have a particular adverse effect
- The higher the NNH, the better the treatment/intervention
- Example: NNH = 50

  Interpretation: for every 50 people receiving Depo-Provera, 1 person suffered from suicidal thoughts.

Table 73.12 Types of epidemiology studies

Type of study	Description	Example
Observational	Relies on surveillance of population	The Confidential Enquiry into Maternal and Child Health (CEMACH)
Analytical observational	Analyses performed on observational studies	Case control, cohort CEMACE analyses
Experimental	Investigates effects of intervention	Randomised controlled trial

4.9 Levels of Evidence

- When interpreting a recommendation from a study it is important to do so in context with the level of evidence. See Tables 73.12 and 73.13.

4.10 Types of study design

- It is also important to be familiar with the different types of study designs – see Table 73.12

74 Principles of Screening

Jane Ding

1 Aim of Screening Programme

- to detect one's predisposition for developing a disease
- done at an early stage when patient is still disease free
- allow for early intervention

2 Requirements for Screening Tests

- simple, safe and acceptable to public
- high sensitivity and specificity
- reproducible
- little overlap between affected and unaffected people
- defined cut-off levels
- cost effective
- Sensitivity is the ability of a test to correctly identify those with the disease (true positive rate).
- Specificity is the ability of a test to correctly identify those without the disease (true negative rate).
- Positive predictive values (PPV) is the proportion of positive results in statistics and diagnostic tests that are true positive.
- Negative predictive values (NPV) is the proportion of negative results in statistics and diagnostic tests that are true negative. See Tables 74.1 and 74.2.

Table 74.1 Critical analyses of investigations

	Sick	Healthy	
Positive test	True positive (TP)	False positive (FP)	**PPV** = $\frac{TP}{FP+TP}$
Negative test	False negative (FN)	True negative (TN)	**NPV** = $\frac{TN}{TN+FN}$
	Sensitivity = $\frac{TP}{TP+FN}$	**Specificity** = $\frac{TN}{TN+FP}$	

Table 74.2 Sensitivity and specificity

Sensitivity	Proportion of patients with disease receiving a positive test	TP / (TP + FN)
Specificity	Proportion of patients without disease receiving a negative test	TN / (TN + FP)
Positive predictive value (PPV)	Proportion of patients with positive test who actually have the disease	TP / (FP + TP)
Negative predictive value (NPV)	Proportion of patients with negative test who do not have the disease	TN / (TN + FN)

3 Diseases for Screening

- should be an important health problem
- has a known natural history
- has a long latent phase
- has an acceptable treatment

4 Forest Plot

Information adapted from Cochrane.org

4.1 Meta-Analysis

If enough similar single studies in a given field are conducted, the results can be combined to generate a more reliable result due to a combined population, bigger than any prior population. This is known as a meta-analysis. Forest plots can summarise almost all the essential information of a meta-analysis.

There are three main things that need to be assessed when reading a meta-analysis:

1. Heterogeneity: the differences in the results, methodology or study populations used in the included studies.
2. The pooled result: the overall combined result derived from combining ('pooling') the individual studies.

3. Publication bias: some studies can be missed because they are not written in English, or because they show non-significant results (so they have a lower chance of being published). A forest plot does a great job in illustrating the heterogeneity and the pooled result, but it cannot display potential publication bias. A funnel plot does that instead.

4.2 How to Read a Forest Plot

There are six columns in a forest plot (see Figure 74.1).

Column 1: studies IDs: the leftmost column shows the identities (IDs) of the included studies. Studies are represented by the name of the first author and the year of publication, often arranged in time order.

Columns 2 and 3: data from the intervention group (n/N) and control group (n/N) from each study are shown. 'n' indicates the number of patients having the outcome of interest, while 'N' represents the total number of patients in that group. For example, in the study of Rowling JK (2000) in Figure 74.1, 1 out of 131 participants in the intervention group has the outcome of interest, compared with 2 out of 133 participants in the control group.

Column 4: relative risk (fixed) 95% confidence interval (CI): the next column visually displays the study results. The boxes show the effect estimates from the single studies, while the diamond shows the pooled result. The horizontal lines through the boxes illustrate the length of the CI. The longer the lines, the wider the CI, and the less reliable the study results. The width of the diamond serves the same purpose. The vertical line is the line of no effect (i.e. the position at which there is no clear difference between the intervention group and the control group).

If result estimates are located to the left, it means that the outcome of interest occurred less frequently in the intervention group than in the control group (ratio <1). If result estimates are located to the right, it means that the outcome of interest occurred more frequently in the intervention group than in the control group (ratio >1). If the diamond touches the vertical line, the overall (combined) result is not statistically significant. It means the overall outcome rate in the intervention group is much the same as in the control group.

Column 5: weight (%): the next column is the weight (in %), which indicates the influence an individual study has had on the pooled result. In general, the bigger the sample size and the narrower the CI, the

Study IDs	Intervention group n/N (1)	Control group n/N	Relative risk (fixed) 95% CI (2)	Weight (3) (%)	Relative risk (fixed) 95% CI (2)
Rowling JK 2000	1/131	2/133		17.8	0.50 (0.05–5.49)
Albus D 2003	7/279	9/290		77.7	0.84 (0.36–1.93)
Hermione G 2005	3/102	1/101		4.5	3.00 (0.12–72.77)
Total	512	542		100.0	0.87 (0.41–1.87) (4)

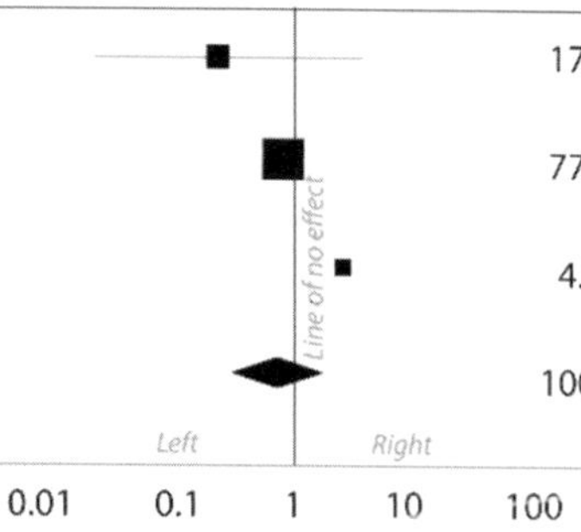

Line of no effect

Left Right

0.01 0.1 1 10 100

Test for herterogeneity Chi-square = 0.79, df = 2, $p = 0.67$, $I^2 = 0.0\%$ (5)
Test for overall effect $z = 0.35$, $p = 0.7$ (6)

(1) N = total number in group, n = number in group with the outcome.
(2) Outcome of interest in picture and in number. Fixed effect model used for meta-analysis.
(3) Influence of studies on overall meta-analysis.
(4) Overall effect.
(5) Heterogeneity (I^2) = 0%. So, we use fixed effect model.
(6) *p* value indicating level of statistical significance

Figure 74.1 How to read a forest plot.

higher the percentage weight, the larger the box and more the influence the study has on the pooled result.

Column 6: relative risk (fixed) 95% CI: the rightmost column contains the same information as is contained in the diagram in column 4, just in numerical format. So, the data can be seen in both in picture and number formats. This can be either the 95% CI of odds ratio (OR) or the 95% CI of relative risk (RR). When the 95% CI does not include 1, the result is statistically significant.

4.2.1 Lower Left Corner of the Plot

The p-value indicates the level of statistical significance. If the diamond shape does not touch the line of no effect, the difference found between the two groups was statistically significant. In that case, the p-value is usually <0.05.

I^2 indicates the level of heterogeneity. It can take values from 0% to 100%. If $I^2 \leq 50\%$, studies are considered homogeneous, and a fixed effect model of meta-analysis can be used. If $I^2 > 50\%$, the heterogeneity is high, and one should use a random effect model for meta-analysis. The difference between homogeneity and heterogeneity therefore lies in the different approaches taken to calculate the pooled result.

4.2.2 Receiver Operating Characteristic (ROC) Curve

The ROC curve is a graphical plot, which illustrates the diagnostic ability of a binary classifier system as its discrimination threshold is varied.

The ROC curve is created by plotting the true positive rate (TPR) against the false positive rate (FPR) at various threshold settings. The TPR is also known as sensitivity, and the FPR can be calculated as (1 – specificity).

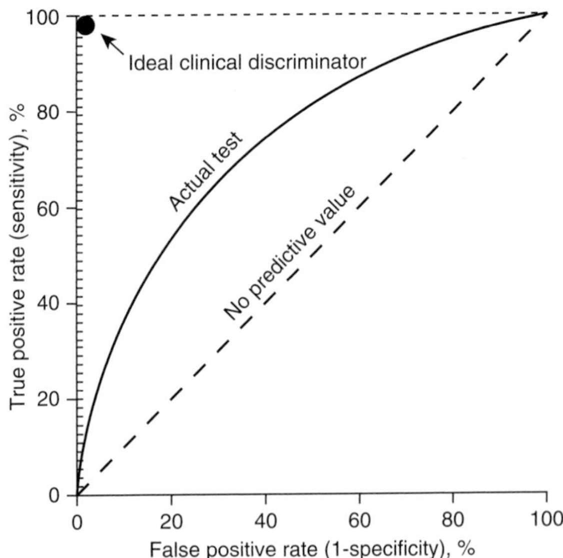

Figure 74.2 The ROC curve.

ROC analysis is related in a direct and natural way to cost/benefit analysis of diagnostic decision-making.

The ROC is also known as a relative operating characteristic curve because it is a comparison of two operating characteristics (TPR and FPR) as the criterion changes.

The ROC curve shows the trade-off between sensitivity and specificity.

Classifiers that give curves closer to the top-left corner indicate a better performance. As a baseline, a random classifier is expected to give points lying along the diagonal (FPR = TPR). The closer the curve comes to the 45-degree diagonal of the ROC space, the less accurate the test. See Figure 74.2.

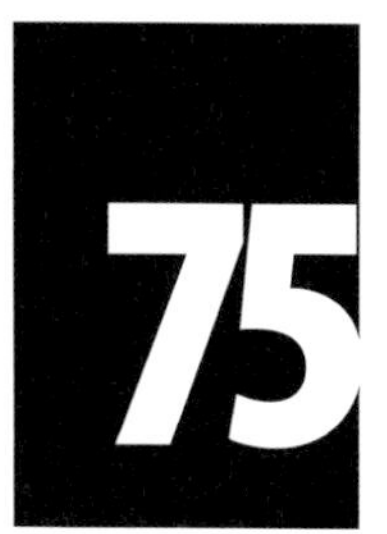

Understanding the Audit Cycle

Jane Ding

1 Audit

- a method to determine whether clinical care is being practised in line with clinical standards; that is, measures practice against performance
- is part of the quality improvement process to improve patient care and outcome
- must have standards to measure against
- standards can be taken from local trust guidelines: NICE, RCOG or other good-quality guidelines
- an important part of clinical governance
- can be performed retrospectively or prospectively
- different from research: audit always involves measurement against standards
- the audit process follows a cycle with six stages and this is outlined in Figure 75.1

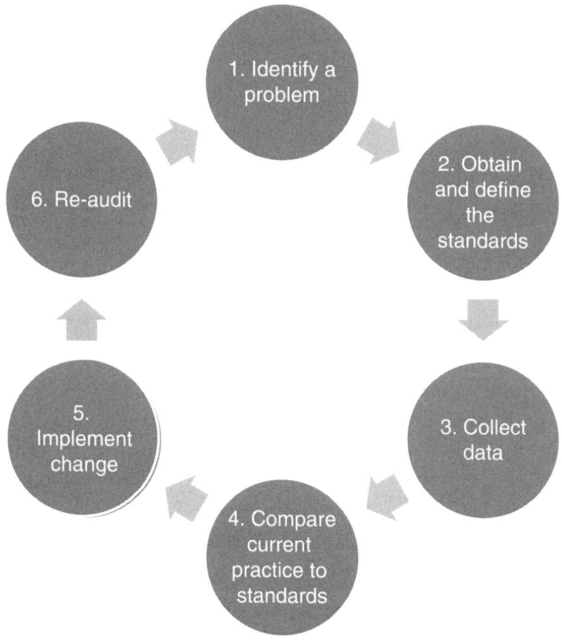

Figure 75.1 Audit cycle.

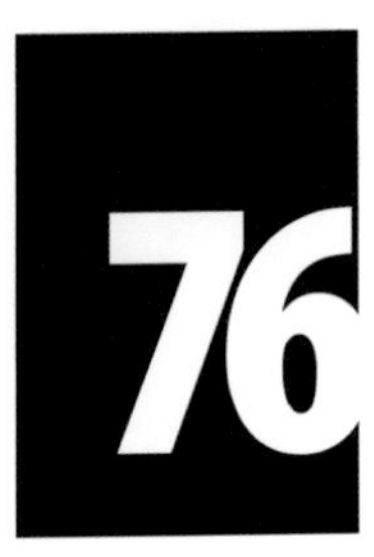

Definition of Maternal, Perinatal and Neonatal Mortality

Jane Ding

1 Maternal Deaths Definitions

- World health Organization (WHO): maternal mortality ratio is the number of maternal deaths per 100 000 live births
- UK: maternal mortality ratio is the number of maternal deaths per 100 000 maternities – see Table 76.1

Table 76.1 Maternal deaths definitions

Maternal death	Death of women when pregnant or within 42 days of end of pregnancy Not from accidental or coincidental causes
Direct maternal death	Deaths due to complications of pregnancy, labour or puerperium; or from interventions, omission or incorrect treatment
Indirect maternal death	Death due to preexisting disease or disease developed during pregnancy, which is not the result of direct obstetric cause
Late maternal death	Death occurring between 42 days and 1 year after the end of pregnancy Direct or indirect cause
Coincidental	Death from unrelated causes, which happened to have occurred during pregnancy or puerperium

2 Perinatal Deaths Definitions

See Table 76.2.

- WHO: measured per 1000 births

Table 76.2 Perinatal deaths definitions

Late fetal loss	Delivery 22^{+0} to 23^{+6} No signs of life Irrespective of when death occurred
Stillbirth	Delivery $\geq 24^{+0}$ No signs of life Irrespective of when death occurred
Antepartum stillbirth	Delivery $\geq 24^{+0}$ No signs of life Known to have died before onset of labour
Intrapartum stillbirth	Delivery $\geq 24^{+0}$ No signs of life Alive at the onset of labour
Neonatal death	Delivery $\geq 20^{+0}$ or birthweight ≥400 g (when gestational age not available) Live-born baby Died before 28 days after birth
Early neonatal death	Delivery $\geq 20^{+0}$ or birthweight ≥400 g (when gestational age not available) Live-born baby Died before 7 days after birth
Late neonatal death	Delivery $\geq 20^{+0}$ or birthweight ≥400 g (when gestational age not available) Live-born baby Died between 7 days and 28 days after birth
Postneonatal death	Delivery $\geq 20^{+0}$ or birthweight ≥400 g (when gestational age not available) Live-born baby Died between 28 days and 1 year after birth
Perinatal death	Stillbirth or early neonatal death
Extended perinatal death	Stillbirth or neonatal death

Appendices: Practice Question Papers with Answers

Neela Mukhopadhaya

Appendix 1

Practice Paper 1: 100 SBAs

SBA Paper 1

- **Duration:** 2.5 hours (150 minutes)
- Number of questions: 100 SBAs

Paper 1 Topics

- Anatomy
- Embryology
- Physiology
- Biochemistry
- Genetics
- Statistics/epidemiology
- Endocrinology

Instructions: This practice paper is laid out in the same style as your examination. Attempt the paper just like you would in an examination setting. Go through your answers and revise any topics you get wrong. This will ensure you revise the topics that you have not mastered or revised yet. Some questions are from topics that have not been covered in this book. Please revise these topics. Most questions adhere to the principles of SBA format, but just for the sake of knowledge, a few questions maybe worded slightly differently. This is to ensure that you study those topics.

Practice Paper 1

1. During menstruation, vasospasm occurs in the arterioles of the secretory endometrium. This is produced mainly by:
   a. Progesterone
   b. Prostacyclin
   c. Prostaglandin E1
   d. Prostaglandin E2
   e. Prostaglandin F2

2. Progesterone has an effect on the growth of breast tissue. Which tissue is mainly affected?
   a. Adipose tissue
   b. Capillaries
   c. Ducts
   d. Glands
   e. Lobules

3. There are two principal types of nuclear estrogen receptors. On which chromosome is receptor ER alpha located?
   a. Chromosome 6
   b. Chromosome 8
   c. Chromosome 10
   d. Chromosome 12
   e. Chromosome 16

4. There are two principal types of nuclear estrogen receptors. On which chromosome is receptor ER beta located?
   a. Chromosome 6
   b. Chromosome 8
   c. Chromosome 10
   d. Chromosome 12
   e. Chromosome 14

5. 98% of the circulating progesterone is bound to proteins. How is this bound?
   a. 10% to albumin and 88% is bound to corticosteroid-binding globulin
   b. 20% to albumin and 78% is bound to corticosteroid-binding globulin
   c. 60% to albumin and 38% is bound to corticosteroid-binding globulin
   d. 80% to albumin and 18% is bound to corticosteroid-binding globulin
   e. 90% to albumin and 8% is bound to corticosteroid-binding globulin

6. What kind of hormone is relaxin?
   a. Glucosan
   b. Liposaccharide
   c. Peptidoglycan
   d. Polypeptide
   e. Polysaccharide

7. A 25-year-old woman is breastfeeding her infant. During suckling, what hormonal response/responses may be triggered?
   a. Decreased secretion of both oxytocin and antidiuretic hormone (ADH)
   b. Decreased secretion of neurophysin
   c. Increased secretion of ADH
   d. Increased secretion of oxytocin
   e. Increased secretion of prolactin

8. During pregnancy, the uterine smooth muscle is quiescent. However, during the ninth month of gestation, the uterine muscle becomes progressively more excitable. What is the main factor that contributes to the increase in excitability?
   a. Activity of the fetus falls to low levels
   b. Increase in maternal prolactin levels
   c. estrogen synthesis by the placenta decreases
   d. Progesterone synthesis by the placenta decreases
   e. Uterine blood flow reaches its highest rate

9. The mere sound of the hungry baby's cry is sufficient to induce milk ejection from the nipples even before the baby is placed to the breast. What is the reason behind this phenomenon?
   a. Increased release of prolactin in the mother that causes milk synthesis
   b. Reflex relaxation of the myoepithelial cells
   c. Secretion of oxytocin from the posterior pituitary, which causes contraction of the myoepithelial cells
   d. Stimulation of the sympathetic nervous system that causes contraction of the myoepithelial cells
   e. Surge of prolactin from the anterior pituitary, which promptly stimulates milk production from the breast

10. Women who are breastfeeding generally have amenorrhoea. What is the physiological basis of lactational amenorrhoea?
    a. Lack of ovarian steroidogenesis during breastfeeding
    b. Oxytocin induced inhibition of GnRH secretion
    c. Oxytocin induced stimulation of GnRH secretion
    d. Prolactin-induced inhibition of GnRH secretion
    e. Prolactin induced stimulation of GnRH secretion

11. What is the nerve innervation of the dartos muscle in males?
    a. Iliohypogastric
    b. Ilioinguinal
    c. Genitofemoral
    d. Lateral cutaneous
    e. Obturator

12. The prostate gland derives embryologically from the:
    a. Cloacal membrane
    b. Genital tubercle
    c. Labioscrotal folds
    d. Urogenital folds
    e. Urogenital sinus

13. Which structure develops embryologically from the paramesonephric ducts in the male?
    a. Appendix of the testes
    b. Lower part of urethra
    c. Prostate gland
    d. Seminal vesicles
    e. Vas deferens

14. Which structure develops embryologically from the mesonephric ducts in a male?
    a. Cowper's gland
    b. Epididymis
    c. Prostatic ducts
    d. Testes
    e. Vas deferens

15. By what factor is the testicular testosterone levels higher compared to blood levels?
    a. 1–5 times
    b. 10–20 times
    c. 20–50 times
    d. 60–80 times
    e. 100–150 times

16. The hydatid of Morgagni is the remnant of which embryological structure?
    a. Gubernaculum
    b. Mesonephric ducts
    c. Müllerian ducts
    d. Urogenital sinus
    e. Utriculus

17. Leydig cell tumours are diagnosed histologically by certain inclusion bodies. What are they called?
    a. Heinz bodies
    b. Henderson Patterson bodies
    c. Howell-Jolly bodies
    d. Negri crystal bodies
    e. Reinke crystal bodies

18. In a woman with known epilepsy, high-dose folic acid is recommended. How long should a pregnant woman continue this for?
    a. Can stop when she has a positive pregnancy test
    b. Until 12 weeks

c. Until 20 weeks
d. Until delivery
e. Continue this until breastfeeding stops

19. Maternal Vitamin K to prevent neonatal haemorrhagic disease of the newborn is recommended in women taking enzyme-inducing antiepileptic drugs. At what gestation would you recommend this?
a. 34 weeks
b. 36 weeks
c. 37 weeks
d. At delivery
e. Not required

20. Which medication should be avoided in women on antiepileptic medication when in labour?
a. Codeine phosphate
b. Diamorphine
c. Halothane
d. Pethidine
e. Remifentanil

21. Physiological hydronephrosis affects the kidneys in a normal pregnancy. What is the average increase in the kidney's longitudinal length?
a. 1 cm
b. 2 cm
c. 3 cm
d. 4 cm
e. 5 cm

22. Isolated microscopic haematuria with structurally normal kidneys can be seen in a pregnant woman. What is the first line of management?
a. Does not need to be investigated during pregnancy
b. Low-dose antibiotics for two weeks
c. PCR
d. Refer to the nephrologist
e. Renal scan

23. What percentage of women with recurrent pyelonephritis have an underlying renal tract abnormality?
a. 10%
b. 20%
c. 30%
d. 40%
e. 50%

24. The commonest cause of acute kidney injury in pregnancy is:
a. Abruption
b. Coagulopathies
c. Eclampsia
d. Fatty liver of pregnancy
e. Septicaemia

25. During wound healing, by what time does the tensile strength of the wound reach that of a normal tissue?
a. Six weeks
b. Three months
c. Six months
d. One year
e. Never

26. Management of an open wound seen 12 hours after the injury is:
a. Debridement and suturing
b. Healing by granulation
c. Should be left open
d. Sterile daily dressing
e. Suturing

27. Many maternal systemic diseases contribute to delayed wound healing. What is the commonest condition that causes delayed healing?
a. Diabetes
b. HELLP Syndrome
c. Hypertension
d. Preeclampsia
e. Pulmonary oedema

28. In a sutured surgical wound, the process of epithelisation is completed within:
a. 30 minutes
b. 24 hours
c. 36 hours
d. 48 hours
e. 4 days

29. In a woman with sickle cell disease, for which blood type should extended phenotype considered?
a. D Punjab type
b. Duffy type
c. Kell type
d. Kidd type
e. O Arab type

30. In a patient with a first-degree heart block, what would be the normal value of the PR interval?
a. 6 seconds
b. 10 seconds
c. 15 seconds

   d. 18 seconds
   e. 22 seconds

31. What is approximate percentage of the mixed venous oxygen saturation in the right atrium?
   a. 10%
   b. 20%
   c. 40%
   d. 60%
   e. 80%

32. In a patient with congestive cardiac failure at 28 weeks of gestation, a decision to check the true mixed venous sample is made by the cardiologist. Where is this blood best sampled from?
   a. Carotid sinus
   b. Left ventricle
   c. Pulmonary artery
   d. Pulmonary vein
   e. Right atrium

33. The QT interval is directly dependent on:
   a. Blood pressure
   b. Cardiac output
   c. Heart rate
   d. Peripheral vascular resistance
   e. Size of the left ventricle

34. By what percentage does the cardiac output increase in pregnancy?
   a. 10%
   b. 20%
   c. 30%
   d. 40%
   e. 50%

35. What condition could reduce the QT interval?
   a. Cardiomyopathy
   b. Digoxin therapy
   c. Hypocalcaemia
   d. Hypokalaemia
   e. Rheumatic carditis

36. Which common factor decreases the SA node discharge?
   a. Atropine
   b. Beta-adrenergic activity
   c. Ischaemia
   d. Pyrexia
   e. Thyroxine

37. Prostacyclin is a vasodilator. Which substrate is it derived from?
   a. Arachidonic acid
   b. Endothelin
   c. Endothelium
   d. L-NMMA
   e. Nitrous oxide

38. Where in the body is angiotensin II synthesised?
   a. Adrenals
   b. Endothelium
   c. Kidneys
   d. Lungs
   e. Platelets

39. Angiotensin II has many effects in the body. Besides being a vasoconstrictor, what is its other main action in the haematological system?
   a. Decreases renal blood flow
   b. Hyperkalaemia
   c. Neutrophilia
   d. Lysis of collagen
   e. Prothrombotic

40. What is the commonest menstrual irregularity caused by hypothyroidism?
   a. Amenorrhoea
   b. Dysmenorrhoea
   c. Menorrhagia
   d. Oligomenorrhea
   e. Polymenorrhoea

41. Thyroid profile of a 25-year-old primigravid woman at 10 weeks of gestation was TSH 10 mIU/L, free T4 2.4 pmol/L, free T3 2.1 pmol/L. What is the most likely diagnosis?
   a. Hyperemesis gravidarum
   b. PIH
   c. Polyhydramnios
   d. Preterm labour
   e. Recurrent miscarriage

42. A young woman presents to your clinic with insomnia and palpitations. You diagnose her to have hyperthyroidism. What is most likely cause?
   a. Grave's disease
   b. Thyroid nodule
   c. Thyroiditis
   d. Toxic multinodular goitre
   e. Toxic thyroid adenoma

43. You are investigating a woman for a pituitary adenoma. What is the first test that you would consider?
   a. Deranged hormonal profile

   b. Fundoscopy
   c. Visual field testing
   d. X-ray of the skull
   e. X-ray of the wrist for bone age

44. Pituitary adenomas can affect any cell type present in the pituitary. What is the most common type of pituitary adenoma?
   a. ACTH-producing tumour
   b. Cystic macroadenoma
   c. Gonadotroph adenomas
   d. Nonfunctional adenomas
   e. Prolactinomas

45. A young girl of 9 years of age presents with thelarche. What structural change best describes changes in mammary gland during puberty?
   a. Appearance of Montgomery tubercles
   b. Breast bud and papilla get elevated and there is enlargement of sides of areola
   c. Fat deposition causes breast bud enlargement
   d. The first noticeable change in the breast occurs during the last phase of menarche
   e. The glandular component increases more in proportion to the ductal system

46. At her booking visit to antenatal clinic, a woman complains of alteration in her breast size. What is the main change in the mammary gland during pregnancy?
   a. Increase in intralobular connective tissue
   b. Increase in myoepithelial cells
   c. Increase in the adipose tissue content
   d. Increase in the number and size of alveoli
   e. Proliferation of the ducts

47. A 35-year-old woman underwent endometrial biopsy. She had a history of regular menstrual cycles of approximately 28 days duration. The biopsy specimen on histological examination showed intact straight uterine glands confined mostly to the superficial part of endometrium and intact surface epithelium. How long before the biopsy did she last ovulate?
   a. 1–3 days
   b. 5–8 days
   c. 7 to 10 days
   d. 14 to 21 days
   e. 42 days

48. Early pregnancy brings about profound changes in the pelvic organs. What is the main change in the cervix during pregnancy?
   a. Appearance of Döderlein's bacilli for the first time
   b. Change in shape of the cervix
   c. Loss of elasticity in the cervix
   d. Softening and cyanosis of the cervix
   e. Uterine body:cervix ratio becomes 3:1

49. What would be the most characteristic structure on histopathological examination in the ovaries of a five-year-old girl?
   a. Corpus luteum
   b. Extensive connecting tissue matrix
   c. Germ cells arrested in prophase of meiosis I
   d. Ovarian follicles containing secondary oocytes
   e. Ovarian follicles in various stages of maturation

50. What are the anatomical layers in the vaginal wall? See table below.

	Epithelium	Muscle	Lamina propria	Adventitial layer
a.	Stratified keratinised squamous	Inner longitudinal and outer circular	Elastic fibres	Loose connective tissue and blood vessels
b.	Stratified squamous	Outer longitudinal and inner circular	Elastic fibres without glands	Dense connective tissue and blood vessels
c.	Columnar	Longitudinal only	Loose connective tissue with glands	Loose connective tissue with lymphatics
d.	Cuboidal	Circular only	Elastic fibres with glands	Dense connective tissue with lymphatics
e.	Tall columnar	Outer longitudinal, and inner oblique	Loose connective tissue without glands	Elastic fibres with lymphatics

51. What is the average weight of a normal adult uterus?
    a. 10–20 g
    b. 30–50 g
    c. 60–80 g
    d. 90–100 g
    e. 120–130 g

52. What are the parts of the anatomical boundaries of the perineum? See table below.

	Anterior	Posterior	Lateral
A	Pubic arch	Anal margin	Ischial rami
B	Pubic symphysis	Coccyx	Sacrotuberous ligament
C	Anterior pubic rami	Pelvic floor	Ischial tuberosity
D	Clitoris	Tip of coccyx	Labia majora
E	Anterior	Fourchette	Sacrotuberous ligament

53. Where are Paneth cells found in the body?
    a. Cerebellar gyri
    b. Large intestine
    c. Oesophagus
    d. Pancreas
    e. Small intestine

54. Cephalic presentation is the most common presentation of fetus at term. What factor is mainly responsible for this?
    a. Gravitation
    b. Power of fetal movements
    c. Power of Braxton-Hicks contractions
    d. Preferential displacement of placenta towards the fundus
    e. Sleeping in left lateral position in pregnancy

55. What is the presenting anterior-posterior diameter of fetus in a completely flexed vertex position?
    a. Biparietal
    b. Mentovertical
    c. Occipitofrontal
    d. Submentovertical
    e. Suboccipitobregmatic

56. What is the attitude of fetal head when the presenting diameter is submentovertical?
    a. Complete extension
    b. Complete flexion
    c. Incomplete extension
    d. Incomplete flexion
    e. Partial flexion

57. Anterior fontanelle is formed posteriorly by the:
    a. Coronal
    b. Frontal
    c. Lambdoid
    d. Mastoid
    e. Sagittal

58. What is the name of the segment of pelvis where internal rotation occurs?
    a. Anatomical outlet
    b. Obstetric outlet
    c. Pelvic cavity
    d. Pelvic inlet
    e. Plane of least pelvic dimension

59. Several nerves can lead to entrapment syndromes in pregnancy. What is the nerve involved in meralgia paraesthetica?
    a. Lateral cutaneous nerve of thigh
    b. Lateral femoral cutaneous nerve of groin
    c. Median nerve
    d. Pudendal nerve
    e. Ulnar nerve

60. Pressure on the genitofemoral nerve can cause pain. Which area is mainly affected?
    a. Anterior abdominal wall
    b. Labia majora
    c. Lower back
    d. Posterior perineum
    e. Outer part of thigh

61. In a patient who has ongoing major obstetric haemorrhage, blood has been requested. How much of crystalloid infusion is required for each litre of blood loss?
    a. 1 litre
    b. 1.5 litres

c. 2 litres
d. 2.5 litres
e. 3 litres

62. Hartmann's solution is commonly used in labour for hydration. What is the main advantage of this solution as compared to normal saline?
  a. Contains electrolytes and bicarbonate
  b. Contains electrolytes and lactate
  c. Contains less chloride
  d. Contains more Na than K
  e. Contains small amount of sugars

63. In the placenta, calcium is transported from the maternal to fetal tissues during pregnancy. Which structure is involved in this transport?
  a. Chorionic cells
  b. Cytotrophoblast
  c. Fibroblasts
  d. Mesenchymal cells
  e. Syncytiotrophoblast

64. There is facilitated transfer of oxygen from maternal to fetal blood during pregnancy. What is the main factor that contributes to this phenomenon?
  a. Increased 2,3 DPG concentration in fetal blood
  b. Increased circulation time of blood in fetal tissues
  c. Increased desaturation of fetal blood
  d. Presence of fetal haemoglobin
  e. Small difference in the pH of maternal and fetal blood

65. fetal haemoglobin (HbF) is different from adult haemoglobin as it binds less avidly to 2,3-diphosphoglycerol. What is the structure of HbF?
  a. 2α and 2β chains
  b. 2α and 2δ chains
  c. 2α and 2θ chains
  d. 2α and 2λ chains
  e. 2α and 2γ chains

66. fetal kidneys have fully developed by the second trimester of pregnancy. What is their main function?
  a. Synthesis of fetal red blood cells
  b. Maintains pH of fetal blood
  c. Regulation of fetal blood pressure by production of angiotensin
  d. Synthesis of fetal haemoglobin by secreting erythropoietin
  e. Synthesis of fetal urine which is excreted in the amniotic fluid

67. After birth, fetal breathing movements are established within a few seconds. What is the main factor responsible for initiation of respiration?
  a. Cooling of fetal skin
  b. Expansion of fetal chest wall
  c. fetal acidosis
  d. fetal hypocapnia
  e. fetal hypoxia

68. A study uses the weight of 100 patients recorded in clinic. How can you best describe this data?
  a. Categorical
  b. Continuous
  c. Discrete
  d. Ordinal
  e. Qualitative

69. Changes in fetal circulation involve functional closure of structures within 2–3 hours of birth. Which structure closes at around 7 days?
  a. Closure of ductus arteriosus
  b. Closure of ductus venosus
  c. Closure of foramen ovale
  d. Closure of umbilical artery
  e. Closure of umbilical vein

70. A multiparous patient presents with placenta accreta and is rushed for an emergency caesarean section. The abdomen is opened through a midline vertical incision to save time. What is the most common immediate complication of a midline vertical incision?
  a. High infection rate
  b. Incisional hernia
  c. Keloid formation
  d. Poor cosmetic result
  e. Wound dehiscence

71. Closure of a Pfannenstiel incision for caesarean section requires good approximation of the rectus sheath. Which nerve is most likely to be entrapped in lateral ends of this transverse incision?
  a. Genitofemoral nerve
  b. Ilioinguinal nerve
  c. Lateral cutaneous nerve of thigh

d. Lateral epigastric nerve
e. Ventral rami of subcostal nerve

72. Prolapse of the uterus and vagina is common in the postmenopausal age group in multiparous patients. Which primary support of the vagina is weakened to cause a prolapse?
a. Cardinal ligament
b. Endopelvic fascia
c. Levator ani muscle
d. Uterosacral ligament
e. Vaginal musculature

73. Culdocentesis is rarely performed in clinical practice. Which structure is pierced last by the needle to reach the pouch of Douglas during this procedure?
a. Mucous membrane of vagina
b. Muscular layer of vagina
c. Parietal layer of pelvic peritoneum
d. Visceral layer of pelvic fascia
e. Visceral layer of peritoneum

74. Cephalopelvic disproportion is an indication for caesarean section. Which type of maternal pelvis is the least favourable for normal vaginal delivery?
a. Androgynaecoid
b. Android
c. Anthropoid
d. Gynecoid
e. Platypelloid

75. The curvature of the spine changes during pregnancy. What is the commonest change seen in pregnancy?
a. Flatback syndrome
b. Kyphosis
c. Lordosis
d. Scoliosis
e. Spondylosis

76. Abnormal fetal presentation may be related to the type of maternal pelvis. What is the most common type of presentation during delivery in an anthropoid pelvis?
a. Brow
b. Direct occipito-posterior
c. Face to pubis
d. Occipito-anterior
e. Occipito-transverse

77. What is the most common cause of red cell antibodies in pregnancy?
a. Idiopathic
b. Previous abruption
c. Previous pregnancy
d. Previous transfusion
e. Previous transplantation

78. What is the commonest encountered antibody in pregnancy?
a. Anti-C
b. Anti-D
c. Anti-E
d. Anti-K
e. Anti-M

79. Which type of antibody causes severe anaemia at low titres?
a. Anti-C
b. Anti-D
c. Anti-E
d. Anti-K
e. Anti-M

80. You performed an audit of 100 patients to check for gestational diabetes. Based on this, you calculated the incidence of gestational diabetes in your patient population. What kind of statistics is this?
a. Advanced statistics
b. Bayesian statistics
c. Descriptive statistics
d. Inferential statistics
e. Probability statistics

81. The standard fetal growth charts use estimated fetal weight plotted on customised charts. What is the main statistical principle in creating this chart?
a. Dispersion
b. Interquartile range
c. Median
d. Range
e. Variance

82. The liver converts the lactate in lactated Ringer's solution to:
a. acetic acid
b. ammonia
c. bicarbonate
d. buffers
e. lactic acid

83. Which vessel does the ureter cross at the pelvic brim?
a. anterior division of the common iliac

b. bifurcation of the common iliac
c. internal iliac artery
d. ovarian artery
e. uterine artery

84. What histological feature is characteristic of invasive carcinoma?
a. Increased nuclear/cytoplasmic ratio
b. Koilocytosis
c. Mitotic figures
d. Nuclear disintegration
e. Poikilocytosis

85. On which histological finding is the diagnosis of moderate dyskaryosis in a cervical smear test made?
a. Nucleus is enlarged >50% of cell size
b. Nucleus is enlarged to <50% of the cell size
c. Nucleus is normal, but cytoplasm is increased
d. Nucleus is normal in shape
e. Nucleus shows increased density

86. The second most common cause of haematological disorder in pregnancy after anaemia is:
a. Deep vein thrombosis
b. Gestational thrombocytopenia
c. Immune thrombocytopenia
d. Iron deficiency anaemia
e. Megaloblastic anaemia

87. The commonest cause of thrombocytopenia in pregnancy is:
a. Gestational
b. HELLP
c. Immune
d. Preeclampsia
e. Sepsis

88. Colloids are used frequently in hypovolaemic shock. What makes it expand the intravascular compartment?
a. High molecular weight
b. Hydrophilic
c. Hygroscopic
d. Lipid soluble
e. Low permeability

89. Several nerves can lead to entrapment syndromes in pregnancy. What is the commonest nerve involved in the thorax and abdomen?
a. Anterior cutaneous nerve
b. Axillary nerve
c. Lateral cutaneous nerve of thigh
d. Lateral femoral cutaneous nerve of groin
e. Phrenic nerve

90. A sick pregnant patient in the ICU has blood gas analysis performed. Her pH is 7.32, pCO_2 is 30 mmHg and HCO_3 is 14 mEq/L. What is the diagnosis?
a. Metabolic acidosis
b. Metabolic alkalosis
c. Normal result
d. Respiratory acidosis
e. Respiratory alkalosis

91. A pregnant patient presents to emergency department with a history of fainting. Her blood gas analysis shows pH of 7.48, pCO_2 of 28 mmHg and HCO_3 level of 13 mEq/L. What is the diagnosis?
a. Metabolic acidosis
b. Metabolic alkalosis
c. Normal result
d. Respiratory acidosis
e. Respiratory alkalosis

92. A pregnant patient with asthma shows a blood gas analysis shows pH of 7.32, pCO_2 of 50 mmHg and HCO_3 level of 30 mEq/L. What do her results indicate?
a. Metabolic acidosis
b. Metabolic alkalosis
c. Normal result
d. Respiratory acidosis
e. Respiratory alkalosis

93. A pregnant patient has taken an overdose of an unknown substance. She is admitted unconscious and her blood gas analysis shows pH of 7.49, pCO_2 of 48 mmHg and HCO_3 of 32. What is the diagnosis?
a. Metabolic acidosis
b. Metabolic alkalosis
c. Mixed metabolic and respiratory alkalosis
d. Respiratory acidosis
e. Respiratory alkalosis

94. The blood gas analysis of a newborn with low Apgar scores shows pH of 7.31, pCO_2 of 50 mmHg and pO_2 of 35 mmHg. What should be the next step in management?
a. Administer high flow oxygen via face mask
b. Breastfeed immediately
c. Give more tactile stimulation
d. Intubate and ventilate
e. Prevent hypothermia

95. Loss of a large portion of the uterine endometrium is initiated at the beginning of the menstrual phase of the uterine cycle each month. This happens due to a change in which structure?
    a. Coiled arterioles of the endometrium
    b. Contractility of myometrial cells
    c. Decidual cells of the endometrial stroma
    d. Helical endometrial gland cells
    e. Straight arterioles of the endometrium

96. Digital vaginal examination is performed to assess the pelvic structures. During digital vaginal examination, which of the following structures is normally palpable through the lateral fornices?
    a. Ischial spine
    b. Ovary
    c. Perineal body
    d. Ureter
    e. Urethra

97. In a female with androgen insensitivity syndrome, testicular cancer is common in an undescended gonad. To rule out metastases of testicular cancer, which group of lymph nodes should be biopsied in the first instance?
    a. Deep inguinal
    b. External iliac
    c. Internal iliac
    d. Lumbar
    e. Superficial inguinal

98. During hysterectomy, brisk haemorrhage is encountered prior to ligation of the uterine pedicle. Which important structure is at risk during the ligation of uterine pedicle near the junction of the uterus and vagina?
    a. Obturator artery
    b. Pudendal nerve
    c. Round ligament of uterus
    d. Ureter
    e. Uterine vein

99. An adolescent girl presents with primary amenorrhoea and is diagnosed to have Mayer-Rokitansky syndrome. Which of the following pelvic organs is always present in this syndrome?
    a. Cervix
    b. Fallopian tubes
    c. Ovaries
    d. Uterus
    e. Vagina

100. The ovary is suspended in the pelvis by the mesovarium. What is the main function of the mesovarium?
    a. It carries ovarian blood vessels from the broad ligament to the ovary
    b. It contains the branches of lumbar nerves
    c. It gives support to the ovary
    d. It has no function
    e. It is a single layered fold of peritoneum suspending the ovary and the fallopian tube

Appendix 2

Practice Paper 2: 100 SBAs

- **Duration:** 2.5 hours (150 minutes)
- Number of questions: 100 SBAs

Paper 2 Topics

- Biophysics
- Clinical Management
- Data interpretation
- Immunology
- Microbiology
- Pathology
- Pharmacology

Practice Paper 2

1. What is a commonly used enzyme-inducing antiepileptic in obstetrics?
   a. Carbamazepine
   b. Eslicarbazepine
   c. Pregabalin
   d. Valproate
   e. Vigabatrin
2. What is a commonly used nonenzyme-inducing antiepileptic in obstetrics?
   a. Carbamazepine
   b. Lamotrigine
   c. Phenobarbital
   d. Pregabalin
   e. Primidone
3. Several medications are contraindicated in pregnancy. In a patient with rheumatoid arthritis, which commonly used drug is absolutely contraindicated due to birth defects?
   a. Azathioprine
   b. Ciclosporin
   c. Mycophenolate
   d. Prednisolone
   e. Tacrolimus
4. Patients with sickle cell disease are hyposplenic and are at risk of infection, in particular from encapsulated bacteria. What is an example of a common encapsulated bacteria?
   a. *Gardnerella vaginalis*
   b. *Legionella pneumophilia*
   c. *Neisseria meningitidis*
   d. *Shigella dysenterae*
   e. *Staphylococcus aureus*
5. Hydroxycarbamide (hydroxyurea) is used in women with sickle cell disease. This reduces sickle cell crises. What is the recommendation for preconception counselling in women on this medication?
   a. Safe in pregnancy
   b. Stop three months before conception
   c. Stop six months before conception
   d. Stop only if breastfeeding
   e. Stop when pregnant
6. Following a vaginal delivery, a 40-year-old woman is noted to have a gaping episiotomy. There are no signs of infection. What factor is very likely to have caused this?
   a. Advanced maternal age
   b. Early ambulation after repair
   c. Inadequate haemostasis
   d. Protein deficiency
   e. Use of absorbable sutures
7. A 32-week-pregnant woman is admitted with severe preeclampsia and signs of HELLP. The plan is an immediate delivery with caesarean section. What is the most life-threatening complication during surgery?
   a. Bleeding within a body cavity
   b. Generalised petechiae and ecchymosis
   c. Haematuria
   d. Postpartum haemorrhage
   e. Wound haematoma
8. A woman presents with deep vein thrombosis of her right leg during pregnancy. What is the commonest acquired cause of venous thrombosis?
   a. Activated protein C resistance
   b. Antiphospholipid syndrome

c. Antithrombin 3 deficiency
d. Hyperhomocysteinemia
e. Protein S deficiency

9. Apoptosis is defined as physiological cell death. What is the most characteristic feature of apoptosis?
a. Cell swelling
b. Cell vacuolation
c. Chromatin condensation
d. Formation of apoptotic bodies
e. Inflammatory response

10. A woman with gestational hypertension presents at 24 weeks of gestation with poorly controlled blood pressures and massive pedal oedema. What would be the most likely diagnosis?
a. High output cardiac failure of pregnancy
b. Hypoalbuminemia
c. Nephrotic syndrome
d. Physiological oedema of pregnancy
e. Preeclampsia

11. A 40-year-old woman presents with itching in her vulva. A biopsy of the skin reveals metaplasia. What characteristic feature of the pathological progression of metaplasia determines treatment?
a. It is a growth disorder
b. It is precancerous
c. It is reversible
d. It causes inflammation
e. It should be surgically removed

12. A 28-year-old nulliparous woman complains of a painless firm lump in her right breast, which tends to grow during periods. The most likely diagnosis is:
a. Blood good's cyst
b. Fat necrosis of the breast
c. Fibroadenoma
d. Intraductal papillary carcinoma
e. Pyogenic abscess

13. Six hours' postvaginal delivery, a woman presents with low blood pressure and hypovolaemic shock. What is the most likely diagnosis?
a. Cardiac failure
b. Dehydration
c. Gram-negative septicaemia
d. Overdose of narcotic medication during labour
e. Postpartum haemorrhage

14. Heparin prevents blood clots. What is the main mechanism of action?
a. It blocks conversion of prothrombin to thrombin
b. It blocks the action of thrombin on fibrinogen
c. It dissolves fibrinogen in the clot
d. It inactivates thromboplastin
e. It reduces platelet adhesiveness

15. Antibiotics act by interfering with the synthesis of bacterial cell wall. What is the commonly used antibiotic that acts on the bacterial cell wall?
a. Clindamycin
b. Fluconazole
c. Gentamicin
d. Metronidazole
e. Vancomycin

16. Methyldopa is commonly used as an antihypertensive in pregnancy. What is its mechanism of action?
a. ACE inhibitor
b. Adrenergic receptor blocking agent
c. Calcium channel blocker
d. Sympathomimetic
e. Vasodilator

17. Diuretics are rarely used in pregnant women. Which condition precludes the use of diuretics in pregnancy?
a. As an adjunct to hydralazine/diazoxide in treatment of hypertension
b. Prior to blood transfusion in severe anaemia
c. Pulmonary oedema
d. Severe anaemia with heart failure
e. Severe hypertension in pregnancy

18. Magnesium sulphate, when used in the management of eclampsia, has effects on the neonate. What is a serious side effect of prolonged use of magnesium sulphate on neonates in pregnant mothers?
a. Hypotonia
b. Muscle wasting
c. Osteopenia with fractures
d. Pulmonary hypertension
e. Respiratory distress

19. Some medications taken by mothers during breastfeeding make them more likely to be excreted through breast milk. What pharmacokinetic property predisposes to this?

a. Ionised
b. Low dose
c. Low molecular weight
d. Short half-life
e. Water soluble

20. The critical time of organ formation is also known as the teratogenic period. With respect to the last menstrual period, which days does this refer to?
    a. Before day 14
    b. Days 14–30
    c. Days 31–60
    d. Days 61–90
    e. Days 91–120

21. Heparin does not cross the placenta and is safe to take during pregnancy. What characteristic feature of the heparin molecule makes this feasible?
    a. High molecular weight
    b. Lipid soluble
    c. Low molecular weight
    d. Negative charged ions
    e. Water soluble

22. Which medication used in pregnancy can cause the 'grey baby syndrome'?
    a. Chloramphenicol
    b. Chlorhexidine
    c. Chloropicrin
    d. Chlorpheniramine
    e. Cimetidine

23. Fetal alcohol syndrome is seen in mothers who consume large amounts of alcohol in pregnancy. What are the three typical facial features that are seen? See table below.

24. Which of the following items describes the middle value in a ranked data set?
    a. Mean
    b. Median
    c. Mode
    d. Range
    e. Standard deviation

25. Which of the following items describes the interval on a frequency histogram within which the greatest number of observations fall?
    a. Mean
    b. Median
    c. Mode
    d. Range
    e. Standard deviation

26. A 75-year-old woman presents with a 6 cm multiloculated ovarian cyst on ultrasound scan. There are solid areas and some ascites seen. No evidence of any metastasis is noted. Her CA125 is 30. What is the risk of malignancy index (RMI)?
    a. 90
    b. 120
    c. 150
    d. 270
    e. 360

27. What are the characteristic features of a normally distributed curve? See table overleaf.

28. The type of information provided in a particular study is anecdotal to practising evidence-based medicine. What is the most superior level of evidence among the following studies?
    a. A well-designed randomised controlled trial
    b. Expert committee reports
    c. Systematic review and meta-analysis of randomised controlled trials
    d. Well-designed descriptive studies
    e. Well-designed quasiexperimental study

29. In a trial, the alternative hypothesis is known to be true. Unfortunately, the trial being small was unable to find a statistically significant difference. What error might be the most likely cause?

	Microcephaly	Thin vermilion	Smooth philtrum	Small palpebral fissures	Sprouting in dental gyrus
a.	✓		✓		✓
b.		✓		✓	✓
c.			✓	✓	✓
d.	✓	✓	✓		
e.		✓	✓	✓	

	Unimodal	Asymptotic	Binomial	Bimodal	Univariate
a.	✓		✓		
b.	✓				✓
c.		✓		✓	
d.			✓	✓	
e.	✓	✓			

a. Distribution error
b. *P*-value error
c. Type I error
d. Type II error
e. Validity error

30. Reliability is often used in statistics. What best describes this?
    a. It can be repeated with minimal variation
    b. It gives the most genuine information about what is being measured
    c. It has a small random error of estimation
    d. It has an interval with a fixed zero
    e. It matches the accepted standard

31. What is a common statistical test used to test the association between groups?
    a. ANOVA
    b. Chi-square test
    c. Linear regression analysis
    d. Student t-test
    e. Wilcoxon test

32. What is the nonparametric equivalent of paired student t-test?
    a. ANOVA
    b. Chi-square test
    c. Kruskal–Wallis test
    d. Mann–Whitney U test
    e. Wilcoxon test

33. What is the most common tumour marker seen with dysgerminoma?
    a. AFP
    b. hCG
    c. Inhibin
    d. LDH
    e. Placental alkaline phosphatase

34. What is the commonest germ-cell tumour of the ovary?
    a. Brenner tumour
    b. Dysgerminoma
    c. Embryonal tumour
    d. Endodermal sinus tumour
    e. Sex cord stromal tumour

35. Calcium level is typically elevated with certain tumours. Which malignant ovarian tumour causes hypercalcaemia?
    a. Small cell carcinoma
    b. Endodermal sinus tumour
    c. Mature cystic teratoma
    d. Metastatic ovarian carcinoma
    e. Sex cord stromal tumour

36. The most common functional cysts in the ovary are:
    a. Corpus luteum cysts
    b. Endometriotic cysts
    c. Follicular cysts
    d. Para-ovarian cysts
    e. Theca lutein cysts

37. Schiller–Duval bodies are characteristic features of:
    a. Endodermal sinus tumour
    b. Epithelial cell cancer
    c. Granulosa cell tumour
    d. Leydig cell tumour
    e. Ovarian fibroma

38. Call–Exner bodies are characteristic features of
    a. Endodermal sinus tumour
    b. Epithelial cell cancer
    c. Granulosa cell tumour
    d. Leydig cell tumour
    e. Ovarian fibroma

39. Reinke's crystals are characteristic features of:
    a. Endodermal sinus tumour
    b. Epithelial cell cancer
    c. Granulosa cell tumour
    d. Leydig cell tumour
    e. Ovarian fibroma

40. Rokitansky protuberance is a characteristic feature of:
    a. Brenner tumour
    b. Dermoid cyst
    c. Endometrioid tumours
    d. Mesonephroid tumours
    e. Serous cyst adenoma

41. Coffee bean nuclei are found in:
    a. Brenner tumour
    b. Dermoid cyst
    c. Endometrioid tumours
    d. Mesonephroid tumours
    e. Serous cyst adenoma

42. Psammoma bodies are calcified structures found in:
    a. Brenner tumour
    b. Dermoid cyst
    c. Endometrioid tumours
    d. Mesonephroid tumours
    e. Papillary serous cystadenoma

43. Hobnail cells are found in
    a. Brenner tumour
    b. Clear cell carcinoma
    c. Endometrioid tumour
    d. Mature cystic teratoma
    e. Mesonephroid tumour

44. What kind of cell is depicted in this slide from an ovarian tumour? See Figure A2.1.
    a. Call–Exner body
    b. Coffee bean nuclei
    c. Hobnail cell
    d. Psammoma Body
    e. Reinke's crystal

45. What is the most common type of vulval cancer?
    a. Adenocarcinoma
    b. Basal cell cancer
    c. Malignant melanoma
    d. Sarcoma
    e. Squamous cell cancer

46. The most common cause of sexually transmitted infection in the UK is:
    a. Chlamydia trachomatis
    b. Hepatitis B
    c. Herpes simplex
    d. Neisseria gonorrhoea
    e. Trichomonas vaginalis

47. The most common cause of viral sexually transmitted infection in the world is:
    a. Chlamydia trachomatis
    b. Hepatitis B
    c. Herpes simplex
    d. HPV
    e. HIV

48. The most common cause of bacterial sexually transmitted infection in the UK is:
    a. Chlamydia trachomatis
    b. Hepatitis B
    c. Herpes simplex
    d. Neisseria gonorrhoea
    e. Trichomonas vaginalis

49. The commonest cause for serious neonatal sepsis is:
    a. Escherichia coli

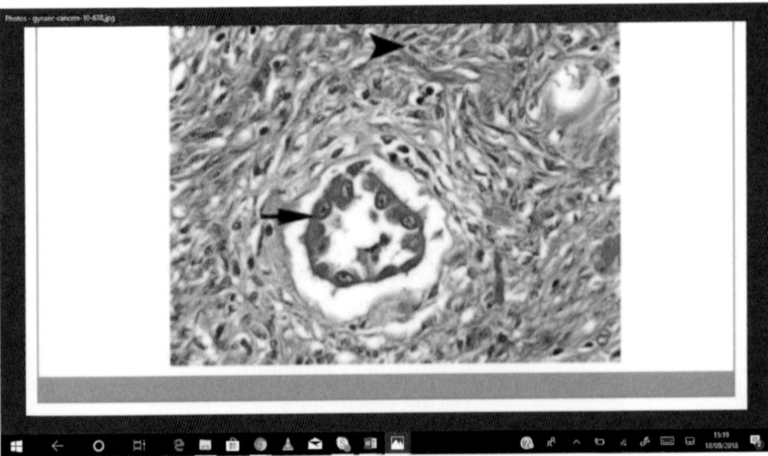

Figure A2.1

b. Group A *Streptococcus*
c. Group B *Streptococcus*
d. Herpes simplex virus
e. Parvovirus B19

50. What is the most common cause of neonatal mortality from sepsis?
a. *Escherichia coli*
b. Group A *Streptococcus*
c. Group B *Streptococcus*
d. Herpes simplex virus
e. Parvovirus B19

51. A 34-year-old woman is admitted with severe vulvar pain. The pain is so severe that she is unable to pass urine and develops urinary retention. On examination, she has multiple ulcerated lesions on the labia minora. What is the most likely cause?
a. *Chlamydia trachomatis*
b. Hepatitis B
c. Herpes simplex
d. *Neisseria gonorrhoea*
e. *Trichomonas vaginalis*

52. A 22-year-old woman complains of vaginal discharge and vulvar pruritis. On local inspection, there is copious greyish discharge with a fishy smell and vulvar erythema and excoriations. On speculum examination, a raw-looking cervix is identified. What is the most likely causative organism?
a. *Chlamydia trachomatis*
b. Hepatitis B
c. Herpes simplex
d. *Neisseria gonorrhoea*
e. *Trichomonas vaginalis*

53. Which infection is the most recognised cause of a midtrimester pregnancy loss?
a. Bacterial vaginosis
b. Group A *Streptococcus*
c. Group B *Streptococcus*
d. HIV
e. Parvovirus B19

54. Which infection is defined by the presence of clue cells?
a. *Chlamydia trachomatis*
b. *Gardnerella vaginalis*
c. Herpes simplex
d. *Neisseria gonorrhoea*
e. *Trichomonas vaginalis*

55. Ison–Hay scoring is used for identification of infections. What kind of infection is this used for?
a. *Bacterial vaginosis*
b. *Chlamydia trachomatis*
c. Herpes simplex
d. *Neisseria gonorrhoea*
e. *Trichomonas vaginalis*

56. Nugent scoring system is used in what kind of infection?
a. *Bacterial vaginosis*
b. *Chlamydia trachomatis*
c. Herpes simplex
d. *Neisseria gonorrhoea*
e. *Trichomonas vaginalis*

57. Clue cell is found in bacterial vaginosis. What kind of structure is this?
a. Collection of bacteria
b. Calcium deposition
c. Degenerated mucosal cells
d. Glandular cells
e. Squamous cells

58. What is the most appropriate treatment for a 28-year-old pregnant woman presenting with vaginal discharge, which shows heavy growth of *Neisseria gonorrhoea*?
a. Azithromycin 1 g single dose orally
b. Ceftriaxone 500 mg intramuscularly single dose with azithromycin 1 g as a single dose
c. Ceftriaxone 500 mg intramuscularly single dose with oral doxycycline 100 mg twice daily and metronidazole 400 mg twice daily for 14 days
d. Ciprofloxacin 750 mg twice daily for 14 days
e. Oral doxycycline 100 mg twice daily and metronidazole 400 mg twice daily for 14 days

59. Strawberry vagina is caused by what kind of infection?
a. *Chlamydia trachomatis*
b. Hepatitis B
c. Herpes simplex
d. *Neisseria gonorrhoea*
e. *Trichomonas vaginalis*

60. Which organism causes fulminant hepatitis in pregnancy?
a. Hepatitis A
b. Hepatitis B

c. Hepatitis C
d. Hepatitis D
e. Hepatitis E

61. Vertical transmission of HIV is maximum at which stage in pregnancy?
    a. Breastfeeding
    b. First trimester
    c. Labour
    d. Second trimester
    e. Third trimester

62. What kind of maternal antibodies cross the placenta to cause haemolytic disease of the newborn?
    a. IgA
    b. IgG
    c. IgD
    d. IgE
    e. IgM

63. Which immunoglobulin is a pentamer?
    a. IgA
    b. IgG
    c. IgD
    d. IgE
    e. IgM

64. Which immunoglobulin is a dimer?
    a. IgA
    b. IgG
    c. IgD
    d. IgE
    e. IgM

65. Regarding cytomegalovirus in pregnancy, what are the commonly presenting features? See table below.

66. What is the most common source of microorganism causing surgical-site infection?
    a. Anaesthetist
    b. Contaminated surgical equipment
    c. Patient
    d. Scrub nurse
    e. Surgeon

67. What is most common microorganism causing surgical-site infections?
    a. Coagulase negative Staphylococcus
    b. Enterococcus
    c. Pseudomonas
    d. Staphylococcus aureus
    e. Streptococcus

68. An 18-year-old girl attends the gynaecology clinic with her mother. She presents with primary amenorrhoea. On examination, her height is 1.78 m with a BMI of 19 kg/m^2. She has no axillary or pubic hair with normal breast development. She has a short, blind vagina. What is the most likely diagnosis?
    a. Complete androgen insensitivity syndrome
    b. Klinefelter syndrome
    c. Mayer–Rokitansky–Küster–Hauser syndrome
    d. Swyer syndrome
    e. Turner syndrome

69. What is the karyotype of a woman with Mayer–Rokitansky–Küster–Hauser syndrome?
    a. 45,XO
    b. 46,XY
    c. 46,XX
    d. 47,XXX
    e. 47,XXY

70. A 50-year-old woman attends the postmenopausal bleeding clinic with her third episode of postmenopausal bleeding. Her haemoglobin is 120 g/L. The pelvic scan shows an endometrial thickness of 2 mm. What is the next step in management?
    a. Cervical smear
    b. Follow-up in six months
    c. Hysteroscopy and biopsy
    d. MRI scan pelvis
    e. Total abdominal hysterectomy and bilateral salpingo-oophorectomy

Options	Microcephaly	Organomegaly	Intracranial calcifications	Cleft lip and palate	Eye defects
a.		✓	✓	✓	
b.	✓	✓	✓		
c.	✓		✓		✓
d.	✓			✓	✓
e.	✓	✓			✓

71. Mirabegron is a treatment for overactive bladder. At which receptor does this drug act as an agonist?
   a. Alpha-2 adrenergic receptor
   b. Beta-3 adrenergic receptor
   c. D-2 receptor
   d. Nicotinic receptor
   e. Muscarinic receptor

72. What is the recommended method of uterine evacuation for a suspected molar pregnancy at 12 weeks in a 40-year-old woman?
   a. Medical evacuation with mifepristone and misoprostol
   b. Medical evacuation with oxytocin drip
   c. Suction curettage with misoprostol priming
   d. Suction curettage
   e. Total abdominal hysterectomy

73. A 55-year-old woman underwent a laparoscopic bilateral salpingo-oophorectomy for a persistent right ovarian cyst and CA125 of 35. Histology showed a well-differentiated ovarian cancer confined to the right ovary. She had a staging laparotomy and lymphadenectomy following the diagnosis. The peritoneal washings were negative and stage was 1a. What chemotherapy is required for her?
   a. Carboplatin
   b. Cisplatin
   c. Etoposide
   d. No adjuvant chemotherapy
   e. Paclitaxel

74. A 55-year-old woman attends the general practitioner surgery with low abdominal pain, abdominal bloating and urinary urgency. Abdominal examination was unremarkable. What is the most appropriate next step?
   a. CA125
   b. CT scan of abdomen and pelvis
   c. MRI pelvis
   d. Reassure and discharge
   e. Refer to gastro-enterologist

75. What proportion of patients will develop a surgical-site infection after a surgical procedure?
   a. 5%
   b. 10%
   c. 15%
   d. 20%
   e. 25%

76. A 36-year-old woman presents to the gynaecology outpatient department with complaints of heavy menstrual bleeding and dysmenorrhoea for three months. The rest of her history and examination are unremarkable. She is not keen on hormonal treatment and she has a coil in situ. What treatment would you initially recommend?
   a. Combined oral contraceptive
   b. Mefenamic acid
   c. Levonorgestrel intrauterine system
   d. Norethisterone
   e. Tranexamic acid

77. A 38-year-old woman with Huntington's disease wishes to know the risk of having an affected child. Her partner is not known to have this condition. What is the risk?
   a. 1 in 2
   b. 1 in 3
   c. 1 in 4
   d. 1 in 8
   e. 1 in 16

78. A 52-year-old woman complains of urinary frequency and nocturia, waking up five times in the night. Urine dipstick shows glucose and nitrites. She drinks 6 L per day. What is the most appropriate next step?
   a. Bladder scan
   b. HbA1c
   c. MSU
   d. Plasma antidiuretic hormone levels
   e. Urodynamic study

79. A patient presents with muscle aches, weakness and fatigue, nausea and occasional vomiting. Routine bloods are done including serum calcium levels. The rest of the bloods are normal.

   Serum calcium: 15 mmol/L (2.25–2.5 mmol/L)

   TSH: 2 (0.4–4.5)

   FT3: 7 (4–8.3)

   FT4: 25 (10–24)

   What could be the possible cause?
   a. Hyperthyroidism
   b. Hypothyroidism
   c. Hyperparathyroidism
   d. Hypoparathyroidism
   e. Renal failure

80. A patient is seen by the general practitioner complaining of excessive thirst and polyuria. The

Full blood count			
White cell count	16.3	10^9/L	4.0–11.0
Haemoglobin	78	g/L	115–165
Platelets	352	10^9/L	150–450
RBC	4.28	10^{12}/L	3.5–5.8
Haematocrit	0.26	L/L	0.35–0.47
MCV	60.1	fl	76–98
Mean cell haemoglobin (MCH)	18.2	pg	27.0–32.0
MCHC	302	g/L	310–360
RDW	19.5	%	11.8–14.8
Neutrophils	11.69	10^9/L	2.0–7.0
Lymphocytes	2.35	10^9/L	1.0–3.0
Monocytes	1.43	10^9/L	0.2–1.0
Eosinophils	0.60	10^9/L	0.0–0.4
Basophils	0.23	10^9/L	0–0.2

RBC: red blood cells; MCV: mean corpuscular volume; MCHC: mean corpuscular haemoglobin concentration; RDW: red cell distribution width

general practitioner arranges a glucose tolerance test. The results are as follows

Fasting 6.5 mmol/L

Two hours 10.0 mmol/L

What does the test indicate?

a. Diabetes insipidus
b. Diabetes mellitus
c. Gestational diabetes mellitus
d. Impaired glucose tolerance
e. Sepsis

81. A couple trying for pregnancy for >1 year is referred to fertility clinic. The woman has regular cycles of 25–29 days. Day 21 progesterone done by the general practitioner shows:
Day 21 progesterone: 37 nmol/L (10–30 nmol/L).
What is the initial diagnosis about ovarian function?
a. Anovulatory cycles
b. Normal ovulatory cycle
c. Polycystic ovarian syndrome
d. Premature ovarian failure
e. Unambiguous findings

82. A couple trying to conceive was seen in fertility clinic. The semen analysis was done:
Semen volume -2.3 mL (1.5 mL)
Total sperm number: 15 million/ejaculate (>39 million/ejaculate)
Sperm concentration: 9 million/mL (15 million/mL)
Progressive motility: 35% (32%)
Sperm morphology (normal): 4% (4%)
Vitality: 60% (58%)
What does this semen analysis suggest?
a. Asthenozoospermia
b. Normozoopermia
c. Oligoasthenozoospermia
d. Oligospermia
e. Teratozoospermia

83. At booking, a 32-year-old woman in her fourth pregnancy presents with chronic constipation and feeling lethargic. She had the blood test results shown in the table above:
What would the next step in management be? See table overleaf.

84. In the above patient, the blood film is shown in Figure A2.2.
What is the diagnosis?
a. Anaemia of chronic disease
b. Iron deficiency
c. Sickle cell anaemia
d. Sideroblastic anaemia
e. Thalassaemia

85. A 28-year-old woman, $G_2 P_1$, comes to triage at 30 weeks of gestation complaining of unsightly dark

Options	Haematinics	Folic acid	Check LDH	Hb electrophoresis	Partner testing
a.		✓	✓	✓	
b.	✓			✓	✓
c.	✓		✓	✓	
d.		✓	✓		✓
e.	✓	✓		✓	

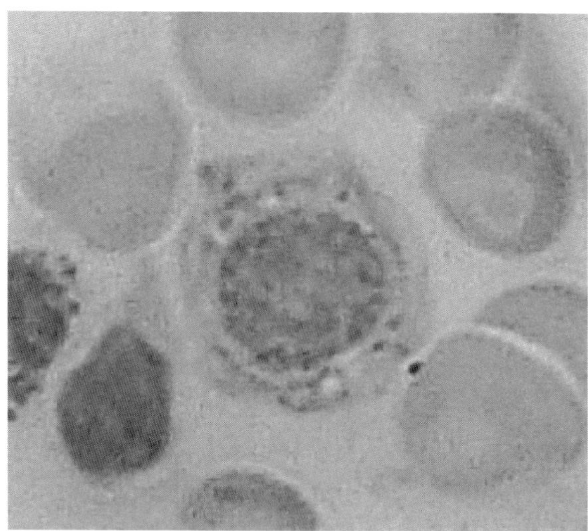

Figure A2.2

marks on her limbs and frequent nose bleeds.
Full blood count results are shown in the first table overleaf.
What is the likely provisional diagnosis?
a. Acute fatty liver of pregnancy
b. HELLP
c. Idiopathic thromobocytopenic purpura
d. Placental abruption with disseminated intravascular coagulation (DIC)
e. Streptococcal infection

86. In the above case, what is the best management plan?
a. IV immunoglobulin
b. Platelet transfusion
c. Start oral steroids
d. Start tranexamic acid IV
e. Urgent haematology referral

87. A 34 weeks' pregnant primiparous woman complains of feeling generally unwell. She noticed some offensive vaginal discharge over last week.
Full blood count results are shown in the second table overleaf.
What is the most likely diagnosis?
a. Bacterial vaginosis
b. Candidiasis
c. Chorioamnionitis
d. Early labour
e. Preterm premature rupture of membranes (PPROM)

88. Normal saline is a secondary choice of fluid replacement in labour. What is the undesirable effect this can cause?
a. Hyperchloraemic acidosis
b. Hypernatraemia
c. Hypokalaemia
d. Hypomagnesaemia
e. Lactic acidosis

89. Amniotic fluid embolism is a rare cause of maternal death. What is the mortality rate related to this?
a. 30%
b. 50%
c. 70%
d. 90%
e. 100%

90. You are requested to review the antenatal bloods taken for a low risk primiparous woman at 28 weeks. See table on page 415. The patient has noticed that her gums are bleeding regularly.
What is the next investigation that you should request?
a. Amylase
b. Blood film
c. Coagulation
d. Liver function tests
e. Thrombophilia

91. In the above scenario, what would the most likely provisional diagnosis be?
a. Chronic anaemia

FBC			
HGB	103	g/L	115–165
WBC	5.7	10^9/L	4.0–11.0
PLT	44	10^9/L	150–450
RBC	4.62	$X10^{12}$	3.50–5.80
HCT	0.322	L/L	0.370–0.470
MCV	69.6	fl	76.0–98.0
MCH	22.3	pg	27.0–32.0
MCHC	321	g/L	310–360
MEAN PV	8.9	fl	7.0–12.0
NEUT #	2.60	10^9/L	2.00–7.00
LYM #	2.40	10^9/L	1.00–3.00
MONO	0.60	10^9/L	0.20–1.00
EOS	0.10	10^9/L	0.00–0.50
BASO	0.00	10^9/L	0.0–0.20

HGB: haemoglobin; PLT: platelets; HCT: haematocrit; MCH: mean cell haemoglobin; MCHC: mean cell haemoglobin concentration; NEUT: neutrophils; LYM: lymphocytes; MONO: monocytes; EOS: eosinophils; BASO: basophils

FBC			
HGB	127	g/L	115–165
WBC	18.9	10^9/L	4.0–11.0
PLT	165	10^9/L	150–450
RBC	4.42	$X10^{12}$	3.50–5.80
HCT	0.385	L/L	0.370–0.470
MCV	86.9	fl	76.0–98.0
MCH	28.7	pg	27.0–32.0
MCHC	330	g/L	310–360
Mean plasma viscosity	10.4	fl	7.0–12.0
NEUT #	12.90	10^9/L	2.00–7.00
LYM #	1.50	10^9/L	1.00–3.00
MONO	0.40	10^9/L	0.20–1.00
EOS	0.10	10^9/L	0.00–0.50
BASO	0.00	10^9/L	0.0–0.20

b. Idiopathic thrombocytopenia
c. Gestational thrombocytopenia
d. HELLP
e. Immune thrombocytopenia

92. A one-day postnatal woman following a caesarean section feels unwell and dizzy.

Blood pressure is 70/40 mmHg

Pulse is 130 BPM (weak and thready pulse)

Full blood count results are given in the table on page 416.

What is the immediate step in management?

a. IV resuscitation/transfusion
b. Oxygen
c. Repeat bloods including coagulation

FBC			
White cell count	7.8	10^9/L	4.0 – 11.0
Haemoglobin	118	g/L	115 – 165
Platelets	100	10^9/L	150 – 450
RBC	3.77	10^{12}/L	3.5 – 5.8
Haematocrit	0.39	L/L	0.35 – 0.47
MCV	81.5	fl	76 – 98
Mean cell haemoglobin	27.1	pg	27.0 – 32.0
MCHC	333	g/L	310 – 360
RDW	13.5	%	11.8 – 14.8
Neutrophils	5.80	10^9/L	2.0 – 7.0
Lymphocytes	1.48	10^9/L	1.0 – 3.0
Monocytes	0.46	10^9/L	0.2 – 1.0
Eosinophils	0.02	10^9/L	0.0 – 0.4
Basophils	0.04	10^9/L	0.0 – 0.2
NRBC	<0.5	10^9/L	<0.5

d. Catheterisation for input and output balance
e. Tranexamic acid IV

93. With laterally extended transverse incisions, the extensions should have sutures placed only in the external oblique fascia. What is the main risk with putting deep sutures in the external oblique muscle?
a. Abscess
b. Haematoma
c. Neuroma
d. Seroma
e. Urinoma

94. What is the lowest temperature at which denaturation of proteins and coagulation occurs during radiofrequency ablation?
a. 40 °C
b. 50 °C
c. 60 °C
d. 70 °C
e. 80 °C

95. What kind of current does radiofrequency ablation use?
a. Alternating current
b. Continuous waveform current
c. Direct current
d. Mixed waveform current
e. Nonelectrical waveform current

96. Vicryl is a commonly used suture in surgery. What material does it contain?
a. Polyglycolic acid
b. Polydioxanone
c. Polyglactin
d. Polyglactin 910
e. Poliglecaprone

97. What kind of current causes the cutting effect in electrodiathermy?
a. Alternating low and high
b. High amplitude
c. High voltage
d. Low duty cycle
e. Low voltage

98. Vicryl rapide is used in suturing the perineum. What is the time needed to dissolve?
a. 7 days
b. 7–14 days
c. 20–40 days
d. 60–90 days
e. 90–120 days

99. Latex allergy is a quite common condition seen in hospitals. What kind of allergic reaction is it?
a. Type I
b. Type 2
c. Type 3
d. Type 4
e. Type 5

FBC			
White cell count	11.3	10^9/L	4.0 – 11.0
Haemoglobin	82	g/L	115 – 165
Platelets	123	10^9/L	150 – 450
RBC	2.83	10^{12}/L	3.5 – 5.8
Haematocrit	0.24	L/L	0.35 – 0.47
MCV	84.9	fl	76 – 98
Mean cell haemoglobin (MCH)	28.9	pg	27.0 – 32.0
MCHC	340	g/L	310 – 360
RDW	14.9	%	11.8 – 14.8
Neutrophils	9.12	10^9/L	2.0 – 7.0
Lymphocytes	1.32	10^9/L	1.0 – 3.0
Monocytes	0.69	10^9/L	0.2 – 1.0
Eosinophils	0.14	10^9/L	0.0 – 0.4
Basophils	0.03	10^9/L	0.0 – 0.2
NRBC	<0.5	10^9/L	<0.5

100. Mersilene tape is used in cervical cerclages. What kind of material does this contain?
   a. Dexon
   b. Nylon
   c. Polyester
   d. Polymethylene
   e. Silk

Appendix 3

Practice Paper 3: 100 SBAs

SBA Paper 3

- **Duration:** 2.5 hours (150 minutes).
- Number of questions: 100 SBAs

Paper 3 Topics

Usually, the questions in the papers are as per the curriculum and blueprinting.

This is a mixed paper with questions from all sections. Use this for practice and self-directed learning on topics that are not covered in the book and those areas that you get wrong.

1. Ergometrine is used in cases of postpartum haemorrhage. How long is the duration of action after intramuscular dose?
   a. 30 minutes
   b. 1 hour
   c. 2 hours
   d. 3 hours
   e. 4 hours

2. Misoprostol is widely used in management of postpartum haemorrhage worldwide. What makes this feasible?
   a. It is inexpensive
   b. It is present in its active form
   c. It is rapidly absorbed
   d. It is widely available
   e. It should be refrigerated

3. Some of the bowel injuries might not be diagnosed at the time of laparoscopy. Roughly how many injuries go undiagnosed at surgery?
   a. 2%
   b. 5%
   c. 10%
   d. 15%
   e. 25%

4. When inserting the Veress needle or the primary trocar, there is a risk of vascular injury. Which group of women are at the highest risk?
   a. Multiparous
   b. With high BMI
   c. With inverted umbilicus
   d. With normal BMI
   e. With well-developed abdominal musculature

5. Hirudin is a specific anticoagulant. What is the mechanism of action?
   a. Acts on circulating antithrombin
   b. Converts fibrinogen to fibrin
   c. Converts prothrombin to thrombin
   d. Direct thrombin block
   e. Hydrophilic interaction

6. Lepirudin is effective in the management of venous thromboembolism (VTE) in patients with thrombosis and heparin-associated thrombocytopenia. What kind of drug is this?
   a. Indirect thrombin blocker
   b. Recombinant apixaban
   c. Recombinant hirudin
   d. Recombinant heparin
   e. Unfractionated heparin

7. Which vein is easily cannulated and lies in the anatomical snuffbox?
   a. Basilic vein
   b. Cephalic vein
   c. Digital vein
   d. Palmar vein
   e. Princeps pollicis

8. While cannulating in the cubital fossae, which nerve and artery are at risk of damage?
   a. Median nerve and basilic artery
   b. Median nerve and brachial artery
   c. Median nerve and median cubital artery
   d. Ulnar nerve and basilic artery
   e. Ulnar nerve and cephalic artery

9. Intraosseous access is generally used in neonates. What is the main site?
   a. Distal humerus
   b. Proximal femur

c. Proximal tibia
d. Sternum
e. Ulna

10. Lumbar epidural injections carry a low risk of injuring the spinal cord. At what level does the spinal cord terminate in an adult?
    a. The disc between L1 and L2
    b. The disc below L5
    c. The disc between L2 and L3
    d. The disc between L3 and L4
    e. The disc between L4 and L5

11. In evidence-based medicine, what level of evidence is provided by a large case control study?
    a. 1a
    b. 1b
    c. 2a
    d. 2b
    e. 3

12. What is the World Health Organization definition of late neonatal death?
    a. Delivery of a 23+6 week live-born baby who died 5 days after birth
    b. Delivery of a 26+6 week live-born baby who died 32 days after birth
    c. Delivery of a 23+6 week live-born baby who died 8 days after birth
    d. Delivery of a 26+6 week live-born baby who died 42 days after birth
    e. Delivery of a 23+6 week baby with no signs of life

13. A new test to assess the risk of preterm labour was developed. The test has a high positive predictive value. What is the definition of positive predictive value?
    a. The proportion of patients with positive test who have the disease
    b. The proportion of patients with the disease who have a positive test
    c. The proportion of patients with negative test who do not have the disease
    d. The proportion of patients without the disease who have a positive test
    e. The proportion of patients with positive test who do not have the disease

14. You were given a set of data with skewed distribution, which cannot be converted to normal distribution. Which of the following tests is suitable to compare the variables?
    a. Analysis of variance
    b. Fisher's test
    c. Pearson's rho test
    d. Student's t-test
    e. Wilcoxon's test

15. What is a requirement for developing a screening programme?
    a. The disease has a short latent phase
    b. The disease has no acceptable treatment
    c. The natural history of the disease is not understood
    d. The screening test has high sensitivity and specificity
    e. The screening test is expensive

16. One-hundred patients are booked at the new high BMI antenatal clinic. The average BMI at booking is 38. The standard deviation is 10. What is the standard error of the mean?
    a. 1.0
    b. 1.2
    c. 2.4
    d. 2.6
    e. 3.8

17. A new test was developed for diagnosing tuberculosis (TB). Fifity patients with TB had positive tests. Five patients with TB had negative tests. Two-hundred patients without TB had negative tests. Three patients without TB had positive tests. What is the specificity of the test?
    a. 86%
    b. 92%
    c. 94%
    d. 96%
    e. 98%

18. A new test was developed for diagnosing early gestational diabetes. Eighty patients with diabetes had positive tests. Twelve patients with diabetes had negative tests. Six-hundred patients without diabetes had negative tests. Twenty patients without diabetes had positive tests. What is the negative predictive value of the test?
    a. 80%
    b. 87%
    c. 91%
    d. 97%
    e. 98%

19. A large case control study was used to determine the association between vulval cancer and

smoking. The odds ratio was 2.1 comparing vulval cancer to controls with 95% confidence interval of 1.7 to 3.1. *P*-value was <0.05. How can this be best described?

a. Smokers are twice as likely to develop vulval cancer compared to controls
b. The confidence interval suggests that there is no significant difference in development of vulval cancer between those who smoke and those who do not
c. The larger the confidence interval the more likely the association between vulval cancer and smoking
d. The *p*-value suggests that the null hypothesis should be accepted
e. The results show that smoking causes vulval cancer

20. A medical student was asked to do an audit on the management of anal sphincter tear. How can the audit methodology be designed?
    a. Audits are the same as quality improvement projects
    b. Audits are the same as research projects
    c. Audits can be performed retrospectively or prospectively
    d. Audits require patients and doctors to be blinded to the intervention
    e. Audits require two people to independently analyse the results

21. A 32-year-old woman has been referred to clinic by her general practitioner for counselling. She is trying for a pregnancy and has had three miscarriages within the last year. She has a 4-year-old child from a previous relationship. She is a smoker, does not drink alcohol and has BMI 38. There is no other medical problem.
    What is the most appropriate advice?
    a. Advise her to stop smoking
    b. Perform a thrombophilia screen
    c. Reassure and continue trying
    d. Start on 75 mg aspirin
    e. Start on progesterone

22. A 38-year-old woman has been referred to clinic by her general practitioner for counselling. She is trying for a pregnancy and has had three miscarriages within the last year. She is a nonsmoker, does not drink alcohol and has BMI 28. There is no other medical problem.
    What is the most appropriate management?
    a. Perform a thrombophilia screen
    b. Reduce weight
    c. Start on 75 mg aspirin
    d. Start on progesterone
    e. Start steroids

23. A baby was born by emergency caesarean section following an antepartum haemorrhage in the mother. The baby had a haemoglobin of 10 g/dL at birth.
    What is the most likely cause of this haemoglobin level?
    a. Fetomaternal bleed
    b. Loss of blood when the cord was cut
    c. Parvovirus
    d. Thalassaemia
    e. Traumatic delivery

24. A 28-year-old woman has just booked at 30 weeks, having just moved into the area. You notice that her fundus is measuring small for dates. On further questioning, she tells you that she has four children and they were all small or born early. She also had a stillbirth at term but does not recall the reason. What is the most useful investigation?
    a. Blood group and antibody screen
    b. Blood pressure profile
    c. Growth scan
    d. Thrombophilia screen
    e. Uterine artery Doppler

25. Midwife shows you some blood results taken from a patient seen in day assessment. She is 30 weeks pregnant and presented with a temperature and suspected food poisoning. Haemoglobin is 11, white cell count is 18, platelets are 160, blood group A negative, but antibody screen positive.
    What is the first appropriate management plan?
    a. Admit patient for rehydration and IV antibiotics
    b. Community midwife follow-up
    c. Growth scan
    d. Refer to haematology
    e. Send stool sample

26. Teratogens are a group of substances like drugs, radiation and viruses that cause aberrant fetal organogenesis. At what gestation is the maximum risk of teratogenicity in the fetus when a mother is exposed to teratogens?
    a. 4–6 weeks
    b. 5–8 weeks

c. 6–10 weeks
d. 10–12 weeks
e. 12–20 weeks

27. A young woman is taking some medication for her acne and has a history of depression. She has come to your clinic for prepregnancy counselling. Which group of drugs should be stopped if she is contemplating a pregnancy?
    a. Alcohol
    b. Antibiotics
    c. Retinoic acid derivatives
    d. Selective serotonin uptake inhibitors
    e. Tricyclic antidepressants

28. Under the effect of high progesterone concentrations during pregnancy, maternal gut motility is reduced. What effect is seen on pharmacokinetics of drugs?
    a. Bloated sensation after consuming any medicine
    b. Immediate onset of action of oral medications
    c. Increase in bioavailability of most drugs
    d. Lower drug levels in maternal circulation
    e. Higher drug levels in maternal circulation

29. Many physiological changes in pregnancy lead to lower drug concentrations in maternal blood during second and third trimesters of pregnancy. What is the main change?
    a. Active transport of drugs by the fetoplacental unit
    b. Increase in basal metabolic rate in the mother
    c. Increase in plasma concentrations of binding proteins
    d. Increase in renal clearance of drug due to 50% increase in GFR
    e. Reduced maternal gut motility

30. A 34-year-old woman is referred to antenatal clinic. She has booked at 10 weeks following a fourth attempt at IVF. She was advised about high natural killer cells. She is anxious. What is the most appropriate management for her pregnancy?
    a. Start fluoxetine
    b. Start immunoglobulins
    c. Start intralipid
    d. Start prednisolone
    e. Start vitamin D

31. A 39-year-old has been referred to gynaecology outpatient department (GOPD) with menstrual irregularities. She is concerned about her fertility. Her BMI is 38. She is a type 1 diabetic and has lupus. There is a strong family history of thyroid dysfunction. What is the most appropriate next step in management?
    a. Check HBA1c
    b. Reassure
    c. Refer to fertility services
    d. Start steroids
    e. Take endometrial biopsy

32. A 34-year-old woman is referred to antenatal clinic. She is now 20 weeks pregnant. This is an IVF pregnancy following six years of unexplained infertility. As part of her fertility investigations she was found to have high natural killer cells. She has heard that steroids can improve her pregnancy outcome and wants to know if you can prescribe. What advice do you give?
    a. Explain there is no evidence that steroids improve pregnancy outcome
    b. Measure serum natural killer cells and if high start on oral steroids
    c. Offer induction of labour at 39 weeks to reduce the risk of stillbirth
    d. Offer prednisolone as there is level 2 evidence that steroids improve pregnancy outcome
    e. Reassure her that she is in the second trimester and therefore not at risk of miscarriage

33. You see a couple referred to recurrent miscarriage clinic. The woman is 18 years old and had a deep vein thrombosis while taking oral contraceptives. There is a strong family history of diabetes and her mother had preeclampsia while pregnant. She has had two consecutive early pregnancy losses before 12 weeks of gestation. What is the next investigation?
    a. Pelvic ultrasound
    b. GTT
    c. Progesterone
    d. Thrombophilia screen
    e. Nothing is required

34. You are asked to review a growth scan report for a 32-week scan for a woman with previous intrauterine growth restriction (IUGR). The scan looks normal and the estimated fetal weight is 2477 g. What is the variance in the estimated fetal weight measured on ultrasound?
    a. +/−5%
    b. +/−10%

c. +/−15%
d. +/−20%
e. +/−25%

35. A scan report on a 58-year-old woman with postmenopausal bleeding shows an endometrial thickness of 5 mm. What would your next step in management be?
a. Offer a hysterectomy
b. Offer a hysteroscopy
c. Reassure and discharge
d. Start progesterone
e. Take a pipelle endometrial sample

36. A 49-year-old woman had a total abdominal hysterectomy/bilateral salpingo-oophorectomy for a fibroid uterus. She developed severe pain on the first postoperative day. A CT scan showed a 2 x 2 cm collection at the vault. Her observations and bloods are normal. What would you do next?
a. Consider an ultrasound guided drainage
b. Consider surgical drainage
c. Keep the catheter in for longer
d. Reassure and watch
e. Repeat CT in three days

37. An MRI scan on a 35-year-old asymptomatic woman shows a 4–5 cm solid ovarian mass suggestive of a mature cystic teratoma. What tumour markers should be requested for? See table below.

Options	CA125	LDH	CA199	AFP	hCG
a.	✓	✓		✓	
b.	✓		✓		✓
c.		✓	✓	✓	
d.		✓		✓	✓
e.	✓		✓	✓	

38. What is the most appropriate management of a 28-year-old woman with an asymptomatic 5–7 cm simple right ovarian cyst?
a. Laparoscopic ovarian cystectomy
b. MRI scan
c. Tumour markers
d. Ultrasound guided drainage
e. Yearly ultrasound scan

39. A 25-year-old woman attends Accident and Emergency with tubo-ovarian abscess and sepsis. She has no other medical problems. She is hyperventilating. You are given the blood gas results. Please select the appropriate diagnosis.

pH	7.36
HCO_3	14 mEq/L
BE	−3 mmol/L
pCO_2	4.2 kPa
pO_2	10.5 kPa
K^+	5.7 mmol/L

a. Acidosis with hyperkalaemia
b. Metabolic acidosis
c. Metabolic acidosis superimposed on alkalosis
d. Mixed metabolic acidosis with respiratory acidosis
e. Respiratory acidosis

40. A 40-year-old pregnant patient presents with hysteria in the postnatal period. She is hyperventilating and blood gases are provided. What is the diagnosis?

pH	7.46
HCO_3	23 mEq/L
BE	3 mmol/L
pCO_2	6 kPa
pO_2	10.5 kPa
K^+	4.1 mmol/L

a. Compensated combined alkalosis
b. Metabolic alkalosis
c. Metabolic alkalosis with respiratory acidosis
d. Metabolic alkalosis with respiratory alkalosis
e. Respiratory alkalosis

41. A 37-year-old pregnant woman with severe asthma has a 3 L blood loss after delivery. Four units of blood are transfused. Blood gases are done. What do the results show?

pH	7.36
HCO_3	14 mEq/L
BE	−3 mmol/L
pCO_2	4.8 kPa
pO_2	10.5 kPa
K^+	5.7 mmol/L

a. Acidosis with hyperkalaemia
b. Metabolic acidosis
c. Metabolic acidosis superimposed on alkalosis
d. Mixed metabolic acidosis with respiratory acidosis
e. Respiratory acidosis

42. A 13-week pregnant woman comes in with high fever, rigours and feeling unwell. She has a blood lactate level of 2.5 mmol/L.
What is the most obvious diagnosis?
a. Flu
b. Liver disease
c. Pyelonephritis
d. Renal failure
e. Sepsis

43. A 35-year-old woman had an IUD insertion two months ago. She now presents with menorrhagia. An ultrasound pelvis is unable to identify an IUD. What will be the next management step in this patient?
a. Book for an EUA under general anaesthetic
b. Hysteroscopy
c. CT scan of the abdomen
d. MRI scan of the pelvis
e. X-ray abdomen

44. A 13-year-old girl presents with pelvic pain localised to the right lower quadrant. Her serum markers for infection are within normal limits.
What will be the next management step for this patient?
a. CT scan
b. Diagnostic laparoscopy
c. MRI pelvis
d. Transabdominal ultrasound of the pelvis
e. Transvaginal ultrasound of the pelvis

45. A 25-year-old woman presents with pelvic pain localised to the right iliac fossa. Her serum markers for infection are within normal limits.
What will be the next management step for this patient?
a. Diagnostic laparoscopy
b. CT scan
c. MRI pelvis
d. Transvaginal ultrasound of the pelvis
e. Transabdominal ultrasound of the pelvis

46. A 25-year-old woman at 24 weeks of gestation presents with chest pain and shortness of breath. What will be the preferred imaging modality to exclude pulmonary embolism in this clinical instance?
a. Chest X-ray
b. MR angiogram of pulmonary arteries
c. CT angiogram of pulmonary arteries
d. Ventilation/perfusion scintigraphy
e. Low-dose ventilation only scintigraphy

47. A 45-year-old woman is suspected to have a ureteric injury after a recent difficult hysterectomy.
What will be the best imaging modality to exclude ureteric injury in this instance?
a. Abdominal X-ray
b. Intravenous urogram
c. CT urogram
d. MR urogram
e. Ultrasound abdomen

48. A pregnant patient is on the list for caesarean section under general anaesthetic and is anticipated to have a difficult intubation. What is the most important step to prevent hypoxia to mother and fetus during general anaesthetic?
a. Attempting nasal intubation
b. Giving a long-acting muscle relaxant to ensure complete relaxation
c. Keeping the patient in the left lateral position
d. Preoxygenating the mother prior to induction of anaesthesia
e. Using a fibreoptic laryngoscope

49. A pregnant patient with gestational diabetes, controlled on insulin, is booked for elective caesarean section. What is the most likely outcome on blood sugars during surgery?
a. Can be variable
b. Go up and then fall sharply
c. Likely to fall due to preoperative fasting
d. Remain stable during surgery
e. Rise due to the stress of surgery

50. Balance of nitric oxide levels is important during pregnancy. Which isoform of the enzyme nitric oxide synthase (NOS) is important during pregnancy?
a. Endothelial NOS
b. Fetal NOS
c. Inducible NOS
d. Neuronal NOS
e. Placental NOS

51. What is the main function of nitric oxide?
a. Endocrinal modifications
b. Increase in cell metabolism
c. Reduction in mRNA synthesis
d. Vasoconstriction
e. Vasodilatation

52. During the process of inflammation, the cell derives energy by:
   a. ATP produced by bacterial cells
   b. Gluconeogenesis
   c. Glycogenolysis
   d. Glycolysis
   e. Krebs cycle

53. The organisms most commonly implicated in puerperal sepsis after a postvaginal delivery include:
   a. Gram-negative and anaerobic bacteria
   b. Gram-negative and gram-positive bacteria
   c. Gram-negative bacteria and H1N1 virus
   d. Gram-negative bacteria and yeast
   e. Gram-positive and atypical bacteria

54. What is the correct order of release of inflammatory substances in the cascade of inflammation?
   a. Complement activation leads to release of interferon γ which causes endothelial damage
   b. Hypoxia causes endothelial cell necrosis and activation of complement system
   c. Release of interferon Υ leads to activation of complement which leads to endothelial damage
   d. Stasis of blood leads to microvascular thrombosis that causes endothelial damage and activation of complement
   e. Bacteria adhere to the endothelial cells, causing their lysis and complement activation

55. What is the systemic hallmark of clinical sepsis?
   a. Hypotension
   b. Increased ATP production in tissues
   c. Increased oxygen supply to inflamed tissues
   d. Release of anticoagulant factors
   e. Vasoconstriction

56. Which cells actively secrete proinflammatory cytokines?
   a. Bacterial cells
   b. Macrophages
   c. Megakaryocytes
   d. Red blood cells
   e. Thymocytes

57. During clinical sepsis, there is release of proinflammatory cytokines. The most important of them is:
   a. Interferon γ
   b. Interleukin 10
   c. Interleukin 4
   d. Interleukin 6
   e. Transforming growth factor β

58. What is the commonest outcome of complement activation?
   a. Drop in body temperature
   b. Increased tissue perfusion
   c. Microvascular thrombosis
   d. Profuse sweating
   e. Vasodilatation

59. Vitamins play an important role in cell metabolism. Which one is a water-soluble vitamin present in the body?
   a. Vitamin A
   b. Vitamin B
   c. Vitamin D
   d. Vitamin E
   e. Vitamin K

60. Which vitamins help in release of energy in the cell?
   a. Vitamin A
   b. Vitamin B
   c. Vitamin C
   d. Vitamin D
   e. Vitamin K

61. Which vitamin is the newborn often deficient in?
   a. Vitamin A
   b. Vitamin B
   c. Vitamin C
   d. Vitamin D
   e. Vitamin K

62. What are the erythropoietic vitamins in the body?
   a. Vitamin A and K
   b. Vitamin B and C
   c. Vitamin B and folic acid
   d. Vitamin C and folic acid
   e. Vitamin D and folic acid

63. Concomitant use of certain drugs requires the supplementation of vitamin B6 during pregnancy. Which one would need Vitamin B6 supplementation?
   a. Gabapentin
   b. Isoniazid
   c. Ondansetron
   d. Phenytoin
   e. SSRI

64. Which B group vitamin plays a very important role during pregnancy and lactation?
   a. B_1 or thiamine
   b. B_2 or riboflavin
   c. B_3 or pantothenic acid
   d. B_5 or niacin
   e. B_6 or pyridoxine

65. Folic acid is supplemented universally to pregnant patients. What does folic acid contain?
   a. Folinic acid
   b. GABA and pyrimidine residues
   c. Histidine residues
   d. PABA and glutamic acid residues
   e. Vitamin B_8

66. Which structure synthesises vitamin D during pregnancy?
   a. Amniotic membrane
   b. Fetal bones
   c. Fetal skin
   d. Osteoclasts
   e. Placenta

67. What might be a likely cause of hypervitaminosis A during pregnancy?
   a. Deficiency of retinol-binding protein
   b. Dehydration due to excessive nausea and vomiting
   c. Excessive intake of carrots
   d. Excessive intake of liver
   e. Increased exposure to sunlight

68. What can be the outcome of vitamin E deficiency in pregnancy?
   a. Brittle bones in the newborn
   b. Haemolysis in the newborn
   c. Jaundice in the newborn
   d. Petechiae
   e. Skin rash in the newborn

69. While performing a Pfannenstiel incision, which muscles may need to be cut?
   a. External oblique
   b. Internal oblique
   c. Lateral abdominis
   d. Piriformis
   e. Pyramidalis

70. Where in the pelvis is the ureter most vulnerable to surgical injury?
   a. As it crosses under the uterine artery
   b. At bifurcation of the internal iliac artery
   c. At its entry into the urinary bladder
   d. At the pelvic brim
   e. Near the ovarian pedicle

71. The trigone of the urinary bladder is involved in trigonitis. What is the trigone?
   a. Area between the urethra and ureteric orifices
   b. Area covered by transitional epithelium
   c. Culminates at the uvula
   d. Posterior aspect of the dome
   e. Structure above the urethra

72. Proinflammatory cytokines are secreted mainly by:
   a. Helper T cells
   b. Leucocytes
   c. Mast cells
   d. Phagocytes
   e. Thrombocytes

73. In electrosurgery, several settings are used for diathermy. Which one uses low voltage, but constant waveform duty cycle?
   a. Blended
   b. Coagulation
   c. Cutting
   d. Desiccation
   e. Fulgurating

74. In electrosurgical system, current passes from the generator to the active electrode through the patient to the patient return electrode and returns to the generator. Which type of system is this?
   a. Alternating current system
   b. Bipolar system
   c. Direct current system
   d. High frequency system
   e. Monopolar system

75. During laparoscopic salpingectomy, the surgeon inadvertently activates the monopolar electrode when it touched the camera. This led to a thermal injury to the nearby bowel. What is this type of hazard called?
   a. Alternate path coupling
   b. Capacitive coupling
   c. Direct coupling
   d. Indirect coupling
   e. Insulation failure

76. Several gases are used in electrosurgery. Which is a commonly used gas, but does not have laser properties?
   a. Argon
   b. Carbon dioxide
   c. Helium
   d. Neodymium-doped yttrium aluminium garnet (Nd:YAG)
   e. Potassium titanyl phosphate (KTP)

77. There is a large area of bleeding on the uterus during laparoscopic surgery. The surgeon wishes to coagulate the entire area by using a larger electrode penetrating deeper into the tissue. Which is the tissue effect he or she intends to create?
   a. Blend
   b. Coagulation
   c. Cutting
   d. Desiccation
   e. Fulguration

78. Which of the following is not a component of the electrosurgery unit?
   a. Active electrode
   b. Generator
   c. Passive electrode
   d. Patient
   e. Return electrode

79. How does a bipolar system close the current circuit?
   a. The current does not enter the patient at all as the entire system is external
   b. The current enters the patient, exits via a patient return electrode, then returns to the generator
   c. The current enters the patient, exits via an external return electrode, then returns to the generator
   d. The current penetrates the tissue from one forceps blade to the other forceps blade, exits via a patient return electrode, then returns to the generator
   e. The current penetrates the tissue from one forceps blade to the other forceps blade, exits into the return electrode inside the generator

80. What is an important advantage of using laser compared to monopolar for electrosurgery?
   a. Laser beams are all visible to the eye
   b. Laser does not cause retinal injury to the surgeon
   c. Laser is cheaper
   d. Laser is safer to use
   e. Laser seals nerve endings

81. Which commonly used diathermy instruments use bipolar energy? See table below.

	Blade	Needle tip	Forceps	Roller ball	Loop
a.	✓		✓	✓	
b.	✓	✓			✓
c.		✓	✓	✓	
d.		✓		✓	✓
e.	✓			✓	✓

82. What is the main function of the electrosurgery unit?
   a. Converts high frequency alternating current to low frequency alternating current
   b. Converts high frequency direct current to low frequency direct current
   c. Converts low frequency alternating current to high frequency alternating current
   d. Converts low frequency direct current to high frequency direct current
   e. Converts low frequency direct current to low frequency alternating current

83. When the cutting mode on the monopolar system is used, what is the characteristic feature of the current?
   a. Amplitude of the waveforms is high
   b. Constant waveform with interruption
   c. High pitzels of current is used
   d. Low voltage current
   e. Passage of high voltage current

84. The intracellular calcium ion concentration is:
   a. 10^{-3} M
   b. 10^{-4} M
   c. 10^{-5} M
   d. 10^{-6} M
   e. 10^{-7} M

85. There are several cell membrane receptors. Which one is the largest family of cell surface receptors?

a. Calcium ion
b. Epidermal growth factor
c. G protein
d. Integrins
e. Tyrosine kinases

86. In the cell, calcium ions are released into the cytoplasm from the:
a. Cytoplasmic membrane
b. Endoplasmic reticulum
c. Golgi bodies
d. Mitochondria
e. Nuclear body

87. Nitrous oxide is an important second messenger in the cells. It has a short half-life and is metabolised to:
a. Ammonia and nitric acid
b. Nitrates and nitrites
c. Nitrates and water
d. Nitric acid and water
e. Nitrites and ammonia

88. Fibronectin is a primary messenger that binds to cell receptors. Which receptor does fibronectin bind to?
a. Ephrin receptor
b. Fibroblast growth factor
c. Hyaluronan
d. Integrin
e. NMDA receptor

89. Enzymes exist in a three-dimensional structure. What kind of bonds maintain the structure?
a. Strong hydrogen bonds
b. Strong peptide bonds
c. Weak carboxyl bonds
d. Weak hydrogen bonds
e. Weak peptide bonds

90. When heated enzymes undergo change of shape and loss of action, what is this feature called?
a. Coagulation
b. Denaturation
c. Fragmentation
d. Oxidation
e. Peroxidation

91. Zwitterions are partially charged molecules in the body. The best example of a zwitterion in the body is:
a. Amino acid
b. Free radicals
c. Glycerol
d. Ions
e. Monosaccharides

92. Enzymes are extremely important in every metabolic process in the body. They increase the reaction rate. How is this achieved?
a. By increasing substrate concentration
b. By increasing the metabolic equilibrium
c. By increasing the surface area of the molecule
d. By lowering the activation energy
e. By reducing the surface tension of the molecule

93. A 38-year-old woman presents in labour for a vaginal birth after caesarean section. She is 6 cm dilated with an occipito-posterior vertex. This is the CTG.
What would the next action plan be? See Figure A3.1.
a. Continue with labour
b. Deliver by caesarean
c. Fetal blood sample
d. Fetal scalp electrode
e. Intravenous hydration

94. An irreversible inhibitor permanently inactivates the enzyme, usually by forming a covalent bond to the protein of the enzyme. What is an example of a common drug that works using this form of inhibition?
a. Bromocriptine
b. Carboplatin
c. Haloperidol
d. Penicillin
e. Teicoplanin

95. In the body, several enzymes work as competitive inhibitors. An example of a drug that acts as a competitive inhibitor is:
a. Amiodarone
b. Methotrexate
c. Metoclopramide
d. Na valproate
e. Omeprazole

96. Which cells in the body secrete pepsinogen?
a. Brunner's cells
b. Chief cells
c. Goblet cells
d. Oxyntic cells
e. Parietal cells

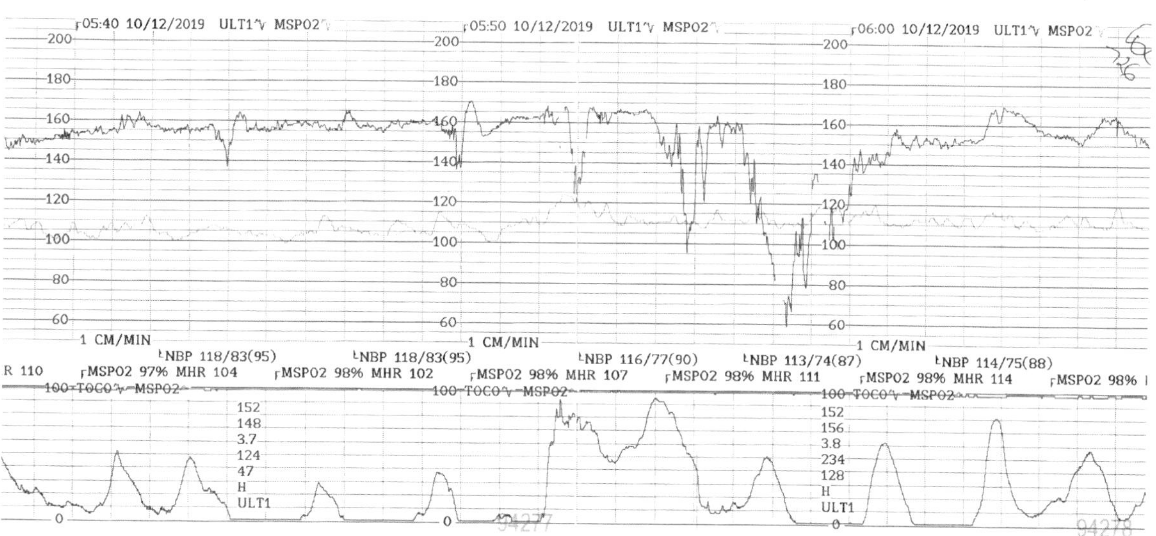

Figure A3.1

97. The lymph produced in the body finally enters the bloodstream. Where does the thoracic duct drain into?
    a. Inferior vena cava
    b. Internal jugular vein
    c. Left subclavian vein
    d. Right jugular vein
    e. Superior vena cava

98. A 46-year-old woman undergoes a total abdominal hysterectomy for heavy periods. The uterus is sent for histological examination. The macroscopic cut section is shown in Figure A3.2.
    What is the diagnosis?
    a. Adenocarcinoma of the uterus
    b. Adenomyosis
    c. Sarcoma
    d. Uterine leiomyoma
    e. Uterine polyposis

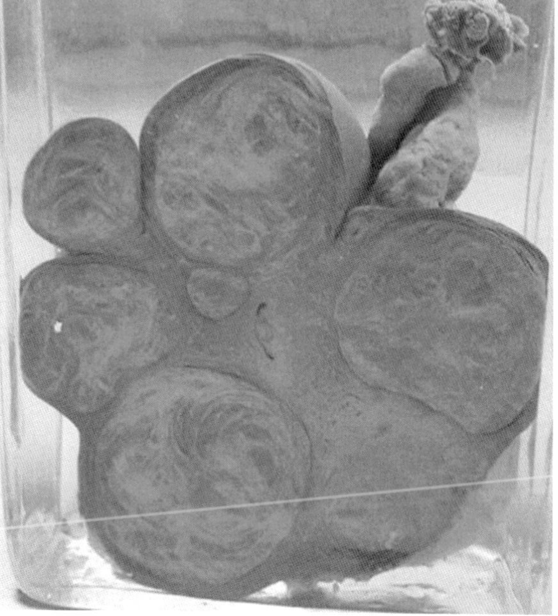

Figure A3.2

99. Figure A3.3 shows the transvaginal scan image in a lady with six weeks' amenorrhoea and slight vaginal discharge. What is the most likely diagnosis based on this image?
    a. Early intrauterine pregnancy
    b. Heterotopic pregnancy
    c. Intrauterine pregnancy with left ovarian cyst
    d. Intrauterine pregnancy with right corpus luteum
    e. Left sided ectopic pregnancy

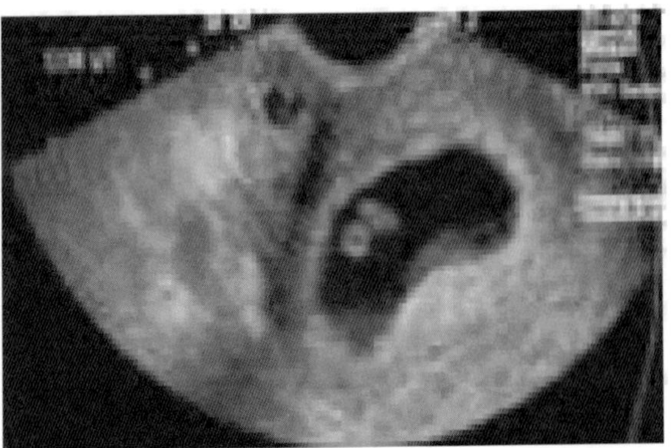

Figure A3.3

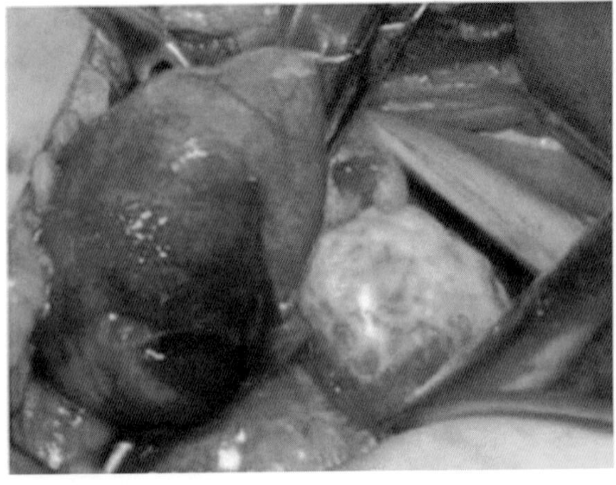

Figure A3.4

100. Figure A3.4 depicts a laparoscopic image of a patient with abdominal pain and irregular periods. Beta hCG is 575 IU/L. Based on this image what is your likely diagnosis?
    a. Left ectopic pregnancy
    b. Right ectopic pregnancy
    c. Fimbrial cyst
    d. Left corpus luteum
    e. Right corpus luteum

Appendix 4

Answers to Paper 1 SBA

1. e
2. e
3. a
4. d
5. d
6. d
7. d
8. d
9. c
10. d
11. c
12. e
13. a
14. e
15. c
16. c
17. e
18. b
19. e
20. d
21. a
22. a
23. b
24. e
25. e
26. a
27. a
28. d
29. c
30. e
31. d
32. c
33. c
34. d
35. b
36. c
37. a
38. b
39. e
40. c
41. a
42. a
43. c
44. d
45. b
46. d
47. c
48. d
49. c
50. b
51. c
52. b
53. e
54. a
55. e
56. c
57. e
58. e
59. a
60. b
61. e
62. b
63. e
64. d
65. e
66. e
67. a
68. b
69. e
70. e
71. b
72. c
73. e
74. b
75. c
76. c
77. d
78. b
79. a
80. d
81. a
82. c
83. a

84. c
85. b
86. b
87. a
88. a
89. a
90. a
91. e
92. d
93. b
94. d
95. a
96. b
97. d
98. d
99. c
100. a

Appendix 5

Answers to Paper 2 SBA

1. a
2. d
3. c
4. c
5. b
6. c
7. d
8. b
9. c
10. e
11. c
12. c
13. e
14. a
15. d
16. d
17. e
18. c
19. c
20. c
21. a
22. a
23. e
24. b
25. b
26. d
27. e
28. c
29. d
30. a
31. c
32. e
33. d
34. b
35. a
36. c
37. a
38. c
39. d
40. b
41. d
42. e
43. b
44. c
45. e
46. a
47. c
48. a
49. c
50. a
51. c
52. e
53. a
54. b
55. a
56. a
57. c
58. b
59. e
60. b
61. c
62. d
63. e
64. a
65. b
66. c
67. d
68. a
69. c
70. c
71. a
72. a
73. c
74. a
75. c
76. c
77. e
78. c
79. d
80. e
81. e
82. c
83. d

84. c
85. e
86. b
87. b
88. d
89. d
90. b
91. a
92. d
93. e
94. d
95. b
96. b
97. c
98. d
99. b
100. a

Appendix 6

Answers to Paper 3 SBA

1. d
2. a
3. d
4. e
5. d
6. c
7. b
8. b
9. c
10. a
11. c
12. c
13. a
14. e
15. d
16. a
17. e
18. e
19. a
20. c
21. a
22. a
23. a
24. c
25. a
26. b
27. c
28. c
29. d
30. e
31. c
32. a
33. d
34. d
35. e
36. d
37. d
38. e
39. b
40. d
41. d
42. e
43. e
44. d
45. d
46. d
47. c
48. d
49. e
50. a
51. e
52. d
53. e
54. c
55. a
56. b
57. a
58. c
59. b
60. b
61. e
62. c
63. b
64. e
65. d
66. e
67. d
68. b
69. e
70. a
71. a
72. c
73. a
74. c
75. e
76. c
77. c
78. e
79. c
80. e
81. e
82. e
83. c
84. d

85. e
86. c
87. b
88. b
89. d
90. d
91. a
92. a
93. d
94. d
95. b
96. b
97. c
98. e
99. b
100. a

Appendix 7

Further Reading

Bier, V. (1990). *Health Effects from Exposure to Low Levels of Ionizing Radiation.* National Academy Press.

Blackburn, S. T. (2012). *Maternal, Fetal, & Neonatal Physiology: A Clinical Perspective*, 4th ed., Elsevier.

Brenner, D. J., Hall, E.J. (2007). Computed tomography–an increasing source of radiation exposure. N *Engl J Med*, 357 (22), 2277–84.

Cook, J.V., Kyriou, J. (2005). Radiation from CT and perfusion scanning in pregnancy. *BMJ*, **331**(7512), 350.

Coursey, C.A., Nelson, R.C., Boll, D.T., et al. (2010). Dual-energy multidetector CT: how does it work, what can it tell us, and when can we use it in abdominopelvic imaging? *Radiographics*, 30(4), 1037–55.

Davison, J. M., Dunlop, W. (1980). Renal hemodynamics and tubular function normal human pregnancy. *Kidney Int*, 18(2), 152–61.

Doll, R., Wakeford, R. (1997). Risk of childhood cancer from fetal irradiation. Br J Radiol, 70, 130–9.

Feghali, M., Venkataramanan, R., Caritis, S. (2015). Pharmacokinetics of drugs in pregnancy. *Semin Perinatol*, 39(7). 512–19.

ter Haar, G. R., Abramowicz, J. S., Akiyama, I., et al. (2013). Do we need to restrict the use of doppler ultrasound in first trimester pregnancy. *Ultrasound in Med. & Biol*, 39(3) 374–80.

Jerome F., et al. (1996) Biology of reproduction. 54, 303–311.

Katzung, B. G., ed. (2017). *Basic & Clinical Pharmacology*, 14th ed. McGraw-Hill.

Kobayashi, H., Yamada, Y., Morioka, S., Niiro, E., Shigemitsu, A. (2014). Mechanism of pain generation for endometriosis-associated pelvic pain. Arch Gynecol Obstet, 289(1), 13–21.

Kurman, R. J. (2013). Origin and molecular pathogenesis of ovarian high-grade serous carcinoma. *Ann Oncol*, 24(10), x16–x21.

Labor, S., Maguire, S. (2008). The pain of labour. Rev Pain, 2 (2): 15–19.

Lax, S. F. (2017). Pathology of endometrial carcinoma. *Adv Exp Med Biol*, 943: 75–96.

Lelubre, C. and Vincent, J. L. (2018). Mechanisms and treatment of organ failure in sepsis. Nature Reviews Nephrology, Sepsis in Pregnancy, Bacterial (Green-top Guideline No. 64a), RCOG.

Loebstein, R., Lalkin, A., Koren, G. (1997). Pharmacokinetic changes during pregnancy and their clinical relevance. *Clin Pharmacokinet*, 33(5), 328–43.

McKeighen, R. A. (1980). Review of gamma camera technology for medical imaging. *Int Urogynecol J*, 27(3): 119.

Medicines and Healthcare Products Regulatory Agency, (2015). *Safety guidelines for magnetic resonance imaging equipment in clinical use.* MHRA.

Moch, H., Humphrey, P. A., Ulbright, T. M., Reuter, V. (2016). *WHO Classification of Tumours of the Urinary System and Male Genital Organs.* International Agency for Research on Cancer.

MSD Manual Professional Version. *Overview of Pain.* (2020). Online article. https://www.msdmanuals.com/professional/neurologic-disorders/pain/overview-of-pain

Murphy, M.M., Scott, J. M., McPartlin, J. M., Fernandez-Ballart, J. D. (2002). The pregnancy-related decrease in fasting plasma homocysteine is not explained by folic acid supplementation, hemodilution, or a decrease in albumin in a longitudinal study. *Am J Clin Nutr*, 76(3), 614–19.

Qasqas, S. A., McPherson, C., Frishman, W. H., Elkayam, U. (2004). Cardiovascular pharmacotherapeutic considerations during pregnancy and lactation. *Cardiol Rev*, 12(4), 201–21.

Radiopaedia. *Ultrasound artifacts* (online). https://radiopaedia.org/articles/ultrasound-artifacts-3

Rakislova, N., Saco, A., Sierra, A., Del Pino, M., Ordi J. (2017). Role of human papillomavirus in vulvar cancer. Adv Anat Pathol, 24, 201–14.

Royal College of Radiologists. (2015). (online). *A guide to understanding the implications of IRMER in diagnostic and interventional radiology.* https://www.rcr.ac.uk/sites/default/files/bfcr152_irmer.pdf

Scheuler, B. A. (1998). Clinical applications of basic X-ray physics principles. *Radiographics*, 18(3), 731–44.

Sharma, H. L., Sharma, K. K. Principles of Pharmacology, 3rd ed., Paras Medical Publisher.

Stratton, P., Berkley, K. J. (2011). Chronic pelvic pain and endometriosis: translational evidence of the relationship and implications. *Hum Reprod Update*, 17(3), 327–34.

Tatiana, N., Buhtoiarova, M. D., Brenner, C. A., Singh, M. (2016). Endometrial carcinoma: role of current and emerging biomarkers in resolving persistent clinical dilemmas. *Am J Clin Pathol*, 145(1), 8–21.

Tripathi, K. D. (2013). *Essentials of Medical Pharmacology*, 7th ed., Jaypee.

Van Eyk, N., van Schalkwyk, J. Infectious Diseases Committee. (2012). Antibiotic prophylaxis in gynaecologic procedures. *J Obstet Gynaecol Can*, 34(4), 382–91.

Vasicka, A., Lin, T. J., Bright, R. H. (1957). Peptic ulcer and pregnancy, review of hormonal relationships and a report of one case of massive gastrointestinal hemorrhage. *Obstet Gynecol Surv*, 12(1), 1–13.

Vercellini, P., Viganò, P., Somigliana E., Fedele L. (2014). Endometriosis: pathogenesis and treatment. *Nat Rev Endocrinol*, 10, 261–75.

Wagner, L., Applegate, K. (2008). *ACR practice guideline for imaging pregnant or potentially pregnant adolescents and women with ionizing radiation*. 1–15.

Wagner, L. K. (1997). *Exposure of the pregnant patient to diagnostic radiations: a guide to medical management*. Medical Physics Publishing.

Waldum, H. L., Straume, B. K., Lundgren, R. (1980). Serum group I pepsinogens during pregnancy. *Scand J Gastroenterol*, 15(1), 61–3.

Woods, R. K., Patchen Dellinger, E. (1998). Current guidelines for antibiotic prophylaxis of surgical wounds. *Am Fam Physician*, 57(11), 2731–40.

- RCOG Green-top Guidelines
- NICE guidelines in obstetrics and gynaecology
- local hospital protocols
- recent updates in molecular biology and genetics
- epidemiological updates in infection screening and microbiology
- physics of the most common radiological investigations and basic principles
- MBRRACE report
- applied anatomy: compare the branches of main arteries, veins and nerves in the abdomen and pelvis with images on other online resources to correlate these visually
- tabulated options
- clinical management and data interpretation including any recently introduced drugs (pharmacology, mode of action, side effects), new investigations (principles, sensitivity, specificity), tests (principles, organisms, physics)
- pathology: changing epidemiological trends in common cancers, infections, common in the UK compared with worldwide prevalence
- biochemistry: enzyme transduction and signalling – any new developments
- pharmacology: newer drugs, placental transfer, effects on fetus, side effects, mode of action at cellular level
- statistics: familiarise yourself with calculating sensitivity, specificity, positive predictive value, negative predictive value, incidence, prevalence, number needed to treat (NNT), odds ratio, relative risk, statistical tests, forest plot and interpretations

Index